Functional neuroimaging in child psychiatry

This unprecedented book reviews the recent rapid development
of functional neuroimaging techniques and their implications for
child psychiatry. It is unique in its focus on children and in
integrating brain mapping with genetics and behavioral testing –
an interface that is likely to become fundamental to functional
neuroimaging. Presenting new imaging techniques in language
accessible to the nonspecialist, this invaluable reference will help
clinicians and investigators to:

- understand through imaging the mechanisms of childhood
  psychiatric disorders
- decide which technique is most appropriate for their purposes,
  with respect to technology, experimental design, data analysis,
  and ethical considerations
- appreciate the role of molecular genetics and neuropsychology
  in planning brain imaging studies.

Coverage includes description of new brain imaging strategies,
recent advances and future applications of neuroimaging for
child psychiatry, and the application to children of imaging
techniques used in adults. As background, an overview is given of
normal brain and cognitive development. Linking the latest
findings from neuroimaging to neurophysiologic models, this
book is an essential resource for researchers and clinicians
concerned with neurodevelopmental disorders.

Monique Ernst is Associate Director of the Brain Imaging Center
at the US National Institute on Drug Abuse.

Judith M. Rumsey is Chief of the US Developmental
Neuroscience of Schizophrenia, Mood and other Brain Disorders
Program, Clinical Neuroscience Branch, National Institute of
Mental Health.

T0213335

Functional neuroimaging in child psychiatry

Edited by

Monique Ernst

Brain Imaging Center,
National Institute on Drug Abuse, Baltimore, MD, USA

and

Judith M. Rumsey

Clinical Neuroscience Branch,
National Institute of Mental Health, Rockville, MD, USA

With a Foreword by

Joseph T. Coyle

Chairman, Department of Psychiatry, Harvard Medical School, Boston, MA, USA

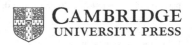

CAMBRIDGE UNIVERSITY PRESS
Cambridge, New York, Melbourne, Madrid, Cape Town, Singapore,
São Paulo, Delhi, Dubai, Tokyo

Cambridge University Press
The Edinburgh Building, Cambridge CB2 8RU, UK

Published in the United States of America by Cambridge University Press, New York

www.cambridge.org
Information on this title: www.cambridge.org/9780521126588

First published 2000
Reprinted 2001
This digitally printed version 2009

A catalogue record for this publication is available from the British Library

Library of Congress Cataloguing in Publication data

Functional neuroimaging in child psychiatry / edited by Monique Ernst and Judith M. Rumsey
   p. ; cm.
Includes index.
ISBN 0 521 65044 5 (hb)
1. Pediatric neuropsychiatry.   2. Brain–Imaging.   3. Developmental neurophysiology.
I. Ernst, Monique, 1953–   .   II. Rumsey, Judith M.
[DNLM: 1. Mental Disorders – diagnosis – Child.   2. Brain Diseases – diagnosis – Child.
3. Diagnostic Imaging – Child. WS 350 F979 2000]
RJ486.5.F865 2000
618.92′890754–dc 21   99–04455

ISBN 978-0-521-65044-1 Hardback
ISBN 978-0-521-12658-8 Paperback

Additional resources for this publication at www.cambridge.org/9780521126588

Contents

Plates between pp. 82 and pp. 83 and between pp. 242 and pp. 243. These plates are available in colour as a download from www.cambridge.org/9780521126588

Contributors

Carl Anderson
Department of Psychiatry, Harvard Medical School,
Boston, MA, USA

L. Eugene Arnold
Professor Emeritus of Psychiatry, Ohio State University,
Columbus, OH 43210, USA

Alessandro Bertolino
Clinical Brain Disorders Branch, National Institute of
Mental Health, NIH, Bethesda, MD 20892, USA

Daniel Buxhoeveden
Medical College of Georgia, Augusta, GA 30910, USA

Lauren Caravella
National Institute of Mental Health, NIH, Bethesda, MD
10892, USA

Manuel F. Casanova
Medical College of Georgia, Augusta, GA 30910, USA

B. J. Casey
Sackler Institute for Developmental Psychobiology, Weill
Medical College of Cornell University, New York, NY
10021, USA

Uttom Chowdhury
Department of Psychological Medicine, Great Ormond
Street Hospital for Children, London WCIN 3JH, UK

Bradley C. Christian
Wright State University and Kettering Memorial Hospital,
Kettering, OH 45429, USA

Diane C. Chugani
Wayne State University and Children's Hospital of
Michigan PET Center, Detroit, MI 48201, USA

Eric Courchesne
Department of Neurosciences and the Children's Hospital
Research Center for the Neuroscience of Autism,
University of California, San Diego, CA 92037, USA

Pablo A. Davanzo
University of California, Los Angeles, CA, USA

Clayton H. Eccard
Department of Psychiatry, University of Pittsburgh,
Pittsburgh, PA 15213, USA

Guinevere F. Eden
Institute for Cognitive and Computational Sciences,
Georgetown University Medical Center, Washington, DC
20007-2197, USA

Graham J. Emslie
Department of Psychiatry, South Western Medical Center
at Dallas, Dallas, TX 75235-9070, USA

Christopher J. Endres
Johns Hopkins University, Baltimore, MD, USA

Monique Ernst
Brain Imaging Center, National Institute on Drug Abuse,
Baltimore, MD 21224, USA

Ronald E. Fisher
Baylor College of Medicine (Houston) and Veterans Affairs
Hospital, Houston, TX, USA

D. Lynn Flowers
Department of Neurology, Bowman Gray School of
Medicine, Winston Salem, NC 27157-1043, USA

Isky Gordon
Great Ormond Street Hospital for Children, London,
WCIN 3JH, UK

Peter Herscovitch
NIH Clinical Center, National Institutes of Health,
Bethesda, MD 20892-1180, USA

Leslie K. Jacobsen
Department of Psychiatry, Yale School of Medicine, West
Haven, CT 06516, USA

Nicole Korbly
National Institute of Mental Health, NIH, Bethesda, MD
10892, USA

Robert A. Kowatch
Department of Psychiatry, South Western Medical Center
at Dallas, Dallas, TX 5235-9070, USA

Bryan Lask
Great Ormond Street Hospital for Children, London
WCIN 3JH, UK

Andy C. H. Lee
Department of Experimental Psychology, University of
Cambridge, Cambridge CB2 3EB, UK

Rona Livnat
Department of Psychiatry, University of Pittsburgh,
Pittsburgh, PA 15213, USA

Monica Luciana
Department of Psychology and Institute of Child
Development, University of Minnesota, Minneapolis, MN
55455, USA

Frank P. MacMaster
Wayne State University School of Medicine, Department
of Psychiatry and Behavioral Neurosciences, Detroit, MI
48201, USA

Gregory J. Moore
Wayne State University School of Medicine, Department
of Psychiatry and Behavioral Neurosciences, Detroit, MI
48201, USA

Gloria Morote
Psychiatric Associates of Alexandria, Alexandria, VA
22314, USA

Evan D. Morris
Sensor Systems, Sterling, VA, USA

Ralph-Axel Müller
Department of Cognitive Science and the Children's
Hospital Research Center for the Neuroscience of Autism,
University of California, San Diego, CA 92037, USA

Raymond F. Muzic Jr
Case Western Reserve University and University Hospital
of Cleveland, OH 44106, USA

Charles A. Nelson
Department of Pediatrics and Institute of Child
Development, University of Minnesota, Minneapolis, MN
55455, USA

Adrian M. Owen
Wolfson Brain Imaging Centre, Cambridge, UK

Daisy M. Pascualvaca
Section on Clinical and Experimental Neuropsychology,
Laboratory of Brain Cognition, National Institute of
Mental Health, Bethesda, MD 20892, USA

David L. Pauls
Child Study Center, Yale University School of Medicine,
New Haven, CT 06150, USA

Lori Anne D. Paulson
Wayne State University School of Medicine, Department
of Psychiatry and Behavioral Neurosciences, Detroit, MI
48201, USA

Bradley S. Peterson
Yale Child Study Center, New Haven, CT 06520, USA

Martin L. Reite
University of Colorado Health Sciences and Denver Veterans Affairs Medical Center, Denver, CO 80262, USA

Perry F. Renshaw
Brain Imaging Center, Belmont, MA 02178, USA

Trevor W. Robbins
Department of Experimental Psychology, University of Cambridge and the MRC Cognitive and Brain Sciences Unit, Cambridge CB2 3EB, UK

Robert D. Rogers
Department of Experimental Psychology, University of Cambridge, Cambridge CB2 3EB, UK

Donald C. Rojas
University of Colorado Health Sciences Center, Denver, CO 80262, USA

David R. Rosenberg
Wayne State University School of Medicine, Department of Psychiatry and Behavioral Neurosciences, Detroit, MI 48201, USA

Judith M. Rumsey
Clinical Neuroscience Branch, National Institute of Mental Health, Rockville, MD 20857, USA

Barbara J. Sahakian
Department of Psychiatry, University of Cambridge, Cambridge, UK

Julie B. Schweitzer
Maryland Psychiatric Research Center, University of Maryland, Baltimore, MD 21228, USA

Gurkirpal S. Sohal
Medical College of Georgia, Augusta, GA 30910, USA

Peter D. Teale
University of Colorado Health Sciences, Denver, CO 80262, USA

Kathleen M. Thomas
Department of Psychiatry, University of Pittsburgh, Pittsburgh, PA 15213, USA

Prakash Thomas
Yale University, New Haven, CT 06520, USA

David J. Vandenbergh
Center for Developmental and Health Genetics and Department of Biobehavioral Health, The Pennsylvania State University, Philadelphia, PA 16802, USA

Tomihisa F. Welsh
Department of Psychiatry, University of Pittsburgh, Pittsburgh, PA 15213, USA

Frank B. Wood
Section of Neuropsychology, Wake Forest University Baptist Medical Center, Winston Salem, NC 27157-1043, USA

Deborah A. Yurgelun-Todd
Brain Imaging Center, McLean Hospital and Harvard Medical School, Boston, MA, USA

Alan J. Zametkin
Division of Intramural Research, Child Psychiatry Branch, National Institute of Mental Health, NIH, Bethesda, MD 20892, USA

Thomas A. Zeffiro
Sensor Systems, Sterling, VA 20164, USA

Preface

"Unprecedented", "revolutionary", "extraordinary" are terms commonly used to describe the promise that the emergence of functional neuroimaging techniques presents for neuroscience. Indeed, until recently, the possibilities that such techniques now provide for the advancement of knowledge fell within the realm of "neuroscience fiction".

Many recent books have been dedicated to various facets of neuroimaging. This volume is unique in its focus on children, as well as in its effort to encompass the fields of genetics and neuropsychology the interface of which with neuroimaging will soon become the state of the art in neuroimaging research. This book is addressed to clinicians and investigators. Clinicians will learn about the basic principles, advantages, and disadvantages of neuroimaging techniques and the advances made in our understanding of the mechanisms underlying childhood psychiatric disorders through neuroimaging research. Investigators may rely on this volume as a reference book to aid them in (i) deciding which technique is most appropriate for a given research question, (ii) evaluating the ethical issues raised by the involvement of children in research in order to weigh them in reference to the progress that has been made in understanding certain childhood psychiatric disorders through the use of neuroimaging, and (iii) considering how the fields of molecular genetics and neuropsychology can be exploited in planning for a brain imaging study.

The book is divided into five sections. Part 1 is dedicated to the description and future potential of the various functional imaging techniques currently used to study the human brain. Readers should come away from this section with an understanding of the relative advantages and limitations of each of these techniques and become fluent in the language of nuclear medicine and neuromagnetic imaging. To this purpose, a glossary of the terms commonly used in functional neuroimaging is provided at the end of the book. In addition, the issues raised by the application of these techniques to pediatric studies are clearly and uniquely addressed. Part 2 comprises the ethical issues raised by the inclusion of children in functional neuroimaging protocols. Part 3 gives an overview of neural development and cognitive development and addresses the issues of controlling for, as well as exploiting, these maturational changes in neuroimaging research, particularly in functional magnetic resonance imaging studies involving cognitive activation. Part 4 reviews the progress made in research on child psychiatric disorders. Because of the paucity of research in children, the review of imaging findings in adults often predominates and provides hypotheses to be tested in children. Each group of psychiatric disorders is described separately, and the specific problems (scientific, technical, and ethical) of studying children with specific disorders using neuroimaging are covered. Finally, Part 5 addresses future

directions. It introduces the important tools of genetics and neuropsychology that are expected to act synergistically to potentiate the yield of neuroimaging research and discusses how neuroimaging findings can be interpreted within the context of neurodevelopmental disorders.

In our concluding remarks, we mention the development of new brain imaging techniques and strategies that were not covered previously. We also express our opinions regarding the most important advances and future applications of this exciting field of research in child psychiatry.

The authors wish to thank Stephen Foote, PhD, Director of the Division of Neuroscience and Basic Behavioral Science, NIMH for his support of this work and to thank Barry Horwitz, PhD, Language Section, Voice, Speech, and Language Branch, National Institute on Deafness and Other Communication Disorders for his helpful review of the final chapter.

Monique Ernst and Judy Rumsey

Foreword

Research is limited by the instruments that it uses: from the telescope came the solar system: from the microscope came the germ theory. A subtext of these discoveries is "seeing is believing". For all too long, psychiatric illness has been defined by what could not be seen: a lesion on autopy transformed a psychiatric disorder into a neurologic disorder. The ken of clinical responsibility of psychiatry has, therefore, been delimited to conditions with behavioral and intrapsychic symptoms without visible neuropathology. This situation, of course, has been fertile ground for the persistence of stigma, as psychiatric disorder was equated with moral weakness among the lay public and derided as "functional" by nonpsychiatric clinicians.

Fortunately, the solution for this seeming oxymoron, *mental illness*, came from technology. Since the mid-1980s increasingly powerful devices have been developed to image the structure, function, neurophysiology, and chemical composition of the living human brain. The impact of these technologies has been informative for brain science but *transformative* for psychiatry. For example, no longer can schizophrenia be considered a political act or psychologic deviance when one can *see* the atrophic cortex, hypofunctional frontal lobe, enhanced release of striatal dopamine and reduced levels of *N*-acetyl-aspartate.

Functional Neuroimaging in Child Psychiatry, edited by Monique Ernst and Judy Rumsey, takes current imaging opportunities and discusses their applicability to the realm of the child and adolescent subject. The power of this important textbook is that it addresses the critical fact that children are not simply miniature adults. Children present unique opportunities but also formidable challenges. The textbook provides superb reviews of the major methods – the use of radioactive tracers in PET and SPECT, fMRI and spectroscopy, and magnetoencephalography – with an eye toward pediatric applications.

Perhaps one of the most difficult barriers confronting pediatric brain imaging is the misperception of the ethical constraints on such studies. Arnold and his colleagues provide a very thoughtful commentary on risks, risk–benefit assessment, informed consent, and patient selection. In particular, they cover in some detail radiation biology in considering the risk of exposure to radioactive ligands in pediatric SPECT and PET studies, making comparisons to other sources of radiation that can be readily understood. This chapter should be required reading for investigators as well as members of Institutional Review Boards (IRBs) involved in pediatric imaging.

The most compelling aspect of brain imaging is the ability to monitor neuronal function with increasingly higher resolution. These technical advances have transformed imaging research from a passive diagnostic method to a strategy for mapping the dynamics of neural systems involved in cognitive function, emotional states, and motor–sensory processing. Cognitive neuroscientists have now become major innovators in developing tasks that illuminate dysfunctional circuits. In this regard, those involved in pediatric functional brain imaging will face the enormously complex but informative unfolding of circuit maturation, plasticity, and cognitive functions during brain development. Consequently, the textbook takes particular care in critically reviewing selected psychological instruments that can be brought to bear on neurocognitive development.

At the time of writing this Foreword, those sequencing the human genome in the Human Genome Project are whirling along with an estimated completion date of 2003 for mapping the entire human genome. Then begins the really exciting biological research aimed at determining how a mere 100 000 genes interact to create the human body and its most complex organ, the brain. Brain imaging during human development will play a major role in this endeavor. For this reason, I believe that *Functional Neuroimaging in Child Psychiatry* is a critically important book: it provides the roadmap to this extraordinary research frontier.

Joseph T. Coyle

Chairman, Department of Psychiatry, Harvard Medical School, Boston, MA, USA

Part 1

Techniques of functional neuroimaging

Since the mid-1980s, there has been a rapid technological development in functional neuroimaging methods that have enabled the study of the human brain in vivo. Positron emission tomography (PET), single photon emission computed tomography (SPECT), functional magnetic resonance imaging (fMRI), magnetic resonance spectroscopy (MRS), and magnetoencephalography (MEG) now offer a diverse array of methods for studying metabolic and neurochemical brain development, as well as the neural systems subserving cognitive and emotional processes.

To provide a foundation for understanding these methods, particularly as applied to the study of brain development and deviance, Part 1 delineates the basic principles, advantages, and disadvantages of these modalities. Herscovitch and Ernst discuss the nuclear medicine techniques of PET and SPECT (Chapter 1) and Morris and colleagues discuss PET methods used to map receptors (Chapter 2). Eden and Zeffiro then describe the recent emergence of fMRI as a technique that can be used with neurophysiologic and neurocognitive probes to define neural circuits and determine their integrity in childhood disorders (Chapter 3). Yurgelun-Todd and Renshaw in Chapter 4 discuss advances in MRS for the study of brain chemistry and the evolution of this technique into a brain mapping technique. Finally, in Chapter 5, Rojas and colleagues describe MEG, a technique with superior temporal resolution that directly measures neuronal electrical activity.

This diversity of functional imaging methods provides the means for mapping a variety of important brain maturational processes. These methods differ in the nature of the recorded signal (radioactive counts, electromagnetic energy), the physiologic variables (e.g., cerebral blood flow, glucose metabolism, receptor density, neurochemical concentration), the temporal and spatial resolution, the health risks, and the availability and cost. The neuroscientist can theoretically choose a best method or combination of methods to address scientific questions relating to normal and aberrant brain development. Furthermore, the integration of these techniques (multimodal imaging) will doubtlessly increase over time, offering a more comprehensive knowledge base from which to study, diagnose, and treat psychiatric disorders.

Functional brain imaging with PET and SPECT

Peter Herscovitch and Monique Ernst

Introduction

Functional brain imaging refers to the use of techniques to obtain images of the brain that are related to its physiology or biochemistry, rather than its structural anatomy. Two nuclear medicine-based approaches to functional brain imaging can be used to study the pediatric population, positron emission tomography (PET) and single-photon emission computed tomography (SPECT). Both will be reviewed in this chapter.

PET is a nuclear medicine technique for performing physiologic measurements in vivo. The PET scanner provides tomographic images of the distribution of positron-emitting radiopharmaceuticals in the body. From these images, measurements such as regional cerebral blood flow (rCBF) and glucose metabolism can be obtained. PET has been widely used as a research tool to study normal brain function and the pathophysiology of neurologic and psychiatric disease in adults (Grafton and Mazziotta, 1992; Volkow and Fowler, 1992). Its role in the management of patients with brain disorders is at an earlier stage (Powers et al., 1991) and its use in children has been limited. Conceptually, PET consists of three components: (i) tracer compounds labeled with radioactive atoms that emit positrons; (ii) scanners that provide tomographic images of the concentration of positron-emitting radioactivity in the body; and (iii) mathematical models that describe the in vivo behavior of radiotracers and allow the physiologic process under study to be quantified from the images. The first tomographs for quantitative PET imaging were developed in the mid-1970s (Ter-Pogossian, 1992). Subsequently, instrument design has become more sophisticated, with improved spatial resolution and sensitivity. Radiotracer techniques have been developed to study regional CBF and blood volume; glucose, oxygen, and protein metabolism; blood–brain barrier permeability; numerous neuroreceptor–neurotransmitter

systems; tissue pH; and the concentration of radiolabeled drugs in brain.

SPECT is another nuclear medicine technique that provides tomographic images of radioactivity (George et al., 1991; Wyper, 1993; Green, 1996). SPECT is simpler than PET because it uses radiopharmaceuticals labeled with conventional radionuclides such as technetium-99m (^{99m}Tc); however, it still has the same three components: radiotracers, scanners, and mathematical models. Its quantitative accuracy is less than that of PET and the range of radiopharmaceuticals for studying the brain is relatively limited; it has primarily been used to map cerebral perfusion. Improvements in instrumentation and radiopharmaceuticals are being actively pursued, especially in the development of radiotracers labeled with iodine-123 (^{123}I) to image neuroreceptors (Holman and Devous, 1992; Juni, 1994), and there is a strong interest in clinical SPECT brain studies.

This chapter will provide an overview of PET instrumentation, radiotracers, and mathematical modeling, emphasizing methods to measure cerebral hemodynamics and metabolism, and the most common applications. In addition, SPECT instrumentation and radiopharmaceuticals are described. The analysis and interpretation of functional brain images and special considerations for the pediatric age group are discussed. Methods for studying neurotransmitter systems are treated elsewhere in this volume (Chapter 2). An abbreviated lexicon of various terms used in nuclear medicine is provided in the glossary (p. 408).

Positron emission tomography

Imaging

PET provides tomographic images of the distribution of positron-emitting radioactivity using rings of radiation

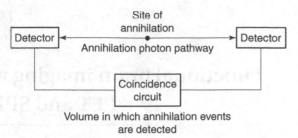

Fig. 1.1. The two high-energy photons resulting from a positron emission and annihilation are detected by two radiation detectors that are connected by an electronic coincidence circuit. A decay event is recorded as a coincidence line between the detectors only when both photons are detected almost simultaneously. A very short time window for photon arrival, typically 5–20 ns, called the coincidence resolving time, is allowed for registration of a coincidence event. This coincidence requirement localizes the site of the annihilation to the volume of space between the detectors.

detectors that are arrayed around the body (or head). Because of the special nature of the positron and the techniques used for image reconstruction, it is possible to obtain absolute radioactivity measurements from these images (Daube-Witherspoon and Herscovitch, 1996).

Formation of the PET image

Certain radioactive atoms, such as oxygen-15 (^{15}O) or fluorine-18 (^{18}F), decay by the emission of a positron from the nucleus. Positrons are the "antimatter" particles to electrons; they have the same mass as electrons but are positively charged. After emission from the nucleus, positrons travel a variable distance in tissue, up to a few millimeters, losing kinetic energy. When almost at rest, they interact with atomic electrons, resulting in the "annihilation" of both particles. Their combined mass is converted into two high-energy (511 keV each) photons that travel in opposite directions from the annihilation site at the speed of light. Detection of these photon pairs is used to measure both the location and the amount of radioactivity in the field of view of the scanner. The two annihilation photons are detected by two opposing radiation detectors connected by an electronic coincidence circuit (Fig. 1.1). This circuit records a decay event only when both detectors sense the almost simultaneous arrival of both photons (the time window for coincidence detection is typically 5–20 ns). The site of the decay event is, therefore, localized to the volume of space between the two detectors, although there is no information about the depth or location of the radioactive source within the volume between the two detectors.

In practice, several rings, each consisting of many radiation detectors, are used. Opposing detector pairs in each

ring are connected by coincidence circuits. With each decay event, the two resulting annihilation photons are detected as a coincidence line; as a result, the number of coincidence lines sensed by any detector pair is proportional to the amount of radioactivity between them. A computer records the coincidence events from each ring. Tomographic images of the underlying distribution of radioactivity are then reconstructed with the same mathematical technique, referred to as filtered back-projection, that is used in conventional X-ray computed tomography (CT) (Hoffman and Phelps, 1986). In addition to filtered back-projection, there are other approaches to image reconstruction. These require considerably more computational time and are used much less frequently.

The intensity of each point or pixel in the reconstructed PET image is proportional to the concentration of radioactivity at the corresponding location in the brain. For the calibration of the scanner to obtain *absolute* radioactivity measurements, a cylinder filled with a uniform solution of radioactivity is imaged. The radioactivity concentration of the solution is then measured with a calibrated well counter, and the scanner calibration factor is calculated to convert PET image counts (in units of cts/s per pixel) to units of radioactivity concentration (e.g., nCi/ml).

Limitations in image quality and quantification

A variety of physical effects, such as attenuation, deadtime losses, scatter, and random coincidences, affect the PET image and are corrected for as part of the image reconstruction process. Other factors such as image noise and spatial resolution also affect image quality and are important considerations in the design and interpretation of PET studies (Hoffman and Phelps, 1986; Karp et al., 1991; Daube-Witherspoon and Herscovitch, 1996).

Attenuation correction

A key step in image reconstruction is correction for the absorption or attenuation of annihilation photons that occurs through their interactions with tissue (Bailey, 1998). This substantially decreases the number of coincidence counts detected. Although the amount of attenuation can be estimated using an assumed value for the attenuating properties of tissue, actual measurements are more accurate. Before the administration of the radiotracer, a separate "transmission scan" is performed with a source of positron-emitting radioactivity positioned between the subject's head and the detector rings. The outside source, filled with germanium-68/gallium-68 (^{68}Ge/^{68}Ga) radioactivity, is a ring or a rod that is rotated around the body. A similar measurement is made with nothing in the scanner field of view. The ratio of the two measurements gives the amount of attenuation between each detector pair and is used in the image reconstruction process to correct for attenuation.

To respond to the demands of some protocols in which there is a long delay between radiotracer administration and subsequent emission scanning, techniques have been devised to calculate the attenuation correction using a transmission scan obtained *after* radiotracer administration, that is, with positron-emitting radioactivity still in the body (Carson et al., 1988). This approach is particularly useful when using (^{18}F)-labeled deoxyglucose (FDG) to measure regional cerebral glucose metabolism (rCMRGlu; see below).

Image noise
The PET image has inherent statistical noise because of the random nature of radioactive decay. The disintegration rate of a radioactive sample undergoes moment-to-moment variation. The resultant uncertainty in measuring the amount of radioactivity decreases as the number of counts recorded increases. Similarly, the statistical reliability of a PET measurement depends on the number of counts. The situation is more complex, however, because the value of radioactivity in any small brain region is obtained from an image reconstructed from multiple views or projections of the radioactivity distribution throughout the entire brain slice. Therefore, the noise in any individual brain region is affected by noise in other brain regions and tends to be greater (Budinger et al., 1978). Excessive noise gives the PET image a grainy, "salt and pepper" appearance and decreases the ability to quantitate radioactivity accurately.

Image noise depends upon the number of counts collected, which in turn depends upon scanner sensitivity, the duration of the scan, and the concentration of radioactivity in the field of view. Scanner sensitivity (measured in units of (counts/s)/(μCi/ml)), is determined by its design features, such as the nature and arrangement of the radiation detectors. For example, the sensitivity is inversely proportional to the diameter of the detector rings. Although increasing scan duration increases counts, this is frequently not possible, either because of the short half-life of the radiotracer or because it would not be compatible with the tracer-kinetic mathematical model that is used. Administering more radioactivity increases counts, but this approach is limited by radiation safety considerations and also by the inability of tomographs to operate accurately at high count rates, that is by count rate performance.

Deadtime losses and random coincidences
Count rate performance refers to the level of radioactivity that can be accurately measured with a PET scanner. It is limited by deadtime loss and by random coincidences.

Deadtime loss is the decreasing ability of a scanner to register counts as the count rate increases because of the time required by the physical processes involved in handling each count. Deadtime loss originates from limitations of the electronic circuitry used to process information from the detectors and from the recovery time of the detectors themselves. Deadtime causes a reduction in measured coincidences as radioactivity increases in the field of view of the scanner. This reduction can be predicted for a given count rate and a correction factor can be applied. This correction, no matter how accurate, does not compensate for the loss in statistical accuracy of the image that occurs because fewer counts were actually collected.

Random coincidences also limit count rate performance. These occur when two photons from two *different* positron annihilations are sensed by a detector pair within the coincidence resolving time; as a result, a false or random coincidence count is collected. The fraction of total coincidences recorded that are random increases linearly with radioactivity. Random coincidences add noisy background to the image. Although corrections can be made that subtract an estimate of these false counts, the contribution to the image noise persists (Hoffman et al., 1981). Therefore, for any given tomograph, the amount of radioactivity administered must be carefully selected to balance the competing effects of improved counting statistics with the "diminishing returns" resulting from deadtime and random coincidences.

Scatter
Another source of background noise in the PET image is scatter. Scatter occurs when an annihilation photon traveling in tissue is deflected in a collision with an electron and its direction changes. This results in incorrect positioning of the coincidence line. Not only is information lost from the affected coincidence line but also a noisy background level is added to the image. This leads to an overestimation of radioactivity, especially in areas containing relatively less radioactivity, e.g., regions with low blood flow or metabolism. The amount of scatter in an image is a function of the distribution of radioactivity, the anatomy of the tissue scattering the photons, and the design of the scanner. It is necessary to correct for scatter because it can contribute up to 20% of the counts in an image. Methods have been developed to correct for scatter that vary in their complexity and effectiveness (Bergstrom et al., 1983; Hoffman and Phelps, 1986).

Spatial resolution
A critical issue in interpreting PET (and SPECT) images is the concept of image resolution. Image resolution is the

minimum distance by which two points of radioactivity must be separated to be perceived independently in the reconstructed image. Limited resolution, which is visually apparent as blurring of the image, has a major effect on the ability to quantify radioactivity accurately, especially in small structures (see below).

In PET, image resolution depends upon the accurate localization of positron-emitting nuclei. This is limited by the physics of positron annihilation and by detector design. Annihilation photons are produced only after the positron has traveled up to several millimeters from the nucleus. This limits the accuracy of localizing the nucleus. The distance the positron travels (positron range) varies and depends on the specific radionuclide and tissue density; it averages 1.2 mm for ^{18}F, 2.1 mm for ^{11}C. In addition, the angle between the two annihilation photons deviates slightly from 180°, causing a slight misplacement of the coincidence line (noncolinearity of the annihilation photons). These effects result in a 1–3 mm resolution loss (Phelps and Hoffman, 1976) and are larger when the detectors are farther apart, as in a body scanner compared with a head scanner. Detector size and shape determine how accurately the position of each coincidence line is recorded; smaller detectors provide better resolution.

Resolution is measured by imaging a thin line source of positron-emitting radioactivity (Fig. 1.2). Because of limited resolution, the radioactivity in the source appears blurred or spread out over a large area; resolution is defined by the amount of spreading. The resolution of current scanners is about 4–5 mm in the image plane (de Grado et al., 1994; Wienhard et al., 1994).

PET Instrumentation

A PET system consists of many components (Hoffman and Phelps, 1986; Council on Scientific Affairs, 1988; Koeppe and Hutchins, 1992). Several rings of radiation detectors are mounted in a gantry. Each detector consists of a small scintillation crystal that gives off light when the energy of an annihilation photon is deposited in it. The detector is coupled to a photomultiplier tube that converts the light pulse to an electrical signal which is fed into the coincidence circuitry. Scanners have numerous rings, each containing up to several hundred detectors (de Grado et al., 1994; Wienhard et al., 1994), with a tomographic slice provided by each ring. In addition, "cross-slices" halfway between the detector rings are derived from coincidences between detectors in adjacent rings. Therefore, 47 contiguous slices can be obtained simultaneously by a 24-ring system. To date, the most sophisticated scanners have 32 rings, which permit the acquisition of 63 slices. A dedicated computer is used to control the scanning process, collect the coincidence count information, and reconstruct and display the images.

During the scan, the subject lies on a special table that is fitted with a head holder to restrain head movement. The gantry has low-powered lasers that project lines onto the subject's head and aid in positioning. Some gantries can be tilted from the vertical to obtain slices in specific planes, for example parallel to the canthomeatal line.

A relatively recent, major advance in scanner design permits coincidence counts to be collected by opposing detectors that do not have to be in the same or adjacent rings (Spinks et al., 1992; de Grado et al., 1994; Bailey et al., 1998). Because more coincidence lines are collected by this three-dimensional (3D) imaging approach, scanner sensitivity is substantially increased. This improves image quality or, alternatively, permits the same number of image counts to be obtained with less administered radioactivity. These factors are a great benefit in pediatric imaging, in which radiation exposure is a particular consideration. The disadvantages of 3D acquisition are an increase in the amount of scatter and contribution from radioactivity outside the field of view (i.e., from other parts of the body) to the counts seen by the detector rings. This can be more of a problem when scanning small pediatric subjects because the rest of the body is closer to the gantry than it is in adults.

Positron-emitting radiotracers

The second requirement for PET is a radiotracer of physiologic interest that is labeled with a positron-emitting radionuclide. A radiotracer can be a naturally occurring compound in which one of the atoms is replaced with its radioactive counterpart or it can be a labeled analog which behaves in vivo similarly to the natural substance. It can also be a synthetic substance, such as a radiolabeled drug, that interacts with a specific biologic system.

The positron-emitting nuclides most commonly used to label PET radiotracers are ^{15}O, ^{13}N, ^{11}C, and ^{18}F with half-lives of 2.05, 10.0, 20.3, and 109.8 min, respectively. (The half-life is the time required for radioactivity to decay to one-half of its original value.) The chemical nature of ^{15}O, ^{13}N, and ^{11}C is identical to that of their nonradioactive counterparts, which are basic constituents of living matter as well as of most drugs. Consequently, they can be incorporated into radiotracers with the same in vivo behavior as the corresponding nonradioactive compound. Fluorine-18 is used to substitute for hydrogen or hydroxyl groups to synthesize analogs with characteristics similar to those of the unsubstituted compound. Drugs that would normally contain fluorine can be synthesized as their ^{18}F-labeled counterparts. Relatively large

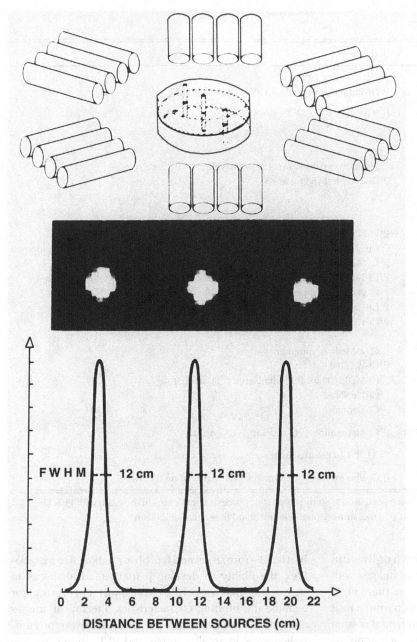

Fig. 1.2. Definition and measurement of the resolution of a PET scanner. Thin line sources of positron-emitting radioactivity perpendicular to the image plane are scanned (upper panel). Because of resolution limitations, the radioactivity in each source appears blurred or spread over a larger area (middle panel). Scanner resolution is defined by the amount of spreading that occurs. A plot of the image intensity along a line through the center of the images (lower panel) shows that this spreading approximates a bell-shaped or Gaussian curve. The width of this curve at one-half of its maximum height (termed the full width at half maximum, FWHM) is the measure of resolution. Here the resolution is 1.2 cm. Another interpretation of the FWHM is that it is the minimum distance by which two points of radioactivity must be separated to be independently perceived in the reconstructed image. (From Ter-Pogossian et al. 1975, with permission.)

Table 1.1. Representative PET radiotracers

Physiologic process or system	Radiotracer
Cerebral blood flow	$H_2^{15}O$
	[^{15}O]-Butanol; [^{11}C]-butanol, [^{18}F]-fluoromethane
Cerebral blood volume	$C^{15}O$; ^{11}CO
Cerebral energy metabolism	
Oxygen metabolism	$^{15}O_2$
Glucose metabolism	[^{18}F]-Fluorodeoxyglucose; [^{11}C]-deoxyglucose, [^{11}C]-glucose
Glucose transport	[^{11}C]-3-*O*-Methylglucose
Neuroreceptor systems	
Dopaminergic	
Presynaptic dopamine pool	[^{18}F]-Fluoro-L-dopa; [^{18}F]-fluoro-L-*m*-tyrosine
Dopamine D_2 receptors	[^{11}C]-*N*-Methylspiperone; [^{11}C]-raclopride; [^{18}F]-spiperone; [^{18}F]-*N*-methylspiperone
Dopamine D_1 receptors	[^{11}C]-SCH23390
Dopamine reuptake sites	[^{11}C]-Nomifensine; [^{11}C]-cocaine; [^{18}F]-labeled 1-[2-(diphenylmethoxy)ethyl]-4-
	(3-phenyl-2-propenyl)piperazine ([^{18}F]-GBR)
Opiate	[^{11}C]-Carfentanil; [^{11}C]-diprenorphine, [^{18}F]-cyclofoxy
Benzodiazepine	[^{11}C]-Flumazenil
Serotonergic (5-HT)	
Presynaptic serotonin pool	[^{11}C]-α-Methyltryptophan
5-HT$_{1A}$ receptors	[^{11}C]-WAY100,635
5-HT$_{2A}$ receptors	[^{11}C]-MDL100,907; [^{18}F]-altanserin; [^{18}F]-setoperone
5-HT reuptake sites	[^{11}C]-McN5652
Monoamine oxidase B	[^{11}C]-Deprenyl
Amino acid transport, protein synthesis	[^{11}C]-Methionine; [^{11}C]-leucine; [^{11}C]-tyrosine
Tissue pH	$^{11}CO_2$; [^{11}C]-Dimethadione
Tissue drug kinetics	[^{11}C]-Phenytoin; [^{11}C]-valproate; [^{13}N]-carmustine (BCNU)

Note: This is a partial listing of radiotracers that have been used to study physiologic processes or systems in the brain with PET. The most commonly used radiotracer methods are those to measure regional cerebral blood flow and metabolism.

amounts of these radionuclides with short half-lives can be administered to provide good-quality images with acceptable radiation exposure because of their rapid decay. The short half-lives, especially of ^{15}O, permit repeat studies in the same subject in one experimental session because of the rapid physical decay after each administration.

The disadvantage of these short half-lives is that the synthesis of PET radiotracers is demanding. On-site production of radionuclides by means of a cyclotron is required (Wolf and Schlyer, 1993), and rapid techniques must be devised for radiotracer synthesis and quality control. These must yield products that are pure, sterile, and nontoxic. The tracer must have the appropriate properties to permit the desired physiologic measurement to be made (Kilbourn, 1991; Dannals et al., 1993). Important factors include its permeability across the blood–brain

barrier, the formation and fate of any radioactive metabolites, the ability to develop a mathematical model to describe the behavior of the tracer, and, for neuroreceptor ligands, the binding characteristics. Preclinical studies are typically performed, using tissue sampling or autoradiography in small animals and PET studies in large ones. The recent development of PET scanners designed to image small animals (e.g., rat), should facilitate the preclinical assessment of new PET tracers (Cherry et al., 1998). A wide variety of positron-emitting radiopharmaceuticals has been synthesized (Table 1.1) (Fowler and Wolf, 1991).

Radiotracer modeling

A mathematical model is required to calculate the value of the physiologic variable of interest from measurements of radiotracer concentration in brain and blood. The model describes the in vivo behavior of the radiotracer, that is the relationship over time between the amount of tracer delivered to a brain region in its arterial input and the amount of tracer in the region. The use of models allows PET to be a quantitative physiological technique rather than only an imaging modality (Huang and Phelps, 1986; Carson, 1991, 1996). Compartmental models are typically used. It is assumed that there are entities called compartments that have uniform biologic properties and in which the tracer concentration is uniform at any instant in time. The compartments can be physical spaces such as the extravascular space, or biochemical entities such as neuroreceptor-binding sites. The model is described by one or more equations, that contain measurable terms (i.e., the brain and blood radiotracer concentrations over time) and unknowns such as blood flow or receptor concentration that are of interest.

Several factors must be considered in developing a model. These include tracer transport across the blood–brain barrier, the behavior of the tracer in brain, the presence of labeled metabolites in blood, the potential for alterations in tracer behavior if there is pathology, and the ability to solve the model accurately for the unknown parameters. Error analysis and model validation are important. Error analysis consists of mathematical simulations to determine the sensitivity of the model to potential sources of measurement error. Validation experiments are usually performed to demonstrate that the method provides reproducible, accurate, and biologically meaningful measurements.

This chapter will describe the PET methods used to measure rCBF and cerebral blood volume (rCBV) and glucose and oxygen metabolism. Measurements of CBF glucose metabolism are widely used as indices of neuronal activity (see below). In addition, SPECT tracer methods for assessing cerebral perfusion will be discussed.

PET radiotracer techniques

Cerebral glucose metabolism

The measurement of rCMRGlu utilizes FDG. The approach is based on the technique used to measure rCMRGlu in laboratory animals with [^{14}C]-deoxyglucose and tissue autoradiography (Sokoloff et al., 1977) and adapted for PET by using ^{18}F as the label (Phelps et al., 1979; Reivich et al., 1979; Huang et al., 1980). FDG is a glucose analog in which a hydroxyl group has been replaced with an ^{18}F atom. FDG is transported across the blood–brain barrier and is phosphorylated in tissue, as is glucose, by hexokinase to form FDG 6-phosphate (FDG-6-P). Because of its anomalous struc-

ture, however, FDG-6-P cannot proceed further along the glucose metabolic pathway. Also, there is little dephosphorylation of FDG-6-P back to FDG. As a result of this "metabolic trapping", there is negligible loss of FDG-6-P. This facilitates the calculation of rCMRGlu from measurements of local tissue radioactivity. Sokoloff's three-compartment model applied to FDG consists of plasma FDG in brain capillaries, free FDG in tissue, and FDG-6-P in tissue (Fig. 1.3a). Rate constants describe the movement of tracer between these compartments. An operational equation permits the calculation of rCMRGlu from the tissue radioactivity concentration, the arterial plasma concentration of FDG over time, and the plasma glucose concentration (Fig. 1.3b). The equation also contains the rate constants and a factor termed the lumped constant (LC). The LC corrects for the differences between glucose and FDG in blood–brain barrier transport and in phosphorylation. Neither the rate constants nor the LC can be routinely determined for each experimental subject or condition. It was found possible, however, to use standard values that can be determined once in separate groups of normal subjects.

To implement the method, images are obtained starting 30–45 min after intravenous injection of 5–10 mCi FDG. Blood is sampled to measure the concentrations of glucose and FDG in plasma over time. The operational equation with standard values for the rate constants and LC is used to generate images of rCMRGlu (Fig. 1.4). Typical normal values of rCMRGlu are 6–7 and 2.5–3 mg/min per g tissue in gray and white matter, respectively. (Sasaki et al., 1986; Hatazawa et al., 1988; Tyler et al., 1988; Camargo et al., 1992).

Measurements of rCMRGlu with FDG reflect the state of the subject primarily during the first 10–20 min after tracer injection (Huang et al., 1981). This means that if a challenge is used, such as cognitive, motor, or pharmacologic activation, it must start slightly before FDG injection and continue for some time. If unwanted subject activity occurs during tracer uptake, such as anxiety or fidgeting, it will affect the results particularly if it occurs during the first 10–20 min.

The accuracy of using standard values for the rate constants and LC has been the subject of considerable discussion (Cunningham and Cremer, 1985; Baron et al., 1989). Their values may change in the presence of pathology, and the use of incorrect values results in inaccurate rCMRGlu calculations (Sokoloff et al., 1977; Sokoloff, 1985). Because the terms in the operational equation containing rate constants approach zero with increasing time (see Fig. 1.3b), a delay of 30–45 min between FDG injection and PET imaging is used to minimize the error associated with using standard values. There can still be substantial error

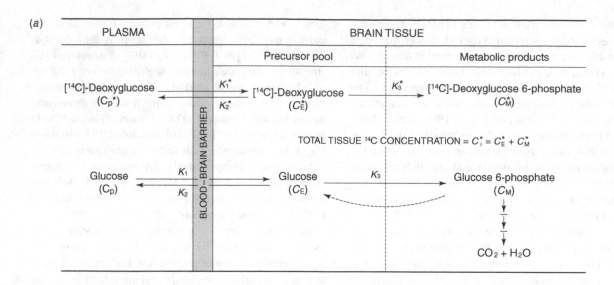

(a)

(b)

$$rCMRGlu = \frac{\text{Plasma glucose}}{\text{Lumped constant}} \cdot \frac{\text{Tissue radioactivity at time } T - \text{Free DG in tissue at time } T}{\text{Total amount of FDG entering tissue}}$$

$$= \frac{C_p}{LC} \cdot \frac{C(T) - k_1^* \exp[-(k_2^* + k_3^*)T] \int_0^T C_p^*(t)\exp[k_2^* + k_3^*)t]\,dt}{\int_0^T C_p^*(t)\,dt - \exp[-(k_2^* + k_3^*)T] \int_0^T C_p^*(t)\exp[(k_2^* + k_3^*)t]\,dt}$$

Fig. 1.3. Measurement of regional cerebral glucose metabolism (rCMRGlu) using deoxyglucose (DG) labeled with ^{18}F (FDG). (a) The Sokoloff three-compartment model used to measure rCMRGlu with DG. The compartments consist of DG in the plasma in brain capillaries, DG in brain tissue, and DG 6-phosphate (DG-6-P) in tissue. Rate constants describe the movement of tracer between compartments, two for the bidirectional transport of DG across the blood–brain barrier between plasma and tissue (k_1^*, k_2^*), and one for the phosphorylation of DG to DG-6-P (k_3^*). In the adaptation of this model to PET, FDG is used and a fourth rate constant, k_4^*, is added to account for the small amount of dephosphorylation of FDG-6-P back to FDG. (From Sokoloff, 1977, with permission.) (b) The operational equation of the DG method. The equation in words aids in understanding the model. The terms that are measured are $C(T)$, the tissue radioactivity concentration at time T, typically 30–45 min after DG administration; $C_p^*(t)$, the plasma DG concentration over time; and C_p, the plasma glucose concentration. The concentration of free DG in tissue at time T is calculated from $[C_p^*(t)]$ and the rate constants. The difference between the two terms in the numerator is the concentration of DG-6-P that has been formed. The denominator equals the amount of DG delivered to tissue. Therefore, the ratio on the right-hand side is the fractional rate of phosphorylation of DG. Multiplying this ratio by C_p would give the rate of glucose phosphorylation if DG and glucose had the same behavior. Because this is not the case, the lumped constant (LC) is included to account for the difference. The adaptation of this equation to PET using FDG is more complex because of the inclusion of a fourth rate constant, k_4^*.

in the presence of cerebral ischemia or a tumor, however (Wienhard et al., 1985; Nakai et al., 1987; Graham et al., 1989). Several investigators reformulated the operational equation to decrease its sensitivity to the rate constants and have refined the methods to measure them from sequential PET images (Brooks, 1982; Lammertsma et al., 1987).

The LC is assumed to be uniform and constant throughout brain under normal physiologic conditions, based on theoretical arguments. Originally, the value for the LC in

humans was selected so that the average whole brain CMRGlu measured with FDG would equal that determined by earlier investigators with the more invasive Kety–Schmidt technique (Phelps et al., 1979). It is possible to measure the LC of whole human brain from the ratio of the brain arteriovenous extraction fraction of FDG to that of glucose (Reivich et al., 1985). A recent study (Hasselbalch et al., 1998) in which great care was taken in the methodologic aspects of the measurement obtained a value for the LC in normal subjects of 0.81, higher than the

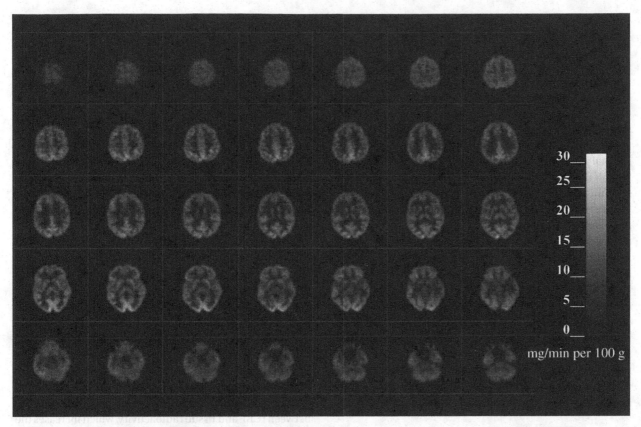

Fig. 1.4. Cerebral glucose metabolic rates. Quantitative images obtained in a normal subject with [^{18}F]-fluorodeoxyglucose and application of Sokoloff's model. Anterior is up and left is to the reader's left. These images start at the level of the superior cortical level (upper left) and proceed down through the brain to the level of the cerebellum. Note the bar scale at the right indicating the correspondence between glucose metabolic rates and gray levels in the image.

values of 0.42–0.52 used in earlier work. The LC does change in pathologic conditions such as acute cerebral ischemia, recent cerebral infarction, and brain tumor (Gjedde et al., 1985; Nakai et al., 1987; Spence et al., 1990; Greenberg et al., 1992). Since calculated rCMRGlu is inversely proportional to the LC (see Fig. 1.3), the use of an incorrect value leads to a corresponding error in the calculation. Consequently, it is necessary to redetermine both the LC and the rate constants to avoid such errors in pathologic conditions where there is a gross abnormality of tissue or an imbalance between glucose supply and demand. This is difficult and has been rarely done in PET studies.

An alternative approach to measure rCMRGlu uses [^{11}C]-glucose, which is transported and metabolized in the same way as glucose (Blomqvist et al., 1990). As a result, the compartmental model does not require a LC correction factor. A disadvantage is that the labeled metabolites of glucose, such as ^{11}CO$_2$, are not all trapped in tissue and the model must account for their egress. [^{11}C]-Glucose may be more widely used in the future, especially in pathologic conditions. For example, it has been recently used to measure cerebral glucose transport and metabolism in preterm infants (Powers et al., 1998).

Cerebral blood volume

Measurement of rCBV uses trace amounts of ^{11}CO or C^{15}O administered by inhalation (Grubb et al., 1978; Martin et al., 1987). The tracer binds to hemoglobin and is confined to the intravascular space. Local radioactivity in brain is proportional to its red cell content; consequently, rCBV can be calculated from the ratio of the radioactivity in brain to that in peripheral blood. However, the hematocrit is less in brain than in peripheral large vessels owing to the behavior of blood in the brain microvasculature, and the ratio of cerebral hematocrit to peripheral hematocrit (R) must be incorporated into the calculation (Grubb et al., 1978; Lammertsma et al., 1984; Martin et al., 1987). Equation (1.1), or a modification (Videen et al., 1987), is used to calculate rCBV in units of milliliters per 100 g tissue, from the radiotracer concentrations in tissue (C_t) and blood (C_{bl}):

$$rCBV = \frac{C_t}{C_{bl}R} \tag{1.1}$$

The use of $C^{15}O$ has practical advantages over ^{11}CO (Martin et al., 1987). The 2 min half-life of ^{15}O permits other PET studies to be performed with little delay and lowers radiation exposure, and the synthesis is more convenient. Normal values for rCBV are 4–6 ml/100 g in gray matter and 2–3 ml/100 g in white matter (Lammertsma et al., 1983; Perlmutter et al., 1987).

In cerebrovascular disease, rCBV reflects vasodilatation in response to decreased cerebral perfusion pressure, as may occur with a narrowed internal carotid artery (Powers, 1991; Heiss and Podreka, 1993). Changes in rCBV can also be seen with elevated intracranial pressure (Grubb et al., 1975). In addition, rCBV data may be required as part of other PET methods (e.g., the measurement of cerebral oxygen metabolism and extraction fraction or some neuroreceptor studies) to correct for radiotracer located in the intravascular space so as to determine the amount of radiotracer that actually enters tissue. Measurement of rCBV has recently been used to determine the vascular response to focal brain activation (Wang et al., 1998).

Cerebral blood flow

Methods to measure rCBF with PET are based on a model developed by Kety to measure rCBF in laboratory animals (Kety, 1951; Landau et al., 1955). The model describes inert tracers that can diffuse freely across the blood–brain barrier. The technique involves infusing a radioactive tracer over a brief time period T, often 1 min. Frequent timed blood samples are obtained during the infusion to determine the arterial time–radioactivity curve $C_a(t)$. The animal is then killed. Regional brain radioactivity at the end of the infusion, $C_t(T)$, is measured by quantitative tissue autoradiography. Tissue blood flow f (units of ml/min per 100 g) is calculated from these measurements using Eq. (1.2):

$$C_t(T) = f \int_0^T C_a(t)\exp[-f/\lambda(T-t)]dt \tag{1.2}$$

Where λ is the brain–blood partition coefficient for the tracer defined as the ratio between the tissue and blood radiotracer concentrations when they are in equilibrium. Its value can be determined from independent experiments or can be calculated as the ratio of the solubilities of the tracer in brain and blood (Kety, 1951; Herscovitch and Raichle, 1985). Equation (1.2) is solved numerically for flow, using measured values for $C_t(T)$ and $C_a(t)$, and a specified value for λ.

Kety's method is the basis for methods to measure rCBF with PET. Although there are different approaches, they all involve administering a diffusible, positron-emitting radiotracer, blood sampling to determine the time–activity curve in arterial blood (typically from the radial artery), and the application of a modification of Eq. (1.2) to generate images of rCBF from PET images of radioactivity. The tracer most commonly used is [^{15}O]-water ($H_2^{15}O$) administered by intravenous injection. Because of the short half-life of ^{15}O, repeat measurements can be performed within 10–12 min.

The steady-state method was the earliest widely used PET method to measure rCBF (Subramanyam et al., 1978; Frackowiak et al., 1980). The subject inhales $C^{15}O_2$ delivered at a fixed rate. The action of carbonic anhydrase in red blood cells results in transfer of ^{15}O to water and the $H_2^{15}O$ constantly generated in the lungs circulates throughout the body. A steady state is reached in which radioactivity delivered to brain tissue equals that leaving by decay and by venous washout. The brain distribution of radioactivity remains constant, and a simple equation can be used to calculate rCBF. This method was convenient with the early, single-ring tomographs, since multiple tomographic slices could be obtained by repositioning the patient during $C^{15}O_2$ inhalation. A limitation is the nonlinear relationship between rCBF and tissue radioactivity, which increases the sensitivity of the CBF calculation to errors in measured tissue and blood radioactivity (Lammertsma et al., 1981; Herscovitch and Raichle, 1983; Baron et al., 1989). Because of this, the long period required for CBF measurement, and the development of multislice scanners, the steady-state method has been largely supplanted.

Alternative approaches use bolus intravenous injections of $H_2^{15}O$ and an adaptation of Kety's equation. Equation (1.2) is not used directly because scanners cannot measure the instantaneous brain radiotracer concentration $C_t(T)$. It has been modified in different ways to allow for performance of the scans over many seconds, summing enough counts to obtain satisfactory images. With the PET/autoradiographic approach, $H_2^{15}O$ is administered by bolus intravenous injection, and a 40 s scan is obtained after the radiotracer arrives in the head (Herscovitch et al., 1983; Raichle et al., 1983). The relationship between tissue counts and rCBF is almost linear and errors in measurement of tissue radioactivity result in approximately equivalent errors in calculated rCBF. Because the PET image obtained with a brief scan (1 min or less) closely reflects flow differences in different brain regions, useful information about relative CBF can be obtained without blood sampling. This approach is widely used in functional brain mapping experiments, in which $H_2^{15}O$ images are used to determine relative rCBF changes during neurobehavioral tasks (Frackowiak and Friston, 1994). Average values for rCBF in normal subjects obtained with either the steady-state method (Leenders et al., 1990) or the PET/autoradiographic method (Herscovitch et al., 1987; Perlmutter et al., 1987) are 40–60 ml/min per 100 g in gray matter and 20–30 ml/per 100 g in white matter.

There are other methods for measuring rCBF based on the Kety model. One approach involves collecting several sequential, brief images after bolus intravenous administration of tracer (Koeppe et al., 1985). Parameter estimation techniques are used to estimate both rCBF and λ from the scan and blood radioactivity data. To simplify blood sampling for these $H_2^{15}O$ rCBF techniques, automated systems have been designed to withdraw arterial blood continuously past a radiation detector (Eriksson et al., 1988).

Methods using $H_2^{15}O$ assume that it is freely diffusible across the blood–brain barrier. However, there is a modest diffusion limitation, which results in an underestimation of rCBF at higher flows (Raichle et al., 1983). There are other tracers without a diffusion limitation, such as $[^{11}C]$- or $[^{15}O]$-butanol (Herscovitch et al., 1987; Berridge et al., 1991). The diffusion limitation of $H_2^{15}O$ is accepted, however, because of the tracer's convenience. Also, in conditions with decreased rCBF, tracer diffusion limitation is less important.

Cerebral oxygen metabolism

The regional cerebral metabolic rate of oxygen (rCMRO$_2$), which is more complex to obtain than cerebral glucose metabolism, is not widely used in research in pediatric disorders. It is measured using inhaled $^{15}O_2$. One method developed in conjunction with the steady-state rCBF technique uses continuous inhalation of $^{15}O_2$ (Subramanyam et al., 1978; Frackowiak et al., 1980). Another, a companion to the PET/autoradiographic rCBF method, uses a brief inhalation of $^{15}O_2$ (Mintun et al., 1984). The principles underlying these methods are similar. Approximately 35–40% of the oxygen delivered to the brain is extracted and metabolized (Perlmutter et al., 1987; Leenders et al., 1990). Both methods measure this oxygen extraction fraction (OEF). There are essentially no stores of oxygen in brain, and all extracted oxygen is metabolized. Therefore, rCMRO$_2$ can be determined from the product of OEF and the rate of oxygen delivery to brain, which equals rCBF multiplied by arterial oxygen content. The tracer models describe the fate of the ^{15}O label following $^{15}O_2$ inhalation. Extracted $^{15}O_2$ is metabolized to $H_2^{15}O$, which is then washed out of brain. The $H_2^{15}O$ that is produced by brain as well as by the rest of the body recirculates to brain and

diffuses into and out of brain tissue. Another component of the measured radioactivity is intravascular $^{15}O_2$ that is not extracted by brain. It is necessary to account for this component so that it is not attributed to radioactivity in tissue. Therefore, an independent measurement of rCBV is needed. Both PET methods require three scans to measure regional oxygen extraction fraction (rOEF) and rCMRO$_2$: an rCBF scan, an rCBV scan, and a scan obtained with $^{15}O_2$.

With the steady-state method, scanning is performed during continuous inhalation of $^{15}O_2$ and rCBF is measured with continuous inhalation of $C^{15}O_2$ and rCBV with $C^{15}O$. The rOEF is computed from these scans and from measurements of blood radioactivity (Lammertsma et al., 1983). An alternative method for measuring rOEF and rCMRO$_2$ uses a brief inhalation of $^{15}O_2$ (Mintun et al., 1984; Videen et al., 1987). A 40 s scan is obtained following $^{15}O_2$ inhalation, and frequent arterial blood samples are collected for measurements of blood radioactivity. It also involves measurement of rCBF with $H_2^{15}O$ and the PET/autoradiographic method, and of rCBV with $C^{15}O$. The method was validated in baboons in a series of experiments that included very reduced rCMRO$_2$ (Mintun et al., 1984; Altman et al., 1991). A different approach has been described to measure rCMRO$_2$ that involves dynamic scanning (i.e., obtaining multiple short scans over time) following only one brief inhalation of $^{15}O_2$ (Ohta et al., 1992). Average normal values for gray matter rCMRO$_2$ are 2.5–3.5 ml/min per 100 g (Perlmutter et al., 1987; Leenders et al., 1990).

Single photon emission computed tomography

Principles

The radionuclides used in SPECT decay by emitting a single photon or gamma ray from their nucleus; radioactivity distribution is estimated by detection of gamma rays. The most commonly used SPECT systems have one or more gamma camera "heads" (Devous et al., 1986; George et al., 1991; Holman and Devous, 1992; Masdeu et al., 1994; Devous, 1995). The gamma camera head has a large, relatively thin (e.g., 3/8 in by 12–20 in (0.96 cm by 30–50 cm) diameter) scintillation crystal of sodium iodide, which gives off a localized pulse of light when it absorbs a gamma ray. The front of the crystal is covered with a parallel-hole collimator, which is typically made up of lead perforated by an array of small hexagonal holes. The collimator limits the gamma rays that strike the crystal to those traveling along parallel lines perpendicular to the crystal face. An array of photomultiplier tubes and position logic circuits behind

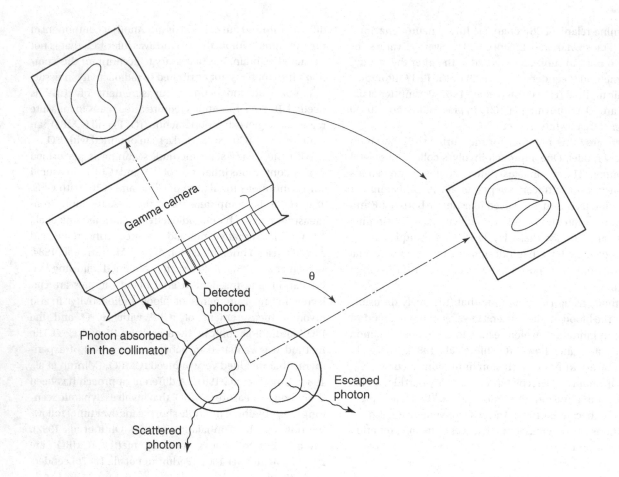

Fig. 1.5. SPECT data acquisition with a gamma camera. The collimator and the thin sodium iodide crystal detector behind the collimator are shown. Gamma rays or photons pass through the parallel holes in the collimator to the crystal and are registered by photomultipliers and electronic circuitry behind the crystal. Some photons strike the collimator septa at an angle and are absorbed, while others escape the body away from the view of the camera head and are not detected. As the head rotates around the patient, images are collected at each scanning angle. Scan profiles from these images are used as input for the SPECT reconstruction algorithm to obtain tomographic images of the distribution of radioactivity in the body. (From Sorenson and Phelps, 1987, with permission.)

the crystal sense the light pulses and determine the location of each pulse in the crystal. This information is used to generate a planar image of the distribution of radioactivity in the body. In order to obtain tomographic images, the camera head is rotated around the body to obtain multiple views (Fig. 1.5). These are combined to reconstruct tomographic images of the radioactivity distribution. To improve sensitivity, modern systems have two or three heads, mounted in a gantry, that surround the body and rotate together. Alternative SPECT designs, which are in limited use, employ either a circumferential array of small detectors or a single continuous cylindrical crystal that surrounds the patient (Holman et al., 1990).

SPECT devices have a spatial resolution of about 15 mm with single heads, and 6–9 mm with multiple heads and different collimator designs. Sensitivity tends to be low, even with multiple head devices, because of the need for collimators; as a result, the imaging time is typically 20–30 min and radiotracers that provide a static unchanging distribution are typically used. Unlike PET, an accurate measured correction for attenuation is not convenient, and in some camera configurations is not possible at all. The methods currently used provide only an approximate attenuation correction (Bailey, 1998), and thus limit the absolute quantification of regional radioactivity. Typically, radioactivity is not quantified in absolute terms, but rather the tomographic images are used to obtain information about the relative concentration of radioactivity in different regions. A major advantage is that single-headed cameras with SPECT capability are ubiquitous in nuclear medicine departments, and multi-headed systems have become more widespread. In addition, a cyclotron is not required to produce SPECT radiopharmaceuticals. The cost of SPECT instruments at the end of the 1990s ranges from $250 000 to $1 000 000, depending primarily upon the number of heads; in contrast PET scanners cost about $2 500 000 (and, additionally, the cyclotron needed to produce PET radionuclides itself costs about $1 500 000).

Radiotracer methods

Most SPECT brain studies are performed with radio-pharmaceuticals that map CBF. Several radio-pharmaceuticals are available for this purpose (George et al., 1991; Holman and Devous, 1992; van Heertum et al., 1993). The most commonly used radiotracer strategy is based on the microsphere method, a technique used to measure local flow in experimental animals (Warner et al., 1987). With that method, radioactive microspheres of a size appropriate to be trapped in capillaries are introduced into the left side of the animal's heart. They are distributed and trapped in tissue in proportion to flow and then local radioactivity is measured in samples of tissue. SPECT uses lipophilic radiotracers with microsphere-like behavior that are administered intravenously. Ideally they are freely diffusible across the blood–brain barrier and are completely extracted and retained by brain in a distribution that is proportional to local flow. The tracers have a stable distribution in the brain, facilitating imaging. Several SPECT perfusion agents are based on this principle, although their extraction or retention by brain is not complete (Gemmell et al., 1992).

The first widely use SPECT CBF tracer was [^{123}I]-iodoamphetamine ([^{123}I]-IMP). It must be prelabeled by the commercial supplier, however, which is logistically difficult. Tracers using ^{99m}Tc are preferable because ^{99m}Tc is more convenient to use: it is obtained from generators that are delivered regularly to nuclear medicine departments; thus on-site labeling is possible. In addition, the physical characteristics of its radioactive decay are more favorable for SPECT imaging. A widely used ^{99m}Tc CBF agent is [^{99m}Tc]-labeled hexamethylpropylene amine oxime (also called [^{99m}Tc]-exametazime, [^{99m}Tc]-HMPAO). Another compound, [^{99m}Tc]-labeled ethyl cysteinate dimer [^{99m}Tc]-bicisate, [^{99m}Tc]-ECD), is replacing HMPAO. ECD provides higher brain-to-background radioactivity ratios because of more rapid blood clearance and is more convenient to employ because of greater in vitro stability. Although there are methods to calculate absolute rCBF with these tracers that use arterial blood sampling and a tracer kinetic model (Greenberg et al., 1990; Murase et al., 1992), they are rarely

used. As a result, SPECT studies typically provide information about relative rCBF, not absolute rCBF.

SPECT studies are relatively easy to perform since the scanners are widely available and they do not require an in-house cyclotron to produce the radiotracer. The distribution of radiotracer in brain reflects the blood flow during the first few minutes after injection of the tracer and remains relatively stable. Therefore, scanning can start up to 30 min after tracer injection and it is not necessary to inject the tracer while the subject is in the scanner. Repeat SPECT studies cannot be performed rapidly because the half-life of ^{99m}Tc is 6 h, unless methods are used to subtract residual radioactivity. SPECT perfusion studies have been performed in the pediatric age group, and even in newborn infants (Borch and Greisen, 1997). It is also possible to measure rCBV with SPECT using [^{99m}Tc]-labeled red cells (Kuhl et al., 1980); the approach is similar to that used for PET. However, there are no SPECT radiotracers to study cerebral metabolism.

Recently, there has been considerable progress in the development of receptor-binding ligands for SPECT, especially for dopamine and benzodiazepine receptors (Holman and Devous, 1992) and for dopamine reuptake transporters (Seibyl et al., 1996) (Table 1.2). Iodine-123 is typically used to label these ligands. The techniques of tracer kinetic modeling described above are applied to analyze image and blood radioactivity data (Laruelle et al., 1994a,b).

Data analysis

After a PET study has been completed, the relevant tracer model is applied to calculate the physiologic variable of interest. For the methods to measure cerebral hemodynamics and metabolism described above, the model is applied on a point-by-point basis and the intensity of the resultant image depends upon the local value of the physiologic measurement (see Fig. 1.4). Although visual inspection of PET images may reveal abnormalities, quantitative analysis and appropriate statistical techniques are required for clinical research. Data reduction, analysis, and interpretation are very demanding. Newer scanners acquire up to 63 slices simultaneously, each containing data from many brain structures. Several scans of the same or different types may be obtained in one session, for example multiple rCBF scans, or rCBF and rCMRGlu scans, and subjects may have repeat studies on different days. The analysis of PET data is greatly facilitated by interactive computer programs. These programs permit regions of interest (ROIs) of arbitrary size and shape to be placed over

Table 1.2. Representative SPECT radiotracers

Physiologic process or system	Radiotracer
Cerebral blood flow	[^{123}I]-Iodoamphetamine ([^{123}I]-IMP)
	[^{99m}Tc]-labeled exametazime ([^{99m}Tc]-HMPAO)
	[^{99m}Tc]-labeled ethyl cysteinate dimer ([^{99m}Tc]-ECD)
Cerebral plasma and red cell volume	[^{99m}Tc]-labeled human serum albumin
	[^{99m}Tc]-labeled red blood cells
Neuroreceptor systems	
Dopaminergic	
Dopamine D$_2$ receptors	[^{123}I]-Iodobenzamide ([^{123}I]-IBZM); [^{123}I]-epidepride
Dopamine D$_1$ receptors	[^{123}I]-SCH23982
Dopamine reuptake sites	[^{123}I]-N-(3-Fluoropropyl)-2β-carbomethoxy-3β-(4-iodophenyl)nortropane ([^{123}I]-β-CIT)
Benzodiazepine	[^{123}I]-Iomazenil
Cholinergic muscarinic	[^{123}I]-Labeled quinuclidinylbenzilate [^{123}I]-QNB; [^{123}I]-iododexetimide
Serotonergic 5-HT$_{2A}$ receptors	[^{123}I]-R93274
Amino acid transport	[^{123}I]-Iodo-α-methyltyrosine

different structures for which the physiologic variable is then computed. Also, whole-brain measurements can be obtained by averaging over several PET slices, or by using a template of ROIs to sample multiple brain regions.

PET measurements must be related to the underlying anatomy. Early approaches to data analysis used PET images obtained in standard planes, for example parallel to the canthomeatal line. The images were visually compared to corresponding anatomic sections in a brain atlas and the ROIs manually drawn. This method, however, is subjective and liable to observer bias. A refinement uses a template of standard regions to sample brain structures of interest, with visual adjustment to fit the template to the images. Alternative approaches have been developed that relate PET images to anatomy more accurately and objectively. A widely used approach uses the principles of stereotactic localization to establish a correspondence between brain areas or volumes in a stereotactic brain atlas and specific regions or pixels in the PET image (Fox et al., 1985; Friston et al., 1989). Other methods are required if there are structural abnormalities. An approach widely used for both normal and abnormal brain is to obtain anatomic images with CT or MRI in the same planes as the PET slices. Methods to achieve this include head holders transferable between imaging modalities, fiducial markers affixed to the head, and, most conveniently, automated computer techniques to register and reslice PET and MR or CT images (Pelizzari et al., 1989; Wilson and Mountz, 1989; Evans et al., 1991; Woods et al., 1993; Ge et al., 1994). After coplanar anatomic and PET images have been obtained,

ROIs can be transferred between them. These automated techniques have also been used to register brain SPECT images with CT or MR images (Holman et al., 1991).

A variety of sophisticated methods have been developed to extract information from functional brain images. One approach consists of calculating the relationship between CBF or metabolism in multiple pairs of brain regions (Horwitz et al., 1992). A high degree of correlation or covariance between the activity in two brain regions is attributed to a high level of functional connectivity or coupling between them during a particular condition (Friston, 1994). This implies that the regions work together, influence each other, or are affected in a similar fashion by a third region. In a refinement of this approach called path analysis, knowledge of the neuroanatomic connections between brain areas is included in the computation of interregional correlations, and functional networks consisting of several brain regions can be identified (McIntosh et al., 1994). An alternative group of approaches, including principle components analysis and scaled subprofile modeling, attempts to identify groups of regions that account for the variability in a dataset and which may be functionally related (Strother et al., 1995).

The technique of statistical parametric mapping (SPM) has become a widely applied method. It is typically used to determine the difference, on a pixel-by-pixel basis, between sets of rCBF images obtained in different study conditions (Friston et al., 1991; Frackowiak and Friston, 1994; Acton and Friston, 1998). This method basically consists of three steps. The first is image normalization in which each pixel is mapped into the same stereotactic space; thus all pixels in the image set are transformed into a common reference brain in a 3D coordinate system. This permits the second step, that is averaging images obtained from different subjects studied during the same condition. This reduces image noise and facilitates the detection of significant differences between conditions. Because image noise in PET images is random, it decreases when images are averaged, while the rCBF pattern, which is consistent across subjects, remains. The final step is to perform statistical tests on a pixel-by-pixel basis between datasets to identify regions of significant rCBF change. The results are displayed as 3D maps or views of the reference brain in which pixels with a significant change in rCBF are highlighted.

SPM was originally designed to determine the changes in local CBF measured with $H_2^{15}O$ in subjects studied during two or more different neurobehavioral tasks in functional brain mapping experiments. It can also be applied in a parametric analysis to see which brain regions covary in a systematic fashion with some parameter related to the performance of a cognitive, sensory, or motor task (e.g., the rate of hand movement). SPM has subsequently been applied to both $H_2^{15}O$ and FDG images in other types of study, for example before and after administration of a drug or to compare a group of patients with a control group. It has also been used to analyze perfusion images obtained with SPECT (Acton and Friston, 1998).

There is variability in both regional and global PET measurements. The coefficient of variation (i.e., the ratio of the standard deviation to the mean value) for measurements of rCBF, rCMRGlu, and rCMRO$_2$ is 15–25% in groups of normal subjects (Perlmutter et al., 1987; Tyler et al., 1988; Camargo et al., 1992; Wang et al., 1994), although the variability in repeat measurements in the same subject is less (Matthew et al., 1993). This may reflect normal physiologic variation or methodologic inaccuracies. Approaches have been developed to facilitate detecting regional changes in spite of this variability. These adjust for the effect of global variations by "normalizing" regional data, thereby decreasing their variance. This can be done by dividing regional values by the global average value or by the value in a structure presumed to be minimally involved in the disease being studied. Such techniques, however, can result in a loss of the information contained in the absolute values, especially if widespread changes occur. If the denominator as well as the numerator differs between groups, erroneous conclusions may be drawn. For example, in a study of Alzheimer's disease (Cutler et al., 1985), normalized rCMRGlu in thalamus was significantly *increased* because of a *decrease* in global metabolism. In other words, the

metabolism in the thalamus may be relatively spared. Therefore, normalized PET data must be carefully interpreted. In spite of the variability of PET measurements, it is possible to demonstrate meaningful physiologic abnormalities with absolute data, for example in cerebrovascular disease (Powers, 1998).

SPECT perfusion studies typically do not involve quantitation of absolute rCBF. Although the image intensity is proportional to flow, it also depends on the amount of tracer reaching the brain, which can vary between patients and even in the same patient because of variations in the peripheral circulation as well as body size. A normalization procedure is performed if regional tissue count data are to be averaged in a patient group or compared with data from normal subjects. This is accomplished by dividing the count data in individual ROIs by the average count value (Goldenberg et al., 1992) or by the value in the cerebellum, assuming that it is not involved in the disease process. There are potential ambiguities with this approach. For example, a region with the appearance of increased perfusion may actually have an elevated flow, but the finding may also reflect reduced flow in other brain regions (Wilson and Wyper, 1992).

Data from control subjects are required to interpret PET or SPECT measurements obtained in patients. Quantitative data obtained in appropriately selected normal subjects are used. Depending on the nature of the study, selection criteria must control for variables such as age, gender, handedness, and condition of general health; in children, sexual and cognitive maturation must also be included. Average data from patients are statistically compared with the same regional measurements made in a group of normal control subjects. It is also possible to analyze regional data obtained in an individual patient, for example by determining whether they are outside the range of normal. In comparing measurements obtained from many brain regions, it is possible that some regions will be found to be significantly different by chance because of the large number of multiple comparisons being made. One approach to avoid this error, which is rather conservative, is to adjust the study p value (typically 0.05) by dividing it by the number of measurements being made (the Bonferroni correction).

One must also consider the possibility of a drift in measurements over years in the case of longitudinal studies, which have a special place in pediatric research. Usually, these changes over time caused by subtle changes in scanner performance can be corrected by covariance analysis. This stresses the importance of systematic and rigorous quality control of scanners and the interleaving of patients and controls over the duration of a study.

If visual analysis of SPECT and PET images is used, it requires a rigorous approach. SPECT images are frequently interpreted visually for abnormalities. The criteria for defining an abnormality are usually subjective, however, and further work must be done to define the sensitivity and specificity for detecting abnormalities (Juni, 1994; Stapleton et al., 1994). In some SPECT studies, there is a clear definition of regional abnormality and scans are graded by agreement among two or more observers (Jacobs et al., 1994), whereas other studies have used less careful methodology. This makes it difficult to compare different studies.

Interpretation of changes in cerebral blood flow and metabolism

Physiologic considerations

To interpret changes in PET and SPECT studies, it is necessary to understand the relationships among CBF, metabolism, and local neuronal activity, and the mechanisms by which CBF and metabolism can become abnormal.

Normally, about 30% of the brain's energy metabolism supports synaptic transmission, 30% residual ion fluxes and transport, and 40% other processes such as axoplasmic transport and macromolecular synthesis (Astrup et al., 1981). In the resting state, the energy needs of the brain are met by the oxidative metabolism of glucose, and there is a proportional relationship, termed coupling, between rCBF and both $rCMRO_2$ and rCMRGlu (Sokoloff, 1981; Baron et al., 1984; Fox and Raichle, 1986; Fox et al., 1988). During increased local neuronal activity, for example with somatosensory or visual stimulation, there are coupled or parallel increases in rCBF and rCMRGlu in the brain regions involved (Sokoloff, 1961; Leniger-Follert and Hossman, 1979; Toga and Collins, 1981; Yarowsky et al., 1983; Fox and Raichle, 1984; Ginsberg et al., 1987; Fox et al., 1988). Within physiologic limits, these increases parallel the stimulus rate and the rate of neuronal firing. Most of the brain's additional glucose consumption during increased neuronal activity is used to maintain ionic gradients across cell membranes, which must be restored after depolarization (Yarowsky and Ingvar, 1981). These observations form the basis for using measurements of rCBF and rCMRGlu as markers of local neuronal function (Raichle, 1987). PET studies in humans have shown, however, that there is only a slight increase in $rCMRO_2$ during functional activation (Fox and Raichle, 1986; Fox et al., 1988). This observation challenged the hypothesis that oxidative glucose metabolism or its products regulate the rCBF changes during neuronal activation. In fact, the processes responsible for

coupling rCBF to rCMRGlu at rest and during activation remain to be elucidated (Lou et al., 1987; Raichle, 1991; Edvinsson et al., 1993b; Jueptner and Weiller, 1995).

Various mechanism can lead to abnormalities of CBF and metabolism. Changes in neuronal activity can result in increases or decreases in local CBF and metabolism. Decreased neuronal activity in coma decreases CBF and metabolism (Obrist et al., 1984), as can drugs and anesthetics that act on synapses or membranes to depress neuronal activity. Abnormalities in blood flow and metabolism in specific brain regions have been found in many neurologic and psychiatric diseases. These may reflect altered neuronal activity either in the area(s) of abnormality or in distant brain regions that project to the area(s). In many diseases, several brain areas are affected, implying an abnormality in underlying brain networks. Both acute and chronic administration of drugs have been shown to change rCBF and metabolism. These changes have been related to the action of the drug on a specific receptor system with a resulting change in activity.

Tissue damage or loss, either gross or through loss of neurons, can decrease flow and metabolism. In addition, coupled decreases in flow and metabolism can be seen in structures *distant* to a lesion. This phenomenon, called diaschisis, is attributed to a decrease in neuronal activity in a brain structure through loss of afferent projections from the damaged region (Feeney and Baron, 1986). For example, decreased flow and metabolism can be seen in the cerebellum contralateral to a cerebral infarct. There are situations when flow and metabolism are not coupled, for example with changes in arterial blood gases (Edvinsson et al., 1993a) and in pathologic conditions such as cerebrovascular disease (Powers, 1988, 1991; Heiss and Podreka, 1993) or elevated intracranial pressure (Grubb et al., 1975).

Effect of limited spatial resolution

Artifactual abnormalities of CBF and metabolism can be observed with PET or SPECT because of the limited spatial resolution of the imaging devices. Limited resolution results in blurring of PET and SPECT images (Fig. 1.6). More important is its effect on the accuracy of radioactivity measurement (Hoffman et al., 1979; Mazziotta et al., 1981). Because the radioactivity appears spread out over a larger area, a brain region in the image contains only a portion of the radioactivity that was in the corresponding brain structure. In addition, some of the radioactivity in surrounding structures appears to be spread into the region. Because of this effect, called partial volume averaging, a regional measurement contains a contribution from both the structure of interest and surrounding struc-

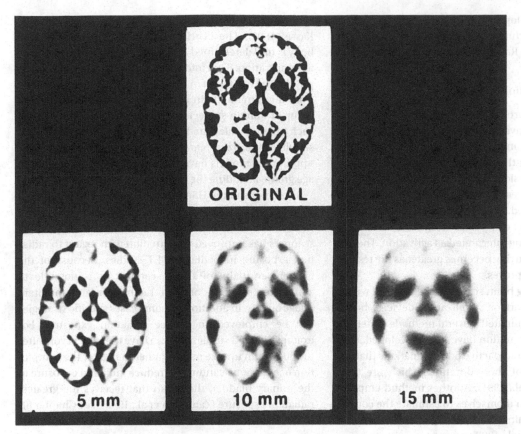

Fig. 1.6. The effect of scanner resolution on the accuracy of images obtained. At the upper center is a simulated "ideal" PET image of regional radioactivity, reflecting the higher metabolic activity in gray matter. Subsequent images simulate the effect of obtaining this image with tomographs of varying spatial resolution, from 5 to 15 mm FWHM (full width at half maximum). Note the blurring or spreading out of radioactivity, with gray matter structures appearing paler. As a result, radioactivity in cortical and subcortical gray matter regions is underestimated. Similar considerations hold for SPECT images. (From Mazziotta et al., 1981, with permission.)

tures. High radioactivity levels surrounded by lower values will be underestimated, while low radioactivity surrounded by high activity will be overestimated. These errors are less when the size of the structure of interest is large with respect to scanner resolution. In a circular, uniform structure with a diameter twice the resolution, the radioactivity concentration will be accurately represented in the center. However, statistical considerations limit obtaining a measurement with a very small ROI. In general, it is not possible to measure pure gray matter radioactivity, especially in thin cortical regions.

Partial volume averaging with cerebrospinal fluid in sulci or ventricles can lead to an underestimation of tissue blood flow and metabolism. If there is cerebral atrophy, PET and SPECT measurements will be further reduced because of partial volume averaging with enlarged, metabolically inactive, cerebrospinal fluid spaces (Herscovitch et al., 1986; Videen et al., 1988). Beyond the border of a circumscribed

region of decreased flow or metabolism, one would observe a gradual transition of the physiologic measurement to the value in surrounding normal tissue, also caused by partial volume averaging (Powers, 1988). This gives rise to the false perception that the PET or SPECT "lesion" is larger than the actual abnormality. Recently, decreased CBF and metabolism in the subgenual prefrontal cortex in patients with familial depression was found to be associated with a focal reduction in gray matter volume of the affected cortical structure. This intriguing observation indicates that altered PET measurements can be found through partial volume averaging in conditions with an unsuspected anatomic abnormality (Drevets et al., 1997).

Methods have been developed to correct for partial volume averaging and recover a more accurate radioactivity measurement from small brain structures (Meltzer et al., 1996), and these should find increasing application. The contribution of partial volume effect is particularly important in the developing brain where size, shape, and homogeneity of structures vary with neural maturation (Giedd et al., 1996a, b; Rajapakse et al., 1996).

Effect of patient motion

Head movement is particularly important when subjects are children who have trouble remaining immobile. Motion between the transmission and emission scans can lead to a mismatch in the attenuation correction factors. Motion during an emission can blur the image in a nonuniform manner and increase partial volume errors. Motion between scans obtained at rest and during performance of a task in a given subject can lead to artefactual differences between the scans being interpreted as activation. The relative impact of this blurring becomes greater as the resolution of the scanner improves.

Head motion during brain scans can be reduced with a variety of head support or stabilization devices, but it cannot be entirely eliminated. Several methods of detecting and correcting for motion have been developed. One technique is based on radioactive fiducial markers that are used to align scans of short duration, which are then summed (Koeppe et al., 1991). Another method employs the images of the brain themselves to estimate the corrections necessary to obtain maximum alignment of the serial images (Minoshima et al., 1992).

Radiation exposure and technical issues in pediatric imaging

Radiation exposure

Although the short half-lives of PET radionuclides favourably affects the radiation exposure to subjects, this exposure is not negligible. Radiation exposure in the context of PET and SPECT is an important consideration when they are used for research rather than diagnostic purposes (Veatch, 1982; Huda and Scrimger, 1989). Limits on radiation exposure to research subjects are set by regulatory bodies such as the US Food and Drug Administration and institutional radiation safety committees. The potential risks associated with low levels of radiation such as those received from PET are carcinogenesis and genetic effects in future generations (Brill, 1987). Although the risk is very low (for review, see Ernst et al., 1998), it is agreed that the least amount of radiotracer necessary to perform an adequate PET study should be administered.

Methods have been developed to determine radiation exposure from internally administered radiopharma-

ceuticals (Cloutier and Watson, 1987; Loevinger et al., 1988; Kassis, 1992). The distribution of the radiotracer in the body is first determined as a function of time following its administration. This information can be calculated using physiologic models of in vivo tracer behavior, extrapolated from measurements in animals, or measured in a small group of human subjects. Then the radiation exposure to each organ is calculated using a model of the body that simulates the size, shape, and properties of body organs. Appropriate models have been designed for the pediatric age group, including the neonate.

Regulations in the USA typically restrict radiation exposure in minors participating in research studies to one-tenth that allowed in adults. The use of newer, 3D PET scanners has improved the situation with regard to radiation exposure in pediatric PET studies. Because of the greater sensitivity of these scanners, it is possible to administer smaller doses of radiotracer and maintain image quality. In addition, in some cases specific strategies can be employed to reduce radiation exposure. For example, in FDG studies one can have the subject void after the 30–45 min uptake period rather than after the completion of emission scanning, to reduce radiation exposure to the urinary bladder, the organ that receives the greatest radiation exposure (Zametkin et al., 1993) (see Chapter 6).

Technical issues

Clinical research with PET is more complex in the pediatric age group than in adults for several reasons.

Measurement of radioactivity in arterial blood is typically required to perform truly quantitative studies. In the adult, arterial catheters can routinely be inserted purely for research purposes (Lockwood, 1985), but this is a major obstacle in minors. In sick infants, arterial samples have been obtained from catheters previously placed for intensive care purposes (Volpe et al., 1983). There are alternatives, however. For FDG studies, venous sampling can be performed from a hand heated to 44 °C to "arterialize" venous blood (Phelps et al., 1979); this does require cooperation from the subject. With certain PET tracer techniques, the image of local radioactivity is approximately proportional to the underlying physiologic variable, for example rCBF with a bolus intravenous injection of $H_2{}^{15}O$, or rCMRGlu with FDG. With appropriate data analysis strategies, information about regional abnormalities can be obtained without blood sampling.

A novel approach to obtaining the arterial time–radioactivity curve involves imaging the heart after injection of tracer. Multiple brief scans are obtained, and the blood curve is measured using an ROI placed over the left ventricle. This approach was originally applied to PET studies of the heart, where both the heart chamber and the tissue of interest (the myocardium) are simultaneously in the field of view of the scanner (Weinberg et al., 1988; Bergmann et al., 1989; Iida et al., 1992). It can also be used with certain radiotracer techniques that are used to study the brain, for example with FDG or [^{11}C]-α-methyltryptophan (Muzik et al., 1998), for which there is a prolonged tracer uptake period that is followed by emission imaging of the brain.

During a PET scan, it is necessary to prevent head movement. In cooperative adults, this is accomplished by means of a specially designed headholder affixed to the scanner couch. Children may find this difficult to tolerate. For the FDG method, it is possible to sedate the subject for the emission image after the 30–45 min tracer uptake period, because the tracer distribution in brain has already been established. Also, for scans that require prolonged imaging, it is possible to collect the data in multiple brief scans that can be spatially registered to each other to correct for head movement.

Although normal adults are frequently scanned to obtain control data for comparison with patient data, it is usually difficult to scan normal children in PET or SPECT studies because of ethical considerations (Chapter 6). Depending upon the research question, some studies do not require control data (e.g., Altman et al., 1989; Perlman and Altman, 1992). For studies that require normal control data, a suboptimal approach can be used: the control group can include retrospectively selected children who had been scanned for appropriate clinical research indications, such as a neurologic event thought not to affect brain development or diagnostic evaluation for a neurologic disease that is ultimately excluded (Chugani and Phelps, 1991; Bentourkia et al., 1998; van Bogeart et al., 1998). Another strategy is to enroll healthy siblings of children affected by the condition being studied because the siblings have the possibility of indirect benefit from increased knowledge of the condition. The issue of studying normal children is discussed further in Chapter 6.

References

Acton, P. D. and Friston, K. J. (1998). Statistical parametric mapping in functional neuroimaging: beyond PET and fMRI activation studies. *Eur. J. Nucl. Med.*, **25**, 663–7.

Altman, D. I., Perlman, J. M., Volpe, J. J. and Powers, W. J. (1989). Cerebral oxygen metabolism in newborn infants measured with positron emission tomography. *J. Cereb. Blood Flow Metab.*, **9**(Suppl. 1), S25.

Altman, D. I., Lich, L. L. and Powers, W. J. (1991). Brief inhalation method to measure cerebral oxygen extraction with PET: accuracy determination under pathologic conditions. *J. Nucl. Med.*, **32**, 1738–41.

Astrup, J., Sorensen, P. M. and Sorensen, H. R. (1981). Oxygen and glucose consumption related to Na$^+$-K$^+$ transport in canine brain. *Stroke*, **12**, 726–30.

Bailey D. L. (1998). Transmission scanning in emission tomography. *Eur. J. Nucl. Med.*, **25**, 774–87.

Bailey, D. L., Miller, M. P., Spinks, T. J. et al. (1998). Experience with fully 3D PET and implications for future high-resolution 3D tomographs. *Phys. Med. Biol.*, **43**, 777–86.

Baron, J. C., Rougemont, D., Soussaline, F. et al. (1984). Local interrelationships of oxygen consumption and glucose utilization in normal subjects and in ischemic stroke patients: a positron emission tomographic study. *J. Cereb. Blood Flow Metab.*, **4**, 140–9.

Baron, J. C., Frackowiak, R. S. J., Herholz, K. et al. (1989). Use of PET methods for measurement of cerebral energy metabolism and hemodynamics in cerebrovascular disease. *J. Cereb. Blood Flow Metab.*, **9**, 723–42.

Bentourkia, M., Michel, C., Ferriere, G. et al. (1998). Evolution of brain glucose metabolism with age in epileptic infants, children and adolescents. *Brain Dev.*, **20**, 524–9.

Bergmann, S. R., Herrero, P., Markham, J., Weinheimer, C. J. and Walsh, M. N. (1989). Noninvasive quantitation of myocardial blood flow in human subjects with oxygen-15-labeled water and positron emission tomography, *J. Am. Coll. Cardiol.*, **14**, 639–52.

Bergstrom, M., Eriksson, L., Bohm, C., Blomqvist, G. and Litton, J. (1983). Correction for scattered radiation in a ring detector positron camera by integral transformation of the projections. *J. Comput. Assist. Tomogr.*, **7**, 42–50.

Berridge, M. S., Adler, L. P., Nelson, A. D. et al. (1991). Measurement of human cerebral blood flow with [^{15}O]butanol and positron emission tomography. *J. Cereb. Blood Flow Metab.*, **11**, 707–15.

Blomqvist, G., Stone-Elander, S., Halldin, C. et al. (1990). Positron emission tomographic measurements of cerebral glucose utilization using [1-^{11}C]D-glucose. *J. Cereb. Blood Flow Metab.*, **11**, 467–83.

Borch, K. and Greisen, G. (1997). ^{99m}Tc-HMPAO as a tracer of cerebral blood flow in newborn infants. *J. Cereb. Blood Flow Metab.*, **17**, 448–54.

Brill, A. B. (1987). Biological effects of ionizing radiation. In *Nuclear Medical Physics*, ed. L. E. Williams, pp. 163–83. Boca Raton, FL, CRC Press.

Brooks, R. A. (1982). Alternative formula for glucose utilization using labeled deoxyglucose. *J. Nucl. Med.*, **23**, 583–9.

Budinger, T. F., Derenzo, S. E., Greenberg, W. L., Gullberg, G. T. and Huesman, R. H. (1978). Quantitative potentials of dynamic emission computed tomography. *J. Nucl. Med.*, **19**, 309–15.

Camargo, E. E., Szabo, Z., Links, J. M. et al. (1992). The influence of biological and technical factors on the variability of global and regional brain metabolism of 2-[^{18}F]fluoro-2-deoxy-D-glucose. *J. Cereb. Blood Flow Metab.*, **12**, 281–90.

Carson, R. E. (1991). Precision and accuracy considerations of physiological quantitation in PET. *J. Cereb. Blood Flow Metab.*, **11**, A45–50.

Carson, R. E. (1996). Mathematical modeling and compartmental analysis. In *Nuclear Medicine*, ed. J. C. Harbert, W. E. Eckelman and R. D. Neumann, pp. 167–93. New York: Thieme.

Carson, R. E., Daube-Witherspoon, M. E. and Green, M. V. (1988). A method for postinjection PET transmission measurements with a rotating source. *J. Nucl. Med.*, **29**, 1558–67.

Cherry, S. R., Chatziioannou, A., Shao, Y., Silverman, R. W., Meadors, K. and Phelps, M. E. (1998). Brain imaging in small animals using MicroPET, In *Quantitative Functional Brain imaging with Positron Emission Tomography*, ed. R. E. Carson, M. E. Daube-Witherspoon and P. Herscovitch, pp. 201–6. San Diego, CA: Academic Press.

Chugani, H. T. and Phelps, M. E. (1991). Imaging human brain development with positron emission tomography [editorial comment]. *J. Nucl. Med.*, **32**, 23–6.

Cloutier, R. J. and Watson, E. E. (1987). Internal dosimetry – an introduction to the ICRP technique. In *Nuclear Medical Physics*, ed. L. E. Williams, p. 143. Boca Raton, FL: CRC Press.

Council on Scientific Affairs (1988). Instrumentation in positron emission tomography. *J. Am. Med. Assoc.*, **259**, 1351–6.

Cunningham, V. and Cremer, J. E. (1985). Current assumptions behind the use of PET scanning for measuring glucose utilization in brain. *Trends Neurosci.*, **8**, 96–9.

Cutler, N. R., Haxby, J. V., Duara, R. et al. (1985). Clinical history, brain metabolism, and neuropsychological function in Alzheimer's disease. *Ann. Neurol.*, **18**, 298–309.

Dannals, R. F., Ravert, H. T. and Wilson, A. A. (1993). Chemistry of tracers for positron emission tomography. In *Nuclear Imaging in Drug Discovery, Development, and Approval*, ed. D. H. Burns, R. E. Gibson, R. F. Dannals and P. K. S. Siegl, pp. 55–74. Boston: Birkhäuser.

Daube-Witherspoon, M. E. and Herscovitch, P. (1996). Positron emission tomography. In *Nuclear Medicine*, ed. J. C. Harbert, W. E. Eckelman and R. D. Neumann, pp. 121–43. New York: Thieme.

de Grado, T. R., Turkington, T., Williams, J. J., Stearns, C. W., Hoffman, J. M. and Coleman, R. E. (1994). Performance characteristics of a whole-body PET scanner. *J. Nucl. Med.*, **35**, 1398–1406.

Devous, M. D., Stokely, E. M., Chehabi, H. H. and Bonte, F. J. (1986). Normal distribution of regional cerebral blood flow measured by dynamic single-photon emission tomography. *J. Cereb. Blood Flow Metab.*, **6**, 95–104.

Devous, M. D. (1995). SPECT functional brain imaging: technical considerations. *J. Neuroimaging*, **5**(Suppl. 1), S2–13.

Drevets, W. C., Price, J. L., Simpson, J. R. et al. (1997). Subgenual prefrontal cortex abnormalities in mood disorders. *Nature*, **386**, 824–7.

Edvinsson, L., MacKenzie, E. T. and McCulloch, J. (1993a). Changes in arterial gas tensions. In *Cerebral Blood Flow and Metabolism*, pp. 524–52. New York: Raven Press.

Edvinsson, L., MacKenzie, E. T. and McCulloch, J. (1993b). Neurotransmitters: metabolic and vascular effects in vivo. In *Cerebral Blood Flow and Metabolism*, pp. 159–80. New York: Raven Press.

Eriksson, L., Holte, S., Bohm, C., Kesselberg, M. and Hovander, B. (1988). Automated blood sampling systems for positron emission tomography. *IEEE Trans. Nucl. Sci.*, **35**, 703–7.

Ernst M., Freed M. E. and Zametkin, A. J. (1998). Health hazards of radiation exposure in the context of brain imaging research: special consideration for children. *J. Nucl. Med.*, **39**, 689–98.

Evans, A. C., Marrett, S., Torrescorzo, J., Ku, S. and Collins, L. (1991). MRI–PET correlation in three dimensions using a volume-of-interest (VOI) atlas. *J. Cereb. Blood Flow Metab.*, **11**, A69–78.

Feeney, D. M. and Baron, J. C. (1986). Diaschisis. *Stroke*, **17**, 817–30.

Fowler, J. S. and Wolf, A. P. (1991). Recent advances in radiotracers for PET studies of the brain. In *Radiopharmaceuticals and Brain Pathology Studied with PET and SPECT*, ed. M. Diksic and R. C. Reba, pp. 11–34. Boca Raton, FL: CRC Press.

Fox, P. T. and Raichle, M. E. (1984). Stimulus rate dependence of regional cerebral blood flow in human striate cortex, demonstrated by positron emission tomography. *J. Neurophysiol.*, **51**, 1109–20.

Fox, P. T. and Raichle, M. E. (1986). Focal physiological uncoupling of cerebral blood flow and oxidative metabolism during somatosensory stimulation in human subjects. *Proc. Natl. Acad. Sci. USA*, **83**, 1140–4.

Fox, P. T., Perlmutter, J. S. and Raichle, M. E. (1985). A stereotactic method of anatomical localization for positron emission tomography. *J. Comput. Assist. Tomogr.*, **9**, 141–53.

Fox, P. T., Raichle, M. E., Mintun, M. A. and Dence, C. (1988). Nonoxidative glucose consumption during focal physiologic neural activity. *Science*, **241**, 462–4.

Frackowiak, R. S. and Friston, K. J. (1994). Functional neuro-anatomy of the human brain: positron emission tomography – a new neuroanatomical technique. *J. Anat.*, **184**, 211–25.

Frackowiak, R. S. J., Lenzi, G.-L., Jones, T. and Heather, J. D. (1980). Quantitative measurement of regional cerebral blood flow and oxygen metabolism in man using ^{15}O and positron emission tomography: theory, procedure and normal values. *J. Comput. Assist. Tomogr.*, **4**, 727–36.

Friston, K. J. (1994). Functional and effective connectivity in neuroimaging: a synthesis. *Hum. Brain Map.*, **2**, 56–78.

Friston, K. J., Passingham, R. E., Nutt, J. G., Heather, J. D., Sawle, G. V. and Frackowiak, R. S. J. (1989). Localisation in PET images: direct fitting of the intercommissural (AC–PC) line. *J. Cereb. Blood Flow Metab.*, **9**, 690–5.

Friston, K. J., Frith, C. D., Liddle, P. F. and Frackowiak, R. S. J. (1991). Comparing functional (PET) images: the assessment of significant change. *J. Cereb. Blood Flow Metab.*, **11**, 690–9.

Ge, Y. R., Fitzpatrick, J. M., Votaw, J. W. et al. (1994). Retrospective registration of PET and MR brain images – an algorithm and its stereotaxic validation. *J. Comput. Assist. Tomogr.*, **18**, 800–10.

Gemmell, H. G., Evans, N. T. S., Besson, J. A. O. et al. (1992). Regional cerebral blood flow imaging: a quantitative comparison of technetium-99m-SPECT with $C^{15}O_2$ PET. *J. Nucl. Med.*, **31**, 1595–1600.

George, M. S., Ring, H. A., Costa, D. C., Ell, P. J., Kouris, K. and Jarritt, P. H. (1991). *Neuroactivation and Neuroimaging with SPECT*. London: Springer-Verlag.

Giedd, J. N., Snell, J. W., Lange, N. et al. (1996a). Quantitative magnetic resonance imaging of human brain development: ages 4–18. *Cereb. Cortex*, **6**, 551–60.

Giedd, J. N., Vaituzis, A., Hamburger, S. D. et al. (1996b). Quantitative MRI of the temporal lobe, amygdala, and hippocampus in normal development: ages 4–18 years. *J. Comp. Neurol.*, **366**, 223–30.

Ginsberg, M. D., Dietrich, W. D. and Busto, R. (1987). Coupled forebrain increases of local cerebral glucose utilization and blood flow during physiologic stimulation of a somatosensory pathway in the rat: demonstration by double-label autoradiography. *Neurology*, **37**, 11–19.

Gjedde, A., Weinhard, K., Heiss, W.-D. et al. (1985). Comparative regional analysis of 2-fluorodeoxyglucose and methylglucose uptake in brain of four stroke patients. With special reference to the regional estimation of the lumped constant. *J. Cereb. Blood Flow Metab.*, **5**, 163–78.

Goldenberg, G., Oder, W., Spatt, J. and Podreka, I. (1992). Cerebral correlates of disturbed executive function and memory in survivors of severe closed head injury: a SPECT study. *J. Neurol. Neurosurg. Psychiatry*, **55**, 362–8.

Grafton, S. T. and Mazziotta, J. C. (1992). Cerebral pathophysiology evaluated with positron emission tomography. In *Diseases of the Nervous System: Clinical Neurobiology*, 2nd edn, ed. A. K. Asbury, G. M. McKhann and W. I. McDonald, pp. 1573–88. Philadelphia, PA: Saunders.

Graham, M. M., Spence, A. M., Muzi, M. and Abbott, G. L. (1989). Deoxyglucose kinetics in a rat brain tumor. *J. Cereb. Blood Flow Metab.*, **9**, 315–22.

Green, M. V. (1996). Single photon imaging. In *Nuclear Medicine*, ed. J. C. Harbert, W. E., Eckelman and R. D. Neumann, pp. 87–120. New York: Thieme.

Greenberg, J. H., Kushner, M., Rangno, M., Alavi, A. and Reivich, M. (1990). Validation studies of iodine-123-iodoamphetamine as a cerebral blood flow agent using emission tomography. *J. Nucl. Med.*, **31**, 1364–9.

Greenberg, J. H., Hamar, J., Welsh, F. A., Harris, V. and Reivich, M. (1992). Effect of ischemia and reperfusion on the lumped constant of the [^{14}C] deoxyglucose technique. *J. Cereb. Blood Flow Metab.*, **12**, 70–7.

Grubb, R. L., Jr, Raichle, M. E., Phelps, M. E. and Ratcheson, R. A. (1975). Effects of increased intracranial pressure on cerebral blood volume, blood flow, and oxygen utilization in monkeys. *J. Neurosurg.*, **43**, 385–98.

Grubb, R. L., Jr, Raichle, M. E., Higgins, C. S. and Eichling, J. O. (1978). Measurement of regional cerebral blood volume by emission tomography. *Ann. Neurol.*, **4**, 322–8.

Hasselbalch, S. G., Madsen, P. L., Knudsen, G. M., Holm S. and Paulson O. B. (1998). Calculation of the FDG lumped constant by simultaneous measurements of global glucose and FDG metabolism in humans. *J. Cereb. Blood Flow Metab.*, **18**, 154–60.

Hatazawa, J., Masatoshi, I., Matsuzawa, T., Ido, T. and Watanuki, S. (1988). Measurement of the ratio of cerebral oxygen consumption to glucose utilization by positron emission tomography: its consistency with the values determined by the Kety–Schmidt method in normal volunteers. *J. Cereb. Blood Flow Metab.*, **8**, 426–32.

Heiss, W.-D. and Podreka, I. (1993). Role of PET and SPECT in the assessment of ischemic cerebrovascular disease. *Cerebrovasc. Brain Metabol. Rev.*, **5**, 235–63.

Herscovitch, P. and Raichle, M. E. (1983). Effect of tissue heterogeneity on the measurement of cerebral blood flow with the equilibrium $C^{15}O_2$ inhalation technique. *J. Cereb. Blood Flow Metab.*, **3**, 407–15.

Herscovitch, P. and Raichle, M. E. (1985). What is the correct value for the brain–blood partition coefficient of water? *J. Cereb. Blood Flow Metab.*, **5**, 65–9.

Herscovitch, P., Markham, J. and Raichle, M. E. (1983). Brain blood flow measured with intravenous $H_2^{15}O$. I. Theory and error analysis. *J. Nucl. Med.*, **24**, 782–9.

Herscovitch, P., Auchus, A., Gado, M., Chi, D. and Raichle, M. E. (1986). Correction of positron emission tomography data for cerebral atrophy. *J. Cereb. Blood Flow Metab.*, **6**, 120–4.

Herscovitch, P., Raichle, M. E., Kilbourn, M. R. and Welch, M. J. (1987). Positron emission tomographic measurements of cerebral blood flow and permeability–surface area product of water using [^{15}O]water and [^{11}C]butanol. *J. Cereb. Blood Flow Metab.*, **7**, 527–42.

Hoffman, E. J. and Phelps, M. E. (1986). Positron emission tomography: principles and quantitation. In *Positron Emission Tomography and Autoradiography*, ed. M. E. Phelps, J. C. Mazziotta and H. R. Schelbert, pp. 237–86. New York: Raven Press.

Hoffman, E. J., Huang, S.-C. and Phelps, M. E. (1979). Quantitation in positron emission computed tomography: 1. Effect of object size. *J. Comput. Assist. Tomogr.*, **3**, 299–308.

Hoffman, E. J., Huang, S. C., Phelps, M. E. and Kuhl, D. E. (1981). Quantitation in positron emission computed tomography. 4. Effect of accidental coincidences. *J. Comput. Assist. Tomogr.*, **5**, 391–400.

Holman, B. L. and Devous, M. S. (1992). Functional brain SPECT: the emergence of a powerful clinical method. *J. Nucl. Med.*, **33**, 1888–904.

Holman, B. L., Carvalho, P. A., Zimmerman, R. E. et al. (1990). Brain perfusion SPECT using an annular single crystal camera: initial clinical experience. *J. Nucl. Med.*, **31**, 1456–61.

Holman, B. L., Zimmerman, R. E., Johnson, K. A. et al. (1991). Computer-assisted superimposition of magnetic resonance and high-resolution technetium-99m-HMPAO and thallium-201 SPECT images of the brain. *J. Nucl. Med.*, **32**, 1478–84.

Horwitz, B., Soncrant, T. T. and Haxby, J. V. (1992). Covariance analysis of functional interactions in the brain using metabolic and blood flow data. In *Advances in Metabolic Mapping Techniques for Brain Imaging of Behavioral and Learning Functions*, ed. F. Gonzalez-Lima, T. Finkenstaedt and H. Scheich, pp. 189–217. Dordrecht, the Netherlands: Kluwer.

Huang, S.-C. and Phelps, M. E. (1986). Principles of tracer kinetic modeling in positron emission tomography and autoradiography. In *Positron Emission Tomography and Autoradiography*, ed. M. E. Phelps, J. C. Mazziotta and H. R. Schelbert, pp. 237–86. New York: Raven Press.

Huang, S. C., Phelps, M. E., Hoffman, E. J., Sideris, K., Selin, C. J. and Kuhl, D. E. (1980). Non-invasive determination of local cerebral metabolic rate of glucose in man. *Am. J. Physiol.*, **238**, E69–82.

Huang, S. C., Phelps, M. E., Hoffman, E. J. and Kuhl, D. E. (1981). Error sensitivity of fluorodeoxyglucose method for measurement of cerebral metabolic rate of glucose. *J. Cerebr. Blood Flow Metab.*, **1**, 391–401.

Huda, W. and Scrimger, J. W. (1989). Irradiation of volunteers in nuclear medicine. *J. Nucl. Med.*, **30**, 260–4.

Iida, H., Rhodes, C. G., de Silva, R. et al. (1992). Use of the left ventricular time–activity curve as a noninvasive input function in oxygen-15-water positron emission tomography. *J. Nucl. Med.*, **33**, 1669–77.

Jacobs, A., Put, E., Ingels, M. and Bossuyt, A. (1994). Prospective evaluation of technetium-99m-HMPAO SPECT in mild and moderate traumatic brain injury. *J. Nucl. Med.*, **35**, 942–7.

Jueptner, M. and Weiller, C. (1995). Does measurement of regional cerebral blood flow reflect synaptic activity – implications for PET and fMRI. [Review] *Neuroimage* **2**, 148–56.

Juni, J. E. (1994). Taking brain SPECT seriously: reflections on recent clinical reports in the *Journal of Nuclear Medicine. J. Nucl. Med.*, **35**, 1891–5.

Karp, J. S., Daube-Witherspoon, M. E., Hoffman, E. J. et al. (1991). Performance standards in positron emission tomography. *J. Nucl. Med.*, **32**, 2342–50.

Kassis, A. I. (1992). The MIRD approach: remembering the limitations. *J. Nucl. Med.*, **33**, 781–2.

Kety, S. S. (1951). The theory and applications of the exchange of inert gas at the lungs and tissues. *Pharmacol. Rev.*, **3**, 1–41.

Kilbourn, M. (1991). Radiotracers for PET studies of neurotransmitter binding sites: design considerations. In *In Vivo Imaging of Neurotransmitter Functions in Brain, Heart and Tumors*, ed. D. E. Kuhl, pp. 47–65. Washington, DC: American College of Nuclear Physicians.

Koeppe, R. A. and Hutchins, G. D. (1992). Instrumentation for positron emission tomography: tomographs and data processing and display systems. *Semin. Nucl. Med.*, **22**, 162–81.

Koeppe, R. A., Holden, J. E. and Ip, W. R. (1985). Performance comparison of parameter estimation techniques for the quantitation of local cerebral blood flow by dynamic positron computed tomography. *J. Cereb. Blood Flow Metab.*, **5**, 224–34.

Koeppe, R. A., Holthoff, V. A., Frey, K. A., Kilbourn, M. R. and Kuhl, D. E. (1991). Compartmental analysis of [^{11}C]flumazenil kinetics for the estimation of ligand transport rate and receptor distribution using positron emission tomography. *J. Cereb. Blood Flow Metab.*, **11**, 735–44.

Kuhl, D. E., Alavi, A., Hoffman, E. J. et al. (1980). Local cerebral blood volume in head-injured patients: determination by emission computed tomography of ^{99m}Tc-labeled red cells. *J. Neurosurg.*, **52**, 309–20.

Lammertsma, A. A., Jones, T., Frackowiak, R. S. J. and Lenzi, G.-L. (1981). A theoretical study of the steady-state model for measuring regional cerebral blood flow and oxygen utilization using oxygen-15. *J. Comput. Assist. Tomogr.*, **5**, 544–50.

Lammertsma, A. A., Wise, R. J. S., Heather, J. D. et al. (1983). Correction for the presence of intravascular oxygen-15 in the steady-state technique for measuring regional oxygen extraction ratio in the brain. 2. Results in normal subjects and brain tumor and stroke patients. *J. Cereb. Blood Flow Metab.*, **3**, 425–31.

Lammertsma, A. A., Brooks, D. J., Beaney, R. P. et al. (1984). In vivo measurement of regional cerebral haematocrit using positron emission tomography. *J. Cereb. Blood Flow Metab.*, **4**, 317–22.

Lammertsma, A. A., Brooks, D. J., Frackowiak, R. S. J. et al. (1987). Measurement of glucose utilization with [^{18}F]2-fluoro-2-deoxy-D-glucose: a comparison of different analytical methods. *J. Cereb. Blood Flow Metab.*, **7**, 161–72.

Landau, W. M., Freygang, W. H., Jr, Rowland, L. P., Sokoloff, L. and Kety, S. (1955). The local circulation of the living brain; values in the unanesthetized and anesthetized cat. *Trans. Am. Neurol. Assoc.*, **80**, 125–9.

Laruelle, M., Baldwin, R. M., Rattner, Z. et al. (1994a). SPECT quantification of [^{123}I]iomazenil binding to benzodiazepine receptors in nonhuman primates. I. Kinetic modeling of single bolus experiments. *J. Cereb. Blood Flow Metab.*, **14**, 439–52.

Laruelle, M., van, Dyck, C., Abi, D. A. et al. (1994b). Compartmental modeling of iodine-123-iodobenzofuran binding to dopamine D$_2$ receptors in healthy subjects. *J. Nucl. Med.*, **35**, 743–54.

Leenders, K. L., Perani, D., Lammertsma, A. A. et al. (1990). Cerebral blood flow, blood volume and oxygen utilization: normal values and effect of age. *Brain*, **113**, 27–47.

Leniger-Follert, E. and Hossman, K.-A. (1979). Simultaneous measurements of microflow and evoked potentials in the somatomotor cortex of rat brain during specific sensory activation. *Pflugers Arch.*, **380**, 85–9.

Lockwood, A. H. (1985). Invasiveness in studies of brain function by positron emission tomography. *J. Cereb. Blood Flow Metab.*, **5**, 487–9.

Loevinger, R., Budinger, T. F. and Watson, E. E. (1988). *MIRD Primer for Absorbed Dose Calculations*. New York: Society of Nuclear Medicine.

Lou, H. C., Edvinsson, L. and MacKenzie, E. T. (1987). The concept of coupling blood flow to brain function: revision required? *Ann. Neurol.*, **22**, 289–97.

Martin, W. R. W., Powers, W. J. and Raichle, M. E. (1987). Cerebral blood volume measured with inhaled C^{15}O and positron emission tomography. *J. Cerebr. Blood Flow Metab.*, **7**, 421–6.

Masdeu, J. C., Brass, L. M., Holman, B. L. and Kushner, M. J. (1994). Brain single-photon emission computed tomography. *Neurology*, **44**, 1970–7.

Matthew, E., Andreason, P., Carson, R. E. et al. (1993). Reproducibility of resting cerebral blood-flow measurements with H$_2$^{15}O positron emission tomography in humans. *J. Cereb. Blood Flow Metab.*, **13**, 748–54.

Mazziotta, J. C., Phelps, M. E., Plummer, D. and Kuhl, D. E. (1981). Quantitation in positron computed tomography. 5. Physical-anatomical effects. *J. Comput. Assist. Tomogr.*, **5**, 734–43.

McIntosh, A. R., Grady, C. L., Ungerleider, L. G., Haxby, J. V., Rapoport, S. I. and Horwitz, B. (1994). Network analysis of cortical visual pathways mapped with PET. *J. Neurosci.*, **14**, 655–66.

Meltzer, C. C., Zubieta, J. K., Links, J. M., Brakeman, P., Stumpf, M. J. and Frost, J. J. (1996). MR-based correction of brain PET measurements for heterogeneous gray-matter radioactivity distribution. *J. Cereb. Blood Flow Metab.*, **16**, 650–8.

Minoshima, S., Berger, K. L., Lee, K. S. and Mintun, M. A. (1992). An automated method for rotational correction and centering of three-dimensional functional brain images. *J. Nucl. Med.*, **33**, 1579–85.

Mintun, M. A., Raichle, M. E., Martin, W. R. W. and Herscovitch, P. (1984). Brain oxygen utilization measured with O-15 radiotracers and positron emission tomography. *J. Nucl. Med.*, **25**, 177–87.

Murase, K., Tanada, S., Fujita, H., Sakaki, S. and Hamamoto, K. (1992). Kinetic behavior of technetium-99m-HMPAO in human brain and quantification of cerebral blood flow using dynamic SPECT. *J. Nucl. Med.*, **33**, 135–43.

Muzik, O., Chugani, D. C., Shen, C. and Chugani, H. T. (1998). Noninvasive imaging of serotonin synthesis rate using PET and α-methyltryptophan in autistic children. In *Quantitative Functional Brain Imaging with Positron Emission Tomography*, ed. R. E. Carson, M. E. Daube-Witherspoon and P. Herscovitch, pp. 201–6. San Diego, CA: Academic Press.

Nakai, H., Yamamoto, Y. L., Diksic, M. et al. (1987). Time-dependent changes of lumped and rate constants in the deoxyglucose method in experimental cerebral ischemia. *J. Cereb. Blood Flow Metab.*, **7**, 640–8.

Obrist, W. D., Langfitt, T. W., Jaggi, J., Cruz, J. and Gennarelli, T. A. (1984). Cerebral blood flow and metabolism in comatose patients with acute head injury. *J. Neurosurg.*, **61**, 241–53.

Ohta, S., Meyer, E., Thompson, C. J. and Gjedde, A. (1992). Oxygen consumption of the living human brain measured after a single inhalation of positron emitting oxygen. *J. Cereb. Blood Flow Metab.*, **12**, 179–92.

Pelizzari, C. A., Chen, G. T. Y., Spelbring, D. R., Weichselbaum, R. R. and Chen, C.-T. (1989). Accurate three-dimensional registration of CT, PET, and/or MR images of the brain. *J. Comput. Assist. Tomogr.*, **13**, 20–6.

Perlman, J. M. and Altman, D. I. (1992). Symmetric cerebral blood flow in newborns who have undergone successful extracorporeal membrane oxygenation. *Pediatrics*, **89**, 235–9.

Perlmutter, J. S., Powers, W. J., Herscovitch, P., Fox, P. T. and Raichle, M. E. (1987). Regional asymmetries of cerebral blood flow, blood volume, oxygen utilization and extraction in normal subjects. *J. Cereb. Blood Flow Metab.*, **7**, 64–7.

Phelps, M. E. and Hoffman, E. J. (1976). Resolution limit of positron cameras. *J. Nucl. Med.*, **17**, 757–8.

Phelps, M. E., Huang, S. C., Hoffman, E. J., Selin, C., Sokoloff, L. and Kuhl, D. E. (1979). Tomographic measurement of local cerebral glucose metabolic rate in humans with (F-18) 2-fluoro-2-deoxy-D-glucose: validation of method. *Ann. Neurol.*, **6**, 371–88.

Powers, W. J. (1988). Positron emission tomography in the evaluation of cerebrovascular disease: clinical applications? In *Clinical Neuroimaging*, ed. W. H. Theodore, pp. 49–74. New York: Alan R. Liss.

Powers, W. J. (1991). Cerebral hemodynamics in ischemic cerebrovascular disease. *Ann. Neurol.*, **29**, 231–40.

Powers, W. J., Berg, L., Perlmutter, J. S. and Raichle, M. E. (1991). Technology assessment revisited: does positron emission tomography have proven clinical efficacy? *Neurology*, **41**, 1339–40.

Powers, W. J., Rosenbaum, J. L., Dence, C. S., Markham, J. and Videen, T. O. (1998). Cerebral glucose transport and metabolism in preterm human infants. *J. Cereb. Blood Flow Metab.*, **18**, 632–8.

Raichle, M. E. (1987). Circulatory and metabolic correlates of brain function in normal humans. In *Handbook of Physiology: The Nervous System*, ed. V. B. Mountcastle and F. Plum, pp. 643–74. Bethesda, MD: American Physiological Society.

Raichle, M. E. (1991). The metabolic requirements of functional activity in human brain: a positron emission tomography study. In *Fuel Homeostatis and the Nervous System*, ed. M. Vranic, S. Efendic and C. H. Hollenberg, pp. 1–4. New York: Plenum.

Raichle, M. E., Martin, W. R. W., Herscovitch, P., Mintun, M. A. and Markham, J. (1983). Brain blood flow measured with intravenous $H_2{}^{15}O$. II. Implementation and validation. *J. Nucl. Med.*, **24**, 790–8.

Rajapakse, J. C., Giedd, J. N., Rumsey, J. M., Vaituzis, A. C., Hamburger, S. D. and Rapoport, J. L. (1996). Regional MRI measurements of the corpus callosum: a methodological and developmental study. *Brain Dev.*, **18**, 379–88.

Reivich, M., Kuhl, D., Wolf, A. et al. (1979). The [18F]fluoro-deoxyglucose method for the measurement of local cerebral glucose utilization in man. *Circ. Res.*, **44**, 127–37.

Reivich, M., Alavi, A., Wolf, A. et al. (1985). Glucose metabolic rate kinetic model parameter determination in humans: the lumped constants and rate constants for [18F]fluorodeoxyglucose and [11C]deoxyglucose. *J. Cereb. Blood Flow Metab.*, **5**, 179–92.

Sasaki, H., Kanno, I., Murakami, M., Shishido, F. and Uemera, K. (1986). Tomographic mapping of kinetic rate constants in the fluorodeoxyglucose model using dynamic positron emission tomography. *J. Cereb. Blood Flow Metab.*, **6**, 447–54.

Seibyl, J. P., Laruelle, M., van Dyck, C. H. et al. (1996). Reproducibility of iodine-123-β-CIT SPECT brain measurement of dopamine transporters. *J. Nucl. Med.*, **37**, 222–8.

Sokoloff, L. (1961). Local cerebral circulation at rest and during altered cerebral activity induced by anesthesia or visual stimulation. In *Regional Neurochemistry*, ed. S. S. Kety and J. Elkes, pp. 107–17. New York: Pergamon Press.

Sokoloff, L. (1981). Relationships among local functional activity, energy metabolism, and blood flow in the central nervous system. *FASEB J.*, **40**, 2311–16.

Sokoloff, L. (1985). Basic principles in imaging of cerebral metabolic rates. In *Brain Imaging and Brain Function*, ed. L. Sokoloff, pp. 21–49. New York: Raven Press.

Sokoloff, L., Reivich, M., Kennedy, C. et al. (1977). The [14C]deoxyglucose method for the measurement of local cerebral glucose utilization; theory, procedure, and normal values in the conscious and anesthetized albino rat. *J. Neurochem.*, **28**, 897–916.

Sorenson, J. A. and Phelps, M. E. (1987). *Physics in Nuclear Medicine*. Orlando, FL: Grune and Stratton.

Spence, A. M., Graham, M. M., Muzi, M. et al. (1990). Deoxyglucose lumped constant estimated in a transplanted rat astrocytic glioma by the hexose utilization index. *J. Cereb. Blood Flow Metab.*, **10**, 190–8.

Spinks, T. J., Jones, T., Bailey, D. L. et al. (1992). Physical performance of a positron tomograph for brain imaging with retractable septa. *Phys. Med. Biol.*, **37**, 1637–55.

Stapleton, S. J., Caldwell, C. B., Leonhardt, C. L., Ehrlich, L. E., Black, S. E. and Yaffe, M. J. (1994). Determination of thresholds for detection of cerebellar blood flow deficits in brain SPECT images. *J. Nucl. Med.*, **35**, 1547–55.

Strother, S. C., Kanno, I. and Rottenberg, D. A. (1995). Commentary and opinion. 1. Principal component analysis, variance partitioning, and functional connectivity. *J. Cereb. Blood Flow Metab.*, **15**, 353–60.

Subramanyam, R., Alpert, N. M., Hoop, B., Jr, Brownell, G. L. and Taveras, J. M. (1978). A model for regional cerebral oxygen distribution during continuous inhalation of $^{15}O_2$, $C^{15}O$, and $C^{15}O_2$. *J. Nucl. Med.*, **19**, 13–53.

Ter-Pogossian, M. M. (1992). The origins of positron emission tomography. *Semin. Nucl. Med.*, **22**, 140–9.

Ter-Pogossian, M. M., Phelps, M. E., Hoffman, E. J. and Mullani, N. A. (1975). A positron-emission transaxial tomograph for nuclear imaging (PETT). *Radiology*, **114**, 89–98.

Toga, A. W. and Collins, R. C. (1981). Metabolic response of optic centers to visual stimuli in the albino rat: anatomical and physiological considerations. *J. Comp. Neurol.*, **199**, 443–64.

Tyler, J. L., Strother, S. C., Zatorre, R. J. et al. (1988). Stability of regional cerebral glucose metabolism in the normal brain measured by positron emission tomography. *J. Nucl. Med.*, **29**, 631–42.

van Bogeart, P., Wikler, D., Damhaut, P., Szliwowska, H. B. and Goldman, S. (1998). Regional changes in glucose metabolism during brain development from the age of 6 years. *Neuroimage*, **8**, 62–8.

van Heertum, R. L., Miller, S. H. and Mosesson, R. E. (1993). SPECT brain imaging in neurologic disease. *Radiol. Clin. North Am.*, **31**, 881–907.

Veatch, R. M. (1982). The ethics of research involving radiation. *IRB: Rev. Hum. Subjects Res.*, **4**, 3–5.

Videen, T. O., Perlmutter, J. S., Herscovitch, P. and Raichle, M. E. (1987). Brain blood volume, flow, and oxygen utilization measured with ^{15}O radiotracers and positron emission tomography: revised metabolic computations. *J. Cereb. Blood Flow Metab.*, **7**, 513–16.

Videen, T. O., Perlmutter, J. S., Mintun, M. A. and Raichle, M. E. (1988). Regional correction of positron emission tomography data for the effects of cerebral atrophy. *J. Cereb. Blood Flow Metab.*, **8**, 662–70.

Volkow, N. and Fowler, J. S. (1992). Neuropsychiatric disorders: investigation of schizophrenia and substance abuse. *Semin. Nucl. Med.*, **22**, 254–67.

Volpe, J. J., Herscovitch, P., Perlman, J. M. and Raichle, M. E. (1983). Positron emission tomography in the newborn: Extensive impairment of regional cerebral blood flow with intraventricular hemorrhage and hemorrhagic intracerebral involvement. *Pediatrics*, **72**, 589–601.

Wang, B., Thompson, C. J., Tremblay, H., Reutens, D., Jolly, D. and Meyer, E. (1998). Measurement of the evoked vascular response (EVR) to cerebral activation due to vibro-tactile stimulation using gated C-11-CO PET acquisition. *IEEE Trans. Nucl. Sci.*, **45**, 1111–16.

Wang, G.-J., Volkow, N. D., Wolf, A. P., Brodie, J. D. and Hitzeman, R. J. (1994). Intersubject variability of brain glucose metabolic measurements in young normal males. *J. Nucl. Med.*, **35**, 1457–66.

Warner, D. S., Kassell, N. F. and Boarini, D. J. (1987). Microsphere cerebral blood flow determination. In *Cerebral Blood Flow: Physiologic and Clinical Aspects*, ed. J. H. Wood, pp. 288–98. New York: McGraw-Hill.

Weinberg, I. N., Huang, S. C., Hoffman, E. J. et al. (1988). Validation of PET-acquired input functions for cardiac studies. *J. Nucl. Med.*, **29**, 241–7.

Wienhard, K., Pawlik, G., Herholz, K., Wagner, R. and Heiss, W.-D. (1985). Estimation of local cerebral glucose utilization by positron emission tomography of [^{18}F]2-fluoro-2-deoxy-D-glucose: a critical appraisal of optimization procedures. *J. Cereb. Blood Flow Metab.*, **5**, 115–25.

Wienhard, K., Dahlbom, M., Eriksson, L. et al. (1994). The ECAT EXACT HR: performance of a new high resolution positron scanner. *J. Comput. Assist. Tomogr.*, **18**, 110–18.

Wilson, J. T. L. and Wyper, D. (1992). Neuroimaging and neuropsychological functioning following closed head injury: CT, MRI, and SPECT. *J. Head Trauma Rehab.*, **7**, 29–39.

Wilson, M. W. and Mountz, J. M. (1989). A reference system for neuroanatomical localization on functional reconstructed cerebral images. *J. Comput. Assist. Tomogr.*, **13**, 174–8.

Wolf, A. P. and Schlyer, D. J. (1993). Accelerators for positron emission tomography. In *Nuclear Imaging in Drug Discovery, Development, and Approval*, ed. D. H. Burns, R. E. Gibson, R. F. Dannals and P. K. S. Siegl, pp. 33–54. Boston: Birkhäuser.

Woods, R. P., Mazziotta, J. C. and Cherry, S. R. (1993). MRI–PET registration with automated algorithm. *J. Comput. Assist. Tomogr.*, **17**, 536–46.

Wyper, D. J. (1993). Functional neuroimaging with single photon emission computed tomography (SPECT). *Cerebrovasc. Brain Metabo. Rev.*, **5**, 199–217.

Yarowsky, P. J. and Ingvar, D. H. (1981). Neuronal activity and energy metabolism. *Fed. Proc.*, **40**, 2353–62.

Yarowsky, P., Kadekaro, M. and Sokoloff, L. (1983). Frequency-dependent activation of glucose utilization in the superior cervical ganglion by electrical stimulation of cervical sympathetic trunk. *Proc. Nat. Acad. Sci. USA*, **80**, 4179–83.

Zametkin, A. J., Liebenauer, L. L., Fitzgerald, G. A. et al. (1993). Brain metabolism in teenagers with attention deficit hyperactivity disorder. *Arch. Gen. Psychiatry*, **50**, 333–40.

2

Modeling of receptor images in PET and SPECT

Evan D. Morris, Raymond F. Muzic Jr,
Bradley C. Christian, Christopher J. Endres,
and Ronald E. Fisher

Introduction

Positron emission tomography (PET) and single photon emission computed tomography (SPECT) are the only noninvasive imaging modalities, currently, that can be used to image specific receptor molecules and to quantify their kinetics. The specificity of these methods results from the use of radiolabeled ligands that are themselves specific for a receptor or transporter molecule. In PET/SPECT studies, the images are a composite of various signals only one of which relates to ligand bound to the receptor site of interest. The component of the image that is from receptor binding is isolated using a mathematical model relating the dynamics of the ligand to the resultant PET image. The mathematical model typically derives from the three-compartment model in which a directly measured blood curve serves as the model's input function. (There are modifications of the model (reference region models) that do not use an independently measured blood curve as input. These models are addressed later in this chapter.) The model contains a number of parameters that are taken to be constants and reflective of inherent kinetic properties of the system and the particular ligand. By formally comparing the output of the model to the experimentally obtained PET or SPECT data, we can estimate values for the kinetic parameters and thus extract information on binding, or any hypothesized process, as distinct from all other processes contributing to the PET signal. In general, the information content of the PET or SPECT data is inadequate to support models of great sophistication, and so adoption of a particular model and the interpretation of its parameters comes with associated assumptions and conditions that must be satisfied.

Kinetic models

The basic compartmental model

The simplest of compartmental models applied to receptor–ligand studies postulates two tissue compartments. These two tissue compartments along with a plasma compartment are arranged in series. (Strictly speaking, the plasma is not a compartment of the model. The concentration of tracer in the plasma is measured independently and applied to the tissue model as a known input function.) The tracer is delivered, typically by intravenous injection, into the plasma and it traverses the "free" compartment on its way to interacting with the receptor. If these three compartments or states of the radioligand are inadequate to describe the data, sometimes a third tissue compartment is introduced (Fig. 2.1) that is termed the nonspecifically bound compartment. The bound and nonspecific compartments are distinguished as follows. Specifically bound ligand, unlike nonspecifically bound ligand is both saturable and displaceable by nonradioactive molecules of the same tracer. The rate of change in *radioactivity* concentration in each tissue compartment in Fig. 2.1 is given by the ordinary differential equations that describe the flux of ligand into the respective compartments:

$$\frac{dF}{dt} = K_1 P - (k_2 + k_3)F + k_4 B - \lambda F \tag{2.1}$$

$$\frac{dB}{dt} = k_3 F - k_4 B - \lambda B \tag{2.2}$$

$$\frac{dN}{dt} = k_5 F - k_6 N - \lambda N \tag{2.3}$$

where F, B, and N are the time-varying concentrations of tracer in the free, bound, and nonspecific tissue compartments, respectively; that is, $F = F(t)$, $B = B(t)$, and $N = N(t)$. The constants $K_1, k_2 \ldots k_6$ are the apparent first-order rate

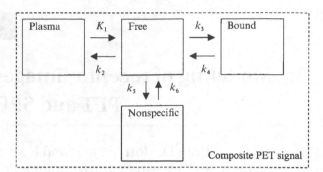

Fig. 2.1. General three-compartment model. Radioactivity in the plasma, free, bound (and nonspecific) compartments sums to give the radioactivity in the PET image. The model parameters K_1 ... k_6 reflect exchange rates for labeled ligand moving between various compartments.

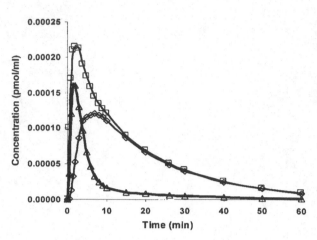

Fig. 2.2. Simulation of [^{11}C]-raclopride dynamics in brain. Equation (2.4) generates the PET activity ($\square$), which is equal to the sum of the activity in the free ($\triangle$) and bound ($\Diamond$) compartments, respectively. The free and bound compartments correspond to the model variables, $F(t)$ and $B(t)$, respectively. Parameters are based on Farde et al. (1989). Data are not decay corrected.

constants relating the transfer of ligand between the various compartments. These constants are the model parameters to be estimated from experimental data. The parameters k_3 and k_4 are apparent first-order rate constants that characterize the binding and dissociation of the ligand to and from the receptor, respectively. The rate constant λ, radioactive decay, refers to the rate of decay of the isotope labeling the ligand. The (measured) concentration of radioactive ligand in the plasma P refers only to the concentration of native ligand molecules and not to any radioactive metabolites. The preceding model, in a slightly different form, was introduced into the PET literature by Mintun et al. in 1984.

One of the innovations of the original Mintun formulation was to "collapse" the nonspecific compartment into the free compartment. Mathematically, this can be justified if the rate constants for nonspecific binding, k_5 and k_6, are fast relative to the other rate constants of the system. In this case, ligand in the nonspecific compartment is defined as being "in equilibrium" with the free compartment. If this condition is satisfied, then at any time a fixed fraction of the free plus nonspecific compartment is the effective free pool available for receptor binding. This fraction, $f_2 = k_6/(k_5 + k_6)$, may not be strictly identifiable (see below) from a receptor-rich region alone, although it may be possible to estimate it from a receptor-free region where only two other parameters (K_1 and k_2) are needed to describe the data.

Output equation

The measured PET data comprise average concentrations over discrete frame times. Once the model has been solved for the instantaneous activity in each compartment (F, B, and N), these concentration curves are summed and inte-

grated to generate the measured PET activity over each acquisition time frame, $[t_i, t_{i+1}]$, as follows:

$$\text{PET}[t_i, t_{i+1}] = \frac{1}{\Delta t_i} \int_{t_i}^{t_{i+1}} (\varepsilon_v V + \varepsilon_f F + \varepsilon_b B + \varepsilon_n N) \, dt \qquad (2.4)$$

The weights ε_i that premultiply each compartment concentration in Eq. (2.4) are the respective volume fractions and V is whole blood activity. Usually the vascular volume fraction ε_v is small, and the tissue volume fractions are set at unity or $(1 - \varepsilon_v)$. We can use numerical methods to solve Eqs. (2.1–2.3) over time. A simulation of the dynamics in the free and bound compartments following bolus injection of the dopamine D_2 ligand, [^{11}C]-raclopride, is shown in Fig. 2.2. The simulation is based on published parameter estimates (Farde et al., 1989) for [^{11}C]-raclopride, in vivo. As in this figure, nonspecific binding is often assumed to be negligible for raclopride.

Measuring the blood curve

The input, or driving function, P represents the amount of tracer ligand that is presented over time to the tissue of interest (i.e., the brain). It is often measured via the radioactivity counted in blood plasma samples drawn from the radial artery. The model given in Eqs. (2.1–2.4) and shown in Fig. 2.1 deals only with the behavior of a unique tracer molecule, such as [^{11}C]-raclopride. The rate constants pertain, specifically, to the defined molecule. Therefore, if metabolism of the radioligand in the periphery leads to labeled metabolites in the plasma, we must invoke at least one correction and one assumption. First, the nonnative species must be removed either physically from the blood samples or mathematically from the resulting radioactivity counts. Second, it must be assumed that the labeled metabolite(s) does not cross the blood–brain barrier. Consequently, one consideration for choosing between candidate tracers may be the generation, or not, of labeled metabolites. In some cases, the production of labeled metabolites may be inevitable. In the case of [18F]-fluorodopa, complicated models have been introduced to account for metabolite species and their contributions to the PET signal (Huang et al., 1991).

Modeling saturability

To this point, the model does not contain a term that reflects the saturable nature of the bound-ligand compartment. That is, there is no explicit upper limit imposed on the size of the bound ligand B. And yet, a unique characteristic of receptor–ligand interactions is that, like enzyme–substrate reactions, they are saturable. The inclusion of an explicit receptor density term, B'_{max}, requires an elaboration of Eqs. (2.1) and (2.2). We expand k_3 from equations (2.1–2.3) as $k_{on}(B'_{max} - B/SA)$:

$$\frac{dF}{dt} = K_1 P - (k_2 + k_5)F + k_6 N - k_{on}(B'_{max} - B/SA)F + k_{off}B - \lambda F \tag{2.5}$$

$$\frac{dB}{dt} = k_{on}(B'_{max} - B/SA)F - k_{off}B - \lambda B \tag{2.6}$$

$$\frac{dN}{dt} = k_5 F - k_6 N - \lambda N \tag{2.7}$$

where k_{off} is equivalent to k_4, above; SA is the specific activity, which declines in time according to the radioactive decay rate λ; k_{on} is the rate constant for a *bimolecular* association of free ligand and available receptors. Therefore, the binding rate is equal to the product of the concentrations of free ligand, F, available receptor sites, $(B'_{max} - B/SA)$, and rate constant, k_{on}. At the time of injection ($t = 0$), the value of B is zero; therefore B'_{max} represents the concentration of available receptors in the absence of exogenous ligand. As additional receptors become bound to ligand molecules, the availability of free receptors drops and saturation is approached asymptotically. Since availability can be affected by either labeled or unlabeled ligand, normalization by SA converts B to concentration of total ligand. This form of the receptor–ligand model, which was first proposed explicitly by Huang and colleagues (Huang et al., 1989, 1986; Bahn et al., 1989) is analogous to the bimolecular interaction between substrate, and available binding sites on an enzyme.

Parameter identifiability: opting for binding potential or other compound parameters

Despite the inclusion of an explicit B'_{max} term in the model representing the baseline level of available receptor sites, this value may not be discernible from the acquired data. In other words, it would not be estimated reliably. Consider that for a single bolus injection of sufficiently *high* SA ligand, the bimolecular binding term in Eqs. (2.5) and (2.6) reduces to $k_{on}(B'_{max})F$; that is, $B/SA = 0$. Since k_{on} and B'_{max} always appear as a product, never separately, they are said not to be identifiable and the model defaults to Eqs. (2.1–2.3). Attempting to estimate both k_{on} and B'_{max} in this case would be akin to trying to estimate m and n from data with the overparameterized model of a line: $y = m*n*x + b$. Mintun and co-authors made this point in their 1984 paper saying that k_{on} and B'_{max} are not separable in a single bolus experiment under tracer (i.e., high SA) conditions. For that reason, they chose to estimate the compound term B'_{max}/K_D, which they referred to as "binding potential". Koeppe et al. (1991) recommend further model simplifications when it is not possible even to identify B'_{max}/K_D, explicitly. Sometimes the data from a receptor–ligand study can be fitted to a two-compartment model (i.e., plasma and free) and inclusion of an explicit bound compartment is not justified. This will be true if the binding and dissociation rate constants for the ligand, k_3 and k_4, are much faster than the influx and efflux constants, K_1 and k_2. When this is true, the estimated k_2 will represent an apparent efflux rate constant, $[k'_2 = k_2/(1 + k_5/k_6 + B'_{max}/K_D)]$. This parameter may still reflect the binding potential, as indicated by the B'_{max}/K_D term, and may be the only reliable index of binding that can be estimated. Koeppe and colleagues have done much work to characterize the kinetics of flumazenil and other muscarinic cholinergic ligands. They point out that quantification is difficult if the dissociation rate constant k_{off} is slow and cannot be reliably distinguished from zero (as is the case with these ligands). Conversely, quantification of binding rate constants of these ligands is difficult and highly sensitive to changes in blood flow when binding is very rapid relative to the rates of transport across the blood–brain barrier (i.e., K_1 and k_2) (Zubieta et al., 1998).

There are many instances in research when binding potential (BP) is a satisfactory indicator of (available) receptor level. In these cases, BP, reported in table form by brain region or as a parametric map, is a reasonable endpoint for a functional imaging study. A number of easy and robust methods for calculating this parameter are discussed below. However, implicit in the adoption of BP as a surrogate B'_{max} is the assumption that the affinity K_D of the

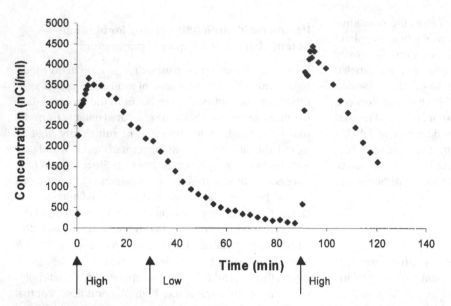

Fig. 2.3. Dynamic PET activity from a region drawn on the striatum of a Rhesus monkey. The three-injection protocol used is described in Morris et al. (1996a). Injections of [^{11}C]-CFT were made at 0, 30, and 90 min (indicated by arrows). Second injection was of low specific activity, causing net displacement of labeled ligand from the receptor by unlabeled ligand. Notice the difference in responses after the first and second *high specific activity* injections because of the presence of residual cold ligand on-board. Data are not decay corrected.

ligand for the receptor is constant across subjects or treatments. For those cases where changes in affinity cannot be excluded or where some other mechanistic question is at stake, more than a single bolus injection is indicated. Delforge et al. (1989, 1990) proposed an experimental protocol involving three sequential bolus injections of varying specific activities. At least one of those injections also contained a nontrace amount of cold (i.e., unlabeled) ligand. In such a protocol, the number of available receptors is significantly perturbed and it is this process of modulating availability over a broad range of values that serves to de-correlate k_{on} from B'_{max}. Delforge and co-authors showed through experiments and simulations that it was possible to estimate unambiguously seven model parameters (including k_{on}, B'_{max} and k_{off}) using a three-injection protocol. In this way, the individual parameters are said to be identifiable. An example of the data from a multiple injection protocol, in which [^{11}C]-CFT (a dopamine transporter ligand) was administered to a rhesus monkey, is given in Fig. 2.3. The authors of the study (Morris et al., 1996a) were able to estimate five parameters simultaneously (nonspecific binding parameters k_5 and k_6 were fixed based on cerebellum data). In designing experiments, one must beware that protocols that rely on nontrace doses of ligand may not be feasible in psychiatric patients – particularly children – because the large mass doses of ligand are likely to have pharmacologic effects.

Modeling multiple-injection data: two parallel models
To analyze data from their multiple-injection experiments, Delforge and colleagues proposed a further modification of the three compartment model. Because these protocols depend on at least one nontrace injection of ligand (nontrace meaning an amount sufficient to have visible biological or pharmacologic effects), the researchers proposed parallel models for the labeled and unlabeled species. The model can be described as follows:

$$\frac{\mathrm{d}F^j}{\mathrm{d}t} = K_1 P^j - (k_2 + k_5)F^j + k_6 N^j - (k_{on}/V_R)(B'_{max} - B^h - B^c)F^j + k_{off}B^j - \lambda^j F^j \tag{2.8}$$

$$\frac{\mathrm{d}B^j}{\mathrm{d}t} = (k_{on}/V_R)(B'_{max} - B^h - B^c)F^j - k_{off}B^j - \lambda^j B^j \tag{2.9}$$

$$\frac{\mathrm{d}N^j}{\mathrm{d}t} = (k_5 F^j - k_6 N^j - \lambda^j N^j) \tag{2.10}$$

where the superscript j refers to either hot (h) or cold (c) ligand; λ^j is the radioactive decay constant for the isotope when j refers to the hot ligand and is 0 when j refers to cold (i.e., there is no radiodecay of cold ligand).

The Delforge nomenclature employs the compound term k_{on}/V_R as the apparent association rate constant, where V_R is the volume of reaction of the receptor but k_{on}/V_R is treated as one indivisible parameter. If the microenvironment surrounding the receptor is unusually inaccessible to the ligand, the apparent binding rate will differ from the true binding rate (see Delforge et al. (1996) for a thorough discussion of the reaction-volume concept).

The number of estimable parameters in the model is seven. No new parameters have been added to the model given earlier (Eqs. (2.4–2.6)) because the hot and cold ligands are identical, biologically.

There is an additional experimental burden in performing multiple-injection experiments. Two plasma input functions must be measured. One, P^h, is the standard curve of radioactivity in the plasma, which has been mentioned previously. The other P^c is the concentration (in picamoles per milliliter) of cold ligand in the plasma. Since this is not readily measurable during the experiment, it must be "reconstructed" from the available plasma radioactivity measurements and knowledge of the specific activities of each injection. (See the appendix of Morris et al., 1996a.) Despite its greater complexity, the Delforge approach maximizes the number of model parameters that can be properly identified (Morris et al., 1996b). This complexity could be justified in the preliminary development and exploration of a new ligand. The result of such a multiple-injection study would then be used to develop a simpler clinical protocol.

Nonconstant coefficients: neurotransmitter changes

Each of the foregoing models, regardless of complexity, is founded on some common assumptions. One is that the model parameters are constant over the duration of the experiment. This is a reasonable assumption if the system itself is at steady state. Whereas [^{11}C]-raclopride levels may rise and fall as it is taken up and eliminated from the tissue following a bolus injection, dopamine levels remain unchanged over the timescale of interest. The rate constants that are determined by the overall state of the system remain unchanged. Anything that violates these assumptions may invalidate the use of the constant-coefficient models given earlier and must be investigated. For example, the consequences of unwanted changes in blood flow and their impact on estimation of raclopride binding have been investigated using both simulations (Frost et al., 1989; Laruelle et al., 1994; Logan et al., 1994) and an experimental perturbation, hyperventilation (Logan et al., 1994). In 1991, Logan and colleagues explored the consequences of changes in dopamine on the measurement of binding parameters of a D_2 receptor ligand, methylspiroperidol.

Of late, there has been growing interest in detecting and quantifying transient changes in neurotransmitter concentrations, which may be useful for understanding the etiology of neuropsychiatric diseases (see Laruelle et al. (1996) and Breier et al. (1997) for evidence that schizophrenia is associated with abnormal amphetamine-induced dopamine release). The potential for such a measurement exists because the endogenous ligand (e.g., dopamine) competes with the exogenous ligand for binding to available receptor sites. Any alteration in the steady-state level of this everpresent competition could alter the PET signal. To model a system in which the neurotransmitter concentration is not constant, we must again extend the models developed above. Just as the Delforge model (Eqs. (2.8–2.10)) extended its antecedents by adding terms for labeled and *unlabeled* exogenous ligand species, the changing-neurotransmitter model must add terms for the *endogenous* ligand species. Morris and co-workers (1995) introduced a differential equation into the receptor–ligand model to describe the binding and release of endogenous species from the receptor:

$$\frac{dB^{en}}{dt} = (k_{on}^{en}/V_R^{en})(B_{max} - B^h - B^c - B^{en})F^{en} - k_{off}^{en}B^{en} \qquad (2.11)$$

where the superscript en refers to the endogenous species. Note that B_{max} is the concentration of *all* the receptor sites (available and not) and the bimolecular binding terms for the other species (hot and cold tracer ligand) must be modified accordingly. The term F_{en} is the time-varying concentration of endogenous chemical available for binding to the receptor and (k_{on}^{en}/V_R^{en}) is the apparent binding rate constant for the endogenous ligand. Equation (2.11) can be solved simultaneously with Eqs. (2.8–2.10). A similar approach was taken by Endres and colleagues (1997) who retained the format of Eqs. (2.1–2.3) but introduced a time-varying binding rate parameter $k_3 = k_3 B_{free}(t)$ where $B_{free}(t)$ is just $B_{max} - B^h - B^c - B^{en}$. Here B_{max} is still constant, but B^h, B^c and B^{en} can all vary with time. This "enhanced model" (as described by Eqs. (2.8–2.11)) is shown in Fig. 2.4.

There have been two experimental approaches to the problem of quantifying neurotransmitter changes. The first, is a natural extension of the studies already mentioned. It is based on the comparison of PET signals from two bolus injections of radiotracer. One bolus study is performed while neurotransmitter is at steady state; a second bolus study is carried out while endogenous neurotransmitter is undergoing an induced change. An alternative experimental approach also involves a perturbation of the neurotransmitter but it is done only after the radiotracer has been brought to a steady state in the tissue by the combination of bolus plus infusion administrations. An approach intermediate between these has been proposed by Friston et al. (1997) but is not discussed further here. In this approach a single bolus study would be performed and any statistically significant deviation in time from the

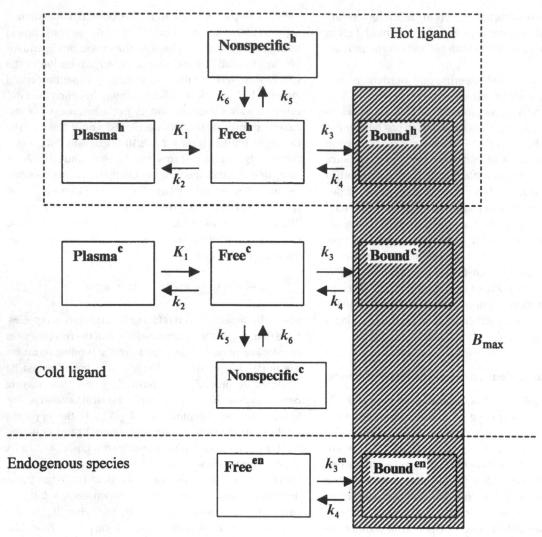

Fig. 2.4. Schematic diagram corresponding to the model described in Eqs. (2.8–2.11). Abbreviations and terms are described in the text.

predicted dynamic curve would be a measure of "activation", in effect detecting a change in k_2. A pharmacologic challenge was used as a test case.

The steady-state technique

The bolus-plus-infusion method was developed for receptor–ligand characterization studies by Carson and colleagues at the National Institutes of Health (Carson et al., 1993). The beauty of this method is that by properly combining a bolus with a constant infusion of radiotracer, the radiotracer level in the brain can be brought to a constant level in a minimum of time. With ligand levels in the tissue no longer varying in time, the derivatives on the left-hand sides of Eqs. (2.1–2.3) disappear and the models reduce to a set of algebraic equations. In fact, no modeling is required. For many ligands, this technique is ideal for

reliably estimating distribution volume (which is a linear function of BP). The steady-state method has been used quite extensively in SPECT studies (Laruelle et al., 1994), which, because of long-lived isotopes, can be applied to data acquired the day following a bolus injection (no infusion needed). The bolus-plus-infusion method is easily extended to neurotransmitter-change experiments by perturbing the endogenous neurotransmitter pharmacologically once the steady-state level of radiotracer has been achieved. The measured parameter that has been used to indicate neurotransmitter alteration is the change in binding potential, ΔBP. Fig. 2.5 shows a change in the steady-state level of raclopride activity in the striatum of a monkey before and after amphetamine perturbation. The activity in the cerebellum (devoid of D_2 receptors) is unaffected (Endres et al., 1997).

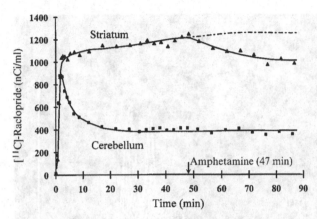

Fig. 2.5. The effect of amphetamine (0.4 mg/kg) on raclopride levels in the brain of monkeys using the bolus-plus-infusion method for detecting a change in neurotransmitter level. The [^{11}C]-raclopride signal in the striatum is depressed following heightened competition between raclopride and dopamine for binding at D$_2$ receptors. The activity in the cerebellum, which has no D$_2$ receptors, is unchanged. The dotted continuation of the top curve shows the model-predicted continuation of the curve in the absence of an amphetamine injection. Data are decay corrected. (Data from Endres et al., 1997.)

Experimental considerations

Whether one chooses the two-bolus or the constant-infusion approach, there are two important questions to be answered. Can the change in PET signal be reliably detected given the inherent variability in the method? Can the apparent change in some parameter of interest be unambiguously linked to changes in neurotransmitter, given the inherent variability and covariability of the parameters? With regard to the former, Endres et al. (1997) used simulations to show that with the bolus-plus-infusion technique, ΔBP is proportional to the integral of the endogenous neurotransmitter curve (i.e., the additional amount of neurotransmitter, released transiently, above the steady state level). Morris, Fisher and colleagues at Massachusetts General Hospital (Fisher et al., 1995; Morris et al., 1995) showed that with the two-bolus method, the sum of squares difference (X^2) between the two dynamic PET curves (with and without perturbation) increases with duration of perturbation. Importantly, the effect of transient neurotransmitter release is distinct from a transient increase in blood flow and the precise timing of the perturbation relative to the tracer bolus can greatly affect the magnitude of the signal change. Endres and Carson (1998) provided a mathematic formalism for understanding the importance of perturbation timing and its relation to the kinetics of the labeled ligand. The implications of these techniques and some recent applications are examined at the end of this chapter.

Limitations to absolute quantification

To this point, we have examined models that describe the concentration of a tracer molecule in various states, or compartments, in the tissue. We have asserted that by summing the concentrations of radioactive tracer in each state postulated by the model, we can predict the measured PET signal, and by comparing the prediction with data we can quantify some useful model parameters. Sometimes, however, for reasons related to the scanner, the measured signal in a region of interest does not reflect the true concentration of tracer in a given tissue. Therefore, before binding or other parameters of interest can be estimated, the *physics* of the measurements must be considered.

Resolution effects

When the structure of interest (e.g., striatum) is small in comparison to the resolution characteristics of the scanner, the radioactivity measured in that structure is a biased estimate of its true radioactivity concentration. This is often referred to generically as the partial volume effect. Figure 2.6 illustrates this point. The radioactivity in the striatum is artifactually reduced from its true value, while it is artifactually increased in adjacent brain regions. How significant is this bias or error in radioactivity measurement? As discussed in Chapter 1, the resolution of PET or SPECT scanners affects the accuracy of the images obtained. This resolution is commonly expressed in terms of the full-width-at-half-maximum (FWHM) (Fig. 2.7). A widely quoted rule of thumb is that the radioactivity in a sphere that is embedded in a nonradioactive background is accurate to within 2% if the sphere's diameter is greater than 2.7 times the FWHM (Kessler et al., 1984). This may be overly optimistic. Chen et al. (1998) observed underestimation of 10 to 20% of true radioactivity for a sphere that was more than three times the FWHM of their modern scanner (FWHM = 4.5 mm, in-plane). Regardless of the specific numbers, the bias is inevitable and will probably be significant in measuring many of the smaller brain structures. The best partial resolution reported to date is approximately 3 mm with PET (Valk et al., 1990). The spatial resolution of SPECT is much worse (typically >10 mm, in-plane).

The important question for the design of quantitative PET/SPECT studies is how will the error in measured radioactivity affect measures of receptor function that are obtained using any of the modeling analyses presented above? The answer, in part, depends on the particular model used to analyze the data and the timing and amount

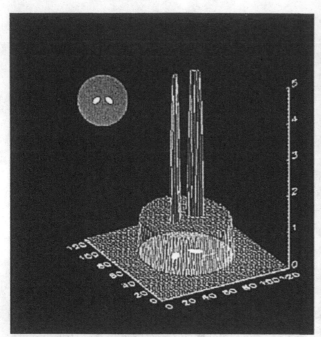
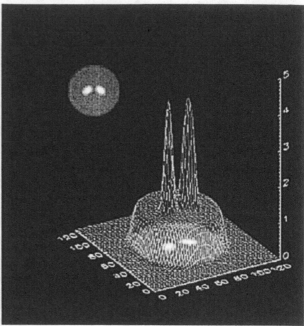

Fig. 2.6. Comparison of images achieved with a perfect scanner (left) and a realistic scanner (right) for the same object. The large circle represents the entire brain while the ellipses represent the striatum. The measured radioactivity concentrations equal the true concentrations in both regions. In the realistic scanner, the radioactivity distribution in the "striatum" is artifactually reduced owing to smearing (spill-over) into the adjacent brain tissue. Conversely, radioactivity in the area of the brain adjacent to the "striatum" is artifactually too high from radioactivity spilling in from the "striatum".

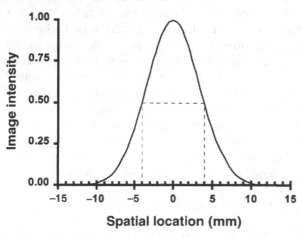

Fig. 2.7. The resolution of a PET or SPECT scanner is often expressed in terms of its full width at-half-maximum (FWHM). The image intensity is plotted as function of position along a line in an image of a point of radioactivity. At half the maximum amplitude, 0.5 here, lines are drawn extending toward the x-axis. The distance between these lines, 8 mm, is the FWHM.

(both in terms of mass and radioactivity) of ligand injected. Figure 2.8 shows results of a simulation study of the effect of striatum size on binding potential estimates. The experimental conditions simulated were similar to those described in the literature (Morris et al., 1999). For simulated striata of sizes comparable to those of a rhesus monkey, the effect was quite pronounced on a PET scanner with 6.5 mm resolution. The estimated binding potential was found to be as little as 35%, and at best 80% of the true value. The error would not be as large for human adult striata but it might still be significant.

By way of example, consider that the age-related decline in striatal D_2 receptor binding has been measured at 1–2% per year in humans (Rinne et al., 1993; Wong et al., 1997) but there is also evidence that the size of the striatum changes (declines) with age (McDonald et al., 1991). Fully one third of the decline in D_2 binding with age in monkeys (measured via PET) can be attributed to size changes with age (Morris et al., 1999). In studies where the difference in the size of an effect between groups is expected to be small and where there may be a *bias* in structure size between subject groups, it would seem prudent to correct for partial volume error. Group biases might be present in develop-

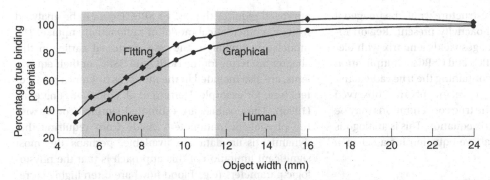

Fig. 2.8. The effect of partial volume (striatum size) on binding potential (BP) estimation studied using computer simulation techniques. Brain and striatum sizes over a wide range of sizes were considered. For sizes that correspond to those of small monkeys, both the fitting and graphical methods of estimating BP produced estimates that were between 35 and 80% of its true value (E. D. Morris and R. F. Muzic, unpublished data). For larger sizes, in the range of adult humans, the BP estimates were much closer to the true value.

mental studies of children or in studies that compare normal subjects with those with brain atrophy. The proper choice of a group of age-matched controls for any PET study requires that researchers consider the possible effects of partial voluming.

Correcting for the partial volume effect

The partial volume effect has been widely recognized as a limiting factor in the ability to quantify the amount of radioactivity in tissue accurately. The challenge has been to formulate a correction that is practical to apply yet accounts for the dependence on the local contrast (which changes with time) and the object size (which does not). Existing correction methods can be divided loosely into two groups: those that require (or make assumptions about) anatomic information and those that do not. Typically, the information is MR or CT data from which the size of the various structures may be determined. When such data are available, it is preferable to use them in the correction since there is the potential to determine the radioactivity concentration accurately in very small structures. In comparison, techniques that do not require or assume anatomic data will have difficulty in distinguishing between a certain amount of radioactivity in a small object and a higher amount of radioactivity in an even smaller object. Hence an inherent limitation of emission tomography is that, below a certain object size, the size of the object and the concentration of radioactivity in that object are intrinsically (inversely) correlated. For a given measurement, size and concentration cannot both be determined. As the size decreases, the degree of correlation worsens. Sometimes it is feasible and convenient to obtain MR or CT data for the purpose of applying a partial volume correction; other times it is not.

Corrections requiring anatomic information

Kessler et al. (1984) presented a seminal paper on a method to correct for partial volume effects. Their work introduced the hot spot recovery coefficient (HSRC) and the cold spot recovery coefficient (CSRC). The measured radioactivity in a structure can be calculated as

$$\text{Measured radioactivity} = (\text{HSRC} \times \text{true structure radioactivity}) + (\text{CSRC} \times \text{true background radioactivity}) \quad (2.12)$$

The HSRC is the fraction of the true activity in the structure that is measured when there is no background radioactivity. The CSRC is the fraction of the background activity that is measured (erroneously) in the structure containing no radioactivity, given a hot background. HSRC and CSRC are dependent on the size of the structure and can be determined either mathematically (i.e., via simulations) or via phantom experiments. They are both independent of contrast. Given an estimate of the structure size, one can determine appropriate values of HSRC and CSRC. With these values and knowledge of the true background radioactivity (often approximated as being equal to the measured background radioactivity), the above equation can be solved to determine a structure's true radioactivity from the measured tissue radioactivity.

A number of studies have extended this method to consider cross-contamination between multiple structures in the image (Rousset et al., 1996, 1998). This is analogous to having HSRC and CSRC values for each structure and 'background' in the image. To determine these values, the structures of interest are defined in the MR or CT images. For each structure, a mask image is created with pixel values inside the structure set to unity, and zero otherwise. A spatial resolution distortion function that models the resolution characteristics of the PET or SPECT scanner is then applied to each. The resultant set of blurred mask images represents how each structure would be imaged if it represented the only radioactivity present. Region-of-interest analysis of these images yields a matrix with elements corresponding to HSRCs and CSRCs. Multiplication of the matrix by the vector containing the true radioactivity concentrations yields a vector of the observed concentrations. Therefore, the true concentrations may be obtained by solving the matrix equation. This is analogous to a generalization of the above equation for a set of n regions:

$$\begin{bmatrix} m_1 \\ m_2 \\ \vdots \\ m_n \end{bmatrix} = \begin{bmatrix} HSRC_1 & CSRC_{12} & \cdots & CSRC_{1n} \\ CSRC_{21} & HSRC_2 & & \\ \vdots & & \ddots & \\ CSRC_{n1} & & & HSRC_n \end{bmatrix} \begin{bmatrix} T_1 \\ T_2 \\ \vdots \\ T_n \end{bmatrix} \quad (2.13)$$

where the left hand side of the equation is the set of measured radioactivities, m_i, in each region i and the elements of the vector on the right hand side are the true radioactivity T_i in each region, respectively. The matrix on the right-hand side consists, on the diagonal, of recovery coefficients for each region. The off-diagonal terms are the spillover fractions $CSRC_{ij}$ indicating the spillover of radioactivity from "background" region j to "foreground" region i. When the region j is far from the region i, then the $CSRC_{ij}$ is zero.

Another group has described a correction technique based on the similar principle except that corrected values are determined directly from the mask images and the measured image (Muller-Gartner et al., 1992). As part of this analysis, the set of blurred masks are then summed together to reconstitute the blurred image. In effect, they are implicitly solving the matrix equations.

The above approaches are quite elegant and use well-accepted principles of scanner performance. Yet, there are caveats to keep in mind. First, and foremost, MR or CT data must be available to create the masks for each structure. Of course the structures of interest must be clearly discernable since small errors in the size of the structures can lead to significant errors in the correction (Herrero et al., 1989). Second, the PET or SPECT data must be accurately registered with the MR or CT data so that mask images can be properly applied to the PET or SPECT data. Third, there is an underlying assumption that the radioactivity concentration within each structure (e.g. all the white matter) is uniform.

Corrections not requiring anatomic information

Corrections that do not require anatomic information can be subclassified into ones that are based on a pharmacokinetic model and ones that are based on a model of scanner (spatial resolution) characteristics. The pharmacokinetic

approach requires the PET or SPECT data to be analyzed using a mathematical model of radioactivity uptake. The models are similar to the one discussed earlier in this chapter but terms for the HSRC and CSRC, or their equivalents, are also included in the model as unknown parameters (see, for example, Herrero et al. (1989) or Feng et al. (1996)). These values are estimated simultaneously with the physiologic parameters. Aside from requiring that dynamic tissue data are available, perhaps the most significant limitation of this approach is that the physiologic parameters (e.g., blood flow) are often highly correlated with HSRC and CSRC parameters (Feng et al., 1996; Muzic, et al., 1998). In other words, estimates of some or all of the parameters may be unreliable.

In the approach based on a model of the scanner, the radioactivity in the structure of interest (e.g., a lesion) is approximated as having a simple geometric shape (e.g., a sphere) containing a uniform concentration of activity (Chen et al., 1999). Likewise, the lesion is assumed to be situated within a much larger "background" region that is also uniform in radioactivity. Parameters representing the size, position, and radioactivity of the lesion along with the radioactivity in the background region are estimated simultaneously. This is accomplished by blurring the sphere with a mathematical model for scanner resolution effects and adjusting the size and activity inside the sphere until the model-predicted image best matches the measured image. This has the advantage of not requiring MR or CT data, although the minimum object size at which both the size and radioactivity can be estimated is limited because the quantities become increasingly correlated as lesion size diminishes. Nevertheless, any anatomic data about the object size, if available, could be used in this model-based method so that only the radioactivity need be estimated.

Model simplifications

It is not always practical to acquire structural data on a patient (e.g., for use in partial volume correction), nor is it always practical, or even permitted, to acquire blood samples for plasma radioactivity measurements. In other words, a kinetic analysis must be attempted without the critical plasma input function P. Luckily, a number of modeling techniques have been developed for such situations.

Eliminating the need for an input function

Although PET receptor studies are promoted as being non-invasive to the patient, this term is often modified to "minimally invasive" when arterial blood sampling is performed. Obtaining arterial blood samples can be a relatively painful experience and carries some risk of arterial damage (Jons et al., 1997). The presence of this risk may preclude the use of quantitative PET and SPECT in pediatric studies. As discussed earlier, determining the proper input function can sometimes be tricky even if blood samples are not proscribed. For these reasons, considerable effort has been spent in eliminating the need for arterial blood samples.

The (metabolite-corrected) radioactivity concentration of tracer in arterial plasma represents the amount of radiotracer that is presented to the tissue of interest over the course of the experiment. In principle, this input function is required to solve any of the systems of equations given earlier (e.g., Eqs (2.1–2.3) or (2.5–2.7)). However, researchers can take advantage of predictable relationships between the input function and activity in either receptor-rich or receptor-poor regions. Because the input to both (receptor-rich and receptor-poor) regions is essentially the same, the equations describing ligand dynamics in one region can be expressed solely in terms of concentration measured in the other. Explicit use of the plasma concentration is not needed. What are the assumptions inherent in this simplification and which parameters can be measured with such techniques?

Reference region techniques

Reference region techniques refer to analysis methods that use scanned measurements in an area in the brain to provide an estimate of the free ligand concentration where specific binding is negligible. The concentration from such a region is then plugged into a tracer kinetic model, either as a dynamic input function or as a static estimate of the free ligand concentration at equilibrium. In order to reduce the degrees of freedom in the estimation problem, these methods typically assume that the free space distribution volume, $DV_F = K_1 / k_2$, is constant across all regions of the brain. That is, at steady state, the ratio of ligand in the free compartment to plasma compartment is assumed to be the same everywhere. The term DV_F describes the volume of tissue into which the free ligand mass present in 1 ml of tissue would distribute with the same concentration as in the blood (P). If the ligand can distribute in only one third of the volume of the tissue, then at steady state, a mass, x, of ligand dissolved in 1 ml blood would distribute in the available space of 3 ml tissue; the distribution volume, DV_F, is 3 (ml tissue)$^{-1}$/(ml blood)$^{-1}$ (Delforge et al., 1996). The assumption of constant DV_F does not mean that K_1 is identical from region to region. Neither is the concentration of free ligand constant across regions except

at steady state. This means that the difference between activities in a target and a reference region cannot be taken as a measure of binding except at equilibrium. This can then be used to modify the model equations.

A model-fitting method
Cunningham et al. (1991) proposed solving for the arterial input function in a reference region in the following way:

$$\frac{dF_R}{dt} = K_1^R P - k_2^R F_R \tag{2.14}$$

Equation 2.14 is rearranged to

$$P = \left[\frac{dF_R}{dt} + k_2^R F_R \right] / K_1^R$$

and substituted into the model to give Eqs. 2.15 and 2.16, which describe dynamics in a receptor-*rich* region:

$$\frac{dF}{dt} = K_1 P - (k_2 + k_3) F + k_4 B \tag{2.15}$$
$$\frac{dB}{dt} = k_3 F - k_4 B \tag{2.16}$$

F_R represents radioligand concentrations in the reference region and F and B represent the (time varying) free and specifically bound activities, respectively, in the target region. We apply the constraint that the free space distribution of the radioligand be equal in the two regions, (i.e., $K_1^R / k_2^R = K_1 / k_2$). Corrections to the technique may be necessary if the reference region is not completely devoid of specific binding (Cunningham et al., 1991). By constraining only the free-space distribution ratio and not K_1 or k_2, individually, the model allows for kinetic differences between regions. The constraint is necessary, however, to guarantee that the remaining parameters, k_3 and k_4, will be identifiable.

This reference region model was originally applied to a μ-opioid receptor ligand, [³H]-diprenorphine (Cunningham et al., 1991) and later modified for use with PET and [¹¹C]-raclopride (Hume et al., 1992) in rats. A comparative study was performed and reported by Lammertsma et al. (1996) examining this method and several others that require arterial blood data for analysis. The goal of the Lammertsma study was to measure the apparent BP, B'_{max}/K_D, accurately. The authors concluded that the most reliable measure of BP was given by the method described above (Eqs. (2.14–2.16)). Because this technique uses an iterative least-squares minimization algorithm, it is presumed to be an unbiased estimator of BP (Hsu et al., 1997). Unfortunately, as an iterative method, it may be too slow for making parametric images. A recent modification of the iterative reference region technique incorporates a further model

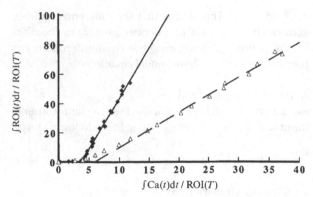

Fig. 2.9. An example of a Logan plot for rapid data analysis. The data are plotted as described in Eq. (2.17) from the cerebellum ($\triangle$) and the straitum ($\diamond$) (Ca is equivalent to P and ROI is equivalent to C_t). The binding potential is determined by the ratio of the slopes (striatum/cerebellum) of the lines regressed to the data.

simplification and uses spectral analysis methods for estimating parameters. It has been used successfully for parametric image generation (Gunn et al., 1997).

Graphical methods: Logan-plot analysis

The method of Logan et al. (1990) was initially developed to provide a technique for rapid data analysis. It uses another rearrangement of the model equations (2.1) and (2.2) that can be solved *noniteratively* to generate a parametric image of BP values at each pixel of a PET/SPECT image. The rearranged operational equation used for this technique is given as:

$$\frac{\int_0^T C_t(t)\mathrm{d}t}{C_t(T)} = DV \frac{\int_0^T P(t)\mathrm{d}t}{C_t(T)} + b \tag{2.17}$$

where $C_t(t)$ is the concentration of the radioligand in the tissue, P is the arterial plasma concentration, DV is the distribution volume, and b is a constant of integration that is a composite function of the rate parameters dependent on the assumed model. Notice the resemblance of Eq. (2.17) to that of a line, $y = mx + b$, with its two estimable parameters. An example of the Logan plot is shown in Fig. 2.9. In essence, the nonlinear "PET" curve in Fig. 2.2, which is made up of bound and free ligand, has been transformed, or linearized, into Fig. 2.9. (By way of comparison, the log function is a common way of linearizing data that demonstrate exponential behavior.) The "free" curve in the earlier figure can be thought of as a reference region; when it is transformed it yields a curve like the lower one in Fig. 2.9. For reversibly bound tracers, a point in time is reached when the change in plasma

concentration is approximately equal to the change in tissue concentration. Beyond this time, the slope of the above function will be constant and will equal DV. On the Logan plot, this time corresponds to a transition point beyond which the plot is linear. (The x axis on the Logan plot represents a sort of "stretched" time.) For a region with no specific binding, DV describes the free space distribution volume K_1/k_2. In regions with specific binding, DV represents the product of free and bound distribution volumes $(K_1/k_2)(1 + B'_{max}/K_D)$. In both regions, slow nonspecific binding (i.e., small values of k_5 and k_6) and plasma volume, ε_v are neglected. Contrary to the modeling approaches discussed at the beginning of the chapter, the transformation underlying the Logan plot cannot accommodate a radioactive decay term. Therefore, it is essential that the data be corrected for radioisotope decay prior to graphical analysis. This method was originally validated for [¹¹C]-cocaine and subsequently for [¹¹C]-raclopride (Logan et al., 1994).

Further work by Logan and co-workers (1996) demonstrated that the above model could be modified to eliminate the need for a measured arterial input function. By substituting reference region data, C_{ref}, for the arterial plasma, Eq. (2.17) becomes:

$$\frac{\int_0^T C_t(t)\mathrm{d}t}{C_t(T)} = DVR \frac{\int_0^T C_{ref}(t)\mathrm{d}t}{C_t(T)} + b' \tag{2.18}$$

where DVR is the ratio of distribution volumes in target to reference region and equals $(1 + f_{NS}B'_{max}/K_D)$, where f_{NS} is equivalent to the free fraction of tracer (f_2), introduced by Mintun, and converts K_D to the effective equilibrium dissociation constant. This equation holds provided that the ratio of C_{ref} to C_t is nearly constant. If this condition is not satisfied, there is still a valid linearization using the reference region concentration but it requires the use of a population-average k_2 value.

The primary merit of this technique, other than obviating the need to sample arterial blood, is its computational ease. The linear function given in Eq. (2.18) can be solved pixel-by-pixel, permitting rapid generation of parametric images; an example of an image of the BP $f_{NS}B'_{max}/K_D$, is shown in Fig. 2.10. The model can also be applied to other reversibly bound radioligands. The application of the model to other radiotracers differs only in choosing the (transformed) time at which the function becomes linear.

The use of [¹¹C]-raclopride has been well validated for determining the BP of D_2 receptors and change in BP (i.e., receptor occupancy). The reference region techniques

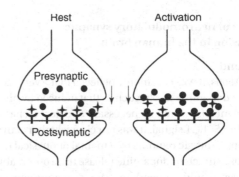

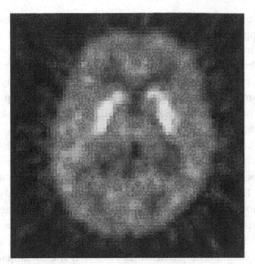

Fig. 2.10. A parametric image of binding potential. A value of binding potential was calculated for each pixel in the image via the reference region technique of Logan et al. (1996).

Fig. 2.11. Schematic diagram of a dopamine (DA) synapse at rest and during activation. At rest, the neuron releases some DA, but there are many free postsynaptic receptors to which the PET tracer (radioligand) can bind. During performance of a task that activates DA neurons (or application of a drug that increases DA release or inhibits reuptake), there is increased DA in the synapse, which causes increased competition for the postsynaptic receptors. Consequently, specific binding of the PET radioligand is decreased.

described above work well for measuring these parameters in a clinical setting.

New clinical and research applications

Armed with an array of both complicated and simple modeling approaches, let us return to the problem of measuring neurotransmitter changes with PET.

Neurotransmitter "activation" studies

Until recently, PET and SPECT brain imaging studies could be divided into two groups: receptor–ligand studies (as discussed above) and tracer studies that included activation. In the latter type, a subject would be asked to perform an activation task, such as speaking words or recalling items from memory, during a brain scan. Images of regional cerebral blood flow (or glucose metabolism) would be obtained and processed to reveal areas of the brain that are involved in the task. This technique, unfortunately, does not reveal the specific neurotransmitter systems that might be activated by the task.

Nevertheless, it has been believed for some time that the competition between endogenous and exogenous ligands (Fig. 2.11) could be exploited to image some aspect of dopamine release in vivo resulting from "activation" of a neuronal pathway or circuit (Dewey et al., 1990, 1991). Through the performance of a task that activates dopaminergic neurons, or the administration of a drug that

increases dopamine levels, extra dopamine can compete with radioligand at dopamine receptors. As mentioned above, to succeed, this competition must reduce the PET signal by a discernible amount. If detectable, the measurement could have applications in the imaging of various neuromodulatory transmitter systems (e.g., dopamine, acetylcholine, serotonin, norepinephrine (noradrenaline)). These systems typically innervate the brain diffusely but constitute only a small fraction of all the synapses in any target brain region (Squire 1987; Cooper et al., 1991). As such, the PET signal from these neurons would probably be overwhelmed by the signal from other neurons in a cerebral blood flow or metabolism study.

In fact, the neurotransmitter activation approach has been used successfully to demonstrate dopamine release induced by a variety of drugs, including amphetamine (Dewey et al., 1991; Laruelle et al., 1995; Carson et al., 1997) and cholinergic antagonists (Dewey et al., 1993). Clinical applications have already begun to appear, including the demonstrations of high dopamine response to amphetamine in schizophrenics (Breier et al., 1997; Laruelle et al., 1996) and the low dopamine response to methylphenidate in cocaine abusers (Volkow et al., 1997). The technique has even been used to visualize task-activated, dopaminergic synaptic transmission in the human brain in vivo (Koepp et al., 1998) *without* a pharmacological stimulus.

Detection of neuromodulatory synaptic transmission in the human brain

Background

Until the 1990s, it was commonly believed that a very large increase in dopamine levels, such as that induced by pharmacologic means, would be necessary to detect a change in the PET or SPECT signal. It was not clear whether activation of dopaminergic neurons by a mental or physical task would cause sufficient dopamine release to be observable. The answer would depend on the concentrations of dopamine and radiotracer in the synapse, affinities of the two molecules for dopamine receptors, and alterations in dopamine neuronal firing rates during activation tasks. The concentration of dopamine in the synapse remains unknown. However, estimates from a variety of sources indicate that it reaches a peak of 10–100 μmol/l following release from the presynaptic terminal and that it clears with a time constant on the order of 2 ms. These numbers suggest an average synaptic concentration of about 100 nmol/l, which rises to at least 200 nmol/l during an activation task (see references and calculations in Fisher et al., 1995).

Given these and other estimates, Fisher and colleagues were willing to predict that such a cognitive activation task would indeed cause a measurable change in radioligand binding (Fisher et al., 1995; Morris et al., 1995). Encouraging preliminary results have been obtained using SPECT with the D_2 receptor antagonist [^{123}I]-IBZM (Ebert et al., 1994): depressed patients that responded to total sleep deprivation showed a decrease in relative radioligand binding in the basal ganglia in the post-sleep deprivation scan compared with the baseline scan. These preliminary results were interpreted as evidence of increased dopamine release induced by sleep deprivation. More definitive experimental support for imaging of behavioral activation was lacking.

New developments

The functional imaging landscape changed after Koepp et al. (1998) observed eight volunteers performing a video game while undergoing an [^{11}C]-raclopride PET scan. The game required players to maneuver a tank through a battlefield, and players received a monetary award depending on their success at the game. On a separate day, the same volunteers underwent another raclopride scan while staring at a blank screen instead of playing the video game. This is the two-bolus protocol discussed earlier in this chapter; the measured parameter that was used as the index of competition was change in binding potential, Δ BP. The researchers found that the binding of [^{11}C]-raclopride in the striatum was significantly decreased during the video game, compared with the level at rest. This indicated that the dopaminergic neurons in the striatum had been activated during the playing of the game and had presumably liberated an increased quantity of dopamine into their synapses. In other words, Koepp and co-workers had witnessed, via PET, the nonpharmacologic activation of the dopamine system in humans.

The results of Koepp et al. (1998) raise several interesting questions. First, what aspect of the video game caused the subjects' dopaminergic neurons to increase their firing rate? The video game is a complex task involving visual perception, decision-making, hand movements, frustration, pleasure, rewards, etc. The game, most likely, was chosen for exactly that reason: it maximized the chances of activating dopaminergic neurons. Now that the investigators have succeeded in demonstrating such activation, an important next step will be to determine what cognitive and/or motor features of physical tasks require the use of dopamine-containing neurons. This new type of PET protocol is exactly what is needed to answer such a question. The fact that the subjects' success in the game correlated significantly with their dopamine outflow (i.e., inversely with radiotracer binding), is intriguing given the role of dopaminergic neurons in pleasure and reward (Robbins and Everitt, 1996; Schultz, 1997). Electrophysiologic studies in animals suggest that dopamine neuron activity is typically triggered by reward stimuli (see Schultz (1997) for review). The hypothesis that this holds true in humans now appears to be testable using PET.

A further question is whether the same results could have been obtained by a conventional regional blood flow study? This appears not to be the case. Koepp et al. (1998) reported a *decrease* in regional blood flow (i.e., a decreased delivery of tracer) to the striatum during the study. This finding underscores the fact that neuromodulatory synapses comprise only a small fraction of all the synapses in any brain region. The striatum is one of the few brain regions where neuromodulatory synapses are relatively concentrated (dopamine synapses may represent up to one third of the synaptic population (Doucet et al., 1986; discussion in Wilson, 1998). And yet, the net neuronal activity in the striatum, as revealed by the blood flow parameter R_i, was seen to decrease despite activation of the dopamine neurons. Had the experiment been performed with conventional blood flow imaging, the results would have provided evidence for *deactivation* of the striatum during the task! The exact *opposite* conclusion regarding striatal (and, by implication, dopaminergic) function might have been reached. It is worth noting that the changes in blood flow from subject to subject had no correlation with the changes in tracer binding, indicating that the dopamine induced decreases in receptor binding were independent of blood flow effects.

The opportunities for dissecting the functional neurochemistry of humans are intriguing. Serotonergic, noradrenergic, and cholinergic systems will surely be probed once radioligands with appropriate neuroreceptor specificity and kinetic properties are identified.

Optimal ligand kinetics

What makes a ligand optimal depends on the conditions and aims of an experiment. If the goal is to estimate the binding properties of a receptor (as Zeeberg (1995) has said, to maximize the "receptor sensitivity" as opposed to "delivery sensitivity") then identifiability of parameters is key. As mentioned earlier, the binding parameters (k_3 and k_4 or k_{on}, and k_{off}) cannot be estimated reliably if they are too fast relative to the influx and efflux parameters (K_1 and k_2). However, if detection of neurotransmitter activation is the goal, then we wish to maximize the magnitude of a particular detection index. Endres and Carson (1998) have shown that for the bolus-infusion protocol there is an optimum range of binding potentials that maximize the detection parameter ΔBP. Morris et al. (1995) demonstrated (also in a simulation study) that irreversible ligands would yield maximal values of χ^2 using the two-bolus protocol.

Possible clinical applications

What are the clinical applications of this new brain imaging paradigm? Our first concern should be with the length of the activation task. The video game, described above, was played continuously for 60 min: from 10 min prior to raclopride injection until 50 min after. This is too long a task for routine clinical examinations, particularly for children and for patients suffering from certain psychiatric illnesses. Children, in fact, will have trouble simply remaining still in the scanner for that long. Fortunately, such a lengthy task is not absolutely necessary to yield a detectable effect. The Koepp study appears to show that release of endogenous dopamine causes a sustained decrease in the PET signal that lasts well beyond the restoration of normal resting dopamine levels. In fact, it had already been predicted that an activation task lasting 7 min could be sufficient to cause a near-maximal effect on raclopride binding using the two-bolus method (Morris et al., 1995).

There is also reason to believe that similar studies will be possible with SPECT which is more widely available. Drug-induced release of dopamine has been demonstrated

using SPECT and the steady-state technique (Laruelle, et al., 1995, 1996). Results were very similar to those of PET. Mental and physical activation of dopamine neurons has not yet conclusively been demonstrated with single photon imaging. However, as mentioned above, Ebert et al. (1994) reported preliminary results of SPECT studies suggesting that sleep deprivation caused depressed subjects to release detectable amounts of dopamine.

Let us assume that quantitative SPECT imaging and analysis is possible without arterial blood sampling, what sort of neurologic or psychiatric patients might benefit from a PET/SPECT neurotransmitter activation study? The first candidates would be those suffering from illnesses that respond to drugs that alter the dopamine system. Some schizophrenics, for instance, are best treated with D_2 receptor antagonists ("typical neuroleptics"), while others respond better to mixed D_2/D_1 antagonists ("atypical neuroleptics"). Clozapine, for example, is an atypical neuroleptic that has been shown to occupy D_1 and D_2 receptors (among others) nearly equally in human subjects (Farde et al., 1992). Theoretically, a PET neurotransmitter activation study using a D_2 receptor ligand (e.g., raclopride) and a D_1 ligand (e.g., SCH23390) could demonstrate that one patient releases too much dopamine at D_2 receptor synapses, while another is overactive at D_1 synapses. Drug therapy could be adjusted accordingly. Related studies have already been performed: schizophrenic patients have been observed to respond to amphetamine with higher elevations of extracellular dopamine at D_2 synapses than normal controls (Breier et al., 1997; Laruelle et al., 1996). These results support the dopamine hypothesis for schizophrenia in that they demonstrate a functional abnormality in the dopamine system in schizophrenics. The results, however, are not yet directly applicable to patient care.

Attention-deficit hyperactivity disorder (ADHD) also may have a strong dopaminergic component (Ernst et al., 1998; Swanson et al., 1998a, b). Given the variety of evidence for pathophysiology of the dopaminergic system in ADHD, there may be an opportunity for a dopamine neurotransmitter-activation scan with a methylphenidate challenge (methylphenidate is commonly used to treat the disorder; it blocks reuptake of dopamine, thereby increasing synaptic dopamine levels). Such a perturbation might be used to predict which children would respond to the drug, as well as to aid in diagnosis in equivocal cases. The noradrenergic and serotonergic systems have been implicated in a variety of psychiatric illnesses, including depression, suicidality, and obsessive compulsive disorder (Jacobs, 1994; Kaplan et al., 1994; Kegeles and Mann, 1997). Again, with the neuroreceptor ligands it might be possible to determine whether patients are hyper- or hypoactive at various classes of synapse; these findings would inform drug therapy decisions.

References

Bahn, M. M., Huang, S. C., Hawkins, R. A. et al. (1989). Models for in vivo kinetic interactions of dopamine D_2-neuroreceptors and 3-(2'-[^{18}F]fluoroethyl)spiperone examined with positron emission tomography. *J. Cereb. Blood Flow. Metab.*, **9**, 840–9.

Breier, A., Su, T.-P., Saunders, R. et al. (1997). Schizophrenia is associated with elevated amphetamine-induced synaptic dopamine concentrations: evidence from a novel positron emission tomography method. *Proc. Natl. Acad. Sci. USA*, **94**, 2569–74.

Carson R. E., Channing, M. A., Blasberg, R. G. et al. (1993). Comparison of bolus and infusion methods for receptor quantitation: application to [^{18}F]-cyclofoxy and positron emission tomography. *J. Cereb. Blood Flow Metab.*, **13**: 24–42.

Carson, R. E., Breier, A., de Bartolomeis, A. et al. (1997). Quantification of amphetamine-induced changes in [^{11}C]-raclopride binding with continuous infusion. *J. Cereb. Blood Flow Metab.*, **17**, 437–47.

Chen, C. H., Muzic, R. F. Jr, Nelson, A. D. and Adler, L. P. (1998). A non-linear, spatially-variant, object-dependent system model for prediction and correction of partial volume in PET, *IEEE Trans. Med. Imaging*, **27**, 214–27.

Chen, C. H., Muzic, R. F. Jr, Nelson, A. D. and Adler, L. P. (1999). Simultaneous recovery of size and radioactivity concentration of small spheroids with PET data. *J. Nucl. Med.*, **40**, 118–30.

Cooper, J. R., Bloom, F. E. and Roth, R. H. (1991). *The Biochemical Basis of Neuropharmacology*. New York: Oxford University Press.

Cunningham, V. J., Hume, S. P., Price, G. R., Ahier, R. G., Cremer, J. E. and Jones, A. K. P. (1991). Compartmental analysis of diprenorphine binding to opiate receptors in the rat in vivo and its comparison with equilibrium data in vitro. *J. Cereb. Blood Flow Metab.*, **11**, 1–9.

Delforge, J. Syrota, A. and Mazoyer, B. M. (1989). Experimental design optimisation: theory and application to estimation of receptor model parameters using dynamic positron emission tomography. *Phys. Med. Biol.*, **34**, 419–35.

Delforge, J., Syrota, A. and Mazoyer, B. M. (1990). Identifiability analysis and parameter identification of an in vivo ligand-receptor model from PET data. *IEEE Trans. Biomed. Eng.*, **27**, 653–61.

Delforge, J., Syrota, A. and Bendriem, B. (1996). Concept of reaction volume in the in vivo ligand–receptor model. *J. Nucl. Med.*, **37**, 118–25.

Dewey, S. L., Brodie, J. D., Fowler, J. S. et al. (1990). Positron emission tomography (PET) studies of dopaminergic/cholinergic interactions in the baboon brain. *Synapse*, **6**, 321–7.

Dewey, S. L., Logan, J., Wolf, A. P. et al. (1991). Amphetamine induced decreases in ^{18}F-*N*-methylspiroperidol binding in the baboon brain using positron emission tomography (PET). *Synapse*, **7**, 324–7.

Dewey, S. L., Smith, G. S., Logan, J. et al. (1993). Effects of central cholinergic blockade on striatal dopamine release measured with positron emission tomography in normal human subjects. *Proc. Natl. Acad. Sci. USA*, **9**, 11816–20.

Doucet, G., Descarries, L. and Garcia, S. (1986). Quantification of the dopamine innervation in adult rat neostriatum. *Neuroscience*, **19**, 427–45.

Ebert, D., Feistel, H., Haschka, W., Barocka, A. and Pirner, A. (1994). Single photon emission computerized tomography assessment of cerebral dopamine D_2 receptor blockade in depression before and after sleep deprivation – preliminary results. *Biol. Psychiatry*, **35**, 880–5.

Endres, C. J. and Carson, R. E. (1998). Assessment of dynamic neurotransmitter changes with bolus or infusion delivery of neuroreceptor ligands. *J. Cereb. Blood Flow Metab.*, **18**, 1196–210.

Endres, C. J., Kolachana, B. S., Saunders, R. C. et al. (1997). Kinetic modeling of [^{11}C]-raclopride: combined PET-microdialysis studies. *J. Cereb. Blood Flow Metab.*, **17**, 932–42.

Ernst, M., Zametkin, A. J., Matochik, J. A., Jons, P. H. and Cohen, R. M. (1998). DOPA decarboxylase activity in attention deficit hyperactivity disorder adults. A [fluorine-18]fluorodopa positron emission tomographic study. *J. Neurosci.*, **18**, 5901–7.

Farde, L., Eriksson, L., Blomquist, G. and Halldin, C. (1989). Kinetic analysis of central [^{11}C]-raclopride binding to D_2-dopamine receptors studied by PET: a comparison to the equilibrium analysis. *J. Cereb. Blood Flow Metab.*, **9**, 696–708.

Farde, L., Nordstrom, A.-L., Wiesel, F.-A., Pauli, S., Halldin, C., Sedvall, G. (1992). Positron emission tomographic analysis of central D_1 and D_2 receptor occupancy in patients treated with classical neuroleptics and clozapine. *Arch. Gen. Psychiatry*, **49**, 538–44.

Feng, D., Li X and Huang, S. C. (1996). A new double modeling approach for dynamic cardiac PET studies using noise and spillover contaminated LV measurements. *IEEE Trans. Biomed. Eng.*, **43**, 319–327.

Fisher, R. E., Morris, E. D., Alpert, N. M. and Fischman, A. J. (1995). In vivo imaging of neuromodulatory synaptic transmission using PET: a review of the relevant neurophysiology. *Hum. Brain Map.*, **3**, 24–34.

Friston, K. J., Malizia, A. L., Wilson, S., Cunningham, V. J., Jones, T. and Nutt, D. J. (1997). Analysis of dynamic radioligand displacement or 'activation' studies. *J. Cereb. Blood Flow Metab.*, **17**, 80–93.

Frost, J. J., Douglass, K. H., Mayber, H. S. et al. (1989). Multicompartmental analysis of [^{11}C]-carfentanil binding to opiate receptors in humans measured by positron emission tomography. *J. Cereb. Blood Flow Metab.*, **9**, 398–409.

Gunn, R. N., Lammertsma, A. A., Hume, S. P. and Cunningham, V. J. (1997). Parametric imaging of ligand-receptor binding in PET using a simplified reference region model. *Neuroimage*, **6**, 279–87.

Herrero, P., Markham, J. and Bergmann, S. R. (1989). Quantitation of myocardial blood flow with $H_2^{15}O$ and positron emission tomography: assessment and error analysis of a mathematical approach, *J. Comput. Assist. Tomogr.*, **13**, 862–73.

Hsu, H., Alpert, N. M., Christian, B. T., Bonab, A. A., Morris, E. and

Fischman, A. J. (1997). Noise properties of a graphical assay of receptor binding. *J. Nucl. Med.*, **38**, 204P.

Huang, S. C., Mahoney, D. K. and Phelps, M. E. (1986). Quantitation in positron emission tomography. 8 Effects of nonlinear parameter estimation on functional images. *J. Cereb. Blood Flow Metab.*, **6**, 515–21.

Huang, S. C., Bahn, M. M., Barrio, J. R. et al. (1989). A double-injection technique for the in vivo measurement of dopamine D_2-receptor density in monkeys with 3-(2'-[^{18}F]fluoroethyl)spiperone and dynamic positron emission tomography. *J. Cereb. Blood Flow Metab.*, **9**, 850–8.

Huang, S. C., Dan-chu, Y., Barrio, J. R. et al. (1991). Kinetics and modeling of L-6-[^{18}F]fluoro-DOPA in human positron emission tomographic studies. *J. Cereb. Blood Flow Metab.*, **11**, 898–913.

Hume, S. P., Myers, R., Bloomfield, P. M. et al. (1992). Quantitation of carbon-11 labeled raclopride in rat striatum using positron emission tomography. *Synapse*, **12**, 47–54.

Jacobs, B. L. (1994). Serotonin, motor activity, and depression-related disorders. *Am. Sci.*, **82**, 457–63.

Jons, P. H., Ernst, M., Hankerson, J., Hardy, K. and Zametkin, A. J. (1997). Follow-up of radial arterial catheterization for positron emission tomography studies. *Hum. Brain Map.*, **5**, 119–23.

Kaplan, H. I., Sadcock, B. J. and Grebb, J. A. (1994). *Kaplan and Sadcock's Synopsis of Psychiatry*. Baltimore: Williams and Wilkins.

Kegeles, L. S. and Mann, J. J. (1997). In vivo imaging of neurotransmitter systems using radiolabeled receptor ligands. *Neuropsychopharmacology*, **17**, 293–307.

Kessler, R. M., Ellis, J. R. J. and Eden, M. (1984). Analysis of emission tomographic scan data: limitations imposed by resolution and background, *J. Comput. Assist. Tomogr.*, **8**, 514–22.

Koepp, M. J., Gunn, R. N., Lawrence, A. D. et al. (1998). Evidence for striatal dopamine release during a video game. *Nature*, **393**, 266–8.

Koeppe, R. A., Holthoff, V. A., Frey, K. A., Kilbourn, M. R. and Kuhl, D. E. (1991). Compartmental analysis of [^{11}C]flumazenil kinetics for the estimation of ligand transport rate and receptor distribution using positron emission tomography. *J. Cereb. Blood Flow. Metab.*, **11**, 735–44.

Lammertsma, A. A., Bench, C. J., Hume, S. P. et al. (1996). Comparison of methods for analysis of clinical [^{11}C]raclopride studies. *J. Cereb. Blood Flow. Metab.*, **16**, 42–52.

Laruelle, M., Wallace, E., Seibl, P. (1994). Graphical, kinetic, and equilibrium analyses of in vivo [^{123}I]β-CIT binding to dopamine transporters in healthy human subjects. *J. Cereb. Blood Flow. Metab.*, **14**, 982–94.

Laruelle, M., Abi-Dargham, A., van Dyck, C. H. et al. (1995). SPECT imaging of striatal dopamine release after amphetamine challenge. *J. Nucl. Med.*, **36**, 1182–90.

Laruelle, M., Abi-Dargham, A., van Dyck, C. H. et al. (1996). Single photon emission computerized tomography imaging of amphetamine-induced dopamine release in drug-free schizophrenic subjects. *Proc. Natl. Acad. Sci. USA*, **93**, 9235–40.

Logan, J., Fowler, J. S., Volkow, N. D. et al. (1990). Graphical analysis of reversible radioligand binding from time-activity measurements applied to [N-^{11}C-methyl]-(−)-cocaine PET studies in human subjects. *J. Cereb. Blood Flow. Metab.*, **10**, 740–7.

Logan, J., Dewey, S. L., Wolf, A. P. et al. (1991). Effects of endogenous dopamine on measures of [^{18}F]-methylspiroperidol binding in the basal ganglia: comparison of simulations and experimental results from PET studies in baboons. *Synapse*, **9**, 195–207.

Logan, J., Fowler, J. S., Volkow, N. D. et al. (1994). Effects of blood flow in [^{11}C]-raclopride binding in the brain: model simulations and kinetic analysis of PET data. *J. Cereb. Blood Flow. Metab.*, **14**, 995–1010.

Logan, J.,Fowler, J. S., Volkow, N. D., Wang, G. J., Ding, Y. S. and Alexoff, D. L. (1996). Distribution volume ratios without blood sampling from graphical analysis of PET data. *J. Cereb. Blood Flow. Metab.*, **16**, 834–40.

McDonald, W. M., Hussain, M., Doraiswamy, P. M., Figel, G., Boyko, O. and Krishnan, K. R. R. (1991). A magnetic resonance image study of age-related changes in human putamen nuclei. *Neuroreport*, **2**, 41–4.

Mintun, M. A., Raichle, M. E., Kilbourn, M. R., Wooten, G. F. and Welch, M. J. (1984). A quantitative model for the in vivo assessment of drug binding sites with positron emission tomography. *Ann. Neurol.*, **15**, 217–27.

Morris, E. D., Fisher, R. E., Alpert, N. M., Rauch, S. L. and Fischman, A. J. (1995). In vivo imaging of neuromodulation using positron emission tomography: optimal ligand characteristics and task length for detection of activation. *Hum. Brain Map.*, **3**, 35–55.

Morris, E. D., Babich, J. W., Alpert, N. M. et al. (1996a). Quantification of dopamine transporter density in monkeys by dynamic PET imaging of multiple injections of ^{11}C-CFT. *Synapse*, **24**, 262–72.

Morris, E. D., Alpert, N. M. and Fischman, A. J. (1996b). Comparison of two compartmental models for describing receptor ligand kinetics and receptor availability in multiple injection PET studies. *J. Cereb. Blood Flow. Metab.*, **16**, 841–53.

Morris, E. D., Chefer, S. I., Lane, M. A. et al. (1999). Decline of D_2 receptor binding with age, in rhesus monkeys: importance of correction for simultaneous decline in striatal size. *J. Cereb. Blood Flow. Metab.*, **19**, 218–29.

Muller-Gartner, H. W., Links, J. M., Prince, J. L. et al. (1992). Measurement of radiotracer concentration in brain gray matter using positron emission tomography: MRI-based correction for partial volume effects. *J. Cereb. Blood Flow. Metab.*, **12**, 571–83.

Muzic, R. F. Jr, Chen, C. H. and Nelson, A. D. (1998). Method to account for scatter, spillover and partial volume effects in region of interest analysis in PET. *IEEE Trans. Med. Imaging*, **17**, 202–13.

Rinne, J. O., Hietala, J. Ruotsalainen, U. et al. (1993). Decrease in human striatal dopamine D_2 receptor density with age: a PET study with [^{11}C]raclopride. *J. Cereb. Blood Flow Metab.*, **13**, 310–14.

Robbins, T. W. and Everitt, B. J. (1996). Neurobehavioural mechanisms of reward and motivation. *Curr. Opin. Neurobiol.* **6**, 228–36.

Rousset, O. G., Ma Y., Marenco, M., Wong, D. F. and Evans, A. C. (1996). In vivo correction method for partial volume effects in positron emission tomography. Accuracy and precision. In *Quantification of Brain Function using PET* ed. R. Myers, V. Cunningham, D. Bailey, T. Jones, pp. 158–165. San Diego, CA: Academic Press.

Rousset, O. G., Ma, Y. and Evans, A. C. (1998). Correction for partial volume effects in PET: principle and validation, *J. Nucl. Med.*, **39**, 904–11.

Schultz, W. (1997). Dopamine neurons and their role in reward mechanisms. *Curr. Opin. Neurobiol.*, **7**, 191–7.

Squire, L. (1987). *Memory and Brain*. New York: Oxford University Press.

Swanson, J. M., Sergeant, J. A., Taylor, E., Sonuga-Barke, E. J. S., Jensen, P. S. and Cantwell, D. P. (1998a). Attention-deficit hyperactivity disorder and hyperkinetic disorder. *Lancet*, **351**, 429–33.

Swanson, J. M., Castellanos, F. X., Murias, M., LaHoste, G. and Kennedy, J. (1998b). Cognitive neuroscience of attention deficit hyperactivity disorder and hyperkinetic disorder. *Curr. Opin. Neurobiol.*, **8**, 263–71.

Valk, P. E., Jagust, W. J., Derenzo, S. E., Huesman, R. H., Geyer, A. B. and Budinger, T. F. (1990). Clinical evaluation of a high-resolution (2.6-mm) positron emission tomography, *Radiology*, **176**, 783–90.

Volkow, N. D., Wang, G. J., Fowler, J. S. and Logan, J. (1997). Decreased striatal dopaminergic responsiveness in detoxified cocaine-dependent subjects. *Nature*, **386**, 830–3.

Wilson, C. J. (1998). Basal ganglia. In *The Synaptic Organization of the Brain*, ed. G. M. Shepherd, pp. 343–63. New York: Oxford University Press.

Wong, D. F., Young, D., Wilson, P. D., Meltzer, C. C. and Gjedde, A. (1997). Quantification of neuroreceptors in the living human brain. III, D_2-like dopamine receptors; theory, validation, and changes during normal aging. *J. Cereb. Blood Flow Metab.*, **17**, 316–30.

Zeeberg, B. R. (1995). Theoretical relationships of receptor and delivery sensitivities and measurable parameters in in vivo neuroreceptor-radioligand interactions. *IEEE Trans. Med. Imaging*, **14**, 608–15.

Zubieta, J.-K., Koeppe, R. A., Mulholland, G. K., Kuhl, D. E. and Frey, K. A. (1998). Quantification of muscarinic cholinergic receptors with [^{11}C]NMPB and positron emission tomography: method development and differentiation of tracer delivery from receptor binding. *J. Cereb. Blood Flow Metab.*, **18**, 619–31.

3

Functional magnetic resonance imaging

Guinevere F. Eden and Thomas A. Zeffiro

Introduction

Investigating the neural basis of cognitive development necessarily requires sensitive measures of brain activity that may be used to obtain repeated observations of subject populations over an extended period of time. MRI methods allow rapid and noninvasive determination of both brain structure and brain function, characteristics that are of particular importance in studies involving children. These imaging techniques employ a combination of static and modulated magnetic fields to obtain local estimates of chemical concentrations in different brain regions. Most commonly, both structural and functional images are derived from proton signals reflecting the local environment of water molecules in various tissue types. The variable environment in different tissue types results in corresponding intensity variations in reconstructed brain images, referred to as tissue contrast. In structural images, the variable tissue contrast provides a means to visualize the spatial distribution of gray matter, white matter, and cerebrospinal fluid throughout the brain. In functional imaging, additional small modulations of signal intensity occur because of changes in tissue blood flow and oxygenation.

Signal intensity changes can be recorded as a function of time and their relation to behavior examined with a variety of signal processing techniques that enhance the behavioral task-related signal change while suppressing undesirable physiologic noise arising from head motion, respiratory artifact, or global changes in cerebral blood flow. In the simplest case, signal intensity in a control condition is subtracted from signal intensity recorded during task performance in order to compute an estimate of task-related brain activity. This process is repeated over the entire brain to derive a "map" of task-related brain activity. In more complex circumstances, the resulting map may reflect the correlation of signal change with some aspect of task performance or behavioral state. The final fusion of these maps with high-resolution structural imaging provides neuroanatomic localization of brain function in a structural context, allowing comparisons of functional neuroanatomy among different individuals or subject groups.

Physiologic basis of fMRI

Most functional MRI (fMRI) studies utilize techniques based on the BOLD-contrast (blood oxygenation level-dependent contrast) effect (Belliveau et al., 1991; Kwong et al. 1992; Ogawa et al., 1992; Turner et al. 1993). This technique utilizes rapid imaging, usually echo planar, of the brain to record the hemodynamic consequences of neuronal activity. Neuronal activity is thought to be associated with concomitant changes in blood flow and oxygenation that result in local changes in the relative proportions of oxyhemoglobin and deoxyhemoglobin, molecules that have differing magnetic susceptibilities. Thus, task-related changes in neuronal activity trigger a series of events that finally result in local changes in magnetic susceptibility that may be captured with rapid MRI techniques. Of note is the fact that these hemodynamic changes are delayed and dispersed in time relative to their neuronal antecedents, properties that limit the temporal resolution of this technique but which may be exploited advantageously in some experimental designs. The goal of analysis of functional MRI (fMRI) time series is to extract the best estimate of neuronal activity from the recorded hemodynamic signal. As discussed below, this process is made difficult by a host of instrumental and physiologic artifacts encountered in fMRI data acquisition and analysis (Cohen, 1996; Turner and Jezzard, 1993). For references concerning the physiologic basis of the BOLD contrast effect see Cohen (1996) and Turner and Jezzard (1993).

Safety considerations

All human structural and functional neuroimaging techniques carry some risk for the individual being studied. Although the hazards associated with fMRI examinations in children and adults are extremely low, it is worthwhile briefly to consider the areas of possible danger to the subject.

The first source of possible hazard is the system's static magnetic field. While there is no evidence of adverse effects from exposure to lower field strengths, whole-body exposure at 5 tesla (T) can affect blood flow through the circulatory system (Tenforde and Budinger, 1985). After being exposed to the even higher field strength of 10 T, some subjects reported discomfort (Beischer, 1962). At the field strengths utilized for most functional neuroimaging studies (1.5–4 T), there have been no reports of significant physiologic effects, with the exception of a sensation of mild dizziness reported by subjects executing rapid head movements in the higher 4 T fields.

Other hazards presented by the static magnetic field involve potentially adverse affects on implanted metallic objects or devices. Cardiac pacemakers become inoperative at field strengths of 0.5 mT or above. Therefore, any patient with implanted cardiac or neural stimulation devices should not be scanned. All persons should be screened prior to entering the magnet room. The first step is to take a careful history, inquiring about the possible presence of cardiac pacemakers, neural stimulators, aneurysm clips, cochlear implants, hip prostheses, hair implants, shrapnel, or a history of metalworking. The interview should be followed by an examination with a magnetometer to confirm the absence of ferromagnetic material on or in the subject. As the static magnetic field may attract metallic objects from a distance, care should also be taken to keep all ferromagnetic materials outside the magnet room. Metallic objects can easily become dangerous projectiles near most commercial MR systems.

The second source of possible biohazard are the cryogens used to maintain the static magnetic field. The liquid nitrogen and helium employed in superconducting magnets are very cold and can cause immediate tissue damage following contact. Under extremely unlikely circumstances, during a "quench", it is possible for the system's cryogen to change state and become gaseous, posing a threat of asphyxiation. Commercial MR systems all have an emergency ventilation system to handle this exigency.

A third source of potential hazard to subjects are the system's gradients, which generate distortions in the static magnetic field allowing spatial localization of the MR signal changes. Echo-planar imaging sequences are accompanied by high-amplitude gradient ringing, characterized by high sound energy in a narrow frequency band. Although there have been no reports of auditory system damage in subjects participating in fMRI experiments, it would seem reasonable to err on the side of caution and equip subjects with attenuating earplugs. Under some circumstances, gradients may also induce electrical currents in the body. During echo-planar imaging experiments, this phenomenon may lead to peripheral nerve stimulation, particularly involving the trigeminal or facial nerves. Limiting the maximal rate and amplitude of gradient field changes can avoid these effects.

The last source of potential hazard stems from radiofrequency energy deposition in the body. Limiting the amount of radiofrequency energy deposition can prevent elevations of body temperature to levels that cause damage to local tissues or systemic physiologic effects (International Non-Ionizing Radiation Committee, 1991). The measure of radiofrequency power used in human imaging systems is called the specific absorption rate (SAR). Safe levels for SAR for infants, adults, and individuals with compromised thermoregulatory systems can be obtained from the MR system manufacturer.

In general, structural and functional brain imaging using commercial MR imaging systems has an excellent safety record. With proper attention to the above cited considerations, investigators should feel comfortable that functional neuroimaging in children and adults poses no significant biohazard.

Pediatric studies using fMRI

Although fMRI has been employed in over 700 studies of the adult brain published to date, its utilization in studying children and human development is only just beginning. Functional MRI was first used in a pediatric study to monitor focal seizures in a 4-year-old boy (Jackson et al., 1994). Here fMRI was used to identify those areas showing activity during clinical seizures. More recently, fMRI has been employed clinically to study language function in children. Hertz-Pannier and colleagues used fMRI to map language dominance in children between ages 8.8 and 18 years with partial epilepsy (Hertz-Pannier et al., 1994, 1997). A word generation task was used to activate the frontal lobes, and the magnitude of signal change was used to calculate language asymmetry indices. The results were in agreement with intra-carotid amobarbital (amobarbitone) testing performed in these children for presurgical evaluation. The data showed clear activation of the left frontal areas of the brain during overt or covert production of words in response to the presentation of letters or words. A further report showed that both a word fluency task and single word reading successfully resulted in task-related signal changes in a 9-year-old boy (Benson et al., 1996). However, more complex tasks, such as generating the opposite meaning of a word or generating the verb form of a noun, were unsuccessful in generating signal changes, thus underscoring the quintessential importance of task selection.

From these early studies, it appeared that children could tolerate the MRI environment for clinical purposes. Whether the same procedures that are applied in cognitive studies of adults can be utilized to study children outside of the clinical setting is of both practical and empirical importance. Casey and colleagues have addressed this issue by studying the same tasks in children and adults (Casey et al., 1997b). One major difficulty in comparing children and adults arises from differences in task performance across the two age groups. A similar problem can also occur in clinical studies when controls may be compared with a group of patients whose task performance is unmatched. Steps can be taken to account for these behavioral differences by controlling for them in the analysis procedures. When differences in task performance are taken into account, neuroimaging studies have shown similar patterns of cortical activity in adults and children during equivalent tasks.

From a developmental point of view, one might expect similar cortical localization for a given task in children and adults. However, should differences be observed between age groups, there is an open question regarding how to best quantify these differences in order to reveal developmental changes. For example, differences might be quantified in terms of spatial extent or amplitude of task-related signal change. Many pediatric studies have focused on frontal areas of the brain (inferior frontal and medial frontal gyri), albeit with different aims and different behavioral tasks. Word generation, working memory, and attention (e.g., continuous performance) tasks have been utilized to activate frontal areas in the brains of children. A study investigating working memory has identified developmental changes measured by greater MR signal (per cent signal change) in children with increasing age (from 9 years and 7 months to 11 years and 7 months) (Casey et al., 1995). As discussed in Chapter 9, the adult data for this same task show a much lower signal compared with that of the pediatric group. This suggests that the age-related

signal increase during development in childhood must be followed by a decrease, producing the lesser signal change associated with this task in adulthood. This initial finding is intriguing because it suggests complex developmental patterns. However, to resolve these changes, a large number of children across a wider age range will need to be studied. Furthermore, other aspects of the data will need to be considered: quantitative measures of developmental changes could involve the number of voxels or the extent of activation. Interestingly, measures of magnitude of activation in frontal cortex have shown that children display a greater volume of activation compared with adults during an attention task (Casey et al., 1997b). It is clear that expansion of these studies to include larger numbers of children will yield important information on the relationship between behavioral performance and physiologic signal changes in the developing brain compared with that of the mature adult brain. This knowledge will provide an understanding of normal development of cognition and sensorimotor processing and the necessary base with which to tackle many serious clinical problems.

Indeed, one of the most important applications of pediatric fMRI studies lies in clinical studies. For example, epilepsy constitutes one of the most common brain disorders (1–2% of the general population). Noninvasive application of fMRI in presurgical planning has already provided a powerful tool for the advancement of preoperative evaluation for epilepsy surgery (Jackson, 1994). It also promises to be of great importance in unraveling the mechanisms of developmental disorders such as dyslexia, as well as other prevalent disorders such as attention-deficit hyperactivity disorder (ADHD). One preliminary report of children with developmental dyslexia undergoing fMRI studies has demonstrated significantly less activation in inferior parietal areas and the inferior frontal gyrus of children with dyslexia compared with those without reading problems (Frost et al., 1997). These findings are in agreement with functional neuroimaging data in adults (Rumsey et al., 1992, 1997b; Shaywitz et al., 1998). Single-subject analysis of such data in larger numbers will eventually contribute substantial information to the understanding of this heterogeneous and complex learning disorder.

Data acquisition

Clearly a number of limitations imposed by the MR environment need to be taken into consideration when conducting functional neuroimaging with MRI. Any equipment utilized for stimulus presentation or recording of the subject's response must be nonferrous. Since the advent of fMRI there have been many advances in equipment design to address this obstacle, and, therefore, this issue will not be discussed in great detail here. However, as a pragmatic aid, an appendix at the end of this chapter lists manufacturers of commercial products that have been optimized for the MRI environment and are commonly used in fMRI experiments. It contains a list of devices used for visual and aural stimulus presentation and response collection and is intended as a guide for those who wish to set up an fMRI experiment.

Practical issues when scanning children

In addition to the already rigorous limitations of the MR environment, further hurdles need to be overcome to ensure that tasks can be presented and responses elicited from young subjects in an uncontrived manner. Making compromises to the ideal experimental situation is an all too familiar situation with fMRI, which often does not allow faithful replication of the "ideal" behavioral or psychophysical situation employed outside of the magnet. With children, tasks that may be suitable for adults may be problematic. Children of younger ages do not have the cognitive and motor skills of adults, and the complexity of their motor responses are more limited. The number and position of buttons available during button-press responses to stimuli should, therefore, be limited; in fact, a maximum of two possible buttons used for response is recommended. Furthermore, while lying down in the scanner, the subject is unable to see his or her hands. This lack of visual guidance during button-press responses adds a further degree of difficulty to the task. The experimenter also cannot expect the child to report accurately whether the stimulus is maximally perceptable, or to give input regarding the necessity of adjustments such as focusing a visual display or increasing the volume of an auditory stimulus. Finally, a child's comfort must be taken into account to a greater degree than required for adult subjects when choosing the mode of stimulus presentation. For instance, a rear-projection screen viewed through a mirror is often used for visual stimulus presentation. It is also possible to project stimuli directly into certain types of goggles. However, we believe that the screen holds a greater advantage than the goggles because it avoids close proximity and hence possible discomfort to the face. Goggles might also require the child to maintain fusion. By maximizing the child's comfort and minimizing apprehension, one hopes to minimize head motion-related artifacts stemming from the child's anxiety-related head movement.

Subject exclusion

It is very common in the USA, and increasingly in other countries, for children and adolescents between the ages of 8 and 18 to be wearing braces on their teeth. While physicians often obtain structural scans of people who wear braces for clinical purposes, the oral cavity causes substantial inhomogeneity effects, resulting in large distortions to the facial area. For fMRI, these artifacts are extensive in the inferior portions of the brain and may result in unusable data. Consequently, children with braces are excluded from fMRI studies. As in adult studies, children with other forms of ferrous material in their body need to be excluded from study participation.

Subject preparation

The probability that a child can successfully complete a scanning protocol with little or no head movement and discomfort can be greatly increased by carefully preparing the individual. Just as in the adult population, if a child is put at ease and has a good understanding of what to expect when placed in the magnet, fewer complications will arise from anxiety, confusion, or discomfort. Having the child first perform the task outside of the magnet will ensure that the child is fairly automated on the task. It is also useful to teach the child what else should be expected during the scan. Listening to a recording of the scanner noise eliminates some of the surprise and anxiety associated with the gradient noise. It is beneficial to have younger children lie in a mock scanner environment prior to the real scan. Some sites have even utilized a magnet for the sole purpose of subject training (Slifer et al., 1993). At some sites, it is feasible to have children visit the scanner before the experiment so that the child can become acclimated. In general, we have found it useful to have children come in for two separate visits. On day one, the child becomes familiarized with the investigators during screening procedures. They are engaged in projects related to the brain (such as coloring pictures of the brain) and they undergo a short anatomic scan at the end of their visit. The child leaves with his first MRI exposure and a picture of his own brain. On day two, the investigator will have acquired relevant behavioral screening data and an anatomic scan used for coregistration with the functional data acquired during the child's visit. Some investigators choose to perform a short functional run during the first visit to be used only for practice purposes and then discarded.

Pediatric protocols often have the option of parental presence in the MR room. While this has the benefit of comforting the child, it increases the likelihood that the child will move his head in order to see the parent, thereby disrupting the imaging protocol. Often it is more useful to assess the situation rather than to follow a strict rule in this regard.

Monitoring of subject responses in the MR environment

The majority of published fMRI studies have employed motivated adults, often investigators, in whom reliable task performance can be obtained throughout the duration of a scan. For children entering this environment, it is important to monitor their behavior during the task in order to ensure task compliance and comfort levels. Pressing a button in response to a stimulus is one useful way of monitoring task performance. This can be practiced before a scan.

As described above, there has been particular interest in language studies using fMRI. In pediatric studies, the commitment of different cortical areas to language and how they change during language acquisition is of great interest. Word pronunciation is often avoided or minimized out of concern that it introduces head motion. Further, there are susceptibility artifacts associated with changes in the size of the oral cavity that occur during articulation. Being located relatively close to the base of the brain, movement of this space can cause artifacts around the base of the temporal lobes. However, particularly in children, there are concerns that failure to respond overtly can lead to noncompliance. There is additional concern about studies that do not allow for pronunciation when studying language, because the signal changes can be modulated by response type. That is, responding overtly or covertly dramatically changes the resulting activation patterns (Bookheimer et al., 1995; Rumsey et al., 1997a). One way to circumvent this problem is to have subjects voice the response very carefully by whispering, or to use acquisition techniques that to some degree minimize this problem (see below).

Minimization of head motion

The scarceness of pediatric fMRI reports in the literature is undoubtedly a consequence, in part, of difficulty of obtaining data free of motion artifact from children. Also, there are concerns with respect to subjecting children to this noisy and confined environment. Studies performed to date report data exclusion or repeated scanning of children because of head motion in 10% (Casey et al., 1997b) to 37% of the children scanned (Hertz-Pannier et al., 1997). One study of children and adults performing the same tasks reported that head motion in children was no greater than that of the adults (Casey et al., 1997b). As might be expected, most investigators' experience has shown that the longer the duration of the scan, the more likely it is that the subject will move their head more frequently and to a larger extent. In studies performed to date, the duration of scans in children lasted about 1 h and were, therefore, not very different to the time engaged during adult protocols.

In general, it is clear that head motion is likely to be one of the greatest obstacles to successful application of fMRI in children; this may be a more serious issue in children with certain clinical conditions. Training children to lie as still as possible in preparation for the scan minimizes interscan head motion. For young children (younger than 10 years), it is beneficial to have them practice lying still in a mock scanner. In this approach, individuals are placed in a device that resembles a magnet or in an old decommissioned magnet. The child can become familiarized to the confined environment of the magnet and practice lying still. This can be achieved either by observing the child or by actually measuring his or her head movement using, for example, a light-emitting diode device. The experimenter should go through a checklist with the child, instructing the child on what will happen through the course of the experiment. Older children might then switch roles with the investigator and "teach" the experimenter how to behave.

Acoustic interference

The gradient noise during fMRI data acquisition causes a measurable signal increase in the auditory cortex. During fMRI experiments, stimulation of the auditory cortex may result from the constant noise (usually around 90 dB) generated by the gradients. While this potent auditory stimulant may result in neuronal activity in the auditory system, it may also cause a reduction of activity in other sensory areas. There is some evidence that modality-specific sensory stimulation causing activation in one sensory cortical area can induce decreases elsewhere. Significant decreases in regional cerebral blood flow have been detected with positron emission tomography (PET) in auditory areas during a visual task (Haxby et al., 1994). In this case, the striking reduction observed in the primary and secondary auditory cortex could result from selective attentional processes, reducing the response to unattended auditory stimuli while enhancing the response in visual areas. It has been demonstrated that these cortical decreases in blood flow are associated with nonselective attention during the performance of a visual task (Shulman et al., 1997). Close examination revealed that this modulation is inconsistently localized across cortical areas and is unpredictable across studies, with the nature of the modulations in the auditory cortex being dependent on the nature of the task. For example, left hemisphere decreases were seen with nonlanguage tasks and right hemisphere reductions were observed during linguistic tasks. While certain areas (auditory cortex, insula, and parietal operculum) appear to show response decreases, it is not currently understood what governs these decreases and why they are not occurring systematically. These findings suggest that the auditory stimulation induced by fMRI is likely to promote modulations in areas not generally thought to be modulated by auditory stimuli. (Fiez et al., 1995; Shulman et al., 1997).

More direct evidence has been obtained from fMRI studies, indicating that the effect of the MRI acoustics is complex. During visual and motor tasks, subjects were exposed to stimuli in noise reduced and noisy conditions (Cho et al., 1998). The resulting task-related BOLD signals differed significantly. During motor activity, the acoustic noise enhanced the motor signal, but during visual stimulation the signal from visual cortex was reduced. These findings emphasize the earlier cautions expressed in the PET literature. In fMRI, the gradient noise can potentially induce such decreases in areas outside of auditory cortex, contaminating estimation of task-related changes in those areas. Such signal modulation has recently been demonstrated to be nonspecific with respect to task and spatial location (Cho et al., 1998).

Investigation into this complex relationship observed in adults has not been extended to pediatric studies. It is not known whether the influence of acoustic stimulation on the brain is the same in children as in adults, regardless of whether it has an attentional or physiologic explanation. Studies involving language or sound processing are especially likely to be polluted by the external noise, and few studies have successfully been able to eliminate the noise by insulation or other approaches. In traditional data acquisition procedures, the gradient noise occurs equally in the control and task conditions. Assuming that the signal change resulting from this gradient noise is linearly additive with task-related signal change, it should be possible to subtract the noise effects. Therefore, data-analysis techniques reliant upon image subtraction, such as the t-test, will be insensitive to this source of noise. Although it is reasonable to assume that linear additivity for gradient noise might hold for many cortical regions, it is less likely that this assumption is reasonable for cortical areas known to be responsive to auditory stimuli.

One way to circumvent the exposure to the gradient noise caused by the magnet is to interleave data acquisi-

tion periods with task performance. This behavior interleaved gradient (BIG) technique takes advantage of physiologic hemodynamic delay and dispersion in order to collect image data under relatively quiet conditions. In our studies, we employ an approach in which the gradients are off during periods of task execution and then immediately switched on to acquire data. Detection of the task-related signal change relies on the presence of a hemodynamic lag of 5–8 s between neuronal activity and the resulting BOLD contrast response. We recently validated this technique using an externally paced finger movement task known to induce large signal changes in motor areas (Eden et al., 1999). Six subjects performed an index finger tapping task with the dominant hand at a rate of 2 Hz paced by a large flashing green star. Finger tapping alternated with periods of rest, during which the subject viewed a red star, flashing at the same rate. Multislice echo-planar image (EPI) acquisition was used (time to echo (TE) 43 ms; time to repetition (TR) 12 s; matrix 64×64; field of view (FOV) 256 mm; 40 axial slices; thickness 4 mm; cubic voxels 4 mm; 50 time points per run). Two runs were performed in each of the following four acquisition modes.

1 Acquired after task, BIG. Data were acquired after the task and involved 8 s of tapping during which no data were acquired, followed by a 4 s interval during which one whole-head volume was acquired.
2 Acquired during task (control). Rest and task were alternated as in the previous condition but the acquisition began during the second half of the task period, thereby providing a control for the assumed hemodynamic lag.
3 Acquired concurrently 1. This employed the traditional block design of continuous task periods alternating with rest periods.
4 Acquired concurrently 2. The same procedure was used as in (3) but it was controlled for differences in the number of movements produced over the total scans by changing the tapping rate.

Fifty time points were collected for each condition. Using MEDx (Sensor Systems, Sterling VA), the image data were corrected for head motion and for global and local intensity variations. Task and rest periods were compared using the t-statistic that was then transformed to a Z-score. The Z-map was then searched for local maxima.

The resulting statistical maps revealed task-related changes in primary motor cortex, primary somatosensory cortex, premotor cortex, the supplementary motor area, the cingulate motor area, thalamus, and anterior cerebellum. Comparisons of the Z-maps generated from the movement minus rest condition for the four acquisition modes listed above revealed that activations in primary motor cortex were similar or higher when data acquisition occurred

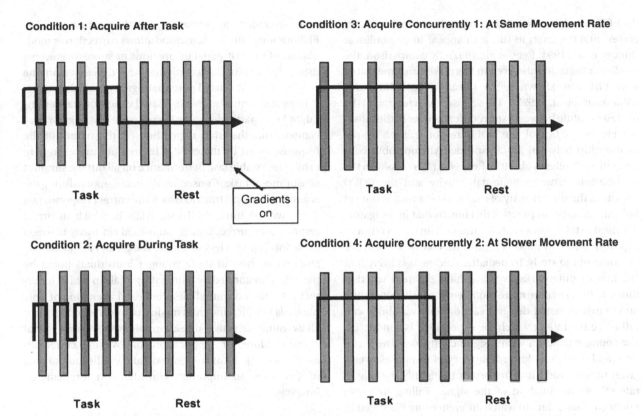

Condition 1: Acquire After Task

Task   Rest

Gradients
on

Condition 2: Acquire During Task

Task   Rest

Condition 3: Acquire Concurrently 1: At Same Movement Rate

Task   Rest

Condition 4: Acquire Concurrently 2: At Slower Movement Rate

Task   Rest

Fig. 3.1. Task description of an experiment assessing the validity of the behavior interleaved gradient (BIG) technique. BIG takes advantage of physiologic hemodynamic delay and dispersion in order to collect image data under relatively quiet conditions (Eden et al. 1999).

following task completion, as is the case for BIG. Figure 3.1 summarizes the experimental procedures for BIG.

Interleaving task performance and data acquisition allows task performance under relatively quiet experimental conditions (Eden et al., 1999; Edmister et al., 1999). Task performance periods of 8s were sufficiently long to yield excellent statistical results. This technique is useful when the experiment requires maximal acoustic isolation of the subject. It is also advantageous when speech is required, as articulation, with its attendant motion artifacts, will not occur during periods of data acquisition.

Rate-related effects

There is now a significant body of literature from the field of PET and MRI describing the effects of stimulus presentation rate or stimulus duration on regional cerebral blood flow (Fox and Raichle, 1984; Price et al., 1994, 1996) or fMRI signal (van Meter et al., 1995; Binder et al., 1997; Dhankhar et al., 1997; Rees, et al., 1997). Rate-related changes have been studied with both types of imaging, but the observations reported vary with the nature of the experiment. The effect

of exposure duration has been systematically studied with PET during oral reading (Price et al., 1994) and listening to words (Price et al., 1992). This latter experiment revealed a linear relationship between the rate of aurally presented words and regional cerebral blood flow bilaterally in portions of the superior temporal gyrus, including primary auditory cortex, and right posterior superior temporal gyrus. However, posterior portions of the left superior temporal gyrus (Wernicke's area) failed to show this linear rate dependence. In a comparison of reading aloud versus lexical decision (Price et al., 1994) bilateral posterior temporal and inferior parietal areas, or Brodmann's area (BA) 39, as well as cingulate gyrus and left hippocampus were significantly more active during reading aloud compared with silent reading (lexical decision). However, this was only the case when words were presented for durations of 150 ms. These differences disappeared when stimuli were presented at a longer duration (1000 ms). Together these findings suggest that responses in these superior temporal and inferior parietal areas are modulated by presentation rates.

Functional MRI studies investigating stimulus response rate have not entirely agreed with the PET studies. While the PET data show a linear dependency on rate in auditory cortex, BOLD signals in this area appear to be nonlinear (Binder et al., 1994; Rees et al., 1997). By comparison, the nonlinear behavior observed in Wernicke's area measured with PET was shown to be linear in an fMRI study (Dhankhar et al., 1997). These discrepancies might be related to subtle between-study differences or to the inherent characteristics of the BOLD response, such as the relationship between BOLD and deoxyhemoglobin concentration (Binder et al., 1994; Rees et al., 1997). As with the relationship between neuronal activity and the BOLD response, the nonlinearity of the BOLD contrast is not yet fully understood. In practice this means that investigators will need to take greater care in situations in which rate and exposure duration make a significant contribution to the outcome of the study. In pediatric studies, it is likely that children of different ages will exhibit different reaction times, as they become more proficient at a task. Depending on the experimental design, reaction time variability can influence the rate at which the experiment is conducted. For younger children with a significantly lower response rate (and, therefore, lower frequency of responses over a given time period), it is important to identify the role of rate-related modulation of the signal. Failing to do so might confound data in which differences are identified in two age groups but obscured by rate effects. One possible solution to this problem is to map the regions that show parametric rate modulation in a group of controls in a separate study. Having determined which brain areas exhibit rate modulation for a given task, it will be possible to interpret more carefully any between-group differences seen in the context of between-group rate differences. If a particular region can be shown to not exhibit rate modulation over the range of rates used in the experiment, then it would be less likely that the performance rate differences between groups accounted for the differing patterns of task-related activation.

Event-related fMRI

Recently, a new experimental approach has been introduced that analyzes the hemodynamic response to single events, cognitive, perceptual or motor. This approach is referred to as event-related or single-trial fMRI (Buckner et al., 1996; Friston et al., 1998). It takes advantage of the fact that averaging of the hemodynamic response to brief events may be used to identify regional changes in task-related brain activity. Among the advantages of event-related techniques is the ability to avoid subject expectancy by randomizing the order of different trial types. During analysis, the trials are sorted by type and

then averaged to enhance signal contrast-to-noise. Elaboration of this basic method allows correction or modulation of the MR signal by previous or successive events using deconvolution techniques first developed in the context of event-related potential signal processing.

In pediatric studies, event-related experimental designs might be of particular value because the investigator may want to sort the trials depending on the nature of the response given by the child. Children are more likely to exhibit less stable task performance on all but the simplest sensorimotor tasks. Consequently, in any epoch during the scanning sessions, trials in which the correct response was made will be intermixed with trials in which incorrect responses occurred, making statistical contrasts between behavioral epochs less sensitive. The greater response variability observed in these younger individuals might be partially ameliorated by eliminating trials in which incorrect responses occurred. Selection and averaging of only the trials in which the child made a correct response might allow more sensitive detection of event-related signal change. Moreover, application of overlap correction methods using deconvolution will allow collection of data in less time, an important consideration for pediatric imaging.

Data analysis

The analysis of functional neuroimaging data may be described as a series of processes beginning with image reconstruction and ending with visualization of fused structure/function for individual subjects and groups of subjects. The outcome of the statistical analysis is greatly determined by the acquisition parameters and experimental procedures described above. In addition, because of the time required to acquire each slice using EPI, there is a trade-off between spatial resolution, temporal resolution, and brain coverage. Therefore, using thinner slices requires a larger number of slice acquisitions to cover the same brain volume. Because the time to acquire each slice is fixed, more time is required for increased spatial resolution orthogonal to the slice orientation. These spatiotemporal constraints on data acquisition have important consequences pertaining to the success of the data analysis phase of experiments.

In the previously described pediatric neuroimaging studies (Hertz-Pannier et al., 1994; Jackson et al., 1994; Casey et al., 1995, 1997a; Benson et al., 1996), all investigators focused their attention on the frontal areas of the brain and, for this reason, restricted data acquisition to the frontal lobes. This was presumably done to achieve shorter data acquisition times, a decided advantage in pediatric studies. A particular disadvantage of this approach is that a partial brain volume makes adequate head motion correction difficult, as the realignment algorithms benefit from the presence of data covering a larger three-dimensional volume.

Image artifacts

Image artifacts can result from both instrumental and physiologic sources. Some of these artifacts can be corrected with improved reconstruction techniques and others require image processing of the reconstructed images. Geometric image distortion is a particularly troublesome artifact, as its degree may adversely affect subsequent stages of data processing. Specifically, low spatial distortion is required for optimal performance of rigid-body head motion correction algorithms. The spatial accuracy of EPI data is strongly influenced by the accuracy of the shimming procedure employed prior to data acquisition. Although most 1.5 T MR imaging systems have adequate facilities for automated shimming, the more profound susceptibility artifacts occurring at higher static field strengths are more difficult to correct using automated procedures.

Rigid-body and parenchymal motion

Despite taking the time to prepare children as described above, it is not possible to completely immobilize subjects during functional imaging procedures. Systems that are best at reducing interscan motion (e.g., bite-bars) are not suitable for use in many pediatric populations. The head motion between scans is the principal source of error variance in fMRI time series. This motion may arise from either translation/rotation of the head or brain parenchymal motion resulting from cardiac or respiratory pulsations.

Translational or rotational motion of the head results in misregistration of sequentially collected brain volumes, resulting in signal intensity changes related to changing partial volume effects. Although the motion is global, the effects of the motion are regionally specific, being most prominent in regions of variable tissue contrast. Examples include boundaries between gray matter and cerebrospinal fluid. This may result in an easily appreciated "rim" artifact around the edge of the brain in statistical maps generated from time series with excessive interscan motion. If peak-to-peak rigid-body motion exceeds 10–30% of the image voxel width, statistical maps are likely to exhibit statistical artifacts. Therefore, assuming constant head motion, statistical map artifact will increase with increasing spatial resolution and decreased voxel width. Linear realignment techniques are effective in correcting this source artifact in statistical images.

Even in the absence of rigid-body head motion, regionally varying parenchymal motion of the brain can produce significant artifacts in statistical parametric maps. This parenchymal motion results from an interaction between the viscoelastic properties of the brain tissue and local pressure changes induced by arterial and venous pressure modulations of cardiac and respiratory origin (Poncelet et al., 1992). This motion is most pronounced in the midline structures and reduces the sensitivity to task-related changes in these areas. Because it varies throughout the brain, parenchymal motion cannot be adequately modeled by rigid-body transformations. An additional complication arises because this motion results in MR signal changes at frequencies above the sampling rates customarily employed in EPI functional imaging, usually one sample each 2 to 5 s. The average heart rate is one per second and therefore it will not be properly sampled. This physiologic aliased noise can be reduced by designing digital filters that attenuate the MR signal at the appropriate frequencies (Biswal et al., 1996). Another promising approach to this problem is to utilize cardiac gating. In this method, MR signal acquisition is synchronized with the cardiac impulse, assuring that each time point is collected in the same phase of the cardiac cycle. This technique has made possible the detection of auditory task-related changes in subcortical structures (Guimaraes et al., 1998).

Motion detection and correction

Prior to attempting any realignment, it is important to assess the magnitude of interscan head motion. This may be accomplished by viewing an animation of the time series, by computing the translational motion of the center-of-intensity of the volumes comprising the time series, or by computing a voxel-wise variance map. Examination of an animated slice from a time-series is an excellent method with which to obtain a rapid qualitative estimate of interscan head motion. Computing the motion of the image volume center-of-intensity is more computationally demanding but results in quantitative estimates of motion. The translational moments in each dimension (x, y, or z) may be further processed to obtain scalar estimates of motion for the entire time series, including mean-square error or three-dimensional path length. Regionally specific motion artifacts may be detected by computing the signal variance across the temporal dimension for each voxel in the image volume. In the resulting map, areas of high variance near tissue boundaries, e.g., the brain surface/cerebrospinal fluid boundary, may identify interscan motion. Translational motion that has a peak-to-peak amplitude of less than 10% of the image voxel width will not usually contribute substantially to variance in the resulting statistical images. Using these methods, it is possible to obtain good estimates of interscan motion to determine the success of subject restraint procedures. They also may be employed before and after corrective procedures are applied to determine their efficacy.

Having determined that sufficient head motion is present to warrant correction, it is possible to employ an automated realignment procedure to determine the coordinate transformation that will bring the members of the time series back into register (Woods et al., 1998a, b). This is usually the most time consuming and computationally intensive part of the entire analysis procedure. For fMRI datasets, a linear realignment algorithm, allowing variation in the translation and rotational degrees of freedom, is usually employed. Having determined the appropriate coordinate transformation to reregister the volumes, a resampling algorithm is employed to generate the realigned image volume. For this procedure, there is a tradeoff between time and accuracy, with the most accurate resampling procedures (sinc interpolation) being significantly slower than the less accurate procedures (nearest neighbor or trilinear interpolation). Most laboratories utilize trilinear interpolation for this step as it provides a reasonable compromise between execution speed and resampling accuracy. An example of the efficacy of head motion correction in children and adults is shown in Fig. 3.2 (p. 82).

Global and local signal variation

There are multiple sources of spatially invariant, global signal intensity changes with time. These variations may be slow, as occurs with instrumental drift, or of mixed frequency, as may occur with physiologically based fluctuations. For example, respiratory activity may have a mechanical effect on the observed MR signal, with intrathoracic pressure modulations causing venous sinus pulsations; it may also have an indirect physiologic effect on the signal by causing changes in the blood partial pressure of carbon dioxide that result in global cerebral blood flow changes. These changes in global cerebral blood flow will be accompanied by changes in the BOLD-contrast signal and will, therefore, confound attempts to measure task-related changes in the BOLD-contrast signal. Whatever their source, global changes in signal intensity may be corrected using the technique of ratio normalization (Friston

et al., 1994), in which the mean value of each volume of the time series is adjusted to a specified mean value. This approach assumes that, as in PET cerebral blood flow images, there is a linear relationship between local and global signal intensity in EPI.

Even after global signal variations are corrected, it is not uncommon to observe regionally specific modulations of the MR signal with time, particularly in areas close to the brain surface. Many of these artifacts result from uncompensated head motion; that is, motion with effects that are not removed by rigid-body transformations. These effects usually occur at frequencies below those of the task of interest and may be removed with linear detrending or high-pass digital filtering. In this instance it is assumed that signal fluctuations occurring at low frequencies are not related to task-related signal changes and may be safely removed.

Statistical map generation

After processing the time series to remove instrumental and physiologic sources of error variance, parametric statistical techniques are employed to detect regionally specific task-related signal changes. These techniques include simple categorical contrasts (t-test), correlation, linear regression, analysis of variance, and many others. A thorough review of these methods is beyond the scope of this chapter and the reader is referred to a number of more detailed reviews of this topic (Bandettini et al., 1992; Bandettini, 1993; Friston et al., 1994, 1998).

Structure–function correlation

One approach for determining the neuroanatomic localization of task-related signal changes in individual subjects involves the coregistration of statistical maps with corresponding high-resolution structural images using intermodality linear spatial registration techniques (Woods et al., 1998a, b). This approach allows direct visualization of the loci of signal change in a neuroanatomic framework and permits labeling of responses according to sulcal or gyral landmarks.

An alternative approach involves transforming the statistical maps into a generalized coordinate system, usually an anatomic atlas (Talairach and Tourneaux, 1988), allowing standardized reporting across experiments and laboratories. An advantage of mapping all scans to a common coordinate system is that it allows intersubject averaging of responses for pixelwise statistical testing (Zeffiro et al., 1997). However, this coordinate system is based on an adult brain, and pediatric counterparts have not been implemented to date. Given the changes in size of cortical and subcortical structures throughout development (Giedd et al., 1996), analogous pediatric templates for the developmental stages will be useful for making accurate standardized maps.

Data interpretation

Statistical maps can be characterized in different ways and currently there is no concensus on which analysis offers the best measure of task-related signal change. Various groups have used the mean Z-score in a cluster of activated voxels, the spatial extent of a cluster, the peak Z-score within a cluster, or the corresponding percentage signal change at this local maximum.

In the pediatric studies described above, it has been reported that frontal activation during a working memory task is very similar between children and adults (Casey et al., 1997a). However, the results show that the percentage increase in MR signal increases with increasing age and yet the activation in children appears to be more diffuse than that in adults (also reported by Hertz-Pannier et al. (1997)). While these response measures may be highly correlated in some circumstances, in others they are not (Eden et al., 1999). Further investigations into the relationships of these measures are needed.

Example of a pediatric language study

Children with developmental dyslexia have difficulties with phonologic processing. The term "phonologic awareness" refers to skills of manipulation and segmentation of the constituent sound of words. For example, rhyme judgement (such as "Hat, cat, dog, mat – which is the odd one out?") can measure phonologic awareness and predict reading outcome (Bradley and Bryant, 1983).

The neuronal mechanisms that subserve phonologic segmentation which are impaired in dyslexia are currently under active investigation (Rumsey et al., 1992; Rumsey and Eden, 1997; Shaywitz et al., 1998). With advances in neuroimaging technology, it is now possible to study an individual subject's performance during a wider variety of tasks than was previously possible because of radiation dosimetry limits. As a result, an effort has begun in our laboratory to study individuals with normal cognitive development to understand the functional organization of the brain for language. These efforts will allow a deeper understanding of the effects of developmental dyslexia on a range of sensory and phonologically related skills. An example of such a study is as follows. We utilized the BIG technique (see above) to investigate phonologic awareness

skills in adults and children with and without dyslexia. The task utilized phoneme elision, which requires an awareness of the sound structure of language in order to be able to delete the first sound of a word. In this study, subjects viewed a series of words and were instructed to either read the word aloud (baseline) or to say the word after omitting the first sound (phonologic manipulation). The sound elision condition was then compared with the word reading condition as well as with a visual fixation condition. As illustrated in Fig. 3.2 (p. 82), fMRI data in individuals typically revealed involvement of temporoparietal areas, the inferior frontal gyri, and cerebellum. This figure also demonstrates that the amount of head movement produced by a child is greater than that of the adult but can be corrected for in the postprocessing procedures.

Conclusions and future directions

Clearly the opportunity to study pediatric populations using noninvasive fMRI has tremendous potential for furthering our understanding of human development in health and disease. Not only does fMRI allow acquisition of physiologic information in children that was previously unobtainable by PET because of restrictions on radiation exposure, but it also allows the information to be sampled at multiple time points. This has implications for longitudinal studies and allows for the observation of physiologic changes at times when behavioral changes may be occurring.

Reorganization of brain function following early brain injury in humans has been studied by making behavioral observations of language and visuospatial development. These behavioral observations have led to theories of functional reorganization across the two hemispheres involving homologous sites. While studies of altered behavioral performance have led to explanations such as crowding (Teuber, 1974), the true reorganization of the brain can only be assessed physiologically. The use of fMRI provides an opportunity to follow individuals in whom large portions of the brain have for some reason become modified. One such case report has been published by Levin et al. (1996), in which an adolescent showed interhemispheric reorganization of visuospatial skills from the right to the left hemisphere that were measured with fMRI.

Utilization of functional neuroimaging techniques is providing new information concerning the neuroanatomic localization of the systems affected in developmental dyslexia (Eden and Zeffiro, 1998). However, the details of how these "altered" brain areas are changed as a result of remediation has not been addressed to date. Rehabilitative recovery of reading functions after stroke has been assessed with fMRI (Small et al., 1996), demonstrating altered brain physiology in the inferior parietal cortex after phonological training in acquired dyslexia. Despite evidence from animal models establishing anatomic and physiologic correlates of recovery or learning, these phenomena have not been investigated in children with developmental disorders. With the ability to scan children repeatedly and noninvasively, in vivo human brain reorganization can be measured. Examination of these physiologic changes will improve our understanding of the plasticity of this disorder; it may also allow the most suitable remediation techniques to be identified and may possibly allow determination of the physiologic predispositions most suited to intervention. The investigation of these questions will further our understanding of the mechanisms of developmental disorders and provide information on the effectiveness of various remediation techniques.

Acknowledgements

We would like to thank Kimberley Noble and Jane Joseph for editing the manuscript. This work was supported by the Charles A. Dana Foundation and the Department of Defense (DAMD17–93–V–3018).

Appendix: suggested sources of equipment for fMRI experiments

LCD projector
  Toshiba LCD products
    http://www.toshiba.com
  Sharp Electronics Corporation
    1-800-BE-SHARP
    http://www.sharp-usa.com, http://www.fei.com
  nView Computer and Video Projection
    http://www.nview.com
Projection lens
  BUHL Optical, USA
    Contact: (412) 321-0076
Rear projection screen
  Da-Lite Screen Company, USA
    (800) 622-3737
    http://www.da-lite.com
Response device (optical)
  Current Designs, Inc.
    (215) 387-5456
    bdugan@netaxs.com

Systems
  Psychology Software Tools
    (412) 271-5040
    info@pstnet.com
  Resonance Technology
    http://mri-video.com/rtc
  Neuroscan Inc.
    (703) 444-7100
    sales@neuron.com
Sensor Systems
  (703) 437-7651
  www.sensor.com

References

Bandettini, P. A. (1993). MRI studies of brain activation: temporal characteristics. In *Proceedings of the First Annual Meeting of the International Society of Magnetic Resonance in Medicine*, pp. 143–51, Dallas, TX.

Bandettini, P. A., Wong, E. C., Hinks, R. S., Tikofsky, R. S. and Hyde, J. S. (1992). Time course EPI of human brain function during task activation. *Magn. Reson. Med.*, **25**, 390–7.

Beischer, D. E. (1962). Human tolerance to magnetic fields. *Astronautics*, **42**, 24–5.

Belliveau, J. W., Kennedy, D. N., McKinstry, R. C. et al. (1991). Functional mapping of the human visual cortex by magnetic resonance imaging. *Science*, **254**, 716–19.

Benson, R. R., Logan, W. J., Cosgrove, G. R. et al. (1996). Functional MRI localization of language in a 9-year-old child. *Can. J. Neurolog. Sci.*, **23**, 213–19.

Binder, J. R., Rao, S. M., Hammeke, T. A., Frost, J. A., Bandettini, P. A. and Hyde, J. S. (1994). Effects of stimulus rate on signal response during functional magnetic resonance imaging of auditory cortex. *Cogn. Brain Res.*, **2**, 31–8.

Binder, J. R., Frost, J. A., Hammeke, T. A., Cox, R. W., Rao, S. M. and Prieto, T. (1997). Human brain language areas identified by functional magnetic resonance imaging. *J. Neurosci.*, **17**, 353–62.

Biswal, B., de Yoe, A. E. and Hyde, J. S. (1996). Reduction of physiological fluctuations in fMRI using digital filters. *Magn. Reson. Med.*, **35**, 107–13.

Bookheimer, S. Y., Zeffiro, T. A., Blaxton, T., Gaillard, W. and Theodore, W. (1995). Regional cerebral blood flow during object naming and word reading. *Hum. Brain Map.*, **3**, 93–106.

Bradley, L. and Bryant, P. (1983). Categorizing sounds and learning to read – a causal connection. *Nature*, **301**, 419–21.

Buckner, R. L., Bandettini, P. A., O'Craven, K. M. et al. (1996). Detection of cortical activation during averaged single trials of a cognitive task using functional magnetic resonance imaging. *Proc. Natl. Acad. Sci. USA*, **93**, 14878–83.

Casey, B. J., Cohen, J. D., Jezzard, P. et al. (1995). Activation of prefrontal cortex in children during a nonspatial working memory task with functional MRI. *Neuroimage*, **2**, 221–9.

Casey, B. J., Cohen, J. D., King, S. W. et al. (1997a). A developmental functional MRI study of cortical activation during a spatial working memory task. *Neuroimage*, 5, S69.

Casey, B. J., Trainor, R. J., Orendi, J. L. et al. (1997b). A developmental functional MRI study of prefrontal activation during performance of a go–no–go task. *J. Cogni. Neurosci.*, 9, 835–47.

Cho, Z. H., Chung, S. C., Lim, D. W. and Wong, E. K. (1998). Effects of the acoustic noise of the gradient systems on fMRI: a study on auditory, motor, and visual cortices. *Magn. Reson. Med.*, 39, 331–6.

Cohen, M. S. (1996). Rapid MRI and functional applications. In *Brain Mapping: The Methods*, ed., A. W. Toga and J. C. Mazziotta, pp. 223–52. San Diego, CA: Academic Press.

Dhankhar, A., Wexler, B., Fulbright, R. F., Halwes, T., Blamire, A. and Shulman, R. G. (1997). Functional magnetic resonance imaging assessment of the human brain auditory cortex response in increasing word presentation rates. *Am. Physiol. Soc.*, 77, 476–83.

Eden, G. F. and Zeffiro, T. A. (1998). Neural systems affected in developmental dyslexia revealed by functional neuroimaging. *Neuron*, 21, 279–82.

Eden, G. F., Joseph, J. E., Brown, H. E., Brown, C. P. and Zeffiro, T. A. (1999). Utilizing hemodynamic delay and dispersion to detect fMRI signal change without auditory interference: the behavior interleaved gradients technique. *J. Magn. Reson. Med.*, 41, 13–20.

Edmister, W. B., Talavage, T. M., Ledden, P. J. and Weisskoff, R. M. (1999). Improved auditory cortex imaging using clustered volume acquisitions. *Hum. Brain Map.*, 7, 89–97.

Fiez, J. A., Raichle, M. E., Miezin, F. M., Petersen, S. E., Tallal, P. and Katz, W. F. (1995). PET studies of auditory and phonological processing: effects of stimulus characteristics and task demands. *J. Cogn. Neurosci.*, 7, 357–75.

Fox, P. T. and Raichle, M. E. (1984). Stimulus rate dependence of regional cerebral blood flow in human striate cortex, demonstrated by positron emission tomography. *J. Neurophysiol.*, 51, 1109–20.

Friston, K. J., Jezzard, P. and Turner, R. (1994). Analysis of functional MRI time-series. *Hum. Brain Map.*, 1, 153–71.

Friston, K. J., Josephs, O., Rees, G. and Turner, R. (1998). Nonlinear event-related responses in fMRI. *Magn. Reson. Med.*, 39, 41–52.

Frost, J. A., Binder, J. R., Newby, R. F. et al. (1997). Phonological processing in developmental dyslexia: an fMRI study. *Neuroimage*, 7, S568.

Giedd, J. N., Vaituzis, A. C., Hamburger, S. D. et al. (1996). Quantitative MRI of the temporal lobe, amygdala, and hippocampus in normal human development: ages 4–18 years. *J. Comp. Neurol.*, 366, 223–30.

Guimaraes, A. R., Melcher, J. R., Talavage, T. M. et al. (1998). Imaging subcortical auditory activity in humans. *Hum. Brain Map.*, 6, 33–41.

Haxby, J. V., Horwitz, B., Ungerleider, L. G., Maisog, J. M., Pietrini, P. and Grady, C. L. (1994). The functional organization of human extrastriate cortex: a PET–rCBF study of selective attention to faces and locations. *J. Neurosci.*, 14, 6336–53.

Hertz-Pannier, L., Gaillard, W. D., Mott, S. et al. (1994). Pre-operative assessment of language by fMRI in children with complex partial seizures: preliminary study. In *Proceedings of the 2nd Annual Meeting of the International Society of Magnetic Resonance in Medicine*, vol. 1, p. 326, Dallas, TX.

Hertz-Pannier, L., Gaillard, W. D., Mott, S. H. et al. (1997). Noninvasive assessment of language dominance in children and adolescents with functional MRI: a preliminary study. *Neurology*, 48, 1003–12.

International Non-Ionizing Radiation Committee (of the International Radiation Protection Association (IRPA/INIRC) (1991). IRPA/INIRC guidelines: protection of the patient undergoing a magnetic resonance examination. *Health Physics*, 61, 923–8.

Jackson, G. D (1994). New techniques in magnetic resonance and epilepsy. *Epilepsia, Suppl.* 6, S2–13.

Jackson, G. G., Connelly, A., Cross, J. H., Gordon, I. and Gadian, D. G. (1994). Functional magnetic resonance imaging in focal seizures. *Neurology*, 44, 850–6.

Kwong, K. K., Belliveau, J. W., Chesler, D. A. et al. (1992). Dynamic magnetic resonance imaging of human brain activity during primary sensory stimulation. *Proc. Natl. Acad. Sci. USA*, 80, 5675–9.

Levin, H. S., Scheller, J., Rickard, T. et al. (1996). Dyscalculia and dyslexia after right hemisphere injury in infancy. *Arch. Neurol.*, 53, 88–96.

Ogawa, S., Tank, D. W., Menon, R. et al. (1992). Intrinsic signal changes accompanying sensory stimulation: functional brain mapping using MRI. *Proc. Natl. Acad. Sci. USA*, 89, 5951–5.

Poncelet, B. P., Wedeen, V. J., Weisskoff, R. M. and Cohen, M. S. (1992). Brain parenchyma motion: measurement with cine echo-planar MR imaging. *Radiology*, 185, 645–51.

Price, C., Wise, R., Ramsay, S. et al. (1992). Regional response differences within the human auditory cortex when listening to words. *Neurosci. Lett.*, 146, 179–82.

Price, C. J., Wise, R. J. S., Watson, J. D. G., Patterson, K., Howard, D. and Frackowiak, R. S. J. (1994). Brain activity during reading: the effects of exposure duration and task. *Brain*, 117, 1255–69.

Price, C. J., Wise, R. J. S., Warburton, E. A. et al. (1996). Hearing and saying: the functional neuro-anatomy of auditory word processing. *Brain*, 119, 919–31.

Rees, G., Howseman, A., Josephs, O. et al. (1997). Characterizing the relationship between BOLD contrast and regional cerebral blood flow measurements by varying the stimulus presentation rate. *Neuroimage*, 6, 270–8.

Rumsey, J. M. and Eden, G. F. (1997). Functional neuroimaging of developmental dyslexia: regional cerebral blood flow in dyslexic men. In *Specific Reading Disability: A View of the Spectrum*, ed. B. Shapiro, P. J. Accardo and A. J. Capute, pp. 35–62. Timonium: York Press.

Rumsey, J. M., Andreason, P., Zametkin, A. J. et al. (1992). Failure to activate the left temporoparietal cortex in dyslexia. *Arch. Neurol.*, 49, 527–34.

Rumsey, J. M., Horwitz, B., Donohue, B. C., Nace, K., Maisog, J. M. and Andreason, P. (1997a). Phonologic and orthographic components of word recognition: a PET–rCBF study. *Brain*, 120, 739–59.

Rumsey, J. M., Nace, K., Donohue, B. C., Wise, D., Maisog, J. M. and Andreason, P. (1997b). A positron emission tomography study of impaired word recognition and phonological processing in dyslexic men. *Arch. Neurol.*, **54**, 562–73.

Shaywitz, S. E., Shaywitz, B. A., Pugh, K. R. et al. (1998). Functional disruption in the organization of the brain for reading in dyslexia. *Proc. Natl. Acad. Sci. USA*, **95**, 2636–41.

Shulman, G. L., Corbetta, M., Buckner, R. L. et al. (1997). Top-down modulation of early sensory cortex. *Cereb. Cortex*, **7**, 193–206.

Slifer, K., Cataldo, M. F., Cataldo, M. D., Llorente, A. M. and Gerson, A. C. (1993). Behavior analysis of motion control for pediatric neuroimaging. *J. Appl. Behav. Anal.*, **26**, 469–70.

Small, S. L., Noll, D. C., Perfetti, C. A., Hlustik, P., Wellington, R. and Schneider, W. (1996). Localizing the lexicon for reading aloud: replication of a PET study using fMRI. *Neuroreport*, **7**, 961–5.

Talairach, J. and Tourneoux, P. (1988). *Co-planar Stereotactic Atlas of the Human Brain: 3-Dimensional Proportional System: An Approach to Cerebral Imaging.* Stuttgart: Thieme.

Tenforde, T. S. and Budinger, T. F. (1985). Biological effects and physical safety aspects of NMR imaging and in vivo spectroscopy. In *NMR in Medicine: Instrumentation and Clinical Applications*, ed. S. R. Thomas and R. L. Dixon, p. 493. New York: American Association of Physicists in Medicine.

Teuber, H. L. (1974). *Why two brains?* Cambridge, MA: MIT Press.

Turner, R. and Jezzard, P. (1993). Magnetic resonance studies of brain function activation using echo-planar imaging. In *Functional Neuroimaging*, ed. R. W. Thatcher, M. Hallett, E. R. John and M. Huerta, pp. 69–78. San Diego, CA: Academic Press.

Turner, R., Jezzard, P., Wen, H. et al. (1993). Functional mapping of the human visual cortex at 4 and 1.5 Tesla using deoxygenated contrast EPI. *Magn. Reson. Med.*, **29**, 281–3.

van Meter, J. W., Maisog, J. M., Zeffiro, T. A., Hallett, M., Herscovitch, P. and Rapoport, S. I. (1995). Parametric analysis of functional neuroimages: application to a variable-rate motor task. *Neuroimage*, **2**, 273–83.

Woods, R. P., Grafton, S. T., Holmes, C. J., Cherry, S. R. and Mazziotta, J. C. (1998a). Automated image registration: I. *J. Comp. Assist. Tomogr.*, **22**, 139–52.

Woods, R. P., Grafton, S. T., Watson, J. D., Sicotte, N. L. and Mazziotta, J. C. (1998b). Automated image registration: II. *J. Comp. Assist. Tomogr.*, **22**, 153–65.

Zeffiro, T. A., Eden, G. F., Woods, R. P. and van Meter, J. W. (1997). Intersubject analysis of fMRI data using spatial normalization. *Adv. Exp. Med. Biol.*, **413**, 235–40.

4

MRS in childhood psychiatric disorders

Deborah A. Yurgelun-Todd and Perry F. Renshaw

Introduction

The application of magnetic resonance spectroscopy (MRS) techniques to the study of neuropsychiatric disorders in childhood provides an extraordinary opportunity to advance our understanding of the neurobiological mechanisms underlying these disorders. Recent developments in imaging technology have afforded researchers the capability to examine in vivo not only brain structure but also neurochemistry and functional architecture. This review will focus on the use of MRS. All MR methods (MRS, magnetic resonance imaging (MRI) and functional MRI, (fMRI)) rely on the same basic principles. In the study of human brain, all three of these procedures use the same hardware. Of these techniques, MRS was the first technology to be developed, exploiting the magnetic properties of nuclei with unpaired protons and neutrons. The earliest observations of NMR signals from bulk matter were made independently by Purcell and colleagues (1946) and by Bloch et al. (1946). However, a number of important technical developments were necessary before the first spectra could be obtained from human brain in the 1980s (Krishnan and Doraiswamy, 1997). A glossary of technical terms used in functional neuroimaging is provided at the end of this book (p. 480).

Methods in MRS

The importance of MRS for understanding neuropathologic processes is derived from the information this technique provides regarding the chemical content of the tissue being studied. The application of this technology allows investigators to acquire data that describe both the chemistry and the physical environment of the tissue. It is, therefore, possible to examine and quantify changes in metabolite levels of chemical substances such as N-acetylaspartate (NAA), phosphocreatine (PCr), creatine plus phosphocreatine (Cr), and cytosolic choline compounds (Cho) and relate them to changes in structural pathology. As with MRI technology, spectroscopic techniques are rapidly evolving.

MR visible compounds give rise to distinct peaks, or resonances. In general, the area of the resonance intensity is proportional to the concentration of molecules that contribute to the resonance. Thus, quantification of resonance intensities may be used to derive tissue concentration estimates for brain chemicals. In practice, these calculations also require knowledge of the relaxation times, T_1 and T_2, of the molecule of interest, the data acquisition parameters, time to repetition (TR) and time to echo (TE), the tissue volume of interest, and the efficiency of signal detection. The collection of these parameters is very time consuming; consequently, it is a common practice to express MRS data as metabolite ratios or in terms of institutional (standardized) units. In addition, the chemical composition of gray matter and white matter are quite different. For many study hypotheses it is important to assess the tissue content of specific brain regions. Quantification of resonance intensities is possible for a number of nuclei, including proton (^1H), carbon (^{13}C), fluorine (^{19}F), and phosphorus (^{31}P). So far, ^{31}P MRS and ^1H MRS have been applied to the study of neuropsychiatric disorders. The aim of these studies has been to characterize the concentrations of metabolites such as NAA, Cr, and Cho in specific brain regions, which may be related to neuropathologic processes.

In general, MR methods are based on the fact that specified nuclei may align with or against a static magnetic field, at slightly different energy levels. Two events are necessary for the generation and observation of MR signals. Two magnetic fields are needed for a signal to be recorded:

first, a stable field (usually in the range 1.5–4.0 T), which is characteristic of the magnetic strength of the MR scanner, and, second, a transient magnetic field that is introduced at a specific frequency, causing a transition of some lower energy spins (aligned with the static magnetic field) to the higher energy level (aligned against the static magnetic field). This second field is typically introduced using a radiofrequency (rf) coil, or antenna. For each magnetic nucleus in the brain, a given static magnetic field is associated with a particular resonance frequency, often called the Larmor frequency. For example, at 1.5 T, the proton resonance frequency is 63.88 MHz. When the second magnetic field is removed, usually by turning off the second rf magnetic field, energy at the resonance frequency is released from the higher energy spins as they align with the first magnetic field and this energy may be detected. This release of energy comprises the MR signal. The process by which the nuclei realign themselves with the static constant field is called relaxation, or recovery (T_1 relaxation is within the longitudinal axis and T_2 is within the transverse axis). More detailed descriptions of the MR method have been published elsewhere (e.g., Krishnan and Doraiswamy, 1997; Mukherji, 1998; see also Chapter 3.)

The design of an MRS experiment requires that study parameters are set to optimize signal-to-noise from a clearly delineated brain region in as rapid a time course as possible. In addition to hardware considerations, and the selection of nuclei to be studied, both localization strategy and relaxation times must be specified. Therefore, the selection of the nucleus to be studied is only the first in a series of important decisions to be made in defining an MRS protocol. Given that MRS techniques have low sensitivity, most study strategies are designed to optimize the available signal.

Nuclei that have been assessed through the application of MRS to the human brain include ^{1}H, ^{31}P, ^{13}C, ^{19}F, lithium-7 (^{7}Li), and sodium-23 (^{23}Na) (Table 4.1). Although psychiatric investigations have generally been limited to the study of lithium, fluorine, hydrogen, and phosphorus, recent studies of neurologic patients have reported interesting findings with ^{23}Na and ^{13}C. Sodium-23 gives rise to a single resonance line, and changes in the sodium MRS resonance have been associated with cerebral ischemia (e.g., Tyson et al., 1996). Carbon-13 is a stable isotope with a low natural abundance, which makes it possible to administer and detect labeled compounds (Mason et al., 1996). At present, ^{13}C-labeled compounds are very expensive, which limits experimentation. Over time, it is likely that ^{13}C MRS methods will be developed that will permit the direct observation of neurotransmitter cycling by introducing a neurotransmitter or its precursor labeled with ^{13}C. Current investigations in children with psychiatric disorders, however, have focused on

Table 4.1. Relative NMR sensitivities

Nucleus	Spin quantum number	NMR resonance at 1.5 T	Relative sensitivity at constant field
^{1}H	1/2	63.87	1
^{19}F	1/2	60.08	0.83
^{7}Li	3/2	24.83	0.29
^{23}Na	3/2	16.89	0.09
^{31}P	1/2	25.88	0.06
^{13}C	1/2	16.07	0.02
^{39}K	3/2	2.99	0.0005

Note: Spin quantum number is a term used to describe the angular momentum of nuclei.

a limited number of metabolites such as NAA, Cr, and Cho. Studies of each nucleus are associated with specific advantages and limitations. From a practical perspective, since each nucleus will have a unique resonance frequency at a given field strength, additional rf coils and amplifiers are usually necessary for each MRS nucleus. Therefore, most clinical studies of patients report findings based on a single nucleus.

Brain ^{31}P, ^{1}H, and ^{13}C spectra give rise to multiple resonance lines, all of which are generated by compounds containing these nuclei. The difference in resonance frequencies for different compounds arises from interactions within molecules (Bovey et al., 1988), making it possible to assess the concentrations of a number of different compounds using these methods. Each nucleus has a different MR sensitivity (Table 4.1), which in turn limits the spatial resolution of the MR experiment. Sensitivity is an important consideration in MRS studies in that the metabolites being observed are typically present at concentrations in the millimolar range. In contrast, the concentration of brain water is of the order of 40 mol/l, the primary reason why MR images of brain water have such striking contrast. At the other end of the sensitivity spectrum, radionuclide imaging (e.g., positron emission tomography (PET) and single photon emission computed tomography (SPECT)) allows the detection of molecules that are present at nanomolar concentrations, and is used to measure, among other applications, brain receptor distributions (Chapters 1 and 2). Parameters for MRS experiments can be adjusted to maximize the detection of metabolites by increasing their "MRS visibility". The most common field strength for human MRS studies at the present time is 1.5 T. However, a number of research centers are currently installing scanners at a field strength of 3 or 4 T. These higher field scanners are particularly valuable for MRS studies, as MR signals increase linearly with field strength, which in turn results in increased sensitivity.

As we have described above, MRS allows for the noninvasive, in vivo visualization and examination of brain metabolites in a manner that was previously not possible. Moreover, MRS offers several advantages over radionuclide neuroimaging techniques (PET and SPECT) for the study of children and adolescents, in particular its absence of ionizing radiation, which allows repeated examinations of a single study subject. MRS data are also acquired with the same basic hardware as structural imaging data, thereby facilitating the collection of both data types within the same scanning session. Several methods are currently used for the acquisition of spectroscopic data and include both single-voxel and chemical shift imaging (CSI). Spectroscopic data may be obtained from either single, predefined tissue volumes (voxels) or from two- or three-dimensional arrays of tissue (spectroscopic images). It is generally easier to perform single-voxel MRS as opposed to spectroscopic imaging as it requires less imaging time for the subject. However, when spectroscopic imaging parameters have been optimized, data sets may be obtained without penalty in terms of data acquisition time or spatial resolution. Therefore, it is usually preferable to obtain spectroscopic imaging data when it is possible. Single-voxel spectroscopy provides information about a specific cube of tissue localized in a particular brain region, defined with help from the magnetic field gradients. CSI is actually a multivoxel method in which a signal is collected from a wide region of tissue that may include up to an entire brain slice. This array of data is later decoded into individual spectra from each of the voxels (Fig. 4.1). In practice, most single-voxel studies of human subjects include anywhere from one to three voxels per imaging session. The resolution of single-voxel spectroscopy is considered superior, as the magnetic field can be optimally homogenized for the volume selected, while CSI has the advantage of being able to acquire data from multiple regions of the brain simultaneously. For clinical investigations aimed at the identification of focal pathology, the single-voxel method may be most advantageous.

Although studies utilizing MRS yield an abundance of information about both the structure and chemical composition of tissue, MR technology is limited by a number of factors. As with any neuroimaging technique, MRS requires that study participants remain completely still for the duration of the examination, which may be difficult for children. Additionally, the signal from one nucleus or from a group of nuclei may be dispersed into two or more through spin coupling. While often used for the identification of specific resonances, this splitting of the signal results in a reduced signal-to-noise ratio and complicates the spectra, making the interpretation of the data more difficult. Perhaps the most significant limitation of

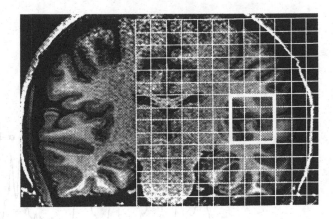

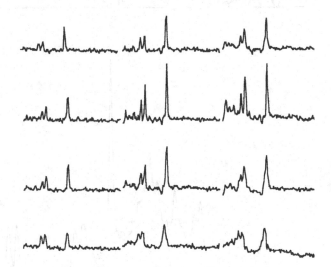

Fig. 4.1. Coronal image through the medial temporal lobe depicting the placement of a multivoxel grid used in chemical shift imaging. Twelve proton spectra are generated from the 12 voxels within the larger volume of interest.

MRS is its lack of sensitivity. The signal strength of a particular nucleus is dependent upon its inherent magnetogyric ratio and the external applied magnetic field strength. The magnetic field needs to be precisely homogenized in order to acquire narrow, clear resonance peaks. The sensitivity of MRS can be increased by altering a number of imaging and study design parameters, for example increasing the applied magnetic field strength.

Measurement of brain metabolites for specific brain regions is accomplished by measurement of the spectrum or spectra after the data collection is complete. An example of a proton spectrum is presented in Fig. 4.2. The MR signal is displayed as a spectrum with characteristic peaks associated with different elements. The area under individual peaks is measured relative to specified reference compounds, although estimation of the area under each peak

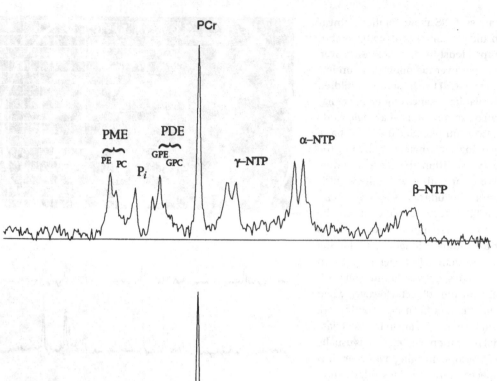

Fig. 4.2. Proton-decoupled, ^{31}P MR spectrum through a 5 cm axial brain slice. The spectrum is displayed both after (top) and before (bottom) removal of a broad phosphodiester resonance that arises from mobile phospholipids. PME, phosphomonoesters; PE, phosphoethanolamine; PC, phosphocholine; PDE, phosphodiesters; GPE, glycerophosphoethanolamine; GPC, glycerophosphocholine; PCr, phosphocreatine; NTP, nucleoside triphosphate. The α-, β-, and γ-NTP resonances arise from different phosphorus atoms within the molecule.

is often confounded by overlapping peaks. Some investigators report their findings as absolute values while others report their data as a ratio of one metabolite to another. Interpretation of spectral data requires that *saturation and relaxation effects* be considered and that the underlying tissue content of the regions of interest are known and examined. Although the MRS procedure requires a thoughtful, detailed approach, this exciting method will

yield in vivo biochemical data that were previously not available for the study of human brain.

Limitations of MRS

In this review, we will consider evidence for abnormal concentrations of various metabolites detected with MRS in the brains of children with psychiatric disorders. Additionally, this chapter will address how these MRS findings fit with data from studies of children with other neurologic pathologies, and how the MRS abnormalities may relate to primary pathology as well as being associated with risk factors and clinical features of behavioral disorders. For example, brain abnormalities found in adult studies of schizophrenic patients have generally been interpreted by investigators as reflective of neuropathology associated with the primary schizophrenic process. However, the meaning ascribed to such cortical changes depends crucially on the theoretical models within which the data are viewed. Caveats in interpreting previous research and suggested directions for new studies will be discussed, along with potential clinical applications for future research.

A critical evaluation of the published research suggests that two major factors may contribute to inconsistency in the results from neuroimaging studies in children with psychiatric disorders. The first involves the nature and extent of potential biases in the selection of both patient and control subjects. Subject selection, sample size, and variables on which patients and controls are matched have all been demonstrated to be important factors for the outcome of neuroimaging studies (Hendren et al., 1995, Jacobsen et al., 1996). In studies of children and adolescents, the effects of age and sex are potent determinants of hemispheric laterality, regional morphometry, metabolite concentration, and cortical activation (Kreis et al., 1985; Witelson, 1985) and may critically affect the ability to identify cortical changes between children from different diagnostic groups. A second factor that restricts the interpretation of neuroimaging studies is the inconsistency in study methods. As with any new technique, there remains debate as to the optimal parameters and procedures for the application of MRS to the study of childhood psychiatric disorders.

Initial studies applying MRS methods to psychiatric populations generally examined a single voxel in the brain. In contrast, recent studies using CSI have provided more extensive, quantitative measurements of metabolite concentrations in multiple brain regions. Findings often vary considerably. Even recent studies using sophisticated MR acquisition techniques are constrained by the absence of completely objective and reliable anatomic landmarks to demarcate precise and specific brain regions of interest. This difficulty in localization results, in part, from an absence of formal agreement as to the cortical landmarks to be used in human MRS studies and the inability to establish isotropic cortical volumes in study subjects. For patient populations that display only small quantitative differences from control subjects in brain structure and chemistry, the inability of imaging techniques to characterize specific cortical regions precisely contributes to the difficulty in reliably detecting group differences. Methodologic limitations also exist both for MR data acquisition and image-analytic techniques. Few investigators, for example, have utilized the same MRS acquisition parameters, postimaging data processing techniques, or statistical approaches to data analyses and hypothesis testing. Finally, conceptual approaches regarding how best to define and demonstrate what is abnormal, and what falls within the spectrum of normal brain variance, has remained a point of debate.

Despite the limitations outlined above, MRS studies of children with psychiatric disorders may have some advantages. It has been hypothesized that children with psychiatric disorders may represent more homogeneous diagnostic subtypes and, therefore, be more likely to yield unique biological correlates for illnesses such as depression and schizophrenia. This would be of considerable clinical importance, as neurobiologic subtypes have been proposed to be related to clinical variables, such as chronicity of illness, poor treatment response, presence of negative symptoms, and neurocognitive function. Studies of children are also more likely to provide data on the etiologic processes as neurobiologic abnormalities are less prone to changes through treatment or to the disease process. To date, brain MRS research has targeted adult populations, in part because of the relative difficulty in obtaining good-quality scans from children. Additionally, children and adolescents are more likely to have imaging data confounded by motion artifact or dental braces and some psychiatric illnesses, such as schizophrenia, are often not diagnosed until the late teens and early twenties.

Metabolites measured by MRS

MRS employs standard MRI devices to make measurements of chemical levels within the brain. MRS-visible compounds that can be measured noninvasively in human brain include psychotropic medications, such as lithium (Sachs et al., 1995; Jensen et al., 1996; Soares et al., 1996; Riedl et al., 1997; Renshaw and Wicklund, 1998) and some fluorinated polycyclic drugs (Komoroski et al., 1991; Renshaw et al., 1992; Miner et al., 1995; Strauss et al., 1997, 1998). Spectra arising from either ^{7}Li or ^{19}F, in drugs that contain fluorine, are typically single lines; however, these lines may also include signal from active and inactive metabolites. These studies have generally reported whole brain drug concentrations because of the relatively low brain concentrations of the therapeutic agents (0.1–1.0

mmol/l for lithium and 1–10–μmol/l for fluorinated drugs). The validity of ^{19}F MRS as a means for assessing brain drug levels has been validated using a primate model (Christensen et al., 1998). To date, ^{7}Li and ^{19}F MRS have not been extensively used to assess the pharmacokinetics of drugs in the brain of children and adolescents. As can be seen in Tables 4.2 and 4.3 a number of investigators have begun to apply MRS methods to the study of children with psychiatric disorders and neurologic abnormalities. The findings to date represent the emergence of unprecedented new data.

Phosphorus

Two different MRS-visible nuclei are evaluated in most studies of brain biochemistry: ^{31}P and ^{1}H. Unlike ^{7}Li or ^{19}F MR spectra, ^{31}P and ^{1}H MR spectra give several resonance lines that arise from well-defined metabolite pools. Phosphorus MR spectra provide information on the concentration of high-energy phosphate compounds (e.g., PCr and nucleoside trisphosphate (NTP, primarily reflecting adenosine trisphosphate (ATP) in the brain) and phospholipid metabolites, which include phosphomonoesters (PME), phosphodiesters (PDE), and inorganic phosphate (P_i). The functional significance of phosphorous and proton metabolite changes are described in Table 4.4. Information on alterations in brain energy metabolism may be gained by measuring the relative levels of PCr ($\sim$1.4 mmol/l), NTP (2.8 mmol/l), and P_i (1.4 mmol/l) (Buchli et al., 1994). The brain PME resonance, which arises primarily from the phospholipid precursors phosphoethanolamine (PE) and phosphocholine (PC), as well as from sugar phosphates, derives from a total metabolite pool of approximately 3.0 mmol/l (Pettegrew et al., 1991). The in vivo PDE resonance has a broad component, arising from membrane bilayers, and a narrow component, which is derived from the phospholipid catabolites glycerophosphocholine (GPC) and glycerophosphoethanolamine (GPE).

At 1.5 T, metabolite information can usually be obtained from brain regions as small as 25–50 cm^3 for phosphorus-31; for example, depth-resolved surface-coil spectroscopy (DRESS). MRS data are typically acquired either from single voxels using spatial localization (e.g., Bottomley et al., 1984) image-selected in vivo spectroscopy (ISIS) (Ordidge et al., 1986), or from low-resolution, two- or three-dimensional spectroscopic images (Brown et al., 1982). If desired, the sensitivity of phosphorus spectroscopy can be increased by applying a proton decoupling technique, which requires a special coil for each metabolite of interest (Luyten et al., 1989; Murphy-Boesch et al., 1993). Proton decoupling will produce line narrowing

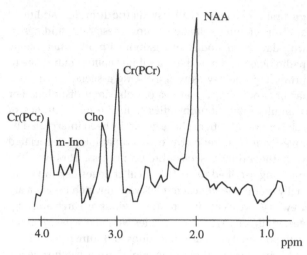

Fig. 4.3. Proton NMR spectrum taken from a 2 cm^3 voxel localized over the anterior cingulate cortex. NAA, *N*-acetylaspartate; Cr(PCr), creatine and phosphocreatine; Cho, cytosolic choline-containing compounds; m-Ino, *myo*-inositol.

effects for improved resolution of the phospholipid precursors PC and PE, in the PME peak and for the phospholipid breakdown products GPC and GPE in the PDE peak.

Protons

In vivo ^{1}H MRS provides a means to detect and quantify a number of cerebral metabolites, including NAA, Cr, cytosolic Cho, and *myo*-inositol (m–Ino) (Fig. 4.3). Approximate gray concentrations of these metabolites are 8–11, 6–7, 0.9–1.4, and 4–5 mmol/l for NAA, Cr, Cho, and m-Ino, respectively (Pouwels and Frahm, 1998). NAA contributes the largest signal to water-suppressed cerebral spectra and is found primarily in neurons (Birken and Oldendorf, 1989; Tsai and Coyle, 1995). Consequently, the NAA resonance has been viewed as a neuronal marker by a number of investigators. However, the exact role of NAA and other in vivo metabolites is not yet known. Phosphocreatine is a high-energy phosphate and the Cr resonance has been used as a reference standard, reflecting the fact that the total concentration of creatine and Pcr is similar in many brain regions, although slightly higher in cerebral cortex than in white matter (Petroff et al., 1989). Most of the Cho in the brain is incorporated in the membrane lipid phosphatidylcholine, which undergoes a restricted range of motion and, therefore, is largely invisible to in vivo MRS (Miller, 1991). The major contributors to the Cho peak are PC and GPC (Barker et al., 1994). Inositol is involved in phospholipid metabolism as well as in the maintenance of osmotic equilibrium (Moore et al., 1999).

Table 4.2. Spectroscopic findings in psychiatric patients

Investigators	Subjects	Age (years)	Method	Location of single voxel	Metabolites/findings in patient groups versus controls
Proton MRS					
Brooks et al. (1998)	Schizophrenics 16M Controls 12M	11 11	Single voxel	Left frontal white matter	Decreased left NAA/Cr
Thomas et al. (1998)	Schizophrenics 13M Controls 11M	14 11	Single voxel	Anterior cingulate; occipital grey matter	Decreased NAA/Cr
Thomas et al. (1998)	Schizophrenics Controls 9	7–17 7–15	Single voxel	No information	Decreased NAA/Cho/Glx
Hendren et al. (1995)	Schizophrenics 12 Controls 13	8–12 8–12	Single voxel	Mesial temporal lobe	Decreased NAA/Cr, decreased Cho/Cr; differences in amygdala volume, callosal area asymmetry
Bertolino et al. (1997)	Schizophrenics 13 Controls 13	– –	CSI	Hippocampus; prefrontal cortex; orbitofrontal cortex; superior temporal gyrus; occipital cortex; thalamus; putamen; cingulate	Decreased frontal NAA/Cr; decreased hippocampus NAA/Cr
Rosenberg et al. (1998)[a]	Obsessive-compulsive disorder 9	8–17	Single voxel	Left caudate	Decreased caudate glutamate concentration caused by paroxetine therapy
Steingard et al. (1998)[a]	Depressed 6M Controls 18M	15 14	Single voxel	Left anterior frontal lobe	Cho/Cr inverse correlation with age; decreased NAA/Cr in orbitofrontal cortex
Bartha et al. (1998)[a]	Obsessive-compulsive disorder 13 Controls 13	– –	No information	Left basal ganglia	Decreased NAA
Phosphorus-31 MRS					
Moss et al. (1997)[a]	Three groups peripubertal children with familial substance use disorder risk	Mean 14.3	CSI (1.5 T)	Frontal/occipital lobes; right and left parietal lobes	Decreased right parietal phosphodiester
Moss et al. (1997)	Controls 29	Mean 12.5	CSI (1.5 T)	Frontal/occipital lobes	Males: increased β-NTP in frontal lobe; decrease in occipital Females: β-NTP decreased in frontal lobe
Rae (1998)[a]	Male adults 26 Male children 42	9–31	CSI (1.5 T)	Frontal/parietal lobes	Significant relationship between cerebral pH and verbal ability in adults and boys

Notes:

NAA, N-acetylaspartate; Cr, creatine plus phosphocreatine; Glx, glutamine + glutamate + gamma-aminobutyric acid; Cho, choline; β-NTP, β-nucleotide trisphosphates; CSI, chemical shift image acquisition.

[a] Results available only in abstract form.

Table 4.3. Spectroscopic findings in neurologic patients

Investigators	Subjects	Age	Method	Location	Metabolites/findings in patient groups versus controls
Proton MRS					
Gadian et al. (1996)	Epileptics, temporal lobe 22	5–17 years	No information	Medial regions, left and right temporal lobes	Left temporal lobe metabolite ratio related to verbal IQ; right side related to performance IQ
Moore et al. (1996)	Sturge–Weber syndrome 5	4 months to 14 years	Single voxel	Cerebrum	Decreased NAA/Cr in gadolinium-enhancing regions
Ende et al. (1996)[a]	Epileptics, temporal lobe 16 Controls 18	No information	No information	Hippocampus	Decreased hippocampal volume and NAA concentration
Holshouser et al. (1997)	CNS injury 82 Controls 24	2 days to 15.9 years	Single voxel	Occipital gray matter	MRS good predictor of neurologic outcome; NAA/Cr lower in infant and child patients; NAA/Cho significantly lower in infants and neonates; lactate significantly higher in patients with poor outcome
Kim et al. (1997)	Encephalopathic 1	Newborn	Single voxel	Parietal white matter; occipital gray matter, basal ganglia	Abnormal basal ganglia
Lee et al. (1997)[a]	Preterm infants 12	28–35 weeks gestation	Single voxel	Parietal white matter	NAA/Cr increases rapidly during preterm, has a linear relationship with age
Vucurevic et al. (1997)[a]	Canavan's disease 3, Alexander's disease 1 Controls 5	11 months to 5.5 years	Single voxel	Parieto-occipital white matter	Patients with Canavan's disease have increased NAA, decreased Cho; patients with Alexander's disease have increased NAA decreased Cho in gray matter and decreased NAA, Cr, Cho in white matter
Tzika et al. (1993)	Neurologic 7 Asymptomatic neurologic 4 Controls 9	2–17 years	No information	Cerebral white matter	Decreased NAA/Cr; increased Cho/Cr; increased glutamate; increased inositol/Cr
Lu et al. (1996)	AIDS 45 Progressive encephalopathy 7 Static encephalopathy 8 Controls 30	2.3 weeks to 17.6 years	Single voxel	Basal ganglia	Decreased NAA/Cr in children with progressive AIDS encephalopathy
Rajanaygam et al. (1997)[a]	Adrenoleuko-dystrophy 31: symptomatic 21, asymptomatic 10	3–19 years	Single voxel	Occipital/frontal white matter	As disease severity increased NAA/Cr, Cr/Cho decreased
Li et al. (1998)[a,b]	Infant encephalopathy 15 Healthy 3 Omphlitis 4	2–5 days	No information	No information	Increased glutamate in patients with severe hypoxic-ischemic symptoms

Table 4.3 (*cont.*)

Investigators	Subjects	Age	Method	Location	Metabolites/findings in patient groups versus controls
van der Grond et al. (1998)[a]	Neonates 27	37–42 weeks	No information	Basal ganglia	NAA/Cr ratio shows largest difference between neonates with good and poor outcome
Kim et al. (1998)[a]	Infants 43: normal outcome 29, mild CNS impairment 4, severe CNS impairment 10	28–43 weeks	Single voxel	Parietal white matter; occipital gray matter	Values of lactate/NAA greater than 2.0 with a decrease in NAA/Cr are early predictors of severe neurodevelopmental outcome
Diklic and Gambarelli (1998)[a]	Neuronal ceroid lipofuscinoses 1	8 years	Single voxel	Frontal/occipital gray matter	Marked neuronal loss and membrane damage in late infantile NCL
Auld et al. (1995)	Infants 30, all acute CNS injury: good outcome 17, bad outcome 10	mean 38 months (good outcome, mean 46 months; poor outcome mean 26 months)	Single voxel	Occipital gray matter parietal white matter	NAA/Cr and NAA/Cho lower in poor outcome group
Phosphorus-31 MRS					
Haseler et al. (1997)	Infants with shaken baby syndrome 3 Control infants 52	5, 24, and 28 weeks –	CSI	Parietal white matter	Loss of integrity of proton MR spectrum appears to signal irreversible damage

Notes:

NAA, *N*-acetylaspartate; Cr, creatine plus phosphocreatine; Cho, choline; CSI, chemical shift image acquisition at 1.5 T.

[a] Results available only in abstract form.

[b] Study carried out with a 2 T magnet.

Proton MRS is complicated by the fact that the signals from most metabolites of interest are five orders of magnitude smaller than the signals arising from tissue water and lipid. However, over the last several years, methods have been developed for the routine suppression of water signals (Ogg et al., 1994) and localized brain spectra do not contain large signals from lipids (Behar et al., 1994). Because of differences in the relaxation times of metabolites, spatial localization methods differ for ^{31}P/^{1}H MRS studies (Moore et al. 1997). Stimulated echo acquisition and pixel-resolved methods (STEAM and PRESS) are often used to collect ^{1}H MRS data (Moonen et al., 1989) and metabolite information can be obtained from brain volumes in the range 1–10 cm^{3}. The relatively high spatial resolution of ^{1}H MRS makes it possible to distinguish metabolite differences in gray and white matter (Pouwels and Frahm, 1998), although relatively few studies to date have reported segmented imaging data in conjunction with metabolite information (Yurgelun-Todd et al., 1996; Renshaw et al., 1997; Lim et al., 1998).

Studies in children with psychiatric disorders

Proton MRS

Childhood-onset schizophrenia/schizophrenia spectrum disorder

Hendren et al. (1995) performed ^{1}H spectroscopy on the frontal lobes of 12 children between the ages of 8 and 12 years who were diagnosed with schizophrenia spectrum disorders and on 13 healthy children who were matched for age, sex, and education. Spectra were obtained from a voxel localized in the left frontal cortex. Although no statistically significant differences were found in metabolite concentrations between patients and control subjects, a

Table 4.4. MRS signals and their functional significance

T_1	Location	Index
Proton MRS		
N-Acetylaspartate (NAA)	Within neurons	Neuronal viability; levels increase with brain maturation
Choline (Cho)	Brain Cho stores from glycerophosphocholine (GPC) and phosphocholine (PC)	Phospholipid metabolism
Creatine + phosphocreatine (Cr)		Cellular energy metabolism
Lactate	Within cells utilizing glycolysis	Anaerobic metabolism
Phosphorus-31 MRS		
High-energy phosphates; phosphocreatine (PCr) peak and polyphosphate regions of the spectrum (primarily ATP)	Specifically measures the level of high-energy phosphates; PCr is the most metabolically labile of the high-energy compounds, falling prior to ATP in situations of rapid energy consumption	Information on the energy status of the brain
Phosphomonoesters (PME) peak: phosphoethanolamine (PE); phosphocholine (PC); α-glycerophosphate (GP) (sugar phosphate)	Levels of small, water-soluble precursors of phospholipid membrane synthesis such as PE and PC, as well as sugar phosphates	Building blocks of membrane phospholipids
Phosphodiester (PDE) peak: GPC; glycerophosphoethanolamine (GPE), mobile phospholipids	Information on both small, water-soluble phospholipid membrane breakdown products (GPE and GPC) and mobile phospholipid vesicles such as synaptic vesicles	Major catabolic products of membrane phospholipid degradation and phospholipids
P_i peak	Final end-product of all of the phosphorus metabolites	

Note: PCr/P_i ratio provides a convenient measure of the energy status of the brain because it is the ratio of the most labile form of high-energy phosphate (PCr) to the ultimate breakdown product of all high-energy phosphate compounds (P_i).

notable reduction of NAA, as well as a reduction in Cho/Cr was found for this region. The investigators concluded that the findings were in agreement with previous findings of decreased NAA in the frontal lobes of adult patients with schizophrenia (Yurgelun-Todd et al., 1996) and suggested that the small sample sizes limited the ability to detect significant metabolite reductions. In addition, this study examined neuropsychologic performance and brain morphometric measures based on MR images. Children with schizophrenia spectrum disorders performed more poorly on neurocognitive tests, particularly on measures of verbal ability and verbal memory, and were characterized by smaller amygdala, reduced mesial temporal cortex volume, and smaller callosal area, without ventricular enlargement. The pattern of MRS, MRI, and neuropsychologic findings identified in the children at risk for schizophrenia led the investigators to propose two etiologic processes as the basis for the cortical changes identified. One developmental process may be related to a global cortical effect that results in alterations of callosal maturation and brain asymmetry. This global process would be associated with a range of neurodevelopmental disorders. In addition, abnormal left and right hemisphere development and changes in the corpus callosum may be related to a number of cognitive and behavioral disorders. The second process would be associated with factors that have greater diagnostic specificity and influence the development of the temporal lobe and the amygdala. This process would be more directly related to the emergence of schizophrenia.

In a subsequent report from the same investigators, ^{1}H MRS data was described for an independent sample of 16 children with schizophrenia spectrum disorders (nine males and seven females, 8–12 years of age, mean age 11 years) (Brooks et al., 1998). The control group consisted of 12 age- and sex-matched subjects (mean age 10.8 years). Single-voxel spectroscopic measurements of the proton metabolites in the left frontal lobe identified a decrease in the NAA/Cr ratio in children with schizophrenia spectrum disorders compared with levels in the control group. As in the earlier study, the authors concluded that these findings provided evidence in support of a neurodevelopmental theory for schizophrenia.

Thomas and colleagues reported similar findings in a recent study focused on the investigation of metabolite concentrations in the frontal lobe (Thomas et al., 1996). Thirteen patients with schizophrenia spectrum disorders, including seven males and six females (mean age 14 ± 3 years), and 12 healthy controls, including six males and six females (mean age 11 ± 3 years), were evaluated with single-voxel ^{1}H MRS. The investigators found a 32% reduction of NAA/Cr ratio in frontal gray matter and a 13% reduction of the ratio of glutamine plus glutamate plus gamma-aminobutyric acid (combined as a "Glx" resonance intensity because of difficulties in resolving these three in spectra) to Cr in occipital gray matter in the children with schizophrenia spectrum disorder. Although not statistically significant, NAA/Cho, Glx/Cho ratios were reduced and Cr/Cho was increased in the frontal lobes of the children with schizophrenia spectrum disorder (Thomas et al., 1996). These findings further confirm that cortical abnormalities are present early in the illness. One unique feature of this study is the quantification of a Glx resonance intensity.

Methods for resolving the resonance lines combined in Glx are currently under active development (Weber et al., 1997; Pouwels and Frahm, 1998). The ability to quantify glutamate, glutamine, and gamma-aminobutyric acid in specific brain regions will provide an important tool for the identification of neurotransmitter dysfunction.

Bertolino et al. (1998) applied CSI techniques to evaluate and measure metabolites in multiple brain regions simultaneously. In this study of 13 children with early-onset schizophrenia (mean age 15.9 years) and 13 healthy control subjects (mean age 14.7 years), both the hippocampus and the prefrontal cortex demonstrated reductions in NAA/Cr. Moreover, the effect size of these metabolite reductions was similar to those reported in previous studies of adult-onset schizophrenia performed by the same group. The consistency in metabolite changes identified for these two age groups is suggestive of a developmental continuum for these abnormalities in schizophrenia. One recent study by Buckley and co-workers (Buckley, 1998) compared children with schizophrenia spectrum disorders and those with autism using ^{1}H MRS. The investigators found a reduction in NAA in the frontal lobes in both study groups (Buckley, 1998). These results were interpreted as reflecting the presence of cortical hypoplasias regardless of diagnostic category.

The extent to which age, gender, duration of illness, and medication influence ^{1}H MRS findings is currently not fully understood. Given that children with schizophrenia spectrum disorders display metabolite changes that are similar to those identified in adults with schizophrenia, it seems likely that these alterations in metabolite concentrations are reflective of a neurodevelopmental process associated with the etiology of this illness. A neurodevelopmental hypothesis is further supported by recent ^{1}H MRS findings by Renshaw et al., (1995) from a series of consecutively referred patients hospitalized with a first episode of psychosis. Compared with normal control subjects, psychotic patients had a significantly lower NAA/Cr ratio, indicating that abnormalities in temporal lobe NAA concentration are present early in psychotic illness.

Obsessive-compulsive disorder

So far, the focus of this section has been on studies examining children with schizophrenia spectrum disorder; however, several recent investigations have applied ^{1}H MRS methods to other psychiatric disorders. Bartha et al. (1998) have investigated metabolite changes in the left basal ganglia in 13 unmedicated children with obsessive-compulsive disorder (OCD) and 13 matched controls. NAA levels were lower in patients than in controls. Proton MRS has also been used to study treatment response in adolescents with OCD. Rosenberg et al. (1998) investigated the relationship between clinical improvement and metabolite concentration in patients treated with paroxetine. Eleven treatment-naive, nondepressed adolescents between the ages of eight and seventeen who met criteria for OCD were treated with paroxetine for 12 weeks. Subjects demonstrated a significant decrease in the concentration of Glx in the caudate nucleus, supporting theories regarding the relationship between OCD and serotonin pathway disruption (Rosenberg et al., 1998).

Depression

In the first application of ^{1}H MRS to the study of depression in adolescents, Steingard et al. (1998) evaluated 14 adolescents diagnosed with depression (mean age 15.6 years) and 26 psychiatrically healthy adolescents (mean age 14.3 years). Using ^{1}H MRS and a 5 in (13 cm) surface coil, investigators collected metabolite data from a 3.4 cm^3 voxel in the orbitofrontal cortex (Fig. 4.4). Depressed subjects demonstrated an increase in the ratio of Cho/Cr in the orbitofrontal cortex compared with the healthy adolescents, while no statistically significant differences were noted for NAA/Cr between the groups. These findings are similar to those reported in adult patients with depression and are suggestive of alterations in cholinergic neurotransmission

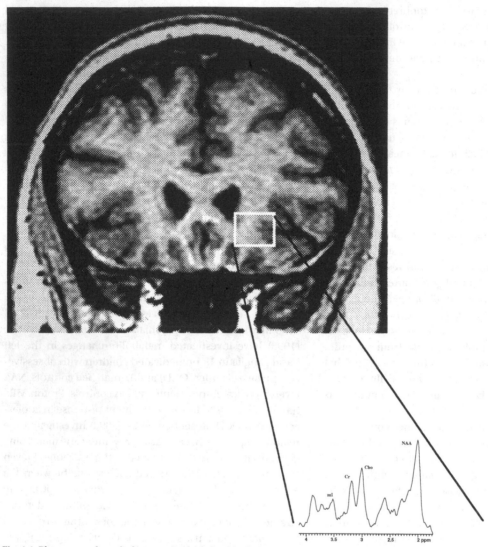

Fig. 4.4. Placement of voxel of interest in the left orbitofrontal cortex (Steingard et al., 1998).

in the orbitofrontal cortex in patients with affective disorders (Charles et al., 1994). An abundant literature exists on the relationship between cholinergic neurotransmission and the expression of clinically significant mood disorders (e.g., as reviewed by Dilsaver (1986) and Fritze (1993)). However, the relationship between cytosolic Cho as detected by ^{1}H MRS and cholinergic activity is by no means direct as Cho is used for multiple purposes within cells and the total cellular Cho pool is quite large.

Phosphorus MRS

Phosphorus-31 MRS has proven useful in the investigation of phosphorus-containing metabolites that are associated with energy and lipid metabolism. With the application of in vivo ^{31}P MRS, detectable phospholipid metabolites include both PME and PDE. As described above, the PME peak consists primarily of PC/PE and metabolites known to be precursors to membrane phospholipid synthesis. The PDE resonance is reflective of breakdown products of membrane phospholipids. Three metabolites are associated with high-energy intracellular metabolism: PCr, P_i, and ATP.

To date, relatively few studies of children and adolescents have utilized ^{31}P MRS. Minshew et al. (1993) used ^{31}P MRS to investigate brain membrane phospholipid and energy metabolism in a region encompassing approximately 15–20 cm^3 of the dorsal prefrontal cortices of 11 adolescents and young adults diagnosed with autism and 11 control subjects matched for age, IQ, race, gender, and socioeconomic status. Subjects in the autistic group demonstrated decreased levels of PCr and esterified ends of ATP, ADP, dinucleotides, and diphosphosugars compared with the control group. The authors hypothesized that this decrease in PCr was likely reflective of an increased utilization of PCr to maintain ATP levels, or a hypermetabolic state (Minshew et al., 1993). Additionally, significant correlations were found for PME, PDE, and PCr levels and measures of cognitive performance. As performance decreased in the autistic subjects, PCr and PME levels fell while PDE levels rose, a pattern that was not detected in the control subjects. The authors concluded that the correlations of phospholipids and declining test performance in autistic subjects were consistent with undersynthesis and enhanced degradation of brain membranes in these subjects.

In a study of children at risk for developing a substance-use disorder, Moss et al. (1997) used CSI (^{31}P MRS) to examine four cortical regions, which included the frontal, occipital, and right and left parietal regions. Subjects at the highest risk for developing this disorder showed a significantly reduced right parietal PDE concentration compared with other voxel locations. In explanation, the authors proposed a heightened degree of right parietal synaptic pruning since the PDE signal is reflective of membrane catabolism.

Moss and Talagala (1997) applied CSI (^{31}P MRS) in a study aimed at examining normal development, with 18 male and 11 female children (mean age 13.4 years), and reported a sex-related difference in the metabolite concentrations of the frontal and occipital lobes (Moss and Talagala, 1997). Male children had a higher concentration of β-NTP in their frontal lobes and lower concentrations in their occipital lobes, while female children showed the reverse pattern. In addition, males had a higher concentration of PDE in their occipital lobes and lower concentrations in frontal lobes (Moss and Talagala, 1997). These results underscore the importance of using age- and sex-matched controls in studies of children and adolescents.

Summary

Interpretation of the findings described above is preliminary because investigations so far have only included small numbers of subjects and results of the spectral data have not been adjusted for the effects of tissue heterogeneity within the brain regions examined. Furthermore, none of the studies utilized absolute quantification of phosphorus or proton metabolites, or adequately determined whether the observed alterations were associated with structural changes in the frontal, parietal, occipital, or subcortical regions. In order to define homogeneous subgroups better within children diagnosed with psychiatric disorders, the

associations between alterations in brain metabolite measures and specific impairments in behavior, neuropsychologic functioning, and clinical symptomatology must be identified. Medication status and duration of illness are important factors in the interpretation of metabolic changes in psychiatric illnesses, although these confounds are minimized in studies of children relative to studies of adults.

Additional studies are needed to examine whether alterations in brain metabolite measures are clinical state or trait markers, and whether they are associated with unique subgroups of patients. Determining how different metabolic alterations relate to specific clinical features and whether these patterns remain stable over the course of development will be an essential part of understanding the pathophysiology underlying the varied clinical presentations.

Neurologic conditions

MRS findings in children with acute or chronic neurologic insults are important because they may clarify the significance of biochemical changes identified in children with psychiatric diagnoses. Furthermore, many etiologic models of psychiatric illness have proposed that multiple neural processes are responsible for the manifestation of psychiatric disorders (Kinney et al., 1994; Brooks et al., 1998). Therefore, metabolite abnormalities, secondary to cortical insults during infancy and in childhood, may represent either risk factors or primary determinants for some behavioral disorders.

In infants, ^{1}H MRS has been useful both as a diagnostic tool and as a predictor of the outcome of injuries sustained. For example, in a study by Holshouser et al. (1997), the outcome of central nervous system (CNS) injury was predicted using ^{1}H MRS in 23 neonates (<1 month), 31 infants (1–18 months), and 28 children (>18 months). A total of 82 patients, all of whom had sustained acute CNS injuries including head injury, hypoxic ischemic encephalopathy, near drowning, and CNS infections, were imaged along with 24 control subjects. Measurements were taken from the occipital region using 8 cm^{3} single-voxel ^{1}H MRS. The authors found that ratios of NAA/Cr were lower in infants and children with poor predicted clinical outcomes, as were ratios of NAA/Cho in neonates and infants with poor predicted clinical outcomes. The reported level of accuracy in prediction of outcome in the neonates was 91%, rising to 100% in the infants and children when ^{1}H MRS and MRI data were combined. This technique may be helpful for clinicians and psychiatrists in predicting clinical outcome of post-CNS injury.

Similar results were found in a study by Auld et al. (1995), who applied single-voxel ^{1}H MRS to examine metabolite ratios in an $8\,cm^3$ area of occipital and parietal white matter in 30 infants with acute CNS injury (mean age 38 ± 52 months). The authors found that the ratios of NAA/Cr and NAA/Cho were significantly lower in the group of infants with poor neurologic outcomes compared with the infants exhibiting good-to-moderate outcomes. Spectroscopic data, including ratios of NAA/Cr, NAA/Cho, and Cho/Cr, correctly classified 81% of patients. The combination of ^{1}H MRS and clinical variables classified all patients into their correct outcome group. These findings suggest that spectroscopic data may be clinically helpful in predicting the neurologic outcome in children who have experienced a neurobiologic insult.

In a study by Lee et al. (1997), ^{1}H MRS was used to examine metabolite ratios of 12 preterm infants, all of a gestational age of 28–35 weeks. Data acquired from parietal white matter was compared with a normal adult spectra. Preterm infants demonstrated lower NAA/Cr ratios and higher Cho/Cr and m-Ino/Cr ratios compared with the adult spectra. Further, the NAA/Cr ratio was found to increase linearly with age, while the m-Ino/Cr ratio decreased linearly with age. The authors concluded that the NAA/Cr ratio increases rapidly during the preterm period when maturation of the brain occurs.

The neurobiologic underpinnings of certain rare childhood diseases have been further clarified through the application of MRS technology. Vucurevic and colleagues (1997) investigated infants with Canavan's and Alexander's diseases, which are typically difficult to differentiate. Both diseases are characterized by megaencephaly and massive leukodystrophy. The study included three patients with Canavan's disease, aged 11, 20, and 21 months, one patient with Alexander's disease, aged 4.5 years, and five normal subjects with a mean age of 5.5 years. It reported an increase in NAA and a decrease in Cho in the subjects with Canavan's disease compared with healthy controls. In the gray matter of the child with Alexander's disease, there was twice the normal amount of NAA and half the amount of Cho; in white matter there was a third less NAA and half the amounts of Cho and Cr (Vucurevic et al., 1997). Although the effects of age have not been fully accounted for in this study, the results highlight the metabolic changes found in the two forms of leukodystrophy.

MRS technology has also been applied to the study of hydrocephalus, another rare childhood disease. Whereas researchers originally hypothesized that the increase in cerebrospinal fluid associated with this disorder produced a decrease in blood flow and a change in energy metabolism, MRS technology has revealed that no metabolic change occurs in this disorder (Bluml et al., 1996). Two other diseases that have been further clarified by the application of MRS technology are adrenoleukodystrophy (Rajanaygam et al., 1997) and Sturge–Weber syndrome (Moore et al., 1996). These diseases, which are progressive, are currently being investigated with ^{1}H MRS. Longitudinal studies will provide objective evidence of the progression and severity of these diseases. Finally, the sensitivity of MRS is illustrated in a study of hypoxic ischemic encephalopathy, where a diagnostic abnormality was detected in the basal ganglia of a 1-day-old infant, whereas structural MR scanning did not detect the abnormality until day 11 (Kim et al., 1998).

Discussion

The interpretation of MR study results must be considered within a neurobiologic framework for understanding psychiatric illness and with an awareness that study methods are often not directly comparable. In general, cortical abnormalities, including MRS findings in psychiatric disorders, are viewed as nonprogressive and are, therefore, interpreted as the result of a neurodevelopmental process (Brooks et al., 1998; Thomas et al., 1998). The direct application of MRS methods to young children and adolescents has allowed this hypothesis to be tested and refined. Future studies will be able to document what brain changes occur in children with schizophrenia *after* the illness, and the extent to which metabolic alteration is associated with treatment. At present the results of cross-sectional brain spectroscopy studies in children have produced promising results, although only a limited number of nuclei and psychiatric diseases have been examined so far.

One important methodologic constraint in interpreting MRS studies is the presence of confounding variables. For example, in studies based on MRI, intracranial volume in patients is frequently compared with that of nonpsychiatric control subjects; however, this comparison is valid only when controls and patients are carefully matched for relevant variables. Significant correlations have been reported between gender and overall head size; consequently, it is necessary to match control subjects and patients for gender. Overall head size has also been correlated with socioeconomic status as well as with level of educational attainment. Studies applying MRS methods will be subject to similar sources of error. Although there has been some dispute regarding these results, matching patients and control subjects for socioeconomic status and educational level when possible is appropriate. Finally, investigators must be cautious in interpreting changes associated with various psychiatric disorders, as there will be abnormalities with etiologic significance and others that may be related to the course of the illness.

Use of adequate sample size and associated statistical power is an important consideration for interpreting past studies as well as in designing new ones. At present, most MRS studies of children with psychiatric illness have been based on small sample size. It is likely that the brain abnormalities in children are subtle, particularly if assessed as a ratio of the concentration of two metabolites. Consequently, the mean differences in regional cerebral metabolites between children with psychiatric disorders and control subjects may well be small relative to the background of normal variation in the general population. In this situation, investigators using small or modest sample sizes risk a high rate of failures to detect true differences between patients and controls.

One important goal of imaging studies is to identify abnormalities central to the development of psychiatric disorders, including the neural substrates of vulnerability or risk factors, as well as the core psychopathology. Identifying brain pathology that distinguishes specific illnesses involves detecting deviances against a background of extensive normal variation in the general population. Given that a considerable portion of this normal variation in brain structure and function results from genetic and other familial factors, choosing appropriate comparison groups to reduce the sources of this normal, familial variance should help to enhance the signal-to-noise ratio. One important comparison group for psychiatric probands is a group of sibling controls of the same sex and similar age. These subjects will reduce multiple familial sources of nonpathologic variance in brain parameters by providing a partial control for genetic sources of variability. Moreover, these subjects control for demographic factors such as race, ethnic background, and parental socioeconomic status, as well as environmental experience.

MR technology, in combination with other brain imaging techniques, offers great promise to the understanding of psychiatric disorders. The clinical utility of MRS studies of children with psychiatric illness has so far been limited as no metabolic findings are diagnostic for a specific illness. Recent findings have related differences in metabolic concentrations to neurobehavioral symptoms, and to treatment response and course of illness in adult psychiatric subjects (D. Yurgelun-Todd, S. Gruber, A. Sherwood, C. Moore, B. Cohen, and P. Renshaw, unpublished data). Similar patterns are beginning to emerge from MRS studies in children. One difficulty with single-voxel spectroscopic studies has been the search for metabolite changes corresponding to a specific location that is presumed to underlie the neuropathology. To address this difficulty, recent investigations have interpreted results in the context of inter-related systems of brain function rather than as isolated focal brain abnormalities.

The application of MRS techniques will facilitate this theoretical perspective, as its noninvasive nature provides the methods necessary for repeated systematic exploration of both brain structure and neurochemistry. Multivoxel methods such as the MRS methods applied by Bertolino (1998) have allowed investigators to examine multiple brain regions simultaneously. The ability to document metabolite changes prospectively will allow investigators to differentiate significant risk factors from CNS changes associated with normal development. In addition, recent techniques have demonstrated that MRS methods may be used to estimate brain concentrations of neurotransmitters. Investigations of this type have been carried out with neurotransmitters such as GABA and glutamate. Proton resonances that arise from GABA and glutamate are difficult to resolve because of their complexity, and spectral editing methods must often be used for this purpose (Keltner et al., 1997; Weber et al., 1997). In addition, the brain concentration of GABA is quite low, approximately 1 mmol/l; consequently, the resonance lines often have limited signal-to-noise ratios at 1.5 T. Although glutamate is present in the brain at much higher concentrations than GABA, only a small fraction of brain glutamate participates in neurotransmission. It is also quite difficult to resolve resonances that arise from glutamate from those that arise from glutamine. Despite these limitations, the increasing availability of high-field MR scanners makes it likely that these methods will be applied to the study of individuals with psychiatric illnesses (Hetherington et al., 1997).

To date, the application of MRS methods to children with psychiatric disorders have been most useful in clarifying processes with etiologic significance in children with schizophrenia. The patterns of decreased NAA concentrations in the dorsolateral prefrontal cortex and mesial temporal lobe have been identified for both adults and children, suggesting a developmental continuum for schizophrenia. The rapid growth in the application of MRI/MRS is beginning to yield new insights into affective illness and OCD. In addition to clarifying the neurobiologic underpinnings of psychiatric illness, MRS methods will ultimately assist in clinical intervention and treatment planning for children with psychiatric disorders.

Acknowledgement

The authors would like to thank Ms Staci Gruber and Ms Norah Janosy for their assistance in preparing this manuscript.

References

Auld, K., Ashwal, S., Holshouser, B. et al., (1995). Proton magnetic resonance spectroscopy in children with acute central nervous system injury. *Pediatr. Neurol.*, **12**, 323–34.

Barker, P., Breiter, S., Soher, B. et al. (1994). Quantitative proton spectroscopy of canine brain: in vivo and in vitro correlations. *Magn. Reson. Med.*, **32**, 157–63.

Bartha, R., Stein, M., Williamson, P. and Drost, D. (1998). Decreased NAA in the left caudate in obsessive-compulsive patients on ^{1}H MRS. *Biol. Psychiatry*, **43**, 9S.

Behar, K., Rothman, D., Spencer, D. and Petroff, O. (1994). Analysis of macromolecule resonances in ^{1}H NMR spectra of human brain. *Magn. Reson. Med.*, **32**, 294–302.

Bertolino, A., Kumra, S., Callicott, J. et al. (1997). Abnormal cortical pattern in early onset schizophrenia as identified by ^{1}H-MRS. [Abstract] In *Proceedings of the 5th Annual Meeting of the International Society for Magnetic Resonance in Medicine*, vol. 2, p. 1227.

Bertolino, A., Callicott, J. H., Elman, I. et al. (1998). Regionally specific neuronal pathology in untreated patients with schizophrenia: a proton magnetic resonance spectroscopic imaging study. *Biol. Psychiatry*, **43**, 641–8.

Birken, D. and Oldendorf, W. (1989). *N*-Acetyl-L-aspartic acid: a literature review of a compound prominent in ^{1}H-NMR spectroscopic studies of the human brain. *Neurosci. Biobehav. Rev.*, **13**, 23–42.

Bloch, F., Jansen, W. W. and Packard, M. E. (1946). *Phys. Rev.* **69**, 127.

Bluml, S., Schad, L. R., Scharf, J., Wenz, F., Knopp, M. V. and Lorenz, W. J. (1996). A comparison of magnetization prepared 3D gradient-echo (MP–RAGE) sequences for imaging of intracranial lesions. *Magn. Reson. Imaging*, **14**, 329–35.

Bottomley, P., Foster, T. and Darrow, R. (1984). Depth-resolved surface coil spectroscopy (DRESS) for in vivo ^{1}H, ^{31}P, and ^{13}C NMR. *J. Magn. Reson.*, **59**, 338–43.

Bovey, F. A., Jelinski, L. and Mirau, P. A. (1988). *Nuclear Magnetic Resonance Spectroscopy*. San Diego, CA: Academic Press.

Brooks, W., Hodde-Vargas, J., Vargas, L., Yeo, R., Ford, C. and Hendren, R. (1998). Frontal lobe of children with schizophrenia spectrum disorders: a proton magnetic resonance spectroscopic study. *Biol. Psychiatry*, **43**, 263–9.

Brown, T., Kincaid, B. and Ugurbil, K. (1982). NMR chemical shift imaging in three dimensions. *Proc. Natl. Acad. Sci. USA*, **79**, 3523–8.

Buchli, R., Duc. C., Martin, E. and Boesiger, P. (1994). Assessment of absolute metabolite concentrations in human tissue by ^{31}P MRS in vivo. Part I: cerebrum, cerebellum, cerebral gray matter and white matter. *Magn. Reson. Med.*, **32**, 447–54.

Buckley, P. (1998). Magnetic resonance spectroscopy and aberrant neurodevelopment. *Biol. Psychiatry*, **43**, 61S.

Charles, H., Lazeyras, F., Krishnan, K. et al. (1994). Proton spectroscopy of human brain: effects of age and sex. *Prog. Neuropsychopharmacol. Biol. Psychiatry*, **18**, 995–1004.

Christensen, J., Babb, S., Cohen, B. and Renshaw, P. (1998).

Quantitation of dexfenfluramine/norfenfluramine in primate brain using ^{19}F NMR spectroscopy. *Magn. Reson. Med.*, **39**, 149–54.

Diklic, V. and Gambarelli, D. (1998). ^{1}H MR spectroscopy in twins discordant for late-infantile neuronal ceroid lipofuscinosis. In *Proceedings of the 6th Annual Meeting of the International Society for Magnetic Resonance in Medicine*, vol. 3, p. 1745.

Dilsaver, S. C. (1986). Cholinergic mechanisms in depression. *Brain Res.*, **396**, 285–316.

Ende, G., Knowlton, R., Laxer, K., Matson, G. and Weiner, M. (1996). NAA is a more sensitive marker of hippocampal disease than atrophy: evidence that NAA is a neuronal marker. In *Proceedings of the 4th Annual Meeting of the International Society for Magnetic Resonance in Medicine*, vol. 1, p. 137.

Fritze, J. (1993). The adrenergic–cholinergic imbalance hypothesis of depression: a review and a perspective. *Rev. Neurosci.*, **4**, 63–93.

Gadian, D., Isaacs, E., Cross, J. et al. (1996). Lateralization of brain function in childhood revealed by MR spectroscopy. *Neurology*, **46**, 974–7.

Haseler, L., Arcinue, E., Danielsen, E. S. B. and Ross, B. (1997). Evidence from proton magnetic resonance spectroscopy for a metabolic cascade of neuronal damage in shaken baby syndrome. *Pediatrics*, **99**, 4–14.

Hendren, R., Hodde-Vargas, J., Yeo, R., Vargas, L., Brooks, W. and Ford, C. (1995). Neuropsychophysiological study of children at risk for schizophrenia: a preliminary report. *J. Am. Acad. Child Adolesc. Psychiatry*, **34**, 1284–91.

Hetherington, H. P., Pan, J. W., Chu, W. J., Mason, G. F. and Newcomer, B. R. (1997). Biological and clinical MRS at ultra-high field. *NMR Biomed.*, **10**, 360–71.

Holshouser, B., Ashwal, S., Luh, G., Shu, S., Tomasi, L. and Hinshaw, D. (1997). ^{1}H-MR spectroscopy in predicting neurologic outcomes in children with acute CNS injury. In *Proceedings of the 5th Annual Meeting of the International Society for Magnetic Resonance in Medicine*, vol. 2, p. 1229.

Jacobsen, L. K., Hong, W. L., Hommer, D. W. (1996). Smooth pursuit eye movements in childhood-onset schizophrenia: comparison with attention-deficit hyperactivity disorder and normal controls. *Biol. Psychiatry*, **40**, 1144–54.

Jensen, H., Plenge, P., Stensgaard, A. et al. (1996). Twelve-hour brain lithium concentration in lithium maintenance treatment of manic-depressive disorder: daily versus alternate-day dosing schedule. *Psychopharmacology*, **124**, 275–8.

Keltner, J. R., Wald, L. L., Frederick, B. D. and Renshaw, P. F. (1997). In vivo detection of GABA in human brain using localized double-quantum filter technique. *Magn. Reson. Med.*, **37**, 366–71.

Kim, K., Lee, J., Kim, S., Pi, S., Auh, Y. and Lim, T. (1997). Early detection of abnormality for hypoxic ischemic encephalopathy (HIE) infant by localized in vivo ^{1}H MR spectroscopy. In *Proceedings of the 5th Annual Meeting of the International Society for Magnetic Resonance in Medicine*, vol. 2, p. 1237.

Kim, K., Pi, S., Kim, E. et al. (1998). Localized ^{1}H MR spectroscopy as early predictor for outcome in infants with birth asphyxia. In

Proceedings of the 6th Annual Meeting of the Society for Magnetic Resonance in Medicine, vol. 1, p. 95.

Kinney, D., Yurgelun-Todd, D., Waternaux, C. and Matthysse, S. (1994). Obstetrical complications and trail making deficits discriminate schizophrenics from unaffected siblings and controls. *Schizophr. Res.*, **12**, 63–73.

Komoroski, R., Newton, J., Karson, C., Cardwell, D. and Sprigg, J. (1991). Detection of psychoactive drugs in vivo using ^{19}F NMR spectroscopy. *Biol. Psychiatry*, **29**, 711–16.

Kreis, R., Suter, D. and Ernst, R. R. (1985). Time-domain zero-field magnetic resonance with field pulse excitation. *Chem. Phys. Lett.*, **118**, 120–4.

Krishnan, R. and Doraiswamy, P. (eds.) (1997). *Brain Imaging in Clinical Psychiatry*. New York: M. Dekker.

Lee, J., Kim, K., Kim, S., Pi, S., Auh, Y. and Lim, T. (1997). Metabolic changes of normal neonatal brain during the preterm period by localized ^{1}H in vivo MR spectroscopy. In *Proceedings of the 5th Annual Meeting of the International Society for Magnetic Resonance in Medicine*, vol. 2, p. 1173.

Li, Q., Pu, Y., Luo, D., Zeng, C., Gao, J. and Gao, J. (1998). An MRS study in newborn infants with hypoxic-ischemic encephalopathy. In *Proceedings of the 6th Annual Meeting of the International Society for Magnetic Resonance in Medicine*, vol. 3, p. 1738.

Lim, K., Adalsteinsson, E., Spielman, D., Sullivan, E., Rosenbloom, M. and Pfefferbaum, A. (1998). Proton magnetic resonance spectroscopic imaging of cortical gray and white matter in schizophrenia. *Arch. Gen. Psychiatry*, **55**, 346–52.

Lu, D., Pavelakis, S., Frank, Y. et al. (1996). Proton MR spectroscopy of the basal ganglia in healthy children and children with AIDS. *Radiology*, **199**, 423–8.

Luyten, P., Bruntink, G., Sloff, F. et al. (1989). Broadband proton decoupling in human ^{31}P NMR spectroscopy. *NMR Biomed.*, **1**, 177–83.

Mason, G. F., Behar, K. L. and Lai, J. C. (1996). The ^{13}C isotope and nuclear magnetic resonance: unique tools for the study of brain metabolism. *Metab. Brain Dis.*, **11**, 283–313.

Miller, B. (1991). A review of chemical issues in ^{1}H NMR spectroscopy: *N*-acetyl aspartate, creatine, and choline. *NMR Biomed.*, **4**, 47–54.

Miner, C., Davidson, J., Potts, N., Tupler, L., Charles, H. and Krishnan, K. (1995). Brain fluoxetine measurements using fluorine magnetic resonance spectroscopy in patients with social phobia. *Biol. Psychiatry*, **38**, 696–8.

Minshew, N., Goldstein, G., Dombrowski, S., Panchalingam, K. and Pettegrew, J. (1993). A preliminary ^{31}P MRS study of autism: evidence for undersynthesis and increased degradation of brain membranes. *Biol. Psychiatry*, **33**, 762–73.

Moonen, C., von Kiellin, M., van Zijl, P., Cohen, J., Gillen, J. and Daly, P. (1989). Comparison of single-shot localization methods (STEAM and PRESS) for in vivo proton NMR spectroscopy. *NMR Biomed.*, **2**, 101–12.

Moore, C., Christensen, J., Lafer, B., Fava, M. and Renshaw, P. (1997). Decreased adenosine trophosphate in the basal ganglia of depressed subjects: a phosphorous-31 magnetic resonance spcctroscopy study. *Am. J. Psychiatry*, **154**, 116–18.

Moore, C., Breeze, J., Kukes, T. et al. (1999). Effects of myo-inositol ingestion on human brain myo-inositol levels: a proton magnetic resonance spectroscopic imaging study. *Biol. Psychiatry*, **45**, 1197–202.

Moore, G., Slovis, T. and Chugani, H. (1996). Proton MRS of Sturge–Weber syndrome in children. In *Proceedings of the 4th Annual Meeting of the International Society for Magnetic Resonance in Medicine*, 1996; **2**, 968.

Moss, H. and Talagala, S. (1997). ^{31}P magnetic resonance spectroscopy of normal peripubertal children: effects of sex and fronto-occipital location. In *Proceedings of the 5th Annual Meeting of the International Society for Magnetic Resonance in Medicine*, vol. 2, p. 1219.

Moss, H., Talagala, S. and Kirisci, L. (1997). Phosphorus-31 magnetic resonance brain spectroscopy of children at risk for a substance use disorder: preliminary results. *Psychiatr. Res. Neuroimaging*, **76**, 101–12.

Mukherji, S. (ed.) (1998). *Clinical Applications of Magnetic Resonance Spectroscopy*. New York: Wiley-Liss.

Murphy-Boesch, J., Stoyanova, R., Srinivasan, R. et al. (1993). Proton-decoupled ^{31}P chemical shift imaging of the human brain in normal volunteers. *NMR Biomed.*, **6**, 173–80.

Ogg, R., Kingsley, P. and Taylor, J. (1994). WET, a T_1- and B_1-insensitive water suppression method for in vivo localized ^{1}H NMR spectroscopy. *J. Magn. Reson. Ser. B*, **104**, 1–10.

Ordidge, R., Connelly, A. and Lohman, J. (1986). Image selective in vivo spectroscopy (ISIS). A new technique for spatially selective NMR spectroscopy. *J. Magn. Reson.*, **60**, 281–3.

Petroff, O., Spencer, D., Alger, J. and Prichard, J. (1989). High-field proton magnetic resonance spectroscopy of human cerebrum obtained during surgery for epilepsy. *Neurology*, **39**, 1197–201.

Pettegrew, J., Keshavan, M., Panchalingham, K. et al. (1991). Alterations in brain high energy phosphate metabolism in first episode, drug naive schizophrenics. *Arch. Gen. Psychiatry*, **48**, 563–8.

Pouwels, P. and Frahm, J. (1998). Regional metabolite concentrations in human brain as determined by quantitative localized proton MRS. *Magn. Reson. Med.*, **39**, 53–60.

Purcell, E. M., Torrey, H. C. and Pound, R. V. (1946). *Phys. Rev.*, **69**, 37.

Rae, C., Scott, R., Lee, M., Hines, N., Paul, C. and Styles, P. (1998). Human brain bioenergetics relate to cognitive ability. In *Proceedings of the 6th Annual Meeting of the International Society for Magnetic Resonance in Medicine*, vol. 3, p. 1743.

Rajanaygam, V., Shapiro, E., Krivit, W., Lockman, L. and Stillman, A. (1997). Childhood adrenoleukodystrophy: an MRS scale to measure disease severity. In *Proceedings of the 5th Annual Meeting of the International Society for Magnetic Resonance in Medicine*, vol. 2, p. 1193.

Renshaw, P. and Wicklund, S. (1998). In vivo measurement of lithium in man by nuclear magnetic resonance spectroscopy. *Biol. Psychiatry*, **23**, 465–72.

Renshaw, P., Guimaraes, A., Fava, M. et al. (1992). Accumulation of fluoxetine and norfluoxetine in human brain during therapeutic administration. *Am. J. Psychiatry*, **149**, 1592–4.

Renshaw, P., Yurgelun-Todd, D., Tohen, M., Gruber, S. and Cohen, B. (1995). Temporal lobe proton magnetic resonance spectroscopy of patients with first-episode psychosis. *Am. J. Psychiatry*, **152**, 444–6.

Renshaw, P., Lafer, B., Babb, S. et al. (1997). Basal ganglia choline levels in depression and response to fluoxetine treatment: an in vivo proton magnetic resonance spectroscopy study. *Biol. Psychiatry*, **41**, 837–43.

Riedl, U., Barocka, A., Kolem, H. et al. (1997). Duration of lithium treatment and brain lithium concentration in patients with unipolar and schizoaffective disorder – a study with magnetic resonance spectroscopy. *Biol. Psychiatry*, **41**, 844–50.

Rosenberg, D., MacMaster, F., Parrish, J. et al. (1998). ^{1}H MRS caudate glutamatergic changes with paroxetine therapy for pediatric obsessive compulsive disorder. *Biol. Psychiatry*, **43**, 24S.

Sachs, G., Renshaw, P., Lafer, B. et al. (1995). Variability of brain lithium levels during maintenance treatment: a magnetic resonance spectroscopy study. *Biol. Psychiatry*, **38**, 422–8.

Soares, J., Krishnan, K. and Keshavan, M. (1996). Nuclear magnetic resonance spectroscopy: new insights into the pathophysiology of mood disorders. *Depression*, **4**, 14–30.

Steingard, R., Renshaw, P., Yurgelun-Todd, D. and Wald, L. (1998). Proton MRS studies of the orbitofrontal cortex of depressed adolescents. *Biol. Psychiatry*, **43**, 28S.

Strauss, W., Layton, M., Hayes, C. and Dager, S. (1997). ^{19}F magnetic resonance spectroscopy investigation in vivo of acute and steady-state brain fluvoxamine levels in obsessive-compulsive disorder. *Am. J. Psychiatry*, **154**, 516–22.

Strauss, W., Layton, M. and Dager, S. (1998). Brain elimination half-life of fluvoxamine measured by ^{19}F magnetic resonance spectroscopy. *Am. J. Psychiatry*, **155**, 380–4.

Thomas, M., Ke, Y., Caplan, R. et al. (1996). Frontal lobe ^{1}H MR spectroscopy of children with schizophrenia. In *Proceedings of the 4th Annual Meeting of the International Society for Magnetic Resonance in Medicine*, vol. 2, p. 1000.

Thomas, M., Ke, Y., Levitt, J. et al. (1998). Preliminary study of frontal lobe ^{1}H MR spectroscopy in childhood onset schizophrenia. *J. Magn. Res. Imaging*, **8**, 841–6.

Tsai, G. and Coyle, J. (1995). *N*-Acetylaspartate in neuropsychiatric disorders. *Prog. Neurobiol.*, **46**, 531–69.

Tyson, R., Sutherland, G. and Peeling, J. (1996). ^{23}Na nuclear magnetic resonance spectral changes during and after forebrain ischemia in hypoglycemic, normoglycemic, and hyperglycemic rats. *Stroke*, **27**, 957–64.

Tzika, A., Ball, W., Vigneron, D., Dunn, R., Nelson, S. and Kriks, D. (1993). Childhood adrenoleukodystrophy: assessment with proton MR spectroscopy. *Radiology*, **189**, 467–80.

van der Grond, J., Groenendaal, F. and de Vries, L. (1998). Prognosis of neurodevelopment in full-term neonates with hypoxia-ischemia, using cerebral ^{1}H MRS with different echo times. In *Proceedings of the 6th Annual Meeting of the International Society for Magnetic Resonance in Medicine*, vol. 3, p. 1734.

Vucurevic, G., Lucic, M., Ivanovic, V. et al. (1997). Possible discrimination between Canavan's and Alexander's disease with localized ^{1}H MRS. In *Proceedings of the 5th Annual Meeting of the International Society for Magnetic Resonance in Medicine*, vol. 2, p. 1205.

Weber, O. M., Trabesinger, A. H., Duc, C. O., Meier, D. and Boesiger, P. (1997). Detection of hidden metabolites by localized proton magnetic resonance spectroscopy in vivo. *Technol. Health Care*, **5**, 471–91.

Witelson, S. F. (1985). The brain connection: the corpus callosum is larger in left-handers. *Science*, **229**, 665–8.

Yurgelun-Todd, D. A., Renshaw, P. F., Gruber, S. A., Ed, M., Waternaux, C. and Cohen, B. M. (1996). Proton magnetic resonance spectroscopy of the temporal lobes in schizophrenics and normal controls. *Schizophr. Res.*, **19**, 55–9.

5

Magnetoencephalography

Donald C. Rojas, Peter D. Teale and Martin L. Reite

Introduction

Although the magnetic fields produced by peripheral nerve action potentials were recorded as early as 1960, the first noninvasive magnetic recordings from the human central nervous system were not performed until late in that decade. David Cohen recorded the first magnetoencephalogram (MEG) in 1968 at the Massachusetts Institute of Technology. Using a one-million turn copper coil in a magnetically shielded room and averaging 2500 samples triggered by a simultaneous electroencephalography (EEG) recording, Cohen (1968) was able to demonstrate evidence of magnetic oscillatory activity in the alpha band in four subjects. Subsequent work in the field of MEG was aided tremendously by the application of superconducting technology, which allowed the recording of spontaneous alpha activity without the use of signal averaging (Cohen, 1972).

From those first years of single-channel, homemade MEG instruments, the field of neuromagnetism has evolved into one of the multichannel recording devices with whole-head sensor coverage. This fact, combined with a larger installed base of MEG systems and increasing sophistication in data analysis techniques, has allowed MEG to take its place in the modern functional neuroimaging community as a technology that has enormous potential for application to psychiatric and neurologic illnesses. In the first 10 years after the seminal Cohen paper, fewer than 25 papers were published on the topic of MEG, but over 800 articles have been published in the last 10 years alone, testament to the rapid growth of the field in the three decades since its inception. Fewer than 15 of those publications, however, deal with the subject of MEG in psychiatry, and none of those articles has studied mentally ill children. (Data obtained with an online *Index Medicus* search from 1966 to present with keywords *magnetoen-* *cephalography, biomagnetism, neuromagnetism, magnetic source imaging,* and *neuromagnetic,* excluding references to *magnetocardiography.*) Therefore although the potential for the application of MEG to problems in child psychiatry is vast, nothing has yet been published on psychiatric disorders apart from a scattering of articles on adult psychiatric patients and most clinical applications of the technology lent toward neurologic disorders such as epilepsy.

Rationale for MEG in pediatric neuroimaging

All currently popular functional neuroimaging strategies have advantages and disadvantages, which taken together argue strongly for their combined use in illuminating brain function. However, given the choice of only one imaging modality, MEG is a good choice as it can provide extremely fine temporal resolution (less than a millisecond) and reasonable spatial resolution (0.5–1.0 cm) within the same recording, which makes it fairly unique among the various imaging strategies. Along with EEG, magnetic recordings provide temporal resolution that, to date, is only constrained by the speed at which the data are sampled by the acquisition hardware and software and by data-storage requirements. For example, a single channel of MEG or EEG data sampled at 1 kHz produces approximately 2 kilobytes of data per second (a 10 min recording of 100 simultaneous channels at the same rate would require at least 120 megabytes of storage capacity). Temporal resolutions of 1 ms or less are commonly seen in both EEG and MEG, but theoretically there are no real physical limitations on the technology, only practical concerns and the limitations imposed by the temporal characteristics of the neuronal activity. This resolving capability is considerably better than those typically achieved with blood-flow techniques such as positron emission tomography (PET), single photon emission computed tomography (SPECT), and functional magnetic resonance imaging (fMRI). Even the high-speed MRI techniques like echo-planar imaging are only currently capable of approximately 40 ms temporal resolution, and they can achieve that resolution through a trade-off in lower signal-to-noise ratios (SNR) (Aine, 1995). As neurophysiologic events occur in the millisecond and sub-millisecond time domain, only EEG and MEG can currently image those events noninvasively as they evolve in real time (George et al., 1995).

Although it can be argued that the spatial resolutions of PET, SPECT, and fMRI are somewhat superior to MEG and EEG, the issue is complicated. The nominal spatial resolution of MRI, unlike the other techniques, is dependent only on the size of the voxels, which is defined a priori by the investigator (Wood, 1992). However, finer spatial resolution in MRI generally results in lower SNR. Currently, most fMRI studies use voxel sizes between 3.75 mm by 3.75 mm by 5–10 mm for the functional image sequence, which is still nominally better than all the other imaging modalities. Some groups report adequate functional activation maps using 3–4 mm^3 voxels on 1.5 T machines. Blood oxygenation level-dependent (BOLD) fMRI, however, may erroneously locate the source of neural activity because of its tendency to image the larger venules, rather than the capillaries, particularly when gradient-recalled echo sequences are employed (Turner and Jezzard, 1994; Sanders and Orrison, 1995). Techniques of fMRI are discussed further in Chapter 3.

Spatial resolution in PET, SPECT, EEG, and MEG, by comparison, is determined by a variety of other factors, foremost among them the SNR (Aine, 1995), which, unlike for MRI, may not be directly controlled by the investigator. Under optimal recording conditions, the error bounds for spatial accuracy of these four imaging techniques are quite comparable (0.5 to 1 cm in all dimensions, with PET at the lower end and EEG and MEG at the higher end of that range (Cohen et al., 1990; Cohen and Cuffin, 1991; Cuffin, 1991; Mosher et al., 1993; Gharib et al., 1995; Krasuski, 1996)). MEG, EEG, and SPECT, however, tend to be less spatially accurate for deeper neuronal sources/structures and are, therefore, generally better suited to recording from shallower, cortical neuronal populations if higher spatial accuracy is desired (Hari et al., 1988; Kullmann, 1993; Gharib et al., 1995; Murro et al., 1995; Krasuski et al., 1996; Braun, 1997).

Of critical concern when children are involved as subjects in neuroimaging procedures is the degree of invasiveness and discomfort. By definition, because of the need to inject radioactive tracers into the bloodstream of the subject prior to imaging, SPECT and PET are more invasive than the other functional neuroimaging modalities, and

their use in children is severely limited (Krasuski et al., 1996). EEG, MEG, and fMRI do not have this disadvantage. Functional MRI is almost certainly more unpleasant for younger subjects than for adults because of the extremely loud noises produced by the magnet (approximately 95 dB sound pressure level (SPL) at the subject's ears in some scanners) and the confinement within the bore of the magnet itself. EEG and MEG recordings do not produce any sound at all, and both can be performed in nonconfining spaces. These two procedures will be compared in greater detail later in the chapter; however, in our experience, MEG is more comfortable for children than EEG since it does not involve scalp abrasion, which is particularly bothersome in studies using high sensor densities. MEG, therefore, provides high temporal resolution and moderate spatial resolution in a relatively comfortable, nonthreatening environment, characteristics that should make it ideal for use in child psychiatry.

Neurophysiologic and neuroanatomic basis of MEG signals

Generation of magnetic fields by electric current

College physics textbooks contain the basic facts of electromagnetism necessary for a conceptual understanding of the basis of neuromagnetic signals. Magnetic fields are generated by current (Ampère's law) and emerge from their source at the speed of light. The direction of the magnetic field is perpendicular to the direction of current flow. This is described easily by the "right-hand rule" (see Fig. 5.1).

Neuronal architectural basis for the externally recorded magnetic field

Just as a length of current carrying wire produces a magnetic field, so do neurons in the brain and spinal cord (as well as other electrically active cells such as muscle). In this case, the moving charges are entire ions instead of just electrons, and as they move across the cell membrane, within, and outside the cell, they produce magnetic fields in the same way as in the wire example. The contribution of action potentials to the externally measured magnetic fields of the brain is probably minimal, since action potentials produce quadrupolar fields which fall off rapidly with the cube of the distance from the source to the detector. The intraneuronal currents, which produce dipolar fields that fall off more gradually with the square of the distance, likely contribute the majority of the externally measureable field (Okada et al., 1987, 1997).

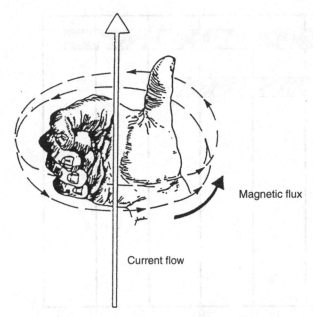

Magnetic flux

Current flow

Fig. 5.1. The right-hand rule of magnetism. If a length of wire is grasped in the right hand with the thumb pointing in the direction of current flow, the fingers wrapped around the wire represent the direction of the magnetic field lines. (With permission from Reeve et al., 1989.)

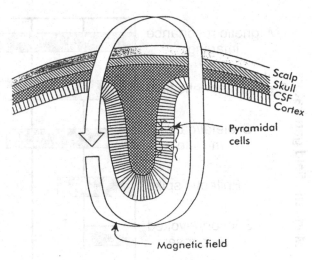

Scalp
Skull
CSF
Cortex
Pyramidal cells
Magnetic field

Fig. 5.3. Source orientation differences in sulcal and gyral cortex. The apical dendrites of pyramidal neurons are oriented approximately normal to the surface of the cortex, which because it folds produces gross differences in source orientations to the scalp and MEG detectors. CSF, cerebrospinal fluid. (With permission from Lewine and Orrison, 1995c.)

Anatomic considerations

One critical constraint on the detectable magnetic fields of the brain is the orientation of the current flow in the volume. In a spherical volume, a source oriented radially to the detector produces no measureable magnetic field (Williamson and Kaufman, 1990; Hamalainen et al., 1993). Even in a nonspherical conductor such as the head, radial sources produce little external magnetic field (Cuffin, 1990). Therefore, MEG is only sensitive to sources oriented tangentially (Fig. 5.2, p. 82). Given that the most superficially located of the largest cortical dendrites (the apical trees of the pyramidal cells) are perpendicular to the surface of the cortex, sulcal cortex is the most likely to contain tangentially oriented cells/sources (Fig. 5.3). This can be viewed as both a disadvantage and an advantage. While it limits the amount of cortex "visible" to MEG, this also allows for greater certainty about the location of source activity. In addition, most primary sensory regions of the brain lie within the sulcal folds of the brain, at least in the visual, auditory, and somatosensory systems. In theory, combined with EEG, which does not have the same orientation sensitivity, subtractive logic could also allow researchers to separate simultaneously active sources with a greater degree of certainty. The comparison of MEG and EEG is discussed below.

Instrumentation and data analysis

Recording environment

The magnetic fields generated by typical currents in the human brain are very small relative to the earth's own magnetic field (Fig. 5.4). In most cases, therefore, it is necessary to conduct neuromagnetic studies inside magnetically shielded environments. Shielded rooms typically consist of multiple layers of eddy-current and ferromagnetic shielding, most often of aluminum and μ-metal (a nickel–iron alloy), respectively. In addition, a strategy termed "shaking" is also sometimes employed, which denotes the application of a strong 60 Hz field to the ferromagnetic layers to increase the magnetic permeability of the layer to other frequencies (Cohen, 1970). Shielding factors of 35 to 50 dB at below 0.1 Hz are common in such rooms (Hamalainen et al., 1993). Today, magnetically shielded rooms suitable for MEG recordings are available from several commercial manufacturers (e.g., Vacuumshmelze GmbH, Amuneal Manufacturing Corp., Sumitomo Metal Industries Ltd.), although some research groups, such as our own, still use custom-built rooms (typical commercial room cost is approximately US$0.5 million). Another strategy for noise reduction, the use of gradiometer sensor configurations, is discussed below.

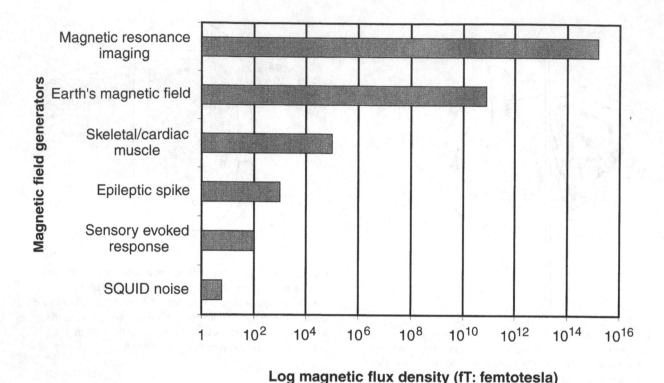

Fig. 5.4. Magnetic field strengths of biological and environmental sources. Note the log scaling of the *x* axis.

Superconducting quantum interference device

Although Cohen's original MEG recording was performed with a room temperature device, practical MEG recordings currently require the use of superconducting electronics to detect the weak fields of the human brain. The only available detector sensitive and reliable enough to detect these fields is the superconducting quantum interference device (SQUID). A low inductance coil (the "sensors" in MEG, analogous to EEG electrodes) positioned near the head is inductively coupled to a SQUID. The SQUID is cooled to 4 K (or −269 °C) by submersion in a thermally shielded dewar (i.e., a specially constructed "thermos" with a vacuum space) containing liquid helium. Some of the newest SQUIDS are capable of operating at liquid nitrogen temperature (77 K) and are known as high-temperature devices (Zhang et al., 1993a, b), but they do not currently have the sensitivities required for recording from the brain and are, therefore, not in wide use. Electronic refrigeration systems have also been tried with very limited success with SQUID systems. At present the liquid helium cryogenic systems still remain the industry standard.

Sensor geometries

The issues of noise (i.e., nonspecific brain signal combined with nonbrain noise) reduction and sensitivity described in the previous two sections also relate directly to the geometric configuration of the flux transformers, or sensors. Several different configurations are currently in use around the world, and each has its own particular advantages and disadvantages. The simplest configuration for magnetic field recordings is the magnetometer, a coil of wire typically made of niobium (Fig. 5.5a). Magnetometers are the most sensitive to magnetic flux of the various types of sensors but as a direct consequence are also sensitive to noise from nonneural sources. As a result, gradiometer configurations (Fig. 5.5b–d) are often adopted for noise cancellation.

The first-order axial gradiometer (Fig. 5.5b) consists of a lower coil called a pickup coil and an upper coil called a compensation coil that is wound in the opposite direction and connected in series. This system is designed so that only differences (gradients) between the coils will be amplified. Consequently, configuration is quite sensitive to nearby field sources, since the high falloff rate for magnetic fields produces a large difference between the two coils. It discriminates effectively against distant (noise) sources, since they will produce a more uniform field at the two

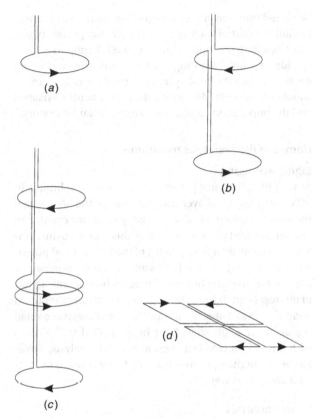

Fig. 5.5. Different geometric configurations of coils:
(*a*) magnetometer, (*b*) first-order axial gradiometer, (*c*) second-order axial gradiometer, (*d*) off-diagonal planar gradiometer, which samples two orthogonal planar gradients (i.e., it is a two-channel device). The arrows indicate directions of winding for coils.

coils. The distance between the pickup coil and the compensation coil is called the baseline and is typically 4–5 cm in most systems.

For even greater noise cancellation, second-order or higher gradiometers may be formed. The second-order configuration shown in Fig. 5.5*c* essentially consists of two first-order gradiometers connected in opposition, which results in even stronger rejection of distant sources. It is important to remember, however, that although distant sources are often unwanted noise (i.e., nonbrain), deeper brain sources are also increasingly discriminated against as higher-order gradiometers are formed, and this is typically seen as a necessary tradeoff in MEG recordings, particularly in noisier environments such as hospitals.

Figure 5.5*d* illustrates a planar, or "figure eight" configured, gradiometer (also called a double D, when the opposing coils are "D" shaped rather than circular). This configuration results in maximal signals being recorded directly over the current source, rather than to each side as

with the axial geometries discussed previously. This has great intuitive appeal when interpreting the underlying current sources of a given magnetic field distribution, particularly when using systems with a small number of sensors. The Neuromag Ltd. MEG systems employ this sensor configuration in their commercial designs, while those of Canadian Thin Films (CTF) Systems and Biomagnetic Technologies Inc. (BTi) rely on various axial configurations. It also has a significant cost advantage over axial systems, since the planar geometry lends itself well to modern thin-film manufacturing techniques.

As digital signal processor technology has evolved, the use of computers to form higher-order-gradients from signals recorded with lower-order sensors has dramatically improved. In these systems, reference sensors are placed some distance from the pickup coils to measure distant source, or noise, activity. Then, either on- or offline, the data acquisition software computes the desired higher-order gradient. CTF Systems was first to use this strategy in their MEG systems, where second- and third-order gradients can be computed from magnetometers or first-order gradiometers. This strategy has two desirable features. First, it allows for extremely sensitive geometries to be employed in the recording while also allowing for good noise cancellation. Second, in some relatively magnetically quiet environments, MEG recordings can be performed in unshielded or poorly shielded rooms (Fig. 5.6).

Sensor arrays

Instrumentation in MEG has evolved significantly since the early 1980s from single channel neuromagnetometer systems to large, high-density whole-head arrays. Several manufacturers (CTF, BTi, Neuromag Ltd.) are currently offering a variety of systems. Figures 5.7 and 5.8 illustrate two generations of MEG systems.

Large arrays like the whole-head systems from each company offer the considerable advantages of patient comfort, short data acquisition times, and simultaneous multisite recordings over the smaller array systems, which must be repositioned multiple times during an experiment to provide similar coverage. These systems are configured with approximately 150 or more sensors around a helmet designed to fit a large number of head sizes (Fig. 5.9). Three caveats to the helmet-based systems exist. First, since they are typically designed to accommodate some percentile of adult head sizes (approximately the 98th percentile of head sizes for the BTi instrument; personal communication to author), some people will not fit well into the helmets. This may be particularly troublesome for studies of individuals with abnormally large heads, such as those with autism

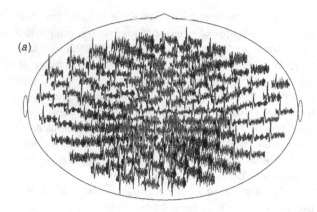

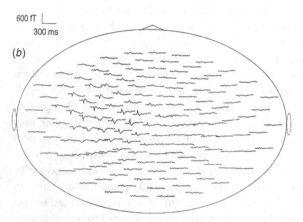

Fig. 5.6. Higher-order gradient formation and recording in unshielded environments. The data illustrate a 100-trial, averaged somatosensory evoked field (SEF) produced from stimulation of the right median nerve. Data were collected with the CTF 143-channel whole-head MEG system configured with first-order gradiometers: (*a*) first-order averaged data (as collected); (*b*) synthetic third-order gradient reconstructed from the lower-order gradiometers (noise cancellation). Note the prominence of the SEF response over the left parietal regions of the image. (Courtesy of Canadian Thin Films, Ltd.)

and fragile X disorder (Davidovitch et al., 1996; Woodhouse et al., 1996; Lainhart et al., 1997). Second, none of the current generation of helmet systems allows for complete coverage of the face, which may be important for recording some brain activities (particularly if the magnetic field extrema were seen over the face). Third, fetal MEG recordings would be nearly impossible on such systems, since the mother's abdomen could not fit into the helmet (specially designed abdominal units are being developed, however). Similarly, infant and nonhuman animal recordings might be extremely difficult because the subject's heads would be too small, leading to large distances between the head and detectors. (However, Fig. 5.10 shows how a young child can

be placed into one of the current generation instruments.) Finally, the cost of such systems is currently prohibitive to most researchers (approximately US$2.0 million with a shielded room). Taken together, the strengths and weaknesses of whole-head versus partial-coverage arrays should be considered based on the experiments envisaged and the populations of interest to a particular laboratory.

Common data analysis techniques

Signal averaging

As with EEG, the most common data analysis technique in MEG involves signal averaging to improve the SNR. When the signal is time-locked to a sensory or motor event, and several hundred trials are averaged, this produces the commonly seen evoked field (analog of the EEG evoked potential; see Fig. 5.11). As with EEG, signal averaging is generally regarded as the sine qua non for extracting neural signals of interest (signal) from the ongoing activity in other brain regions (noise). Other techniques for extracting these small signals from single trials have been applied to EEG data with limited success (e.g., neural network analysis, wavelets, etc.) but their promise is slowly being realized in MEG data analysis as well.

Source analysis

In MEG, as in EEG, in order to understand the relationship between the measured data and the actual neurophysiology of the brain, one must have a model of how one is produced by the other. For MEG and EEG, the most commonly applied model is the single equivalent current dipole (ECD; see also anatomic considerations, above, and Fig. 5.2). As previously described, intraneuronal current flow in the dendritic tree of a single neuron produces a dipolar magnetic field distribution (at least when measured some distance away from the source). Similarly, a small region of tissue with parallel dendritic trees produces a superposition of the dipolar fields generated by the individual neurons. Therefore, the *equivalent* part of the ECD model indicates that the single ECD really represents the superimposed activity of many individual dipoles.

The current dipole in the ECD model is characterized as a short length (L) of current (I), and the strength of the dipole, Q, is the product of length and current ($Q = IL$, in ampere-meters). The magnetic field B (in SI units of tesla) produced by Q at any given point in space is described by:

$$B = \frac{\mu_0 Q \sin \psi}{4\pi r^2}$$

where μ_0 is the permeability of free space, ψ is the angle between field point and current, and r is the distance to the

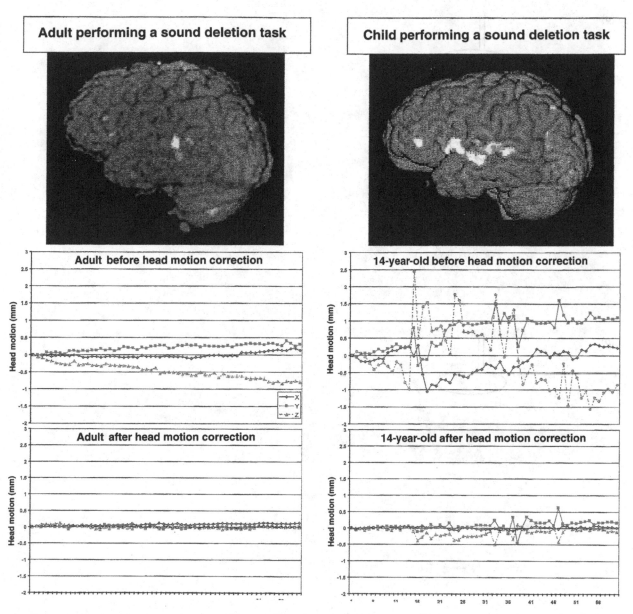

Fig. 3.2. Feasibility of fMRI studies in pediatric populations. Task-related signal change in a child and in an adult during a phonologic awareness task. The graphs show the amount of head motion generated in both individuals and correction after processing of the data.

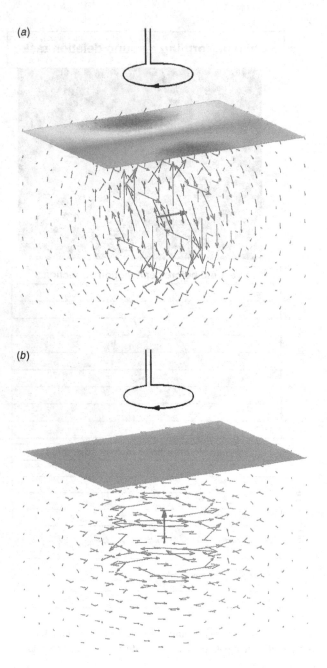

Fig. 5.2. Magnetic field distribution to a current dipole in a homogeneous conductor. Vector plots of the magnetic fields to tangential (*a*) and radial (*b*) orientations of a current dipole to the detector are shown. The length of the arrows is proportional to the field amplitude (high field amplitudes near the source have been left out for overall figure clarity). Contour plots of the sampled field distributions in a single plane are also shown (measurements made normal to the surface and outside of conductor). Red indicates outgoing field and blue the in-going field. Note that the magnetic fields of the radially oriented dipole close inside the conductor; this produces no measurable field at the detectors (shown to illustrate general relationship between dipole and detector).

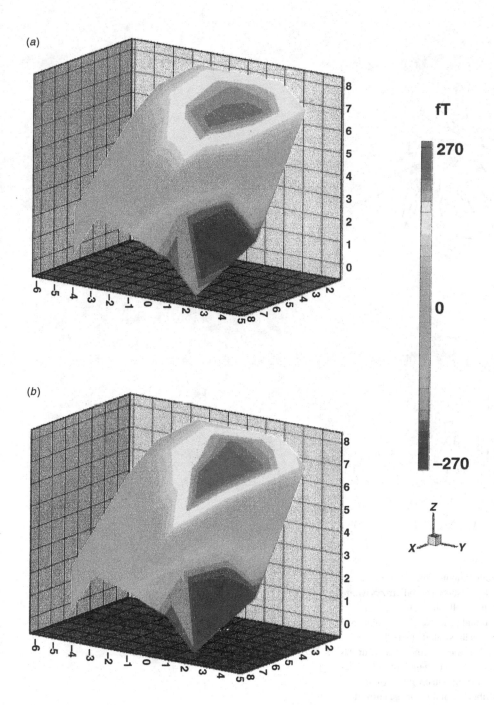

Fig. 5.13. Contour plots of the sensory evoked field data in Fig. 5.12. The three-dimensional topography of the M20 response (the first large deflection seen in Fig. 5.12*b*) is illustrated. Positive values indicate outgoing magnetic flux (red) and negative numbers indicate ingoing flux (blue). (*a*) The theoretical field produced by the final iteration of the forward solution in a single equivalent current dipole (ECD) model; (*b*) the actual measured data. The scaling is the same for both (*a*) and (*b*) and is shown to the right of the figure. The *x, y, z* coordinate system (scaled in centimeters) is also illustrated to the right of the figure and shows the orientation of the two plots in the figure. The *x* axis is defined as the line connecting the two preauricular points (positive *x* exits near the right ear); the *y* axis is the line normal to the *x* axis through the nasion (positive *y* exits the bridge of the nose), and the *z* axis is formed normal to *x* and *y* at their intersection (positive *z* exits the top of the head). The point 0, 0, 0, is the center of the head. Note the close correspondence between the theoretical field and measured field, which is predicted from the low residual error for this component in Fig. 5.12*a*.

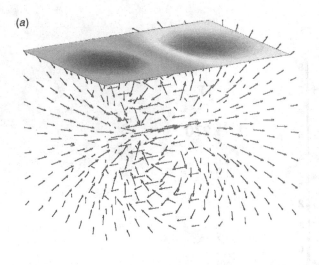

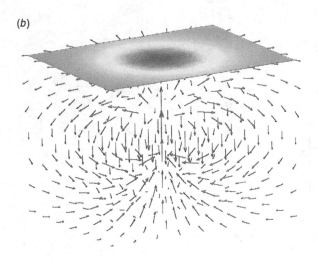

Fig. 5.15. Current density in a homogeneous volume conductor. Two orientations of current dipole are shown as red arrows where the arrows show the direction of intracellular current flow: (*a*) tangential to the surface and (*b*) radial to surface. Vector plots of the current density (blue arrows) are illustrated inside the rectangular volume conductor: this is the "volume current" and is responsible for the scalp-measured EEG. The length of the arrows is proportional to the $\log_{10}$ of the current density magnitude. Contour plots of the surface distribution of the normal current density are shown at the same slice plane through the top of the volume conductor. Compare these figures with those in Fig. 5.2. Note that the radially oriented MEG source produces no externally measurable field, but the same orientation is seen as a single electric potential extremum in this figure. Note also that while the EEG potential distribution appears to have the same spatial resolution as the MEG field distribution in Fig. 5.2, the blurring effects of the skull are not illustrated here. Consequently, this figure would be a more accurate depiction of the potential distribution measured directly from the pial surface of the cortex.

therefore, not detected by coils with axes radial to that surface.

The calculation of the magnetic field strength at a given point in space is referred to as the forward solution. Just as one may calculate the forward solution for a given current, one may attempt to solve backward from the measured data to determine the current source (the so-called inverse solution, or problem). This is currently the most common data analytic technique employed for MEG data. Unfortunately, the inverse problem is ill posed; it is not possible to solve for the current distribution inside a conductor uniquely from knowledge of the magnetic (or electric) fields outside that conductor. An infinite number of source configurations can produce the same electromagnetic field distribution. However, knowledge of the likely origins of the measured field can be used to restrict the possibilities, rejecting biologically implausible solutions. Typically, the inverse solution is realized as an iterative process of changing a dipole's parameters (e.g., strength, orientation, and location) and minimizing the residual error between the forward solution (theoretical field) and the measured data through a least-squares minimization or similar technique (see Figs. 5.12 and 5.13 (p. 82)). A priori hypotheses can be implemented during the fitting process to reject unlikely source configurations. One exciting possibility in MEG/EEG source analysis is that fMRI, SPECT, and/or PET activation regions could be used to restrict the possible locations when such data are available in the same person under the same or similar experimental paradigm (George et al., 1995).

Although the single ECD model is superficially quite simple, several issues make MEG source analysis complex, including, but not limited to, the model for the conducting medium (also known as the head model). In MEG source analysis, the head is usually modeled as a simple sphere with a single, homogeneously conductive compartment. In reality, of course, the head is not a perfect sphere, and there are at least three or four important layers of differing conductivity to be considered: brain, meninges, skull, and skin. For superficial sources, the effects of the nonhomogeneous medium and skull shape appear to be minimal, but deeper sources, especially those in basal frontal and temporal sites, may need to be modeled in a realistically shaped head model (Hamalainen and Sarvas, 1987, 1989; Menninghaus et al., 1994). Such models are readily available, particularly if MRI data are also available for the subject. In those cases, a realistic head shape with different conductivities can be constructed from boundary element modeling or other similar techniques (Menninghaus et al., 1994).

The single ECD model is often criticized as an oversimplification of the true current distribution within

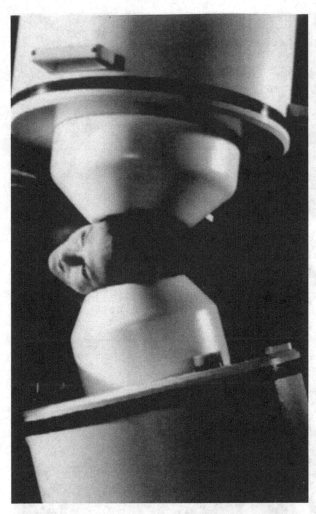

Fig. 5.7. The BTi Magnes II system, configured with two 37-channel, first-order gradiometer units. The gantry system for the overhead unit of this particular device allows five degrees of freedom of movement, but the dewar can only be tilted 45° from vertical to keep the liquid helium from spilling. (Courtesy of Biomagnetic Technologies, Inc.)

point of measurement. This formula indicates that the magnetic field is strongest perpendicular (i.e., $\psi = 90°$) to the current flow and diminishes with the square of the distance from the current source (r). The formula is limited in that it describes the magnetic field produced by the dipole alone (e.g., as if it were located in a nonconducting space). In fact, there are also extracellular currents (see section on EEG/MEG comparison) that maintain charge equilibrium in the volume. The magnetic fields associated with these currents, in volumes that exhibit spherical or cylindrical symmetry, are tangential to the surface of the volume and,

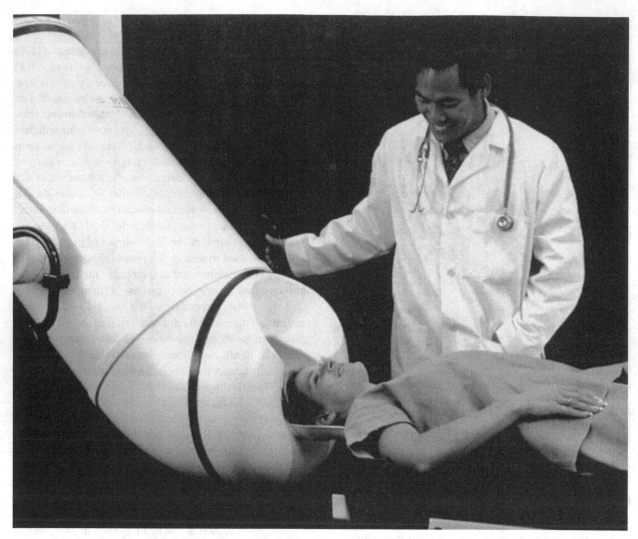

Fig. 5.8. The BTi WH2500 whole-head MEG system. The gantry for this system allows subjects to be recorded both seated and fully inclined and provides coverage over most of the head. (Courtesy of Biomagnetic Technologies, Inc.)

the brain. Multiple brain regions are most likely involved for even the simplest cognitive processes. If these regions are sequentially activated, this may pose no particular problem for the standard moving dipole model discussed above, since a single ECD can be fit across a time epoch point by point. However, to the extent that the multiple sources overlap temporally, the single ECD model will tend to produce more serious errors. Even if the sources do overlap in time, however, a single ECD model may suffice if the sources are separated by a large enough distance in space (this minimum distance is empirically unknown and depends on the sensor array density, geometry of the sources and detectors, as well as the SNR for the sources). For example, auditory stimuli, even when monaurally pre-

sented, produce near simultaneous activation in both temporal lobes. However, the magnetic field distributions from the two hemispheres do not overlap, and a single ECD can be used for each hemisphere to produce satisfactory results. If the sources overlap in time and space, a multiple dipole model may need to be employed. The spatiotemporal dipole model is one such approach that has been adapted to include multiple dipole modeling (e. g. Scherg et al., 1989).

Several other variations of the source analysis scheme have been employed in MEG, such as distributed source modeling, but are well beyond the scope of this chapter because of their complexity. The reader is referred to Sarvas (1987), Hamalainen et al. (1993), Williamson and Kaufman (1990), and Romani (1987) for further information on MEG

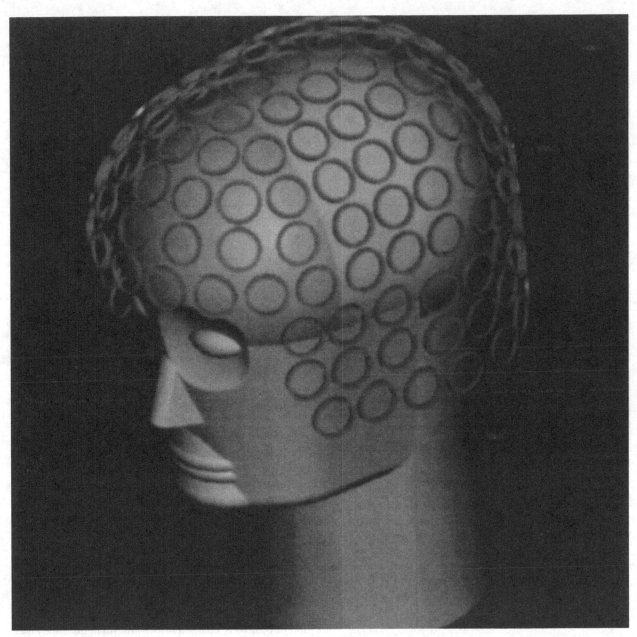

Fig. 5.9. Sensor array for the BTi WH2500 system shown in Fig. 5.8. Each circle represents a magnetometer coil. There are 148 such magnetometers in this system. (Courtesy of Biomagnetic Technologies, Inc.)

and source analysis and to Mosher et al. (1992) for an overview of multiple source modeling in MEG.

Magnetic source imaging

One often wants to know not only the three-dimensional coordinates of the current source underlying the magnetic field distribution but also where that point is in relation to the anatomy of the brain. Therefore, source locations are

often coregistered onto anatomically detailed MRI from the same subject. This is accomplished by transforming the coordinate system from MEG into the MRI system, or vice versa, a procedure that is eloquently described by Rezai et al. (1995). The combination of information from MEG source analysis with MRI data is often referred to as magnetic source imaging (Gallen et al., 1993, 1995; Chuang et al., 1995; Lewine and Orrison, 1995b). Figure 5.14 illus-

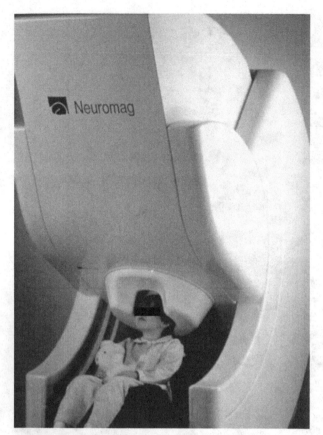

Fig. 5.10. The Neuromag, Ltd Vectorview whole-head system with child subject in special chair insert. This system, like the one shown in Fig. 5.9, is capable of recording in seated and fully inclined positions. The Vectorview system employs 204 off-diagonal planar gradiometers (see Fig. 5.5.*d*) and 102 magnetometers (Fig. 5.5*a*) in 100 sensor locations (i.e., three orthogonal channels per location). (Courtesy of Neuromag, Ltd.)

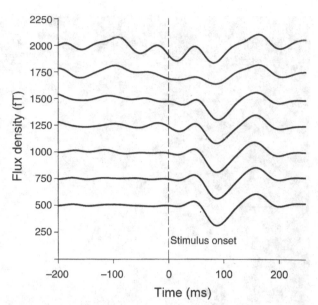

Fig. 5.11. The effect of signal averaging on the auditory evoked field. The topmost waveform is a two-trial averaged evoked response from a gradiometer channel located over the left anterior magnetic extremum of the M100 evoked field. From top to bottom, the rest of the waveforms are 4, 6, 8, 16, 32, and 64 trial averages from the same data set. Note the reduction in amplitude of the prestimulus baseline with the inclusion of more trials in the average, and the approximately 100 ms latency auditory evoked response in the poststimulus window.

trates a typical magnetic source imaging result for MEG data obtained from auditory evoked field (AEF) study.

Comparison of magneto- and electroencephalography

Differences in recorded signal

MEG is related to EEG in a complex way. The most important difference between the two techniques is the measured signal from neuronal activity: EEG reflects primarily extracellular current and MEG measures intracellular current. The origin of the magnetic signals of the brain was discussed above. EEG signals are also generated by the same ionic events that produce magnetic fields. As an example, the major contribution to depolarizing currents at the synapse is a brief increase in sodium ion permeability, typically induced by ligand gating of a protein ion channel on the postsynaptic membrane. This allows sodium ions to move freely along their chemical and electric gradients, usually producing a net inflow of sodium ions into the cell (transmembrane current). This local accumulation in turn causes intracellular current flow away from the open ion channels, causing an accumulation of positively charged ions some small distance away from the original inflow and triggering an outward transmembrane current flow. Since positive ions are now accumulating locally just outside the outward flow (called a current source), displacement of like charges occurs just as it did inside the cell. This time, the extracellular current will be drawn back to the original inflow because a local extracellular depletion of positive charge (called the current sink) will be present there. The extracellular component of this event is commonly referred to as volume conduction and is largely responsible for the observed potential distribution seen at the scalp in EEG. Since the entire brain and

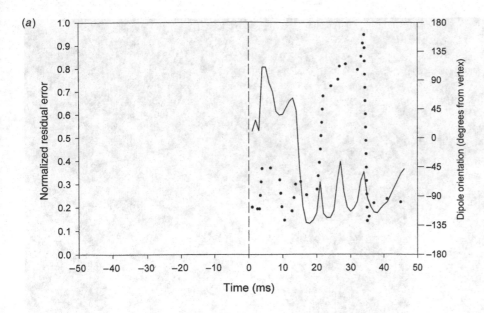

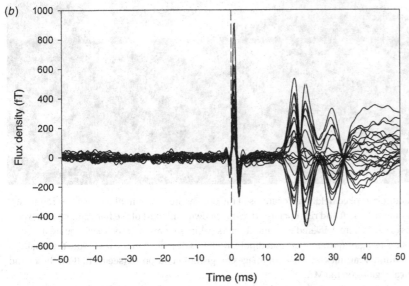

Fig. 5.12. Moving dipole model fit for a somatosensory evoked field (SEF) elicited by contralateral median nerve stimulation. The SEF was measured over the right hemisphere to electrical stimulation of the left median nerve, averaged over 500 stimuli. The time window illustrates 50 ms of prestimulus activity and 50 ms of poststimulus activity. (*a*) Model error and dipole orientation plotted across the poststimulus time window. A single equivalent current dipole (ECD) moving dipole model was used, where the single ECD was fitted to the mean amplitude data from three time points (i.e., the plotted point indicates the result for the mean time point indicated, as well as the points immediately preceding and following that point). Note that the residual error curve (solid black line) has four distinct minima, indicating four sequentially active sources. Using root mean squares (RMS), residual error equals $(RMS_{measured} - RMS_{calculated})/RMS_{measured}$. The dipole orientation curve (dotted line) plots the rotation of the dipole in degrees from the vertex (line exiting the top of the head), where positive numbers indicate anterior tilt and negative numbers indicate posterior tilt. (*b*) Overlapping SEF waveforms used as input for the model in (*a*). Note the prominent stimulus artifact around time zero from the magnetic field produced by the electrical stimulus. Note also the correspondence between the peaks in the waveform and the best fit to the model in (*a*). SEF data were collected with a seven-channel, second-order gradiometer system.

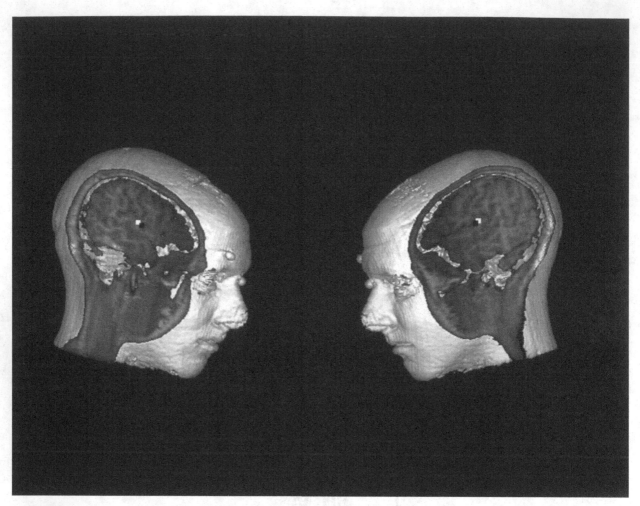

Fig. 5.14. Magnetic source imaging of the M100 auditory evoked field. The locations of the dipoles are shown in black on a 3-D rendering of the head from the subject's MRI data (17-year-old male). Left and right perspectives are shown, with part of the hemisphere removed to illustrate the internal MRI anatomy. Pure tones of 1 kHz were delivered monaurally at 1 s (white squares) and 6 s (black squares) interstimulus intervals. Sources were localized using a single equivalent current dipole model, as described in the text. Note the small bump visible on the nasion, which is one of the vitamin A capsules attached for image coregistration purposes (see text). Both the 1 s and the 6 s sources are well localized to auditory cortical regions on the MRI.

to some extent the meninges, cerebrospinal fluid, and scalp are all reasonable current conductors, strong volume currents may be seen quite some distance from the neuronal activity that produced them. This contrasts directly with MEG, which because it is primarily measuring the magnetic field produced by the intracellular current, is likely to see a more focal field distribution. In addition, the skull, a relatively nonconductive medium, can seriously attenuate and distort the electric potential distribution (seen in EEG) of neuronal sources, whereas the magnetic fields of the brain (as in MEG) pass through the skull with no distortion (van den Broek et al., 1998). These two factors

are, at least in theory, likely to confer a slight spatial resolution advantage to MEG over EEG (see below).

Another key difference between MEG and EEG in the recorded signal is that, although MEG is highly sensitive to source orientation since radially oriented sources produce no external magnetic field (Fig. 5.2, p. 82), both radial and tangential sources contribute to the scalp EEG (Fig. 5.15, p. 82). This can be seen both as an advantage and a disadvantage for EEG: advantage because there is more cortex visible to EEG, and disadvantage because of the resulting increase in complexity of sources contributing to the potential distribution at the scalp, which in turn requires more complex source models and increasing ambiguities about model accuracy. While it seems readily apparent that combining the two technologies could yield richer interpretation of the data than either alone can, the two techniques have rarely been combined in any systematic way (see, however, Diekmann et al., 1998).

Finally, there is always the problem of reference in EEG measurements. The potential measurements made in EEG are, by definition, difference measurements and require the use of two electrode inputs into each amplifier channel. Since the difference (potential) between the two electrode sites is what is recorded in EEG, the locations of and distances between the paired electrodes are critical for interpreting the nature of the recorded signal. This problem has been discussed in detail elsewhere (Lewine and Orrison, 1995a) and will not be elaborated here. Suffice to say that MEG measurements are truly reference-free, and, therefore, signals detected by a single coil can be more easily interpreted with respect to their origin. EEG researchers are, however, able to reduce the impact of the reference problem, usually by computing an average potential reference from all the recording electrodes (which requires a large number of electrodes for accuracy) or by computing the second spatial derivative of the potential distribution (the Laplacian), which is reference-free.

Potential for source localization

There are few direct empirical comparisons of the localization capability of MEG and EEG that can be considered fair. A legitimate direct comparison would have to be for a known source with a tangential orientation, since the point is moot for radial sources in MEG (EEG will always be superior in that case). In addition, a fair comparison would need to have comparable intersensor distances and adequate coverage of the magnetic and electric topographies, both of which are acquired simultaneously with identical stimulation/recording parameters. Only three studies published to date appear to fulfill most of these criteria (with the exception of simultaneity in the first case). Cohen et al. (1990) studied an implanted dipole source in a surgical patient, measuring the activation of this dipole from 16 different sites with both EEG and MEG. The average localization errors for different conditions were 8 mm for MEG and 10 mm for EEG, and the authors suggested that MEG offered no significant advantage over EEG in localizing accuracy. The most recent comparison of MEG and EEG localization was not directly of accuracy; instead, localization replicability was compared in five subjects who underwent repeated high-density, simultaneous EEG/MEG

recording of auditory evoked responses (Virtanen et al., 1998). Localization errors reported over the repeated recordings were 2 mm for MEG and 4 mm for EEG (average standard deviation for x, y, and z coordinates). Computer simulations and theory offer similar conclusions (Cohen and Cuffin, 1991; Lopes da Silva et al., 1991; Mosher et al., 1993; Haueisen et al., 1997). However, MEG source modeling can usually be done satisfactorily with simpler head models, whereas accurate EEG source modeling may require more sophisticated head models that take head shape and conductivity layers into account (Lopes da Silva et al., 1991). It should also be mentioned that for some real-world applications of source localization, MEG may still offer better spatial resolution, as may be the case for the localization of seizure foci (Nakasato et al., 1994). In any case, MEG may not have as great an advantage in localization accuracy over EEG for a single ECD as was once proposed (e.g., Cuffin and Cohen, 1979). Differences might exist for more complex source geometries, but this will need to be empirically evaluated. As it currently stands, the main advantage of MEG may be its sensitivity to source orientation. The most significant disadvantage of MEG compared with EEG remains its significant cost (see Table 5.1 for comparison of MEG/EEG features).

Pediatric research applications

Auditory evoked magnetic fields of the human fetus

One potential advantage of MEG over all other functional imaging modalities is its ability to record the brain's magnetic responses prenatally. Blum and colleagues (Blum et al., 1984, 1985, 1987) were the first to report AEF from the fetus. In these studies, the position of the fetus in utero was determined through ultrasound imaging, and the ear canal of the fetus was projected onto the mother's abdomen, where the authors centered the MEG device, a single-channel, second-order gradiometer. They delivered acoustic stimuli (1 kHz sine waves) from 40 to 100 dB HL (mother's threshold) via a speaker located 1 m away from the mother, and averaged the responses from 300 stimuli to produce AEF waveforms. Two subjects were studied prenatally, and one was recorded again after birth. Both subjects showed a small (<200 fT) AEF component at approximately 140 ms poststimulus, which was also present in the single subject followed up after delivery. Polarity reversals in this component were seen from anterior to posterior across the ear canal, consistent with adult AEF data indicating an auditory cortical source. Wakai et al. (1996) have

Table 5.1. *Comparison of magneto- and electroencephalography*

	Magnetoencephalography (MEG)	Electroencephalography (EEG)
Measurement	Magnetic field	Electric potential
Common measurement units	Femtotesla (fT)	Microvolts (μV)
Measured current source	Intracellular	Extracellular
Source orientation to detector sensitivity	Tangential	Tangential and radial
Visible cortex (based on orientation sensitivity)	Mostly sulcal	Sulcal and gyral
Temporal resolution (ms)	<1	<1
Spatial resolution (cm)[a]	<1.0	<1.0
Minimum modeling complexity for source analysis	Simple (single sphere, single dipole)	Complex (realistic head shape model with multiple conductivity layers, multiple dipoles)
Cost of instrumentation[b] (US$)	~2.0 million for whole head array plus shielding	~150 000 for 128 electrode array system plus cap
Single largest operational cost (personnel costs and optional maintenance contracts excluded)	Liquid helium: $4.00/$l$, 100$l$/week = $20 800/year (costs are typical for users in the USA; they may be substantially higher for other countries)	Replacement of electrode cap/net as elasticity degrades: estimated cost for 128-channel cap is $2000. Estimated need for replacement is every 100 patients
Time to prepare and record patient[c] (min)	~30	~90
Risks to subjects[d]	No known risks	Infectious disease transmission and electric shock

Notes:

[a] Spatial resolution cannot be directly compared between EEG and MEG in any simple fashion, since it depends so strongly on source geometry, sensor density, modeling, experimental paradigm, etc. (see text).

[b] All necessary instrumentation for MEG and EEG is included in estimate (e.g., electrode caps, gels, computers, helium transfer tubes, etc.).

[c] Time is estimated for a completely cooperative subject participating in a simple auditory evoked response study with a whole-head MEG or 128-channel EEG system. Digitization with magnetic digitizer to establish head frame coordinate system and sensor positions is included in estimate. Post-hoc (offline) analyses not included in estimate but should be similar.

[d] Risks listed for EEG are extremely small but are usually required to be stated on informed consent forms as a possible, but slight risk. Most caps can be safely chemically sterilized before use, and modern EEG systems are very safe electrically when properly grounded and the patient is not attached to another electrical device such as a separate heart monitor. Both MEG and EEG, when properly used, should be completely safe for use with children.

replicated these findings in recordings from 14 fetuses between 36 to 40 weeks gestational age (Fig. 5.16).

Auditory evoked magnetic fields in children

Three studies have been published to date concerning AEF development in children. Paetau et al. (1995) were the first to report AEF values in children between the ages of 4 months and 15 years ($n=23$). Using pure tone and phonemic stimuli, they reported a lack of the M100 (100ms latency magnetic field; also termed N100m) AEF waveform in children up to 12 years of age. The M100 waveform, the magnetic analog of the electric vertex N100 auditory evoked potential, is the most prominent AEF component (i.e., largest amplitude) seen in adult magnetic recordings. Paetau et al. (1995) also reported that for longer interstimulus intervals (>1 s), the M100 component appeared in most of the younger children's recordings. The authors interpreted this as possible evidence of a refractory period change in the underlying neuronal population for the M100. In two separate studies conducted in our laboratory, this hypothesis was tested systematically by varying the interstimulus interval between pure tone stimuli (Rojas et al., 1998, 1999). In the first study, six children aged between 8 and 9 years of age participated, and 22 children between 6 and 18 years of age participated in the second. Both studies

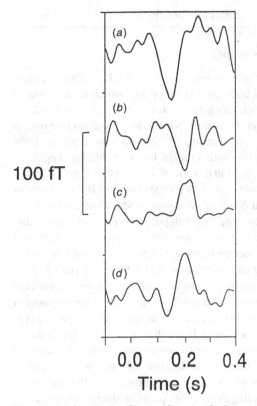

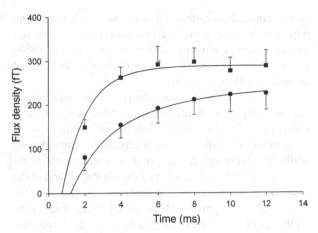

Fig. 5.17. The 100 ms latency magnetic field refractory period in children. Each data point (mean and SEM) represents average amplitude for both left and right hemispheres taken from the anterior magnetic extremum of the M100 auditory evoked field in younger (●, 6–8 years of age) and older (■, 15–17 years of age) children. Data were fit to a standard exponential decay equation (regression lines), and the time constant of decay from the regression was compared between the two groups. The time constant was significantly longer in the younger subjects, indicating longer neuronal trace duration in younger children. (Data from Rojas et al., 1998.)

Fig. 5.16. Fetal MEG recording. Auditory evoked magnetic fields AEF from four different fetal subjects: (a) 37, (b) 34, (c) 35, and (d) 36 weeks gestational age. The placement of the MEG device was determined by ultrasound. Sounds were delivered via a loudspeaker mounted in the recording chamber. The AEF responses are averages of 100 epochs. Stimulus onset is at time zero. (With permission from Wakai et al., 1996.)

provided evidence supportive of the refractory period change hypothesis (Fig. 5.17). These studies, taken together, suggest that one reason the EEG evoked potential recordings in children typically do not find evidence for the N100 may be that the interstimulus intervals used are too short to accommodate the longer refractory period in younger children. One recently published EEG study on the N100 that used intervals of up to 4393 ms in 15 children aged 7–9 years did find evidence supporting the longer refractory hypothesis (Ceponiene et al., 1998). The M100 may be a physiologic index of auditory sensory memory (Lü et al., 1992), and these MEG data may, therefore, imply that the phonologic store duration gets shorter as children mature.

Future research directions

Although there has been some effort to study AEF development in children, no data have yet been reported concern-

ing visual, somatosensory, or motor evoked responses, or responses in any other neurologic domain in younger subjects. Such normative developmental data will be critically important before meaningful studies using MEG in clinical developmental research populations are undertaken. Several potentially exciting applications of MEG lie with the study of sensory/cognitive processing disorders, including childhood-onset schizophrenia, attention-deficit hyperactivity disorder (ADHD), developmental dyslexia, and other developmental disabilities.

Childhood-onset schizophrenia

To date, the only published MEG data on any psychiatric disorder is on adults with schizophrenia. Reite et al. (1988) were the first to use MEG in schizophrenia, reporting that the normal interhemispheric axial plane asymmetry of the M50 AEF (analog of the electric P50) generators was not found in six males with schizophrenia, but was found in six nonpsychiatric control subjects. This report was followed by a study of M100 asymmetry in six schizophrenic males and six nonpsychiatric controls in which this atypical symmetry in the schizophrenic patients was also present (Reite et al., 1989). A subsequent study with a new sample including both men and women has revealed a prominent sex difference in the expression of this anomalous functional asymmetry, with ten male patients showing a lack of M100 asymmetry and ten female patients showing either normal or enhanced asymmetry compared with age- and sex-matched control subjects (Reite et al., 1997).

Hemispheric anatomic asymmetry in the supratemporal auditory areas is typically present at birth (Witelson and Pallie, 1973), but the extent of functional laterality is presently unknown. Critically, one study of 21 schizophrenic adults and 24 controls has shown that the functional asymmetry of the M100 response in adults is independent of the underlying gross anatomy in both groups (Rojas et al., 1997). The development of functional lateralization of the auditory cortex could be studied in normally developing children and in those with early onset of psychotic symptoms. Such an application of MEG would be a natural extension of the earlier work in adults.

Dyslexia

Two MEG studies have been published on the topic of dyslexia (Salmelin et al., 1996; Vanni et al., 1997). Salmelin et al. (1996) in a study of six adult subjects with developmental dyslexia and eight controls found that visually presented words failed to elicit the normal electrophysiologic response from the left inferior temporo-occipital region in the dyslexic subjects. The normal word-specific response, which has also been identified by intracranial recording at approximately 200 ms poststimulus (Nobre et al., 1994), was absent or significantly delayed in all six dyslexic subjects, suggesting a role for this region in the pathophysiology of dyslexia. In the second study, Vanni et al. (1997) reported that visual motion does activate area V5/MT of the visual cortex in dyslexic adults, superficially contradicting two previous findings from the fMRI literature (Eden et al., 1996; Demb et al., 1997). The difference between the MEG and fMRI results raises some important methodological issues that illustrate the potential advantage of combining the two techniques. In the Salmelin et al. study (1996), for example, the MEG responses were delayed in the dyslexics, and fMRI would not be sensitive to this delay because of its coarser temporal resolution. Moreover, while the stimuli used in these experiments were somewhat different, a combined fMRI and MEG study of visual motion addressing the correlation of electrophysiology to blood flow in dyslexia might best resolve the apparently discrepant findings; it is possible, albeit speculative, that reduced blood flow to V5/MT could cause the delayed latency of the MEG responses (or vice versa). Children with dyslexia have not yet been studied in this manner (either with MEG alone or MEG in combination with other imaging modalities).

Pediatric clinical applications

Pediatric epilepsy

The most common application of MEG to pediatric populations has been in neurology, for source localization of epileptic foci. Much research on MEG in source localization of epileptic spikes has been done in adults (see review by Lewine and Orrison, 1995d), but several papers have been published with a special focus on childhood epilepsy (Paetau et al., 1994; Minami et al., 1995, 1996; Zupanc, 1997; Kamada et al., 1998). Of special note is the interest in the Landau–Kleffner syndrome (LKS), a childhood disorder characterized by epileptiform spike and wave discharges and progressive loss of previously acquired language function (manifesting most commonly as verbal auditory agnosia). Paetau et al. (1991) reported localization of spikes in one patient with LKS to the left perisylvian auditory cortex, and a follow-up study of seven patients aged 5–12 years revealed that acoustic stimuli evoked epileptiform discharges from the auditory cortex (Paetau, 1994). Interestingly, although the sounds triggered spikes from the patients with LKS, the AEFs to the same sounds were absent or abnormal in all the subjects. In some cases, the sounds triggered spikes peaking at approximately 100 ms poststimulus, the same latency range for the typical M100 (see above). The sound-evoked spikes were 10–15 times the amplitude of the normal M100, and the authors suggested that the pathophysiology of the LKS spikes might closely correspond with the neuronal population responsible for the M100 (ie., that the seizure activity may represent the disinhibition of normal auditory processing).

Conclusions and future directions

Aside from the small number of clinical applications of MEG currently in place, several of the research directions discussed could lead to the development of important diagnostic capabilities for this imaging strategy. For example, the ability to perform intrauterine electrophysiologic evaluations of fetal brain development might lead to important early diagnostic capabilities with respect to sensorineural hearing impairments and developmental disabilities, as well as a number of other neurologic conditions. Before such applications are possible, more basic research is needed on MEG in clinical, as well as normal, samples, particularly pediatric groups.

MEG instrumentation and data analysis have become increasingly sophisticated since the early 1980s, but the high cost to researchers and clinicians has prevented extensive application to pediatric, as well as adult, clinical populations. As clinical applications for MEG become more widely accepted within the medical community, more instruments are likely to be ordered/installed, and this will certainly have a beneficial effect on system prices. Meanwhile, currently operational research groups have published some promising initial results using MEG in combination with anatomic MRI. As with other functional neuroimaging technologies, MEG is likely to benefit from combined use with multiple imaging modalities, particularly the widely popular fMRI, where the advantages and disadvantages of the two technologies are complementary. To the best of our knowledge, however, at the date of this writing there are only 33 whole-head MEG systems installed worldwide (six in the USA), as well as an unknown, but most likely lower, number of operational partial array systems. This small number of MEG systems has severely limited the ability of the MEG community to collaborate with their other neuroimaging colleagues. As the installed instrument base of MEG increases, collaborative efforts such as these will become more likely, and the future of electrophysiological imaging in pediatric psychiatry will get correspondingly brighter.

Acknowledgements

Funding for this work was provided by USPHS grants MH56601, MH47476, MH15442, and HD35468, and by the Developmental Psychobiology Research Group Endowment Fund at the University of Colorado Health Sciences Center, provided by the Grant Foundation. The authors thank Jeanelle L. Sheeder and Jennifer B. Lopez for their assistance with data collection and analysis related to this manuscript.

References

Aine, C. J. (1995). A conceptual overview and critique of functional neuroimaging techniques in humans: I. MRI/fMRI and PET. *Crit. Rev. Neurobiol.*, 2, 3, 229–309.

Blum, T., Saling, E. and Bauer, R. (1984). Fetal magnetoencephalography I: 1st prenatal registration of auditory evoked neuromagnetic fields. [German] EEG EMG *Z. Elektroenzephalogr. Elektromyogr. Ver. Geb.*, 15, 34–7.

Blum, T., Saling, E. and Bauer, R. (1985). First magnetoencephalographic recordings of the brain activity of a human fetus. *Br. J. Obst. Gynaecol.*, 92, 1224–9.

Blum, T., Bauer, R., Arabin, B., Reckel, S. and Saling, E. (1987). Prenatally recorded auditory evoked neuromagnetic field of the human fetus. In *Evoked Potentials*, Vol. 3, eds. C. Barber and T. Blum, pp. 136–42. Boston, MA: Butterworth.

Braun, C., Kaiser, S., Kincses, W. E. and Elbert, T. (1997). Confidence interval of single dipole locations based on EEG data. *Brain Topgr.*, 10, 31–9.

Ceponiene, R., Cheour, M. and Näätänen, R. (1998). Interstimulus interval and auditory event-related potentials in children: evidence for multiple generators. *Electroencephalogr. Clin. Neurophysiol.*, 108, 345–54.

Chuang, S. H., Otsubo, H., Hwang, P., Orrison, W. W. Jr and Lewine, J. D. (1995). Pediatric magnetic source imaging. *Neuroimaging Clin. N. Am.*, 5, 289–303.

Cohen, D. (1968). Magnetoencephalography: evidence of magnetic fields produced by alpha-rhythm currents. *Science*, 161, 784–6.

Cohen, D. (1970). Low-field room built at high-field magnet lab. *Phys. Today*, 23, 56–7.

Cohen, D. (1972). Magnetoencephalography: detection of the brain's electrical activity with a superconducting magnetometer. *Science*, 175, 664–6.

Cohen, D. and Cuffin, B. N. (1991). EEG versus MEG localization accuracy: theory and experiment. *Brain Topogr.*, 4, 95–103.

Cohen, D., Cuffin, B. N., Yunokuchi, K. et al. (1990). MEG versus EEG localization test using implanted sources in the human brain [see comments]. *Ann. Neurol.*, 28, 811–17.

Cuffin, B. N. (1990). Effects of head shape on EEG's and MEG's. *IEEE Trans. Biomed. Eng.*, 37, 44–52.

Cuffin, B. N. (1991). Moving dipole inverse solutions using MEGs measured on a plane over the head. *Electroencephalogr. Clin. Neurophysiol.*, 78, 341–7.

Cuffin, B. N. and Cohen, D. (1979). Comparison of the magnetoencephalogram and electroencephalogram. *Electroencephalogr. Clin. Neurophysiol.*, 47, 132–46.

Davidovitch, M., Patterson, B. and Gartside, P. (1996). Head circumference measurements in children with autism. *J. Child Neurol.*, 11, 389–93.

Demb, J. B., Boynton, G. M. and Heeger, D. J. (1997). Brain activity in visual cortex predicts individual differences in reading performance. *Proc. Natl. Acad. Sci. USA*, 94, 13363–6.

Diekmann, V., Becker, W., Jurgens, R. et al. (1998). Localisation of epileptic foci with electric, magnetic and combined electromagnetic models. *Electroencephalogr. Clin. Neurophysiol.*, 106, 297–313.

Eden, G. F., van Meter, J. W., Rumsey, J. M., Maisog, J. M., Woods, R. P. and Zeffiro, J. A. (1996). Abnormal processing of visual motion in dyslexia revealed by functional brain imaging [see comments]. *Nature*, 382, 66–9.

Gallen, C. C., Sobel, D. F., Schwartz, B., Copeland, B., Waltz, T. and Aung, M. (1993). Magnetic source imaging. Present and future. *Invest. Radiol.*, 28, S153–7.

Gallen, C. C., Hirschkoff, E. C. and Buchanan, D. S. (1995). Magnetoencephalography and magnetic source imaging. Capabilities and limitations. *Neuroimaging Clin. N. Am.*, 5, 227–49.

George, J. S., Aine, C. J., Mosher, J. C. et al. (1995). Mapping function in the human brain with magnetoencephalography, anatomical magnetic resonance imaging, and functional magnetic resonance imaging. *J. Clin. Neurophysiol.*, **12**, 406–31.

Gharib, S., Sutherling, W. W., Nakasato, N. et al. (1995). MEG and ECoG localization accuracy test. *Electroencephalogr. Clin. Neurophysiol.*, **94**, 109–14.

Hamalainen, M. S. and Sarvas, J. (1987). Feasibility of the homogeneous head model in the interpretation of neuromagnetic fields. *Phys. Med. Biol.*, **32**, 91–7.

Hamalainen, M. S. and Sarvas, J. (1989). Realistic conductivity geometry model of the human head for interpretation of neuromagnetic data. *IEEE Trans. Biomed. Eng.*, **36**, 165–71.

Hamalainen, M., Hari, R., Ilmoniemi, R. J., Knuutila, J. Lounasmaa, O. V. (1993). Magnetoencephalography – theory, instrumentation, and applications to noninvasive studies of the working human brain. *Rev. Mod. Phys.*, **65**, 413–98.

Hari, R., Joutsiniemi, S. L. and Sarvas, J. (1988). Spatial resolution of neuromagnetic records: theoretical calculations in a spherical model. *Electroencephalogr. Clin. Neurophysiol.*, **71**, 64–72.

Haueisen, J., Ramon, C., Eiselt, M., Brauer, H. and Nowak, H. (1997). Influence of tissue resistivities on neuromagnetic fields and electric potentials studied with a finite element model of the head. *IEEE Trans. Biomed. Eng.*, **44**, 727–35.

Kamada, K., Moller, M., Saguer, M. et al. (1998). Localization analysis of neuronal activities in benign Rolandic epilepsy using magnetoencephalography. *J. Neurolog. Sci.*, **154**, 164–72.

Krasuski, J., Horwitz, B. and Rumsey, J. M. (1996). A survey of functional and anatomical neuroimaging techniques. In *Neuroimaging: A Window to the Neurological Foundations of Learning and Behavior in Children*, eds. G. R. Lyon and J. M. Rumsey, pp. 25–52. Baltimore, MD: Paul H. Brookes.

Kullmann, W. H. (1993). Separation of sources of neuromagnetic examinations. *Physiol. Meas.*, **14**, A27–34.

Lainhart, J. E., Piven, J., Wzorek, M. et al. (1997). Macrocephaly in children and adults with autism. *J. Am. Acad. Child Adolesc. Psychiatry*, **36**, 282–90.

Lewine, J. D. and Orrison, W. W. Jr (1995a). Clinical electroencephalography and event-related potentials. In *Functional Brain Imaging*, eds. W. W. Orrison, J. D. Lewine, J. A. Sanders and M. F. Hartshorne, pp. 327–68. St Louis, MO: Mosby.

Lewine, J. D. and Orrison, W. W. Jr (1995b). Magnetic source imaging: basic principles and applications in neuroradiology. *Acad. Radiol.*, **2**, 436–40.

Lewine, J. D. and Orrison, W. W. Jr (1995c). Magnetoencephalography and magnetic source imaging. In *Functional Brain Imaging*, eds. W. W. Orrison, J. D. Lewine, J. A. Sanders and M. F. Hartshorne, pp. 369–418. St Louis, MO: Mosby.

Lewine, J. D. and Orrison, W. W. Jr (1995d). Spike and slow wave localization by magnetoencephalography. *Neuroimaging Clin. N. Am.*, **5**, 575–96.

Lopes da Silva, F. H., Wieringa, H. J. and Peters, M. J. (1991). Source localization of EEG versus MEG: empirical comparison using visually evoked responses and theoretical considerations. *Brain Topogr.*, **4**, 133–42.

Lü, Z.-L., Williamson, S. J. and Kaufman, L. (1992). Behavioral lifetime of human auditory sensory memory predicted by physiological measures. *Science*, **258**, 1668–70.

Menninghaus, E., Lutkenhoner, B. and Gonzalez, S. L. (1994). Localization of a dipolar source in a skull phantom: realistic versus spherical model. *IEEE Trans. Biomed. Eng.*, **41**, 986–9.

Minami, T., Gondo, K., Yanai, S., Yamamoto, T., Tasaki, K. and Ueda, K. (1995). Rolandic discharges and somatosensory evoked potentials in benign childhood partial epilepsy: magnetoencephalographical study. *Psychiatr. Clin. Neurosci.*, **48**, S227–8.

Minami, T., Gondo, K., Yamamoto, T., Yanai, S., Tasaki, K. and Ueda, K. (1996). Magnetoencephalographic analysis of rolandic discharges in benign childhood epilepsy. *Ann. Neurol.* **39**, 326–34.

Mosher, J. C., Lewis, P. S. and Leahy, R. M. (1992). Multiple dipole modeling and localization from spatio-temporal MEG data. *IEEE Trans. Biomed. Eng.*, **39**, 541–57.

Mosher, J. C., Spencer, M. E., Leahy, R. M. and Lewis, P. S. (1993). Error bounds for EEG and MEG dipole source localization. *Electroencephalogr. Clin. Neurophysiol.*, **86**, 303–21.

Murro, A. M., Smith, J. R., King, D. W. and Park, Y. D. (1995). Precision of dipole localization in a spherical volume conductor: a comparison of referential EEG, magnetoencephalography and scalp current density methods. *Brain Topgr.*, **8**, 119–25.

Nakasato, N., Levesque, M. F., Barth, D. S., Baumgartner, C., Rogers, R. L. and Sutherling, W. W. (1994). Comparisons of MEG, EEG, and ECoG source localization in neocortical partial epilepsy in humans. *Electroencephalogr. Clin. Neurophysiol.*, **91**, 171–18.

Nobre, A. C., Allison, T. and McCarthy, G. (1994). Word recognition in the human inferior temporal lobe. *Nature*, **372**, 260–3.

Okada, Y., Lauritzen, M. and Nicholson, C. (1987). MEG source models and physiology. *Phys. Med. Biol.*, **32**, 43–51.

Okada, Y. C., Wu, J. and Kyuhou, S. (1997). Genesis of MEG signals in a mammalian CNS structure. *Electroencephalogr. Clin. Neurophysiol.*, **103**, 474–85.

Paetau, R. (1994). Sounds trigger spikes in the Landau–Kleffner syndrome. *J. Clin. Neurophysiol.*, **11**, 231–41.

Paetau, R., Kajola, M., Korkman, M., Hamalainen, M., Granstrom, M. L. and Hari, R. (1991). Landau–Kleffner syndrome: epileptic activity in the auditory cortex. *Neuroreport*, **2**, 201–14.

Paetau, R., Hamalainen, M., Hari, R. et al. (1994). Magnetoencephalographic evaluation of children and adolescents with intractable epilepsy. *Epilepsia*, **35**, 275–84.

Paetau, R., Ahonen, A., Salonen, O. and Sams, M. (1995). Auditory evoked magnetic fields to tones and pseudowords in healthy children and adults. *J. Clin. Neurophysiol.*, **12**, 177–85.

Reeve, A., Rose, D. F. and Weinberger, D. R. (1989). Magnetoencaphalography. Applications in psychiatry. *Arch. Gen. Psychiatry*, **46**, 573–6.

Reite, M., Teale, P., Zimmerman, J., Davis, K., Whalen, J. and Edrich, J. (1988). Source origin of a 50-msec latency auditory evoked field component in young schizophrenic men. *Biol. Psychiatry*, **24**, 495–506.

Reite, M., Teale, P., Goldstein, L., Whalen, J. and Linnville, S. (1989). Late auditory magnetic sources may differ in the left hemisphere of schizophrenic patients. A preliminary report. *Arch. Gen. Psychiatry*, **46**, 565–72.

Reite, M., Sheeder, J., Teale, P. et al. (1997). Magnetic source imaging evidence of sex differences in cerebral lateralization in schizophrenia. *Arch. Gen. Psychiatry*, **54**, 433–40.

Rezai, A. R., Hund, M., Kronberg, E. et al. (1995). Introduction of magnetoencaphalography to stereotactic techniques. *Stereotactic Funct. Neurosurg.*, **65**, 37–41.

Rojas, D. C., Teale, P., Sheeder, J., Simon, J. and Reite, M. (1997). Sex-specific expression of Heschl's gyrus functional and structural abnormalities in paranoid schizophrenia. [see comments] *Am. J. Psychiatry*, **154**, 1655–62.

Rojas, D. C., Walker, J. R., Sheeder, J. L., Teale, P. D. and Reite, M. L. (1998). Developmental changes in refractoriness of the neuromagnetic M100 in children. *Neuroreport*, **9**, 1261–5.

Rojas, D. C., Sheeder, J. L., Teale, P. et al. (1999). MEG measurement of auditory sensory memory persistence via the M100 in children and adults. In *Advances in Biomagnetism Research: Biomag96*, eds. C. Aine, Y. Okada, G. Stroink, S. Swithenby and C. Wood, New York: Springer–Verlag.

Romani, G. L. (1987). The inverse problem in MEG studies: an instrumental and analytical perspective. *Phys. Med. Biol.*, **32**, 23–31.

Salmelin, R., Service, E., Kiestla. P., Uutela, K. and Salonen, O. (1996). Impaired visual word processing in dyslexia revealed with magnetoencephalography. *Anna. Neurol.*, **40**, 157–62.

Sanders, J. A. and Orrison, W. W. (1995). Functional magnetic resonance imaging. In *Functional Brain Imaging*, eds. W. W. Orrison, J. D. Lewine, J. A. Sanders. and M. F. Hartshorne, pp. 239–326. St Louis, MO: Mosby.

Sarvas, J. (1987). Basic mathematical and electromagnetic concepts of the biomagnetic inverse problem. *Phys. Med. Biol.*, **1**, 11–22.

Scherg, M., Hari, R. and Hamalainen, M. (1989). Frequency-specific sources of the auditory N19–P30–P50 response detected by a multiple source analysis of evoked magnetic fields and potentials. In *Advances in Biogmagnetism*, eds. M. Hoke, G. Stroink and M. Kotani, pp. 97–100. New York: Plenum.

Turner, R. and Jezzard, P. (1994). Magnetic resonance studies of brain functional activation using echo-planar imaging. In *Functional Neuroimaging Technical Foundations*, eds. R. W. Thatcher, M. Hallet, T. Zeffiro, E. R. John and M. Huerta, pp. 69–78. San Diego, CA: Academic Press.

van den Broek, S. P., Reinders, F., Donderwinkel, M. and Peters, M. J. (1998). Volume conduction effects in EEG and MEG. *Electroencaphalogr. Clin. Neurophysiol.*, **106**, 522–34.

Vanni, S., Uusitalo, M. A., Kiesila, P. and Hari, R. (1997). Visual motion activates V5 in dyslexics. *Neuroreport*, **8**, 1939–42.

Virtanen, J., Ahveninen, J., Ilmoniemi, R. J., Näätänen, R. and Pekkonen, E. (1998). Replicability of MEG and EEG measures of the auditory N1/N1m-response. *Electroencaphalogr. Clin. Neurophysiol.*, **108**, 291–8.

Wakai, R. T., Leuthold, A. C. and Martin, C. B. (1996). Fetal auditory evoked responses detected by magnetoencephalography. *Am. J. Obst. Gynaecol.*, **174**, 1484–6.

Williamson, S. J. and Kaufman, L. (1990). Theory of neuroelectric and neuromagnetic fields. In *Auditory Evoked Magnetic Fields and Electric Potentials*, Vol. 6, eds. F. Grandori, M. Hoke and G. L. Romani, pp. 1–39. New York: Karger.

Witelson, S. F. and Pallie, W. (1973). Left hemisphere specialization for language in the newborn: neuroanatomical evidence of asymmetry. *Brain*, **96**, 641–6.

Wood, M. L. (1992). Fourier imaging. In *Magnetic Resonance Imaging*, eds. D. D. Stark and W. G. Bradley, St Louis, MO: Mosby Year Book.

Woodhouse, W., Bailey, A., Rutter, M., Bolton, P., Baird, G. and Le Couteur, A. (1996). Head circumference in autism and other pervasive developmental disorders. *J. Child Psychol. Psychiatry*, **37**, 665–71.

Zhang, Y., Tavrin, Y., Muck, M. et al. (1993a). High temperature RF SQUIDS for biomedical applications. *Phsyiol. Meas.*, **14**, 113–19.

Zhang, Y., Tavrin, Y., Muck, M. et al. (1993b). Magnetoencephalography using high temperature rf SQUIDs. *Brain Topogr.*, **5**, 379–82.

Zupanc, M. L. (1997). Neuroimaging in the evaluation of children and adolescents with intractable epilepsy: II. Neuroimaging and pediatric epilepsy surgery. *Pediatr. Neurol.*, **17**, 111–21.

Part 2

Ethical foundations

Critical to the application of these exciting technologies within child psychiatry are ethical considerations. Ethics is central to all research, but special issues arise when dealing with subjects who are particularly vulnerable by virtue of their age and dependence, as well as by virtue of impairments resulting from psychiatric disorders. In this section, Arnold and colleagues outline the guiding ethical principles in research with children and address the challenges specific to functional neuroimaging studies of both normal control children and those with psychiatric disorders. Specific risks imposed by functional neuroimaging and informed consent/assent issues are examined, and methods for minimizing such risks are described.

6

Ethical issues in neuroimaging research with children

L. Eugene Arnold, Alan J. Zametkin,
Lauren Caravella and Nicole Korbly

Introduction

The "Decade of the Brain" has witnessed a burgeoning of neuroimaging in psychiatric research with children and adolescents. A 1994 survey of the research use of various biological procedures reported in five major journals over a 5-year period revealed 18 reports based on brain imaging, constituting 15% of the reports of biological procedures (Arnold et al., 1995, 1996). Nine of these reports (8%) employed procedures utilizing ionizing radiation. The use of such procedures has increased and has become more frequent in children and adolescents. As with much other research technology, neuroimaging was initially used only in adults and is being extended to minors. Its application to children and adolescents raises additional ethical issues involving both risks and benefits, which will be reviewed here.

Children have often been "research orphans" whose exclusion from research has limited their ability to benefit from it. With the recent adoption by the National Institutes of Health (NIH) of a policy encouraging the inclusion of children in research, their role in neuroimaging research is now entering a new era. Similar to the NIH policy on the inclusion of women and minorities in research, the new policy for the inclusion of children requires explicit justification whenever minors are to be excluded from research. Both policies are designed to extend the benefits of research to groups that have been historically neglected by the scientific community.

Throughout this review, the three principles for the protection of human subjects of scientific research, established in the Belmont report (1979), will be honored. They include:

1 *Respect for persons*, which recognizes the dignity and autonomy of individuals and requires protection for people with diminished autonomy (such as young chil-

dren). This principle is honored through the use of informed consent and assent.

2 *Beneficence*, which requires optimizing benefits and minimizing risks. This principle is reflected by the careful assessment of benefit–risk ratio and the requirement of a favorable ratio to allow research to proceed.

3 *Justice*, which refers to the "fairness of distribution" of the burdens and benefits of research. This principle needs to be considered in the selection of subjects. In fact, the recent NIH initiative regarding the need to justify excluding minors in research stems in part from this principle. The controversial inclusion of healthy children as control subjects in research is also to be examined in light of this principle.

Of these three principles, that of beneficence, with the assessment of benefit–risk ratio, poses the most complex issues.

Benefit–risk ratio: principle of beneficence

Human subjects protections and children

As in any research endeavour, neuroimaging research must minimize the experimental risks to the participants. A given experimental procedure may carry a risk of different magnitude in children than in adults, because of children's additional vulnerabilities. These vulnerabilities include sensitivity to novelty, few previous experiences, incompletely developed ability to understand the altruistic nature of research, and such physiologic vulnerabilities as smaller size, faster metabolism, and potentially altered sensitivity to some medication side effects.

Because of children's special vulnerabilities, society has established special legal and ethical protections for them, including protection from research risk. This generally adds to the safeguards afforded by the natural protection of parents. In fact, society sometimes implies that parents' judgment may not be adequately protective of their children. To insure protection, society may act as a superparent by limiting the rights of parents to make decisions for their children. For example, in some settings the legal concept of *in loco parentis* is invoked to justify societal authorities making decisions that ordinarily would fall to a parent. The US federal research safeguards for children (45 Code of Federal Regulation (CFR), Subtitle A, Part 46, Subpart D, 10-1-91 Edition) indicate that parents' or guardians' permission for research on their children may not be solicited or accepted for research with substantially greater than *minimal risk* unless there is direct benefit to the child with a benefit–risk ratio at least as good as available alternatives. Therefore, the concept of "minimal risk" is crucial for research in children.

Definition of minimal risk

There is much debate over the definition of minimal risk, which Kopelman (1989) characterizes as pivotal. "Risk" invokes a measure of both the probability and the magnitude of potential harm. The threshold defining "minimal risk" can vary greatly among institutional review boards (IRBs) because of its ambiguous meaning. A definition is suggested by 45 Code of Federal Regulation (CFR), Subtitle A, Part 46, Subpart A, 46.102(g) 10-1-91 Edition: "'Minimal risk' means that the risks of harm anticipated in the proposed research are not greater, considering probability and magnitude, than those ordinarily encountered in daily life or during the performance of routine physical or psychological examinations or tests." This definition seems to accept as minimal the risks that are comparable to the risks of everyday activities that parents and society routinely approve for children, such as bike riding, riding in a car, and even seasonal activities such as swimming or sled riding. However, authorities are not clear about this nor about the definitions of "ordinary" or "routine".

Unfortunately, there are many ways to interpret the official definition of minimal risk above. Kopelman (1989) points out that the phrase "ordinarily encountered in daily life" can be interpreted as (i) all the risks ordinary people encounter, (ii) the risks all people ordinarily encounter, (iii) or the minimal risks all ordinary people ordinarily encounter. We should note that research is not considered an ordinary daily risk, but rather an additional risk.

Another problem is that what is routine for one child may not be routine risk or discomfort for another child. A question to be resolved is whether a given procedure represents minimal risk for both patients and health controls. How do the daily risks experienced by a patient with a disorder compare with the daily risks of a control subject? On the one hand, it might be argued that a patient who has daily exposure to electrolyte imbalance or malnutrition from an eating disorder, or a patient who clinically requires daily administration of risky medications, may encounter more risks in daily life than control subjects. On the other hand, it could be argued that the state of vulnerability from these risks makes a patient less able to tolerate additional research risks.

Nicholson (1986) has proposed a list of examples of ordinary daily risks to which research risks can be compared to determine minimal risk. Such a list may be helpful as long as it is used only for guidance and not interpreted rigidly.

Risk and aversiveness

The process of defining minimal risk requires clarification of the relationship between aversiveness and risk. Both are negative outcomes and one may cause the other. A procedure can be risky without being aversive or uncomfortable, or can be aversive without being risky (at least physically). However, extreme aversiveness constitutes a psychologic risk (e.g., adjustment disorder or post-traumatic stress disorder), especially if subjects are not provided careful support. For some anxiety-prone children, the experience of being enclosed in a magnetic resonance imaging (MRI) scanner could conceivably be psychologically traumatic, especially without adequate preparation.

The obvious need for individual evaluation of aversion-driven psychologic risks is partly met by the requirement for child assent in addition to parent permission. By definition and federal statute, minors are required to "assent" to participate in research and only adults (i.e., parents) can consent to their own or their children's participation. If the procedure is extremely aversive or perceived as aversive, assent will presumably not be forthcoming. The same procedure may be less aversive as part of a research protocol than when conducted under routine clinical necessity. Research investigators typically invest time and effort in psychologic preparation to maintain participant cooperation. The pressure of clinical emergencies and stringencies of cost containment often prohibit the same degree of preparation for clinical patients. Several authors (Jay et al., 1982; Castellanos et al., 1994; Rosenberg et al., 1997) have documented that there is an opportunity to minimize the psychologic risk of aversiveness by preliminary rehearsal or role playing.

Risks of neuroimaging

A literature search yielded few systematic studies of the physical or psychologic risks of biological research procedures in general, and none on neuroimaging in children. The relevant clinical literature about risks and side effects is somewhat richer. The risks involved in neuroimaging research in children include those associated with radiation exposure, electromagnetic fields, sedation or anesthesia, and psychologic stress (e.g., claustrophobic reaction, exposure to a hospital setting).

Techniques for studying the brain in vivo have evolved rapidly during the past decades, beginning with X-ray computed tomography (CT) in the late 1960s to early 1970s. Each type of imaging carries its own special risks. The history of CT scan use illustrates the potential of research to reduce risks. Before systematic neuroimaging research, many clinicians routinely obtained CT scans as part of their assessment of developmental disorders such as autism. A benefit–risk assessment, promoted by research studies, suggested this practice to be inappropriate and led to its discontinuation.

Radiation exposure

The health risks of radiation exposure at the doses used in positron emission tomography (PET) and single photon emission computed tomography (SPECT) studies have been extensively reviewed by Ernst et al. (1998). The major concerns lie with the question of whether the levels of radiation exposure involved in these techniques increase a subject's risk for developing cancer.

The review by Ernst and co-workers (1998) of the largest studies of radiation risks, measured as the probability of excess rates of cancer among populations exposed to low-dose radiation (defined as less than 20 or 10 rems), concluded that an excess risk could not be detected in association with low-level radiation exposure. The highest research radiation dose used in imaging studies of healthy children 12 years of age and older has been 0.06 rem to the whole body. The rem is a unit of dose equivalent that accounts for the cellular and subcellular differences in the energy deposition pattern of various ray (1 rem = 0.01 Sv (sievert, the SI unit)). This dose is approximately one-tenth of the dose limit recommended by the US Food and Drug Administration (FDA) for adult volunteers in research.

Because children may be more vulnerable to the effects of radiation than are adults, the FDA restricts the use of radioactive drugs in research involving minors to a cumulative dose per year of 0.5 rem (0.3 rem in single dose) to whole body, active blood-forming organs, lens of the eye, and gonads, and 1.5 rem (0.5 rem in single dose) for other organs, which is one tenth of the limit for research use in adults. The International Commission on Radiological Protection (IRCP) sets general public involuntary risk guidelines at 1 mSv per year (approximately 0.1 rem),

which is slightly above most background levels from soil radioactivity and cosmic radiation at sea level. The IRCP sets occupational limits or whole body exposure at 5 rem per year in adults. In addition, a 3 rem limit for exposure to any individual organ or tissue has been established by 21 Code of Federal Regulations Ch. 1 Part 361.1. In children, the limit is set at one tenth that for adults.

The radiation effect that confers biological risk is that of unrepaired genetic mutation. While such unrepaired mutations increase risk, it is important to note that genetic mutations are common events that are corrected physiologically by powerful cellular repair mechanisms. An average of 240 000 genetic mutations occur spontaneously daily in the human body. Radiation exposure of 1 rem adds about 100 more genetic mutations to this number (Billen, 1990). Although debated, there is some evidence that previous low-level radiation can have a protective effect from subsequent high-dose radiation exposure by stimulating chromosomal repair mechanisms (for review, see Ernst et al., 1998).

Studies that expose human subjects to ionizing radiation must be reviewed by the local Radiation Safety Committee (RSC) or Radioactive Drug Review Committee (RDRC) and the IRB throughout the research. RDRCs or RSCs are composed of members with expertise in radiation biology who are competent to assess the risk of exposure. IRBs often lack this degree of expertise and must be educated both by members of the RSC and by the review of materials addressing these risks. A process of careful collaboration and consultation among researchers, RDRC, and IRB members is essential for a logical, unfragmented risk assessment, with each party contributing their specific expertise and taking the appropriate responsibility. The expertise of RSC and RDRC members should be sought during the conceptualization and design of the protocol, and members of the RSC and RDRC should attend IRB meetings to consult on the use of ionizing radiation. The lay perception of risk from radiation often greatly exceeds the risk measured in controlled research studies of large samples, and this bias is often harboured by members of the IRB despite otherwise excellent scientific credentials.

Electromagnetic field exposure

Functional MRI (fMRI), magnetic resonance spectroscopy (MRS), and magnetoencephalography (MEG) all use conventional MRI scanners. Although MRI does not expose subjects to ionizing radiation risk, the potential risk of exposure to a high magnetic field (>1.5 T) cannot be measured accurately. Some of the inherent risks in MRI studies at any magnet strength include the rare complication of scanning a patient who has had metal clips or pacemakers inserted or has ingested scraps of metal (see Chapter 3). Movement of such materials induced by the magnetic field can have serious consequences. To prevent such occurrences, a medical history with explicit questioning of caretakers about prior surgeries and the possibility of any metallic implants should be systematically included as part of a screening. Histories that raise concern can be followed up with X-rays or other appropriate medical examinations.

Heating of tissue is a theoretical and practical concern at high field strengths. However, with the magnetic fields currently used (up to 4 T), adverse effects from heating are unlikely.

In MRI-related studies, sedation probably remains the greatest risk for those who require it. At present, many IRBs have not allowed minors to participate in studies at the high magnetic field strengths (3–4 T) that permit the fast acquisition of whole-brain fMRI scans with adequate spatial resolution and the analysis of various components of the MRS signal (e.g., the differentiation in MRS of the glutamatergic from the GABAergic components of the composite Glx signal).

Sedation or anesthesia for brain imaging

Sedation of minors for imaging is a routine part of pediatric practice and is associated with very low risk (Williams et al., 1997). For patients, the use of sedation in situations of no direct or immediate benefit requires careful justification but should not be categorically rejected given the low risk. For example, after review of the complication rate associated with deep sedation (propofol) of severely impaired children, an IRB approved the use of this method in PET studies of minors with autism and with Lesch–Nyhan disease, despite the lack of direct benefit to the patients. There was no complication in those studies (Ernst et al., 1996, 1997a). In view of the catastrophic nature of pervasive development disorders, childhood-onset schizophrenia, and similarly crippling disorders, this adjunct to imaging should not stand as a rigid impediment to brain imaging. Although anesthesiologists often argue that general anesthesia with intubation is safer than deep sedation, investigators as well as IRB members will need to be better educated to decide whether the risks of general anesthesia are, in fact, lower than those of deep sedation. In some instances, sedation may be obviated by familiarizing the subjects to the research procedures. Such approaches have been used successfully in several laboratories (for example, see Chapter 13). It may be possible to enhance the benefit–risk ratio by adding clinically indicated tests to a research procedure, such as performing a clinical MRI in the context of a brain imaging study while the participant is sedated.

Hospital/clinic setting as a stressor

Although not technically a neuroimaging procedure, an additional "intervention" to be considered when weighing the risks of research is the hospital visit that is sometimes necessary. Two studies have assessed whether hospitalization of pediatric subjects was related to subsequent psychiatric morbidity. Douglas (1975) found that a single hospitalization of 1 week or less of children below an age of 5 years was not associated with later behavior disturbance or poor reading in adolescence. Similarly, Quinton and Rutter (1976) found no association between one-time hospitalization of a week or more regardless of age with emotional or conduct disturbance at age 10 years. Furthermore, visits to medical centers for children and adolescents may serve to demystify this setting, particularly if the experience is positive, thus making future visits to doctors and hospitals less stressful.

Unexpected or unwanted knowledge about individuals: confidentiality

Much like genetic studies, another problem for neuroimaging procedures is the handling of unexpected or unwanted knowledge gained in the course of research. This is especially relevant for control subjects. It appears advisable to discuss with the child and parents their wishes about possible contingencies before the results are known. Wertz et al. (1994) suggest that the child or adolescent should be the primary decision-maker about being told things with no direct health benefits (i.e., no treatment or prevention possible) but which might be useful to the minor in making future decisions. Others advise that the parents decide whether and how to communicate the information to their child. Consent and assent forms should be explicit regarding any baseline ancillary studies to be performed, such as HIV or pregnancy testing, and should specify who will be informed in the event of positive test results. Such a pre-test discussion must be handled skillfully and reassuringly because it may create risks by arousing unnecessary anxiety. It may also be useful to solicit general policy guidance from nonresearch sources such as self-help groups. Such groups might help to formulate general guidelines about when and what individuals in various scenarios would like to be told.

The risk of breach of confidentiality between children and parents needs to be carefully evaluated and is particularly salient in research with adolescents. For example, most functional neuroimaging protocols require research participants to have no history of illicit substance use. How the investigators will deal with this type of information needs to be carefully delineated in the protocol, and in the consent and assent forms.

A risk of unwanted knowledge increasingly noted by IRBs is an economic one. Evidence of previously undiagnosed chronic disease or genetic vulnerability that may be found in the course of research could prevent the subject from getting medical insurance and possibly life insurance in the future if this information became accessible. Reportedly, some IRBs have interpreted this economic risk as more than minimal and have denied approval of some protocols on this basis even though the other risks were acceptable.

Minimizing risks

Risks can be minimized by limiting the number and type of research procedures to prevent research days from being unduly long, tiresome, or anxiety provoking. In longitudinal studies, deciding the appropriate number and frequency of serial tests requires careful balancing of the incremental value of additional knowledge against incremental risk for each repetition.

Investigators have an obligation to do no more invasive tests than necessary to answer the central research questions and to devise designs that minimize the number and invasiveness of tests. Can a blood draw replace a spinal tap, or can blood be drawn while starting an intravenous line, thus minimizing the number of needle punctures? In the absence of allergy, the application of a local anaesthetic cream (e.g., one containing lidocaine (lignocaine) such as Emla cream) can be used systematically in children prior to a needle puncture. Less-invasive tests should be sought and technology devised to yield the same information for which a more invasive test might have been needed.

Another approach to minimizing risks is to modify the methodologic paradigms. For example, duration of sedation can be shortened in PET imaging by giving the sedative agent only after the uptake of the tracer in the brain has been completed (40 min for fluorodeoxyglucose, 90 min for fluorodihydroxyphenylalanine (fluoro DOPA)). This strategy requires using a sedative with a short and reliable onset of action (like propofol). An additional advantage of this technique is that the study results, which reflect the uptake period of the tracer, are not influenced by the sedative agent; in this case, minimization of risk maximizes the science.

To minimize risk during the PET scanning of minors, Ernst et al. (1997b) modified their procedure for adults to reduce radiation exposure in minors (below the guideline for minors of 10% of the dose limit established for adults). This was accomplished by (i) reducing the amount of tracer injected; (ii) lengthening the scan acquisition time, thus recovering image resolution lost as a result of the lower injected dose; (iii) using measures to avoid artifacts secondary to repositioning subjects in the scanner and (iv) allowing subjects to void during the study, thus removing the tracer from the bladder, which is the organ with the highest level of exposure during fluorodeoxyglucose PET scans.

Another strategy to minimize risk in PET studies has recently become available with the advent of highly sensitive whole-body PET scanners. Prior to the availability of these large-bore cameras, any measurement of absolute levels of brain metabolism required the insertion of a radial arterial catheter for acquisition of an arterial input curve of the tracer. The insertion of arterial catheters in healthy minors for research purposes was considered by most IRBs to be "above minimal risk". Actual risks of arterial catheterization have been reviewed in a follow-up NIH study of 106 subjects with arterial catheterization for PET protocols (Jons et al., 1997). This study identified only minor abnormal signs (e.g., transient haematoma, local redness) that would not have attracted medical attention otherwise. With large-bore PET cameras (whole-body cameras), the arterial input data can be replaced by cardiac input data obtained noninvasively by imaging the left ventricle of the heart (see Chapter 1).

Since risk and discomfort may be inversely proportional to the skill of the technician or clinician performing the procedure, the most skilled clinician should be recruited. Arranging for presence of parents, family, or peers during the procedure may be useful to allay the child's anxiety.

Another minimization of risk, or at least discomfort, involves carefully determining the value and hazards of preparatory procedures (e.g., fasting, special diets, resting, caffeine restrictions, and medication withdrawal). Are these necessary for subject safety? Or are they merely necessary for quality of test results? If the latter, is the increment of knowledge worth the increment of subject discomfort?

Risk can be further minimized by implementation of procedures to prepare the subject and monitor consequences and after-effects (Jay et al., 1982; Kruesi et al., 1988; Castellanos et al., 1994). For example, Amiel (1985) used videotape movies to keep children comfortable while they remained in a supine position after a spinal tap, which reduced the risk of postspinal tap headache. Children may have a lower (or higher) threshold for aversive stimuli than adults, or the after-effects of aversive stimuli may last a longer or shorter time. Studies to establish such thresholds and perceptions of aversive procedures could be useful.

A final point about preparing subjects for imaging procedures is that more preparation is not necessarily better.

Particularly for some developmentally disabled children or individuals with thought disorders, visits to the scanner ahead of time may only serve to increase anxiety or even allow time for paranoid delusions to develop. Each individual situation requires careful assessment informed by advice from parents, who may have previous experience with the child in similar situations.

Assessment of benefit–risk ratio

Assessment of the benefit–risk ratio should consider the entire study. It should evaluate risks comprehensively and consider the known in vitro effects (for example, the effects of a drug on enzymatic processes identified in cell preparation) and in vivo effects (in animals, adults, and children), as well as potential effects of the technician's or clinician's skills on the risks. The database utilized for judgment about risk should also include noncontrolled clinical findings and other observations. It should also evaluate benefits comprehensively and consider the health and welfare of the subject in general, as well as the advancement of medical knowledge that would benefit the subject in the long run. Finally an assessment should consider possibilities for improving the benefit–risk ratio by increasing benefits, decreasing risk, or both (see above).

A problem in extrapolating reports of adverse effects from clinical samples is that the clinical experience is often confounded by complicating factors, including the illness for which the clinical procedure was carried out. Since a research procedure is undertaken on a voluntary basis rather than under clinical necessity, it is less likely to involve those individuals who anticipate the most distress from it. This probably reduces the psychologic risk for the sample as a whole, although there still may be individuals who assent/consent despite negative anticipation. An interesting related question concerns the subsequent effect on the child's later psychologic reaction to the same test if it is clinically indicated. Will the child weather it better because of success in the research administration or experience greater stress because of being sensitized to the risks? Systematic follow-up of child and adolescent research subjects regarding both physical and emotional consequences would be of great value for future formal risk estimation. For example, Kruesi et al. (1988) reported that lumbar punctures for research purposes were rated by child subjects as equivalent in both acceptability and side effects/discomfort to procedures such as blood sampling, electroencephalography, and attending school in the research setting, thus providing a comparison with which to gauge psychologic risk.

The benefit–risk ratio usually differs for patients who can directly benefit from the research through an increase in knowledge about their disorder and for healthy controls, who do not directly benefit from the study of a disorder that they do not have. In this case, the US Code of Federal Regulation (CFR), Subtitle A, Part 46, clearly indicates that studies carrying higher than minimal risk with no direct benefit for the subjects are generally disallowed for children. However, when the risk is "a minor increase above minimal risk", this regulation allows children to participate if the benefits to society are sizable. Just as "minimal risk" is subject to the interpretations of an IRB, so is "minor increase". Therefore, healthy children can participate in brain imaging studies if the risk can be judged to be "minimal' or "just above minimal". Whether this describes the risk from radiation exposure from PET/SPECT is difficult to determine. Although excess health hazards from low-level radiation exposure have not been detected in any large studies so far (Mossman et al., 1996; Ernst et al., 1998), the concept of radiation exposure carries overriding emotional freight that can distort the objective assessment of radiation risks.

A benefit usually not addressed and highly dependent on the way research is conducted by the investigators is the potentially positive experience a child may experience by participating as an autonomous individual in an adult enterprise with the purpose of helping society at large. Examination of this aspect of research with children might identify strategies that could promote the development of altruism.

To insure that the risk experienced by healthy normal controls is not "wasted", it is important to insure they are indeed normal and, therefore, able to yield the needed normative data. This can be done through a multistage screening analogous to that used to insure that patients who are subjects have the relevant disorder. Parents return standard behavior ratings and questionnaires. If no pathology is noted on the paper-and-pencil screen, the parent is interviewed by phone. If no pathology is evident from the phone interview, the parent and child/adolescent are invited to the clinic and observed and interviewed with structured instruments. If no relevant pathology is detected here, the child/adolescent is declared "normal" and offered an opportunity to participate in the study as a healthy control.

Informed assent and consent principle of respect for persons

Although a favorable benefit–risk ratio is likely in the study of severe mental disorders where potential benefits usually outweigh the experimental risks, an issue remains, that of informed consent/assent. In fact, some of the concerns about validity of assent in a mentally impaired population similarly apply to very young children.

By definition and US federal statute, minors cannot actually consent but are permitted "and, above certain ages required", to assent to participate in research, whereas their parents are required to give permission in order for the child to participate. As a reminder, valid informed consent (assent) requires (i) disclosure of relevant information, (ii) comprehension of the information, and (iii) voluntary agreement to participation, free of coercion and undue influences.

Developmentally sensitive consent

As children mature, they concurrently develop a better capability of understanding the risks of research and acquire a better ability to consent (Laor, 1987; Leikin, 1993), that is, as cognitive ability increases gradually, so may consent ability. A considerable amount is now known about minors' understanding of the consent process. The basic work of Piaget and Inhelder (1958) suggests increments of cognitive ability around 7 years of age and when adult-like formal operations are attained during puberty. Lewis et al. (1978) found significant increases by grade level (elementary school) in awareness of risk, understanding of future consequences, wariness of individuals with vested interests, and need for independent professional advice. Keith-Spiegel and Maas (1981) (quoted by Leikin, 1993) found that children, particularly those under age 9 years, had difficulty understanding the scientific purposes of research, failed to recall their role in research, and were unaware of their freedom to withdraw. Those 9 years and under tended to focus on only one or two salient pieces of information, while those above age 9 were more similar to adults in their reasoning about research. Weithorn and Campbell (1982) found that 14-year-olds show the same benefit–risk reasoning as 21-year-olds, and that 9-year-olds reach the same conclusions albeit through a different reasoning strategy. Lewis et al. (1978) found that children aged 7–9 years (but not those aged 6 years) asked all the relevant questions needed for an informed consent. Leikin (1993), after reviewing the literature, concluded that by age 9 children have enough cognitive capacity to participate in the decision. Weithorn and Scherer (1994) concluded that school-age children have the capacity to assent and that children aged 14 years, on average, have the capacity to consent in the same manner as adults. Therefore, enough seems to be known about children's understanding and judgment to justify more empowerment in the consent process, including the right to make some altruistic decisions.

Laor (1987), in fact, offers this resolution: ". . . every individual can achieve, and exercise, different levels of autonomy at different times. . . . The question as to who is or is not autonomous should be replaced by the questions of how much autonomy can/should be ascribed to/required of the individual in different circumstances, be the individual a child or an adult. . . ." He proposes that children age 12 years and above be able to consent to research on their own (like adults); that between ages 7 and 12 years they can consent but parents' assent is also needed (the reverse of the current rules); and below age 7 parental consent is needed, whenever possible coupled with the child's assent. The participation of children under 7 years of age without their assent is a thorny issue, but, given the severity of certain early childhood disease (leukemia, autism), parents could be empowered to make decisions for young children when the research is critical to the understanding of severe illness. Laor's recommendation was not adopted in 1977 by the American National Committee for the Protection of Human Subjects of Biomedical and Behavioral Research because of a lack of public consensus at the time (Grisso and Vierling, 1978; Melton, 1980; Laor, 1987). Is it time to reconsider the recommendation, perhaps with some modification (for example, age 14 rather than 12 years for adult-like consent)?

Motivation

Motivation varies widely among children as a function of their cognitive maturity, individual circumstances, and personality. Motivation to participate in research may be altruistic or may be driven by the compensation offered for participation (see below). A child may find that missing a day of school is rewarding enough to induce participation in a research study. The opportunity to impress peers or to feel special may influence another child. Other motivations may include unconscious seeking of punishment to assuage guilt feelings. For example, healthy siblings of a patient might feel guilty about not sharing the patient's problems. Therefore, the investigator needs to be alert to the motivation of children during the process of informed assent. Particularly, the investigators have the responsibility to insure the absence of coercion or undue influences. Therefore, the assent with children should be conducted separate from the parents, though the child could be present at the parental consent.

Inducements (incentives, coercion, undue influences)

The possibility of coercion (i.e., real or perceived negative consequences of refusing to participate in the research) or coercive inducement (e.g., excessive reward to obtain compliance) needs to be carefully monitored. A generally acceptable incentive may become an undue influence if the individual is particularly vulnerable. Deciding how much is too large a compensation for the risk, discomfort, inconvenience, and lost time of subjects and their parents requires some thought. Paradoxically, the greater the risk, the harder it may be to justify a large compensation. The inducement of compensation should not be so large as to override judgment about the potential risks.

A complication in determining appropriate compensation is the varying economic status of the families. The same payment may be much more of an inducement for a poor subject than a wealthy one. However, it is unfeasible (and unfair) to equalize inducement by varying the compensation with economic status. The child's view of dollar amounts also needs to be considered. For example, Keith-Spiegel and Maas (1981) found that minors ages 9 to 15 years were interested in compensation of any amount, whereas adults were mainly interested in higher amounts.

Parents need to be compensated for lost time from work and transportation costs. How generously parents are compensated may be an issue. Would a poor parent be tempted to coerce the child into research for the compensation? Such exploitation would run counter to the usual expectation that the parent's judgment about the best interests of the child would protect the child from undue inducement. Working middle-class parents should be reimbursed fairly for lost time from work, but this rate may verge on coerciveness for some poor families and yet it is inconceivable to pay poor or unemployed parents less.

Some IRBs and even some ethics experts are tempted to avoid such thorny decisions by banning compensation in child research, at least for the children themselves. However, it is difficult to justify this to the subjects and their parents. It is the practice in some places to reimburse only transportation for the child and one parent, particularly where treatment is part of the study. However, a reasonable approach could be to offer fair compensation at middle-class levels when the study budget can afford it; in high-risk studies where there is a concern about the compensation becoming an undue influence for the poor subjects, some provision could be made for a neutral clinician to monitor the consent/assent process.

Other suggested solutions have not elicited enthusiasm or general acceptance. For example, some ethicists suggest that there be no discussion about compensation until after consent in order to preclude any inducement. However, others feel that this might unfairly exclude some families who could not afford to take time off from work and pay transportation without some reimbursement. In practice, most IRBs take the position that knowledge about compensation is part of a fully informed consent and many even require it to be in the consent form, at least for parents. Some IRBs prohibit the information about parents' compensation to be given to the child. Another controversial recommendation not commonly followed is that none of the funding comes from pharmaceutical companies or other interested parties (Small et al., 1994).

When the IRB's policy is to reimburse the child, then arises the question of who receives the compensation and how. Is the cash given to the parents or the child? Is the check made out to the adolescent's name or parent's name? Is compensation given as a gift certificate for children's stores? The alternatives are many and should be carefully chosen and, unless against the IRB's policy, clearly outlined in protocol and the consent and assent forms.

Paradoxically, insurance for injury during research, to which no one would object ethically, is an inducement not universally used despite general agreement about its desirability. This particular inducement, in fact, would make any research more ethical by reducing economic risk to the subject.

A nonmonetary inducement may occur when the sibling of a patient is used as normal control. Is the sibling psychologically coerced by guilt and by the expectation of taking responsibility to help the ill family member? A partial answer can come from observations such as those reported by Amiel (1985), who found that siblings of patients were enthusiastic about volunteering for a procedure involving two indwelling venous lines for a day because it allowed them to share the attention the sick sibling had been getting and to satisfy their curiosity about what the patient had been going through.

Another nonmonetary inducement is the wish to please the investigator, especially if the investigator is also the child's therapist. Where is the line between cultivating an alliance and seductive trading on friendship? In a longitudinal study, what is too much pressure for retention? Where is the line between healthy, respectful expectation of fulfilling the agreement and manipulating guilt? As already mentioned above, a therapist, case manager, or neutral clinician not involved in the research can be one safeguard against undue inducement of this type.

Neutral clinician to insure understanding

Within the consent/assent empowerment remains an obligation to make sure the child or adolescent understands the information provided. Because of wide individual variation, one cannot depend on the subject's age to insure adequate understanding; even some adults have difficulty understanding consent information. When the investigator is not the child's regular clinician, it would be desirable for the investigator and the child's clinician to join in making sure the child understands the information provided. When the investigator is the child's regular clinician, Weithorn and Scherer (1994) suggest that consent be obtained by another clinician. The participation of a neutral clinician whose only interest and responsibility are the child's welfare could help to justify consent (assent) empowerment for children younger than those currently allowed to consent. The neutral clinician would act as a counterbalance to the investigator's bias, as well as to the potential, perceived or real, parental coercion or undue influence.

It is tempting for researchers to believe that children should be free to participate in research to a greater degree. The possibility of self-serving blind spots within the investigator's assessment makes a dialogue with noninvestigator clinicians and other neutral parties essential, at least for policy-making. These neutral clinicians may need to be recruited from outside the research institution to insure neutrality. They should be paid for their time, perhaps through the IRB from the study budget. This expense would be justified if it makes a valuable but more than minimal risk study ethically possible. Of course, cost and effort considerations suggest that involvement of an additional clinician in day-to-day consent with individual child subjects is necessary and advisable only for research deemed more than minimal risk by the IRB. More-than-minimal risk research is permissible under certain carefully specified situations (see Code of Federal Regulations as cited above).

An example of using an independent clinician to insure that children were not being coerced can be found in a recent National Institute of Mental Health PET study that recruited normal siblings of patients with autism, Tourette's disorder, and Lesch–Nyhan disease. A member of the Bioethics Program of the NIH Clinical Center interviewed each sibling control teenager (minimum age 12 years), alone without investigators or parents present, to screen for understanding of the study, coercion, and undue influence.

It is also critical to make sure that children understand that they have a choice. Weithorn and Scherer (1994) reviewed the development of locus of control (internal in 40% of prepubertal children, >80% of late adolescents) and other relevant psychologic dimensions. They list several ways to help the child to feel more autonomous (e.g., ask them to choose which chair to sit in; ask assent neutrally). They note that this not only promotes valid consent/assent but also improves compliance with the research procedures.

Selection of subjects (principle of justice)

Patients versus healthy controls

A highly controversial question remains as to whether the principle of justice is served or violated by excluding healthy children from research because they may not benefit directly from the research that studies a disorder they do not have and because the research procedure is estimated to be more than minimal risk, because it is one they are not commonly exposed to (for example, an intravenous line). Should the individuals already suffering from a disorder also be the ones to bear the burden of research? True, they are the ones who can mostly benefit from the research directly. However, society at large may also benefit from advanced knowledge and potential prevention of costly diseases. Each research protocol needs to be assessed individually in an effort to respect all three principles of ethics, including justice.

Socioeconomic status and ethnic issues

An important goal in recruiting subjects is to achieve a sample that represents the general population. Control subjects should be representative of the general population, and a clinical sample should reflect the clinical population. This condition requires some attention to the socioeconomic status and ethnic composition of the sample. Cultural and socioeconomic preferences, biases, opportunities, and confounds with exclusion criteria may skew a sample. If major ethnic groups are not represented in the sample, important findings may be missed that might be useful to the absent or under-represented ethnic groups and to the advancement of clinical science. There has been official recognition of the need to insure equal access to research and its benefits (Ellis, 1994; Varmus, 1994) for both minorities and minors (defined in the USA as below 18 years of age). Recent initiatives mandate the participation of minorities, women, and minors in all US NIH-funded research unless their exclusion is explicitly and well justified.

Underrepresentation of ethnic or socioeconomic groups poses a safety and statistical dilemma. Stratifying a sample by ethnicity or socioeconomic group can reduce statistical power and require a larger sample, thus exposing more children to research-related risks. The investigator must make an informed decision as to whether ethnicity is likely to affect the question under study. If not, then all subjects can be pooled with no special recruitment or exclusion criteria other than equal access. If ethnicity is likely to make a difference, then a decision has to be made whether (i) to initially concentrate efforts on one ethnic group to minimize the number who need to be exposed to the risk of the procedure, and then study other groups later if the results warrant it; or (ii) to increase the sample size sufficiently to provide the statistical power for ethnic stratification.

Conclusion

Literature review and recent experience in neuroimaging research suggest that the degree of risk (including aversiveness of neuroimaging procedures to children) is often assumed to be higher than indicated by the data. The available data suggest that, in normal circumstances, the degree of discomfort associated with most neuroimaging studies is comparable to that associated with children's everyday experiences. Likewise, the degree of physical risk appears to be less than commonly assumed (e.g., Huda and Scrimger, 1989). Furthermore, many of these risks can be minimized by appropriate sensitivity and planning.

Despite popular notions to the contrary, available evidence suggests that adolescents can meaningfully evaluate risks and benefits in a fashion similar to adults. Younger children, while cognitively less able, nonetheless reach sensible conclusions concerning risks and benefits, albeit through rationales somewhat different from those used by adolescents and adults. Current regulations may excessively limit children's opportunities both to contribute altruistic service and to benefit as a group from research. Developmentally enlightened revisions of current regulations and research practices could ensure that children and adolescents reap the full benefits of neuroimaging research on their neuropsychiatric disorders. When a study is considered to pose more than minimal risk and does not offer equivalent benefit for the subject, a neutral clinician could insure that the child is not psychologically coerced or unduly influenced by parent or investigator. The risks of neuroimaging research with children and adolescents should be carefully balanced against the risks of depriving them of the benefits of state-of-the-art knowledge concerning the severe neuropsychiatric illnesses that afflict many of them. This delicate balance requires the collaboration of investigators with physicists, ethicists, and patients and their parents.

Acknowledgement

This chapter is adapted and expanded from an article in the *Journal of the American Academy of Child and Adolescent Psychiatry*, (1995) **34**, 929–39.

The opinions expressed herein are the views of the authors and do not necessarily reflect the official position of the National Institute of Mental Health or the US Department of Health and Human Services.

References

Amiel, S. A. (1985). Pediatric research on diabetes: the problem of hospitalizing youthful subjects. *IRB Rev. Hum. Subjects Res.*, **7**, 4–5.

Arnold, L. E., Stoff, D., Cooke, E. et al. (1995). Ethics of biological psychiatric research with children and adolescents. *J. Am. Acad. Child Adolesc. Psychiatry*, **347**, 929–39.

Arnold, L. E., Stoff, D., Cooke, E. et al. (1996). Ethical issues in biological mental health research with children and adolescents. In *Ethical Issues in Mental Health Research with Children and Adolescents*, eds. K. Hoagwood and P. S. Jensen, pp. 89–111. Mahwah, NJ: Lawrence Erlbaum.

Belmont Report (1979). *Ethical Guidelines for the Protection of Human Subjects of Research.* (OPRR Reports). Washington, DC: NIH Office for Protection from Research Risks and The National Commission for the Protection of Human Subjects of Biomedical and Behavioral Research.

Billen, D. (1990). Spontaneous DNA damage and its significance for the "negligible dose" controversy in radiation protection. *Radiat. Res.*, **124**, 242–5.

Castellanos, F. X., Elia, J., Kruesi, M. J. P. et al. (1994). Cerebrospinal fluid monoamine metabolites in ADHD boys. *Psychiatr. Res.*, **52**, 305–16.

Douglas, J. W. B. (1975). Early hospital admissions and later disturbances of behavior and learning. *Dev. Med. Child Neurol.*, **17**, 456–80.

Ellis, G. B. (1994). *Inclusion of Women and Minorities in Research* (OPRR Reports 94–01). Bethseda, MD: NIH Office of Protection from Research Risks.

Ernst, M., Zametkin, A. J., Matochik, J. A. et al. (1996). Presynaptic dopaminergic deficits in Lesch–Nyhan Disease. *N. Engl. J. Med.*, **334**, 1568–1604.

Ernst, M., Zametkin, A. J., Matochik, J. A., Pascualvaca, D. and Cohen, R. M. (1997a). Low medial prefrontal dopaminergic activity in autistic children. *Lancet*, **350**, 638.

Ernst, M., Cohen, R. M. Liebenauer, L. L., Jons, P. H. and Zametkin, A. J. (1997b). Cerebral glucose metabolism in adolescent girls with attention-deficit/hyperactivity disorder. *J. Am. Acad. Child Adolesc. Psychiatry*, **36**, 1399–1406.

Ernst, M., Freed, M. E. and Zametkin, A. J. (1998). Health hazards of radiation exposure in the context of brain imaging research: special consideration for children. *J. Nucl. Med.*, **39**, 689–98.

Grisso, T. and Vierling, L. (1978). Minors' consent to treatment: a developmental perspective. *Professional Psychol.*, **9**, 412–27.

Huda, W. and Scrimger, J. W. (1989). Irradiation of normal volunteers in nuclear medicine. *J. Nucl. Med.*, **30**, 260–4.

Jay, S. M., Elliot, C. H., Ozolins, M., Olsen, R. A. and Pruitt, S. D.

(1982). Behavioral management of children's distress during painful medical procedures. *Behav. Res. Ther.*, **23**, 513–20.

Jons, P. H., Ernst, M., Hankerson, J., Hardy, K. and Zametkin, A. J. (1997). Follow-up of radial catheterization for positron emission tomography scans. *Hum. Brain Map.*, **5**, 119–23.

Keith-Spiegel, P. and Maas, T. (1981). Consent to research: are there developmental differences? In *Proceedings of American Psychological Association, 1981*. Washington, DC: American Psychological Association.

Kopelman, L. M. (1989). When is the risk minimal enough for children to be research subjects? In *Children and Health Care: Moral and Social Issues*, eds. L. M. Kopelman and J. C. Moskop, pp. 89–99. Boston, MA: Kluwer.

Kruesi, M. J. P., Swedo, S. E., Coffey, M. L., Hamburger, S. D., Leonard, H. and Rapoport, J. L. (1988). Objective and subjective side effects of research lumbar punctures in children and adolescents. *Psychiatr. Res.*, **25**, 59–63.

Laor, N. (1987). Toward liberal guidelines for clinical research with children. *Med. Law*, **6**, 127–37.

Leikin, S. (1993). Minors' assent, consent, or dissent to medical research. *IRB Rev. Hum. Subjects Res.*, **15**, 1–7.

Lewis, C., Lewis, M. and Ifekwunigue, M. (1978). Informed consent by children and participation in an influenza vaccine trial. *Am. J. Public Health*, **68**, 1079–82.

Melton, G. (1980). Children's concepts of their rights. *J. Clin. Child Psychol.*, **9**, 186–190.

Mossman, K., Goldman, M., Masse, F. et al. (1996). Radiation risk in perspective. Health Physics Society Position Statement. *Soc. Nucl. Med.* Newsletter.

Nicholson, R. (1986). *Medical Research with Children: Ethics, Law, and Practice*, pp. 82–6. Oxford: Oxford University Press.

Piaget, J. and Inhelder, B. (1958). *The Growth of Logical Thinking from Childhood to Adolescence*, New York: Basic Books.

Quinton, D. and Rutter, M. (1976). Early hospital admissions and later disturbances of behavior: An attempted replication of Douglas' findings. *Dev. Med. Child Neurol.*, **18**, 447–59.

Rosenberg, D. R., Sweeney, J. A. Gillen, J. S. et al. (1997). Simulation for desensitization of children requiring MRI. *J. Am. Acad. Child Adolesc. Psychiatry*, **36**, 853–9.

Small, A. M., Campbell, M., Shay, J. and Goodman, I. S. (1994). Ethical guidelines for psychopharmacological research in children. In *Ethics and Child Mental Health*, ed. J. Hattab, Jerusalem, Israel: Gefen Publishing.

Varmus, H. (1994). NIH guidelines on the inclusion of women and minorities as subjects in clinical research. *Fed. Reg.*, **59**, 14508–13.

Weithorn, L. and Campbell, S. (1982). The competency of children and adolescents to make informed decisions. *Child Dev.*, **53**, 1589–98.

Weithorn, L. A. and Scherer, D. G. (1994). Children's involvement in research participation decisions: psychological considerations. In *Children as Research Subjects: Science, Ethics, and Law*, ed. M. A. Grodin and L. H. Glantz, Cary, NC: Oxford University Press.

Wertz, D. C., Fanos, J. H. and Reilly, P. R. (1994). Genetic testing for children and adolescents. *J. Am. Med. Assoc.*, **272**, 875–81.

Williams, K. S., Hankerson, J. G., Ernst, M. and Zametkin, A. (1997). Use of propofol anesthesia during outpatient radiographic imaging studies in patients with Lesch–Nyhan syndrome. *J. Clin. Anesth.*, **9**, 61.

Part 3

Normal development

Neuroimaging studies of children, whether cross-sectional or longitudinal, are developmental in nature. This aspect requires the careful consideration and evaluation of maturational changes over time. In addition, the basis for understanding aberrant brain development rests with an understanding of normal maturation. Consequently, this section outlines brain and cognitive development and critically discusses the use of cognitive and behavioral probes in developmental imaging studies. Casanova and his colleagues provide a thoughtful and thorough review of brain development from the level of the cell to the level of gross functional anatomy and discuss the impact of genes and environment on brain organization and its evolution (Chapter 7). Pascualvaca and Morote provide an overview of the developmental trajectories of specific cognitive and neuropsychological functions (Chapter 8). Casey and her colleagues address the important themes of age-appropriate tasks for use in functional neuroimaging studies of children, illustrating these themes with paradigms used to explore prefrontal cortical functioning (Chapter 9). Together, these chapters provide an overview of brain development and cognitive development and illustrate how the two come together in study designs appropriate for mapping human brain functional development.

7

Brain development and evolution

Manuel F. Casanova, Daniel Buxhoeveden and
Gurkirpal S. Sohal

Introduction

The neocortex is a thin layer about 2 to 4mm thick that covers the surface of the cerebrum. Neuronal elements occupy 30% of the neocortex, the remainder being accounted for by glial, vascular, and pericytal elements. Only 10% of the neural somata belong to the Golgi type I cells, the source of cortical efferents. Interneurons (Golgi type II cells) account for the majority of cells in the cortex as well as for a majority (80%) of total cortical synapses. In humans, enlargement of the neuronal somata and its dendritic arbor is no longer detectable after the 6th year of life (Scammon, 1932; Caviness et al., 1997).

The brain achieves its maximum volume by the middle of the second decade of life (for both males and females), reaching a plateau by the 12th year (Dekaban and Sadowsky, 1978). According to Wilmer (1940), brain weight comprises 21% of total body weight at 6 months (fetal period), 15% at term, and only 3% in the adult. The brain is dominated by the cerebrum, which occupies 90% of its volume, and 60% of the cerebrum is gray matter. Most of the gray matter is neocortex. It is 60 times the volume of the diencephalon, the second largest cerebral gray matter structure. A weight difference between the brains of males and females is usually the result of a greater volume of central white matter and a larger cerebellum in the male (Caviness et al., 1997).

The neurons and glial cells of the cortex are anatomically grouped according to a vertical and horizontal organization. The horizontal configuration is known as lamina, and the neocortex generally contains six such layers. When utilizing cell-stained slides, each layer has a different appearance that results from the cell types and their arrangement. Each layer has a specific type of input and output as well. Layer IV is always the sensory input layer, receiving incoming connections from the thalamus. The other form of organization, the one which is actually hierarchical to the lamina, is the vertical organization of the cortex. The vertical array of cells and fibers unifies the neurons and laminae into units of function that are known as cell columns.

The first recognition of the anatomic cell column was described by Lorente de No in 1938. Mountcastle (1957) was the first to offer a general hypothesis of columnar organization. Since then, it has become increasingly clear that the mammalian cortex is organized both anatomically and functionally into discrete units called columns. The word "columnar" has acquired multiple meanings. Columns can be recognized by histologic examination, physiologic studies, and immunocytochemistry. A general definition that applies to all forms is that they are an arrangement of operations, neurites, and cell bodies perpendicular to and extending as units through the six laminae of the cerebral cortex.

The smallest unit of columnar organization, the anatomic minicolumn, is based on the ontogenetic cell column (Szentagothai, 1968, 1978; Hubel and Wiesel, 1972, 1974; Mountcastle, 1978; Goffinet, 1984; Leise, 1990). This is a line of cells that arises in the fetal brain and is the first anatomic organization of the cortex, well before the horizontal lamination, which begins around 24–28 weeks. A minicolumn contains approximately 80–120 neurons which extend from the lowest layer VI all the way through layer I and are readily identified under the microscope, especially in areas that are cytoarchitecturally defined as columnar. Larger units of function are known as macrocolumns. The ocular dominance and orientation of columns in the primary visual cortex are examples of macrocolumns. These large units of function are made up of hundreds of co-activating minicolumns and can range from about 300mm to 1500mm in width.

The beauty of columnar organization is the plasticity and dynamic interaction it offers. Individual minicolumns can inhibit their direct neighbors (lateral inhibition), which serves to enhance the localization of function for a particular column unit. A column may also activate immediate neighbors or columns that are farther away. The combination of these individual units creates larger units of function that can be detected by physiologic or metabolic activities. A column may send connections to other areas that are distributed throughout the cortex. Columns receive excitatory input from the thalamus and callossal connections from the other hemisphere as well. Global activation of hundreds of columns is possible by vast arrays of excitatory interconnections. Columnar organization of function has been documented throughout the sensory and association areas (Mountcastle, 1997). Work in recent years has allowed precise descriptions of the working of neurons within a single cell column (Favorov and Kelly, 1994a,b).

Anatomically, the single cell minicolumn can be identified by both the vertical array of neuronal bodies and the dendritic clusters that weave through the center of them. The outer edge of cell columns is the space utilized by the long-distance axonal fibers. Dendrites from large pyramidal cells of layer V form clusters that ascend through layer IV. These are joined in the supragranular layers of cortex by apical dendrites from layers III and II. Each dendritic bundle is the center of a module of pyramidal cells; they arise in the same area where the cell bodies are located and weave through them. The horizontal distance between these cell columns is said to range from 20 to 80 μm and the average modules are 30 μm in diameter. Importantly, these dendrite clusters appear early in ontogenesis as the cortical plate is forming, and before it receives afferent axonal input. They are found in many mammal brains in every cortical area so far studied.

Embryologic studies demonstrate that cell columns have a strong genetic basis. The earliest cell columns arise as ontogenetic units from the ventricular zone, which is the area that gives rise to what will become the mature neurons of the cortex. They start out as discrete units even before they climb up the glial scaffolding into the cortex (Rakic, 1978). The surface area of the neocortex is determined by the number of ontogenetic units, which, in turn, is based on the number of symmetric cell divisions of progenitor cells in the neural epithelium before migration occurs (Rakic, 1988a,b). An extra cycle of cell division would have the effect of roughly doubling the area of neocortex. Therefore, expansion of the neocortex in evolution may be a consequence of mutational changes in the number of symmetric divisions in regional zones of the epithelium (Rakic et al., 1991); alterations in development during this phase have serious consequences for brain development.

An expanding cortex against a rigid cranium provides a mechanical need for folding and consequent gyrification (see below). The process providing uniformed guidance to this striking feature of the primate brain is not known. Recent research suggests that it is the result of intrinsic cortical factors (Armstrong et al., 1991). Elements like maintenance of columnar length and laminar thickness (Smart and McSherry, 1986a,b), ratio of subplate to cortical thickness (Kostovic and Rakic, 1990), and sizes of axonal bundles lying within gyri (Goldman and Galkin, 1978) have been proposed as causal factors.

Gyrification is not equally distributed between the hemispheres. The sylvian fissure is apparent at 14 weeks of gestation, followed successively by the rolandic (24 weeks) and the calcarine (26 weeks) fissures. Gyrations are present throughout the hemispheres by 32 weeks of gestation (Friede, 1989). The amount of folding accrued to gyrification follows a rostro-caudal gradient and varies in relation to the amount of space occupied by the supragranular layers compared with the lower ones (Armstrong et al., 1991). One can usually estimate maturity by counting the number of convolutions crossed by a line joining the frontal and occipital poles above the insula and adding 21 weeks (Friede, 1989). The resultant number is a reliable guide to maturity despite low birth weight or the presence of edema (Pryse-Davies and Beard, 1973).

Embryogenesis

Development of the human central nervous system (CNS) begins around 3 weeks after formation of the zygote. It is then that the embryo takes the form of a flattened disk. Initially the disk is bilaminar and consists of two cell layers, the epiblast and the hypoblast. Proliferation and migration of the epiblast ultimately leads to the formation of the trilaminar embryonic disk and the completion of gastrulation. The three layers derived from the epiblast are: the embryonic mesoderm formed from the migrated epiblast cells, the ectoderm formed from the original epiblast cell layer, and the endoderm formed from epiblast cells replacing the original hypoblast cell layer. These three layers will give rise to all subsequent body structures. Specifically, the ectoderm will give rise to the nervous system.

The next important step in nervous system development involves the formation of a solid notochord, which runs in the midline of the trilaminar disk in the cranial to caudal axis. Slightly earlier in development, a structure known as the primitive streak appears along the longitudinal midline of the embryonic disk. Mesoderm cells migrate through this streak to form a tube called the notochordal process. This structure undergoes several transformations and ulti-

(a)

Neural plate

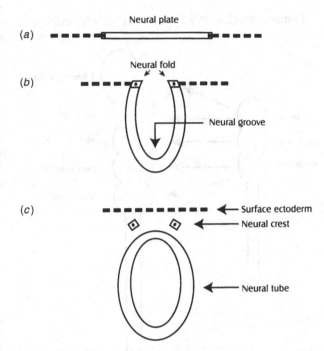

(b)

Neural fold

Neural groove

(c)

Surface ectoderm

Neural crest

Neural tube

Fig. 7.1. Conversion of the neural plate into neural tube. The lateral edges of the flat neural plate (a) begin to rise (b) and eventually meet to form the neural tube (c).

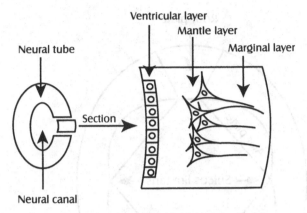

Ventricular layer
Mantle layer
Marginal layer
Neural tube
Section
Neural canal

Fig. 7.2. Three layers become identifiable in the wall of the maturing neural tube.

mately becomes a solid cylinder residing in the mesoderm. The solid cylinder is called the notochord.

Formation of the nervous system is brought about by the process of induction. Induction involves one tissue influencing the development fate of another, by direct or indirect contact, through the release of inducing substances. Mesoderm induces the overlying ectoderm to become the neuroectoderm. After induction, the neuroectoderm is called the neural plate. The neural plate is a flat structure that is broad in the cranial portion and narrow in the caudal portion of the embryo.

The neural plate is transformed into neural tube by the process of neurulation (Fig. 7.1). Neurulation involves changes in cell shapes and is dependent on forces intrinsic to the neuroepithelial cells as well as those exerted by the surrounding cells (Schoenwolf and Smith, 1990). A depression called the neural groove develops in the middle of the neural plate and the lateral edges of the neural plate begin to elevate. The lateral edges are called the neural folds and these continue to elevate and eventually meet in the dorsal midline. The closure of the neural tube first occurs at about the mid level of the embryo and then proceeds simultaneously in the cranial and caudal directions. Failure of neural tube closure or secondary reopening of the neural tube results in neural tube defects, the severity of which varies

with the length of involvement of the neural tube and the region involved (Campbell et al., 1986; Campbell and Sohal, 1990).

As a result of neurulation the surface ectoderm is separated from the neural plate, the cells located between the surface ectoderm and neural plate are separated (these are called neural crest cells), and the neural plate is converted into neural tube. The surface ectoderm gives rise to the skin. The neural crest cells contribute to the formation of the peripheral nervous system and a wide variety of non-neural structures throughout the body (Le Douarin, 1982). Specialized regions of the ectoderm called placodes also contribute to the formation of the peripheral nervous system. The neural tube cells give rise to the CNS. However, this is not the exclusive fate of these cells. Recent studies have shown that some neural tube cells migrate and contribute to the formation of structures developing outside the CNS, both neural and non-neural structures (Sharma et al., 1995; Sohal et al., 1996, 1998a,b, 1999; Bockman and Sohal, 1998).

Initially, the neural tube is composed of a single layer of epithelial cells. As the neural tube matures, three distinct layers become apparent (Fig. 7.2). The layer adjacent to the neural canal is called the ventricular layer. Cellular proliferation occurs in the ventricular layer. After proliferation, the maturing neurons and glial cells begin to migrate away from the ventricular layer and gather in the mantle layer, which in the mature nervous system forms the gray matter. The processes of neurons in the mantle layer form the marginal layer, which becomes the white matter of the mature CNS.

As the neural tube thickens, two regions of increased density of cells become distinct in the wall of the neural tube (Fig. 7.3). These regions are separated by a longitudinal groove called the sulcus limitans. This is present in the spinal cord and the brainstem and it divides the wall of the

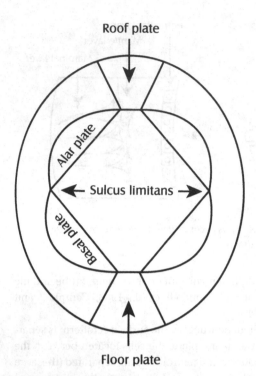

Fig. 7.3. Basic organization of the developing neural tube of the spinal cord and brainstem.

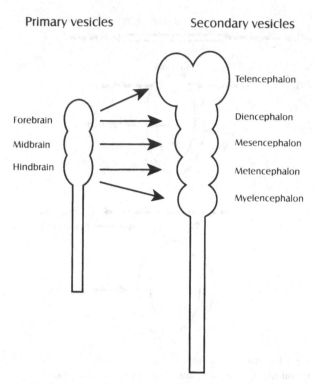

Fig. 7.4. Formation of the primary and secondary vesicles in the rostral neural tube.

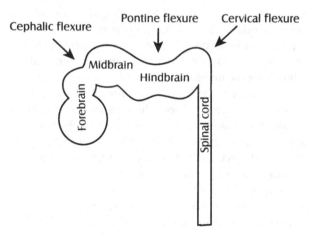

Fig. 7.5. A series of flexures occur in the rostral neural tube.

neural tube into dorsal and ventral portions. The dorsal portion is called the alar plate which gives rise to sensory cells and represents the future sites of afferent structures. The ventral portion is called the basal plate, derivatives of which are motor structures. The dorsal midline of the neural tube is called the roof plate and the ventral midline is called the floor plate (Fig. 7.3). This organization is present in the spinal cord and the brainstem and absent in the telencephalon. The roof plate and the floor plate do not provide neurons for the developing nervous system. Although the functional significance of the roof plate is not yet established, the floor plate plays an important role in morphogenesis. The floor plate is induced by the underlying notochord and both structures provide signals for the differentiation of specific types of neuron; the floor plate attracts nerve fibers that cross the midline (Placzek et al., 1990; Hirano et al., 1991; Yamada et al., 1991).

The pattern of development of the rostral neural tube is different from that of the caudal portion, which forms the spinal cord. Three swellings become apparent in the rostral potion of the neural tube, which will form the brain and the brainstem (Fig. 7.4). These dilated regions are called primary vesicles: the forebrain or presencephalon, the midbrain or mesencephalon, and the hindbrain or rhombencephalon. The forebrain vesicle subdivides to form the

telencephalon and diencephalon. The midbrain vesicle does not divide. The hindbrain vesicle subdivides to form the metencephalon and myelencephalon. These five vesicles are called secondary vesicles.

The rostral portion of the embryo bends at several places and these foldings are called flexures (Fig. 7.5). The first flexures formed are the cervical and the cephalic. The cervical flexure is located at the junction of the hindbrain with

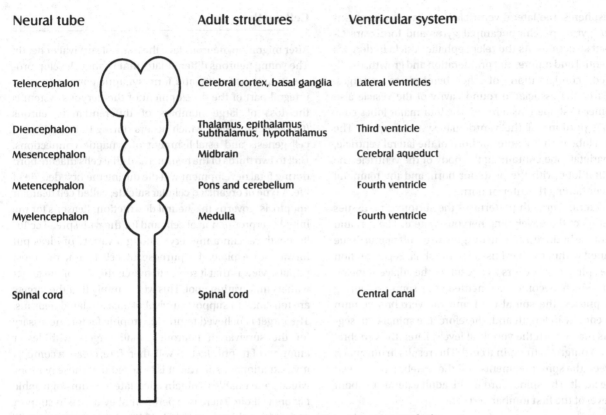

Fig. 7.6. Adult structures and the ventricular system are derived from the embryonic neural tube.

the spinal cord. The cephalic flexure is located between the forebrain and midbrain. Later, the cervical flexure straightens out. The persistence of the cephalic flexure results in the longitudinal axis of the forebrain being at 90° to that of the brainstem and the spinal cord. A third flexure, the pontine flexure, forms later and is located in the dorsal portion of the hindbrain. As a result of this flexure, the dorsal portion of pons and rostral medulla is flattened and the dorsal structures end up in a more lateral position.

Different portions of the neural tube give rise to different structures; the fluid-filled cavities become the ventricular system (Fig. 7.6). The telencephalon forms the cerebral cortex and the basal ganglia and the cavity develops into lateral ventricles. The diencephalon forms the thalamus, epithalamus, subthalamus, and hypothalamus and contains the third ventricle. The mesencephalic vesicle forms the midbrain and the cerebral aqueduct. The metencephalon differentiates into pons and cerebellum and the myelencephalon forms the medulla. The cavities in the metencephalon and myelencephalon become the fourth ventricle. The neural tube caudal to the myelencephalon develops into the spinal cord and its cavity becomes the central canal. The cerebrospinal fluid (CSF) moves through

the ventricular system. It is produced by the choroid plexus in the ventricles and eventually absorbed into the venous system.

The size and the shapes of the various portions of the mature nervous system result from a variety of developmental processes such as cellular proliferation, cellular migration, and cell death, and also from the constraints imposed by the surrounding non-neural tissues.

Cellular proliferation

The cell division in the neural tube takes place in the ventricular zone. The rate of cell division is not uniform throughout the rostrocaudal extent of the neural tube. In general, the rate of cell division is greater in those portions of the neural tube that will eventually form large structures. The time a cell stops dividing is called its "cell birthday", which corresponds with the time of the final DNA synthesis. Cell birthday is important in determining the final destination and the fate of a cell. The differential cellular proliferation and growth results in a number of structures in the mature brain resembling the letter C. The cerebral hemispheres, the lateral ventricles, caudate nucleus, cingulate gyrus, parahippocampal gyrus and fornix are C-shaped structures. As the telencephalic vesicle undergoes sequential and differential proliferation and growth, the C-shaped configuration of the hemisphere emerges. Similarly, the associated round cavity of the vesicle also becomes C-shaped. As a result, the four major lobes containing portions of the ventricular system appear. The frontal lobe with the anterior horn of the lateral ventricle, the parietal lobe containing the body of the ventricle, the occipital lobe with the posterior horn, and the temporal lobe containing the inferior horn.

Differential growth patterns of the surrounding tissues also impact the developing nervous system. The gyri and sulci of the brain result from the growth of soft neural tissue confined within the hard tissue of the skull. Segmentation of the spinal cord occurs as a result of the adjacent mesoderm, which becomes segmented into somites. During early phases, the spinal cord and the vertebral column grow equally in length and, therefore, the spinal cord segments match with the vertebral levels. Later, the vertebral column outgrows the spinal cord. This results in mismatch between the spinal segments and the vertebral levels seen in the adult. The spinal cord in the adult extends to about the level of the first lumbar vertebra.

Cellular migration

After birth, cells begin to migrate from the ependymal layer to their final destination. It is not clear how cells know where to go. Their migration is aided by specialized cells called radial glial cells, which stretch the entire width of the neural tube. Cellular migration is a very important developmental event because where a particular cell ends up will dictate its function. For example, if a cell migrates into the ventral horn of the spinal cord, it will become a motor neuron. If it migrates into the dorsal horn, it will be involved in processing sensory information.

One region where cellular migration has been extensively studied is the cerebral cortex. As cells begin to migrate from the ventricular zone, which occurs around 13 weeks in humans, they form an intermediate zone. The cells in the intermediate zone begin to differentiate and form the cortical plate. From the cortical plate, cells migrate into different layers of the cortex. This migration is dependent on the cell birthday. For example, cells born early migrate least and end up in the deepest layers of the cortex. Similarly, cells born later migrate past the earlier born ones, migrate longer distances, and occupy the more superficial layers of the cortex. Thus, cortical migration occurs in an inside-out fashion.

Cell death

After migration, neurons face the issue of survival or death. The young neurons differentiate, that is, they develop processes and organelles and form synaptic connections. An integral part of the development of the nervous system is the loss of large numbers of differentiated neurons (Oppenheim, 1991), which occurs during both periods of cell genesis and establishment of synaptic connections. Half to two thirds of the neurons and glial cells that are born during fetal development will die during the first decade of life. A type of organized cellular suicide, called cell death or apoptosis, governs this neural destruction. Reasons for the initial overproduction of cells and for the widespread cellular death remain a mystery. Among a variety of ideas put forward to explain the purpose of cell death, the most popular view is that it serves to match the size of the target with its innervation pool. This would imply that the targets are too small to support survival of all associated neurons. The target is believed to provide trophic factors necessary for the survival of neurons. Small targets with lesser amounts of trophic factors will, therefore, create a competitive situation for survival. It is believed that those neurons which were unable to obtain adequate amounts of trophic factors will die. There is experimental evidence in support and against this view (Sohal, 1992). A number of trophic factors, such as the nerve growth factor, ciliary neurotrophic factor, brain-derived neurotrophic factor, and neurotrophins, have been shown to rescue neurons from death. Cell death also affects the neurons of the proliferative zones of the developing brain (ventricular and subventricular zones). Because these neurons have not yet migrated, their cell death may result from errors in cell division or differentiation.

Both extrinsic (e.g., changes in local environment) and intrinsic cellular conditions can induce cell death. In addition to the determining factors mentioned above, the huge extent of neuronal overproduction and neuronal death has to involve serendipity. Chance events in neuronal development, just as in genetic variation (chance mutations and recombinations), are likely to play an important role in interindividual anatomic, physiologic and behavioral differences (evident in monozygotic twins), and, in a larger perspective, in evolution.

Brain growth

The immature cortical plate is apparent by 10.5 weeks of gestation and precedes the appearance of the fetal subplate at 13.5–15 weeks of gestation. This subplate has more

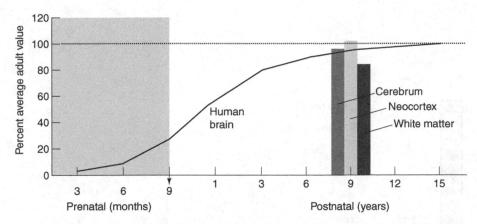

Fig. 7.7. The growth of the human brain presented from two perspectives. For both perspectives, brain weight or volume is expressed as a percentage of the mean adult volume or weight (ordinate: 1 g = 1 cm³). The first perspective is that of the full profile of brain growth, based upon brain weights obtained at autopsy (curve). This is expressed as a continuous change with growth continuing through the fetal months and the first 15 years of postnatal life. (Adapted from Lemire et al., 1975.) The second perspective is based upon volumetric analyses of magnetic resonance images of the cerebrum, the neocortex, and the cerebral central white matter taken from a cross-sectional analysis in the school-age child. The mean volumes for males plus females (15 males and 15 females) over an age range of 6 to 11 years (mean age 9 years) are plotted as histograms at the average age. At school age, the overall cycle of growth is approximately 95% of the corresponding adult volume. By contrast with adults, the neocortex is a relatively greater while the cerebral central white matter is a relatively smaller percentage of the corresponding adult values. (From Caviness, V. S., Kennedy, D. N., Bates, J. F., and Makris, N. (1997). The developing human brain: a morphometric profile. In *Developmental Neuroimaging: Mapping the Development of the Brain and Behavior*, eds. R. W. Thatcher, G. Reid Lyon, J. Rumsey and N. Krasnegor, pp. 3–14. San Diego, CA: Academic Press. Reprinted with kind permission of the publisher.)

mature neurons and undergoes intensive differentiation between 17 and 25 weeks. At that point, intensive dendritic differentiation of the cortical plate simultaneously occurs with the invasion of the thalamocortical fibers of the cortical plate at 26–34 weeks, during which synapses accumulate within the cortical plate. At 27 weeks, pyramidal neurons in the future layers III and V of the cortical plate show a rapid increase in length of basal dendrites as a result of an increase in the number of bifurcations and the growth of terminal segments. In the rhesus monkey, the next rapid phase of synaptogenesis begins at 2 months before birth and ends approximately 2 months postnatally. This process of overproduction and pruning back is a consistent motif in the CNS and is very clearly demonstrated by observing the kinetics of synaptogenesis in the primary visual cortex, where synapses reach a density of about 90 synapses per 100 μm by the third postnatal month. Between the ages of 2.6 and 5 years, the pruning rate peaks with a 40% loss in the density of synaptic contacts. Premature stimulation did not affect the rate of this process and these processes, in fact, proceed in relation to the time of conception and not in relation to birth. Visual experience matures the synapses through strengthening, eliminating, or modifying existing synapses, but the growth or volume will no longer increase.

The brain develops at a roughly sigmoidal rate over a span of about 15 years (Fig. 7.7). The brain undergoes maximal growth during fetal and early postnatal life, enlarging from approximately 100 g at 20 weeks of gestation to 400 g at 40 weeks. The growth rate peaks perinatally at approximately 6% of the adult weight/month. There is a rapid increase in brain volume until 2 years of age and then a gradual increase until 12 years. At 18 months, brain weight is 800 g, or about 60% of adult weight, and at 3 years it is 1100 g or about 80% of adult weight. The brain has attained 95% maximal weight at 9 years of age and reaches an average of 1312 ml at normal adult weight. Of this volume, 86% is cerebral hemispheres, 11% is cerebellum, 2% brainstem, and only 1% ventricular system (Fig. 7.8). The cerebrum is 90% of total brain volume and has a ratio of total gray matter to central white matter of 3:2. Males have a 9% larger brain volume than females (Giedd et al., 1997). When adjusted for cerebral volume, the caudate is larger in females and the globus pallidus is larger in males (Giedd et al., 1997).

Hamano et al. (1990) conducted a study of 32 neurologically normal children, seven children with mental retardation alone and 15 children with mental retardation and motor disturbance. In the neurologically normal children, head circumference and total brain volume increased from

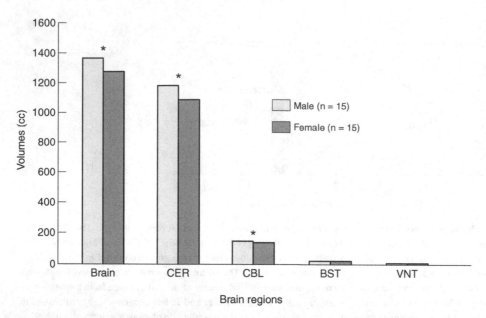

Fig. 7.8. Volumes of principal brain regions of the male and female school-age child. CER, cerebrum; CBL, cerebellum; BST, brainstem; and VNT, ventricular system. *Significant ($p < 0.05$). (From Caviness, V. S., Kennedy, D. N., Bates, J. F., and Makris, N. (1997). The developing human brain: a morphometric profile. In *Developmental Neuroimaging: Mapping the Development of the Brain and Behavior*, eds. R. W. Thatcher, G. Reid Lyon, J. Rumsey and N. Krasnegor, pp. 3–14. San Diego, CA: Academic Press. Reprinted with kind permission of the publisher.)

723 ml to 1407 ml as a function of age. Actual intracranial brain volume was determined by three-dimensional computed tomographic (CT) scans. Mental retardation alone was not denoted by total brain volume. However, in 10 out of 15 children with mental retardation and motor deficit, brain volume was under 2 SD (standard deviations) of the average for the neurologically normal children. Interestingly, only 7 of those 15 had an averaged cerebral volume (combined volume of cerebellum, midbrain, pons, and medulla) 2 SD smaller than that of the neurologically normal children. While head circumference was directly correlated with brain volume in normal children, in many children with mental retardation, head circumference was larger than indicated for their brain volume. This may have been a result of the thickening of the cranium that occurs with cerebral atrophy, and it indicates that head circumference may be insufficient in determining brain development in terms of volume.

Reiss et al., (1996) similarly found that total cerebral volume was the significant predictor in the variance of volumes of all constituent tissue and CSF variables. In this study, 79 children of normal IQ using standard cognitive testing (60 female and 19 male) were analyzed by magnetic resonance imaging (MRI). This study further elucidated a pattern of decreased ratio of gray to white matter with increased age, regardless of gender. This pattern of

increased white matter persisted throughout childhood. Their results further indicated that there was an increase in prefrontal white matter volume with increasing age in addition to the age-related changes of the total white matter. The Reiss study (1996) found no significant gender-by-hemisphere-associated symmetry differences. However, consistent with other studies, modest but statistically significant asymmetries revealed a rightward prominence of cortical and subcortical gray matter and a leftward prominence of ventricular and nonventricular CSF relative to whole brain volumes. A 7–10% greater cerebral volume in male compared to female brains has been reported in many studies, mostly contributed by increased volume of neocortex (males average greater than 700 ml and females average about 680 ml) and central white matter (males averaging about 460 ml and females averaging 420 ml). Although Reiss et al. (1996) determined that IQ is positively correlated with total cerebral volume in children, especially with the volume of cortical gray matter in the prefrontal region (prefrontal gray matter volume predicted almost 20% of the variance in IQ) and subcortical gray matter (gray matter volume predicted 15% of the variance in IQ), there was no gender associated statistical differences in mean (± SD) full scale IQ scores (113 ± 15 for females and 105 ± 17 for males).

Chugani et al. (1987) observed neurofunctional development in terms of metabolism. Twenty nine children were studied with respect to developmental changes in local cerebral metabolic rates for glucose (1CMRGlu). In neonates younger than 5 weeks 1CMRGlu was highest in sensorimotor cortex, thalamus, brainstem, and the cerebellar vermis; and at 3 months, 1CMRGlu was increased in temporal, parietal, and occipital cortices, basal ganglia, and cerebellar cortex. Actual values of 1CMRGlu for various gray matter regions were low at birth, rapidly rose to reach adult values by 2 years and continued to rise until 3 or 4 years, were maintained until 9 years, then declined back to adult rates by the latter part of the second decade. The highest increases occurred in cerebral cortical structures; lesser increases were seen in subcortical structures and in the cerebellum. This timeline, of course, matches that describing the process of overproduction and subsequent elimination of excessive neurons, synapses, and dendritic spines known to occur in the developing brain.

Development of cortical gyri and sulci

The cortical surface of the adult human brain consists of a complex, yet relatively consistent, pattern of gyri and sulci. This pattern is the result of a cortical folding process that begins in the fifth gestational month (Richman et al., 1975; Worthen et al., 1986). According to Smart and McSherry (1986a,b), the floors of sulci are relatively fixed in relation to the deep surface of the cortex and to each other during the folding process. They state that gyri are formed by expansion of intersulcal tissue.

There has been debate over whether cortical folding occurs as a result of intracortical events or because of compression of the cortex by neighboring structures (Jacobson, 1991). In 1950, Barron demonstrated that cortical folding results primarily from intracortical events: after surgically isolating the developing cerebral cortex of sheep from subcortical structures in utero, the normal pattern of cortical folding was still observed. Richman et al. (1975) also have supported the idea of an intracortical mechanism. They further propose that cerebral convolutions result from mechanical stresses produced by the faster growth of the three outer cortical layers with respect to the three inner layers.

Differential growth rates can explain the buckling of the cortex but does not account for the relatively fixed positions of sulci and gyri. Jacobson (1991) postulates that the geometry of dendrite growth and fiber trajectory determine the positions of sulci and gyri. This hypothesis is based on the fact that neuronal genesis and migration are completed by the fifth gestational month and cortical folding occurs simultaneously with the growth of the den-

drites of cortical neurons (Richman et al., 1975; Jacobson, 1991).

Although the exact mechanism of cortical folding has not been elucidated, the sequential development of sulci and gyri has been well documented by several authors. Primary sulci, for example the calcarine sulcus on the medial hemispheric surface (Dorovini-Zis and Dolman, 1977; Worthen et al., 1986) are visible at 20–24 gestational weeks. The lateral sulcus appears earlier but results from gross evagination and rotation of the brain rather than from convolution of the cortical surface (Richman et al., 1975).

Secondary sulci first appear at 26–28 weeks. Between 28 and 30 weeks, a growth spurt occurs with the formation of many new gyri and sulci (Dorovini-Zis and Dolman, 1977; Friede, 1989). Few convolutions develop between 30 and 40 weeks (Dorovini-Zis and Dolman, 1977). By the eighth gestational month, the precentral and postcentral gyri are prominent and all primary and secondary sulci are present (Noback and Demarest, 1981) (Table 7.1). The emergence of tertiary sulci occurs during the last two gestational months (Smith, 1974; Dorovini-Zis and Dolman, 1977; Noback and Demarest, 1981; Worthen et al. 1986; Jacobson, 1991). In the first 6 months after birth, the number of tertiary convolutions increases dramatically, and the convolutional pattern reaches adult complexity at about 2 years of age (Smith, 1974). Tertiary sulcation may continue throughout life (Noback and Demarest, 1981).

Primary sulci are relatively invariant while secondary sulci show some variability even between identical twins (Noback and Demarest, 1981; Jacobson, 1991). Primary sulci include the calcarine, parieto-occipital, central, hippocampal, and cingulate sulci (Smith, 1974; Richman et al., 1975; Jacobson, 1991). Temporal and frontal sulci, as well as the precentral, postcentral, and intraparietal sulci, are considered secondary sulci (Smith, 1974; Jacobson, 1991). Individual authors differ slightly on the classification of sulci, but all generally adhere to this scheme.

Myelinogenesis

Myelinogenesis, the development of myelin sheaths in the fibers of the nervous system, occurs gradually and at varying rates. Flechsig (1876) proposed that nerve tracts become myelinated in the order in which they become functional, and this idea is now widely accepted and supported. Myelinogenesis commences in the fourth gestational month (Lucas Keene and Hewer, 1931; Langworthy, 1933; Smith, 1974; Friede, 1989). Spinal nerve myelination is completed in the second or third year of life (Langworthy, 1933) but the process of myelination continues in the brain

Table 7.1. Gestational age for the appearance of sulci

	Time of appearance (weeks)			
	Smith (1974)	Dorovini-Zis and Dolman (1977)	Friede (1989)	Noback and Demarest (1981)
Calcarine	24	22	24–26	20
Parieto-occipital	24	22		20
Central	24	24	24–26	20
Hippocampal	24			
Cingulate	24	24		
Superior temporal	28	28	26	
Superior frontal	33			
Precentral	33		26	32
Postcentral	33	24	26	32
Middle temporal	33			
Middle frontal	37			
Inferior temporal	37			
Intraparietal	37			

and spinal cord until puberty (Langworthy, 1933; Friede, 1989).

Myelin sheaths first appear in the ventral roots of the spinal cord; this is soon followed by myelination of the dorsal roots and ventral commisure (Langworthy, 1933; Smith, 1974; Friede, 1989). The myelination process is markedly accelerated at 22–24 weeks (Lucas Keen and Hewer, 1931). By the sixth month of gestation, all cranial nerves except I (olfactory) and II (optic) show some myelination. The cuneate and spinocerebellar tracts and the descending pathways have begun myelinating by the sixth to seventh gestational months (Langworthy, 1933; Smith, 1974). Myelination in the 7-month fetus is limited to the medulla and midbrain (Langworthy, 1933).

The 8-month fetus shows little progress in myelination over the 7-month fetus, except for some myelination of the corpus striatum (Langworthy, 1933). Birth speeds the myelination process considerably (Lucas Keene and Hewer, 1931; Langworthy, 1933). At term, the optic nerve and tracts, internal capsule, medial and lateral lemnisci, ascending pathways, and thalamus all show some myelination (Lucas Keene and Hewer, 1931; Langworthy, 1933; Smith, 1974; Nelson et al., 1993). During the first 6 months after birth, myelination increases rapidly in the primary projection zones. Some long association fibers and a few short association fibers are myelinated (Smith, 1974). Myelination of the cerebral hemispheres commences gradually during the first 2 years of life (Friede, 1989). Yakovlev and Lecours (1967) state that hemispheric

myelination first appears in the prepyriform cortex, subiculum of Ammon's horn, and septum pellucidum. Figure 7.9 is a generalized schedule of myelination given by Yakovlev and Lecours (1967).

MRI allows for visualization of myelogenesis and recapitulation of previous histological studies. The long T_1 and T_2 relaxation times of the immature brain make it necessary to use adjusted pulse sequences with a long time to repetition (TR) in order to obtain sufficient tissue contrast (van der Knaap and Valk, 1990). The technique allows the process of myelination in regions of interest to be examined. The total myelination of the brain from neonates to adulthood has been studied by three-dimensional estimations of volumes using MRI (Iwasaki et al., 1997). The results of the study suggest that the volume of the cerebral white matter increases more slowly than the total volume for the cerebral hemispheres (Iwasaki et al., 1997) (Fig. 7.10).

Neurotransmitters and hormones

During brain development, neurons are dependent on external factors for guidance and survival. These factors include biochemical influences such as neurotransmitters (e.g., dopamine, serotonin, acetylcholine) and steroid hormones. The mechanisms involved are complex and require appropriate spatiotemporal relationships and feedback loops. Some of these mechanisms act at a local level, while

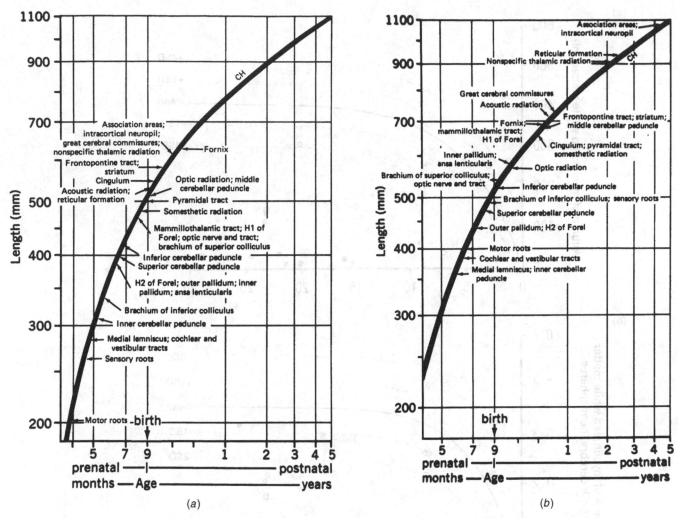

Fig. 7.9.(*a*) Approximate onset of myelination in various parts of the nervous system as observed by light micrsocopy. (*b*) Approximate times at which myelination of the structures shown in (*a*) has progressed to 50% completion as observed by light microscopy. The ordinates depicts crown–heel (CH) length and the abscissae approximate ages. (Reprinted from Lemire, R., Loeser, J., Leech, R. and Alvord, E. (1975). *Normal and Abnormal Development of the Human Nervous System*. Harper Row, publishers, with permission.)

others result in more widespread effects. An example of regional interactions is the effect of glia on neurotransmitters through the production of glial-derived neurotrophic factors. Glial receptors have been involved in the development of several neurotransmitter systems, most notably the serotonergic system. In turn (depending on the target and fetal time period), the development of the neuropil, the myelination of axons, and decreases in the branching of neurites can be stimulated by neurotransmitters such as serotonin (Emerit et al., 1992). It is suggested that the earlier neurotransmitter-specific cells appear (e.g., cells specific for gamma-aminobutyric acid (GABA) before cortical plate formation), the more important is their role in organizing the cerebral cortex. Global factors such as these

neurochemical influences have similarly evoked long cascades of effects that overflow into adulthood and influence ingrained behavioral responses. For example, although cortical development may proceed differently in the two sexes, levels of estrogens and androgens during brain development may be primary in determining future sexual orientation. The differential expression of gonadal steroid hormones during early critical periods of brain development has been linked to differences between the sexes in brain morphology, which are believed to be responsible for a number of behavioral differences. It has been shown in rats that sex differences in circulating androgens early after birth are responsible for sex differences in programmed cell death. Similarly, stress hormones (i.e., glucocorticoid

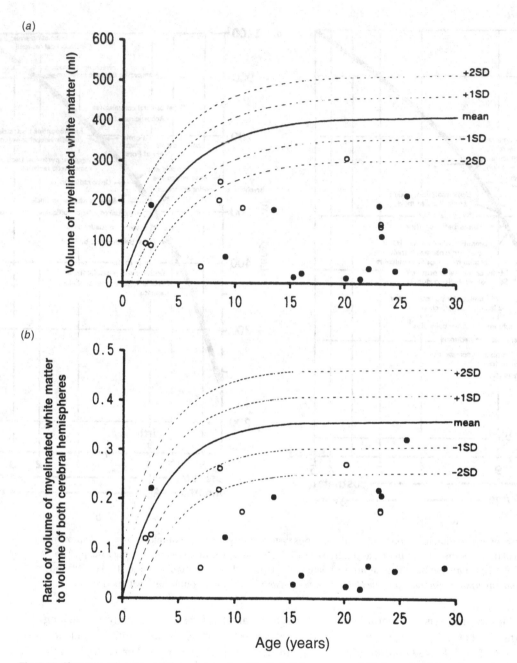

Fig. 7.10. Changes with age in (*a*) the volume of myelinated white matter and (*b*) the ratio of the volume of myelinated white matter to the volume of both cerebral hemispheres in groups 2 (●) and 3 (○). The curves show the mean and the 1 SD and 2 SD ranges for group 1. (Reprinted from Iwasaka, N., Hamano, K., Okada, Y., Horigome, Y., Nakayama, J., Takeya, T., Takita, H. and Nose, T. (1997). Volumetric quantification of brain development using MRI. *Neuroradiology*, 39, 841–6, with permission.)

hormone, hydrocortisone) may have long-lasting effects. Other global effects may be iatrogenic or nutritional. It has been hypothesized that centrally acting drugs that are used during pregnancy may interfere with neurotransmitters, resulting not in gross physical malformations but rather in subtle behavioral symptoms such as hyperactivity and

sleep disturbances. Similarly, dietary variations in choline intake during pregnancy may influence the memory performance of offspring, as shown by Zeisel (1997).

The fact that early changes in the levels of neurotransmitters may have lasting effects into adulthood may be a consequence, in part, of the absence of neuronal stem cells surviving the developmental period. The mature brain cannot regenerate damaged neurons. However, recent work with fetal transplants have shown a capacity for the mature brain to repair itself. The basis for this adult plasticity may relate to the regional grouping of neurotransmitters. For example, in the cerebellum, choline acetyltransferase (ChAT) activity is 10-fold higher in the fetus than in adults. In contrast, ChAT activity in the hippocampus is minimal or absent during the development but rises postnatally to reach a maximum in middle age. According to Perry and co-workers (1993), vulnerability of the hippocampus to age-related pathology may relate to the extended period of cholinergic synaptic sculpturing in this brain region. Pathoclisis (selective vulnerability of certain cells to insults) may also be related to the developmental profile of different neurotransmitters. Glycine, GABA, glutamic acid, aspartic acid, and their key metabolic enzymes progressively increase up to the mid portion of the third trimester of pregnancy (Das and Ray, 1997). Their levels may correlate with the rapid increase in nerve processes and myelination during this period.

Functional neuroimaging may offer some insights into brain development and help to visualize temporal windows of selective vulnerability to damage (see Chapter 20). N-Acetyl-L-aspartic acid (NAA) can be assessed in the human fetal brain by high-resolution proton magnetic resonance spectroscopy (^{1}H MRS, see Chapter 4). It is detected in the cerebral cortex and white matter by 16 weeks of gestation and increases gradually from 24 weeks of gestation to 1 year of age (Kato et al., 1997). Development abnormalities may result in NAA/creatine (Cr) decreases colocalized to structural malformation and extending into normal-appearing regions (Li et al., 1998). Functional imaging may help to define the extent of putative developmental lesions and provide guidance in future therapeutic interventions (Johnston, 1995).

Cortical organization acts like a distributed function system

It is important to realize that the historical and common perception of the brain as a collection of rigidly parceled and discrete areas, each of which is selectively associated with a particular behavior, is most likely a false one. Evidence from many sources, including functional neuroimaging with fMRI and positron emission tomography (PET), have shown that this notion is oversimplistic. While cellular anatomy is necessarily fixed in place, columns allow for regional interactions that result in great dynamic properties and distribute the functions of the cortex throughout many regions. Cross-talk between distant brain areas is the norm. The brain is not locked into self-contained little units.

The columnar organization of the cortex permits a fixed anatomic substrate to act as a flexible distributed system. A distributed system is a collection of processing units, separated in space, that communicate by exchanging messages. A system is distributed if the message-transmission delay is a significant fraction of the time between single events in a processing unit (Mountcastle, 1997).

Higher functions seem especially distributed and not locked into a localized region. There is a hierarchial distribution for multiple functions in a given region that serve to make local regions more complex and more plastic than previously thought. In the macaque monkey brain, researchers have so far identified in a single hemisphere 72 areas that are linked to each other by 758 connections. In addition, many of these connections are reciprocal. Columns can be seen both as structural units having a fixed anatomy with specific cell properties and as dynamic units created by specific behavioral requirements for which multiple columns are recruited. Sensory discrimination and categorization are distributed in wide areas of the brain. How these sensory processes are unified and become part of the conscious experience is still a mystery.

Brain evolution and behavior

A striking outcome of comparative neurology is the general finding that, aside from size, nothing is strikingly unique about the human brain. Yet, it has always been assumed that the human brain contained some special area related to the unique level of consciousness in humans. Most anthropologists contend that human brains are basically ape brains that have undergone numerous small but highly significant changes.

Like everything else in biology, human brains appear to be products of evolutionary mechanisms such as selection and genetic variation. Anatomic differences are ones of degree and do not represent totally new structures. The brain is conservative, and anatomic changes are often subtle rather than gross. Evolution has been likened to a tinkerer that builds upon existing structures rather than creating something entirely new and different. In other areas of anatomy, seemingly small and insignificant alterations in anatomic structures may often give rise to large differences in function and behavior. The same mechanisms that brought about the evolution of all other biological systems can be applied to the study of the anthropoid brain.

The anatomy and physiology of the human brain differ from that of other primates only in a limited fashion because the human brain is built upon a basic mammalian template. It is the same with human behavior. The extent to which human behavior differs from that of other animals, especially higher primates, is a matter of degree. Language and tool use among primates are sometimes matters of degree and specialization rather than novel in themselves. Claims have been made that apes have been taught American Sign Language (ASL) with varying success, and that vervet monkeys used verbal calls signals to refer to objects in their environment (Rumbaugh, 1977). The fact that apes could learn a novel form of communication such as ASL, outside of their evolutionary development, suggests that the primate brain already contains the basic design that could lead to a much more sophisticated mode of language. Both language and tool use in chimpanzees are not merely a product of the brain, however. The chimpanzee has a pharynx and tongue with characteristics that limit the number of sounds to about a dozen, prohibiting spoken language. Likewise, the upper limb of apes are primarily "designed" for locomotion (some form of suspensory or knucklewalking), which results in a very poor precision and power grip. For ape behavior to become human-like, it is not only the brain that must undergo change, but also the body.

Perhaps the most significant aspect of primate behavior is socialization. Many researchers feel this represents the selective push for human-like intelligence. Many animals use tools, and birds have extensive forms of vocalization and communication, but the complexity involved in human societal interaction is perhaps more unique and may have led to greater intelligence, which is manifested in technology and art. Chimpanzee social behavior is complex. Like humans, chimpanzees use bodily touch to communicate feelings of comfort and re-assurance. They can display aggression and have been shown to be capable of murder and even warfare. They are adept at using politics to obtain advantages in their society, gain favors and build alliances. Unlike more primitive mammals, the dominant chimpanzee is not necessarily the strongest one but often is the most "clever" one. The list of similarities to human behavior in all areas including sex (the sexual behavior of the bonobo chimpanzee is especially human-like) is remarkable and suggests that human behavior is not unique and arises from the anthropoid model.

Political and social manipulation require a brain that is capable of hiding its true feelings. Neurologically, this means acquiring a degree of control over the limbic system. "Simpler" animals are unable to mask their emotions such as anger, fear, or excitement. The dominance of

the cortex in higher primates, especially chimpanzees and humans, has created the ability to be deceitful. A smile may hide actual discontent but may fit the complex political or social demands on the animal at a given time. Furthermore, socialization requires the ability to recognize feelings and emotional reactions in self and others. It is easy to see why socialization is such a strong force in the evolution of the mind.

Reorganization of the nervous system: from internally programmed behavior to sensory domination

During the evolution of the nervous system, certain general trends seem to have occurred. One of these is the movement away from internalized central programs (e.g., motor programs) to brains that rely heavily on sensory modulation. "Primitive" nervous systems are more restricted in the amount of data they receive from the environment and in the processing of this information. Mammalian and especially primate evolution has been characterized by an increase in the input and processing of sensory data, which influenced the development and the working of the brain itself.

Central programming refers to the ability of the nervous system to generate behavioral output without the benefit (or with limited use) of sensory information (Fig. 7.11). It is most often associated with motor programs but actually extends to nearly every type of animal behavior. Present in utero, many of these programs are genetically controlled (Hamburger, et al., 1966; Nottebohm, 1970, 1971; Berman and Berman, 1973; Taub et al., 1975; Landlesser, 1976; Taub, 1976). Invertebrate brains are noted for their centrally generated motor activity (Shik et al., 1966; Davis, 1969; Szekely et al., 1969; Davis and Davis, 1973; Dorsett, et al., 1973; Kashin, et al., 1974; Mayeri et al., 1974; Gardner, 1976). Central motor patterning was first described in insect nervous systems and is a basic strategy for a spectrum of behaviors. Examples include song patterns in crickets (Bentley and Hoy, 1972), neural circulation in *Aplysia* (Mayeri, 1974), swimming in leeches and lobsters (Davis, 1969; Davis and Davis, 1973), wing beat of locusts, and escape behavior in *Tritonia* (Dorsett et al., 1973). Central motor programs are usually run by a command neuron that may trigger anything from a few interconnected neurons to a complex set of neuronal connections, utilizing interneurons, lateral inhibition, gamma efferents, and Renshaw cells (Davis, 1976; Grillner, 1985). Invertebrates exhibit a wide variety of behavioral programs ranging from ones that are completely internalized (endogenous bursting cells,

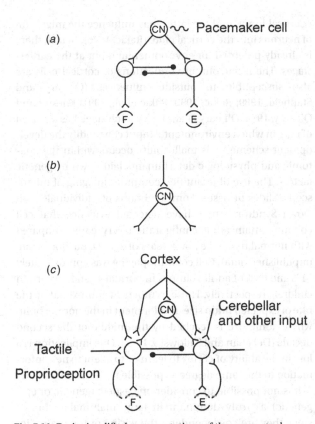

Fig. 7.11. Basic simplified representations of the conceptual operations of some central motor programs. (*a*) This model does not require input or even a triggering device. It is based on a leaky sodium channel (pacemaker cell) that activates the neurons. Each neuron has an inhibitory connection to the other. As the depolarized neuron weakens, its inhibition also weakens and the other cell then fires and inhibits the first. One cell is connected to a flexor (F) and the other to an extensor (E) muscle. This represents a truly internalized mechanism. (*b*) One way of building on this model is to have some kind of input to the command neuron (CN). This serves to make the system less autonomous. (*c*) Now the basic model receives input from many sources. The command neuron is no longer a pacemaker cell, and the system has lost its autonomy. Input circuits come from somatosensory regions, muscle spindles and Golgi tendon organs, and direct or indirect cerebellar input. Therefore, while the basic central mechanism has not disappeared, it cannot be easily detected because it has become heavily modulated by the rest of the brain. In essence, the brain has taken control of the central mechanism.

also known as pacemakers) to those that require some sensory input to modulate the program to the demands of the environment (Bullock, 1961; Willis, 1974; Barker and Gainer, 1975; Anderson, 1976).

In the evolution of mammalian brains, the mechanism of centrally generated programs did not disappear. Evidence of motor programming is found in *Felis* (cats) and primates, including humans (Bossom and Ommaya, 1968; Arshavsky et al., 1972; Pearson, 1976; Taub, 1976; Nashner, 1981; Grillner, 1985). However, they did lose their predominance, especially in the higher primates. Sensory systems have become more abundant and increasingly necessary to the normal operation of mammals. The shift to the larger primate brains (relative to body size) resulted in a new role for central programs. While still present for many behaviors, internalized programs became subordinate to the massive amount of sensory input that took over much of the control. Anthropoid brains have modulated the operation of the central programs to such an extent that it is difficult to discern the presence of pattern generators. In mammalian brain evolution, sensory systems did not trigger the development of novel mechanisms but instead were integrated gradually into the existing protocols of genetic programs. The nervous system is conservative and generally has not invoked radical and abrupt changes; instead it has built up upon existing structures (Strumwasser, 1975).

In humans and other primates, there are direct corticospinal controls over the motor neurons of the spinal cord. Humans have monosynaptic contacts between the primary cortical motor area and the alpha motor neurons of the spinal cord (Carpenter and Sutin, 1983). The corticospinal tract in anthropoids has assumed an increasingly dominant role, especially compared with other primates (Nudo and Masterson, 1990). Central generators have a greater autonomy in organisms that lack a well-developed cerebrum. In encephalized mammals, the generators seem to get buried among the modulating sensory–motor systems (e.g., spinal motor units). Jerison (1977) considers the brains of some vertebrates as adapted to fixed action patterns (in response to environmental stimuli) and to lack the plasticity of those in mammals with more complex sensory motor systems.

The development away from central programming was the result of the proliferation and complexity of sensory systems, which must have presented adaptive advantages. Kaas (1987) concluded that major evolutionary advances in the brain are marked by an increase in unimodal sensory areas but not an increase in association areas as often thought. Considerably more specific sensory information is being channeled into the existing association areas. It has been shown that humans do not have more association cortex than expected for a primate of our brain size

(Armstrong, 1990). In advanced brains, stimuli activate multiple cortical areas that are interconnected, and cortical areas tend to receive more direct sensory inputs (Kaas, 1987). For example, in the owl monkey, each field in the visual cortex, of which there are about 10, are interconnected with three to six other fields in the same hemisphere. The individual fields are also connected callosally with their counterparts in the other hemisphere. Added to this are subcortical connections to the pulvinar complex, the lateral geniculate nucleus, the claustrum, the basal ganglia, the superior colliculus, and the pontine nuclei (Weller and Kaas, 1983). Similar, if not more complex, interconnections are found in the temporal lobes of the primate (Galaburda and Pandya, 1983; Pandya et al., 1988). Based on clinical studies, the areas subserving Wernicke's speech area include Brodmann's area 13, 14, 15, 22, 39, 40, 41, 42, 44, and 45 (Kreig, 1963). Kaas (1987) further states that in less-advanced to moderately advanced mammals, sensory processing is the dominant cortical function, but most processing involves a single modality. In advanced mammals, there is co-activation from many cortical fields (5–20) for even simple stimuli.

Plasticity and a prolonged maturation process

An event that seems to be occurring in the evolution of the human brain is the prolongation of maturation, which is not to be confused with neoteny. (Neoteny refers to the retention of fetal anatomy in development. For example, during the fetal stages the skulls of humans and monkeys are very similar, but whereas the adult human skull remains similar to its fetal anatomy, the skulls of monkeys and apes continue to change.) This prolongation of development might be part of the mechanism that allows the environment to interact with the "hardware" of the brain. The cortex does not develop simultaneously, but rather in stages. A cortical area is characterized by the types of cell that it contains, its external connections with other cortical and subcortical areas, and its internal connections. Laminar differentiation occurs first, callosal and efferent connections are next, thalamocortical connections follow, and the last is the microcircuitry of intracortical connections (Sur et al., 1990). This plasticity is manifested anatomically as well as functionally and, therefore, may be detected by various forms of neuroimaging.

One feature of the cortex that demonstrates anatomic plasticity is the radial column. These columns develop in the cortical plate (Rakic, 1978, 1988a,b) before lamination and are the first anatomic organization of the cortex. There is overlap between the completion of lamination and thalam-

ocortical input, and the latter may influence the migration of neurons into the cortical plate (Rakic, 1976). In fact, there is already potential for environmental input at the earliest stages. The input/output connections of cortical cells are also susceptible to outside influences (O'Leary and Stanfield, 1989; Rakic, 1990; Rakic et al., 1991; Koester and O'Leary, 1992; O'Leary et al., 1992). Each stage has a period of time in which environmental input can modify the development scheme. This malleability occurs within the anatomic and physiologic determinants laid down by genetic factors. The use of quantified computer imaging of microscopic slides of tissue from the brains of individuals with Down Syndrome may have detected evidence that cell columns attain adult configuration very early compared with normal tissue, i.e., by 4 years of age (D. Buxhoeveden, unpublished data). Cell column spacing was approximately 71% and 83% of adult volumes in normal 4- and 6-year-old children, respectively. These numbers fit approximately the rate of expected brain size development in the normal brain where adult size is reached by the middle of the second decade (Dekaban and Sadowsky, 1978). One implication is a loss in the ability of cortex to learn or to adapt to new information to the same degree as possible in the normal brain.

It is not possible to consider one aspect (genetic or epigenetic) as truly dominant in large mammalian brains since they are co-dependent: the wiring of the brain dictates the nature, amount, and temporality of the sensory information input, which sets the range within which environment can act. The environment affects cortical circuitry through afferent inputs. Indeed, the plasticity of circuits has been demonstrated by rerouting sensory projections (Lund and Mustari, 1977; Jaeger and Lund, 1981; Chang et al., 1984, 1986), which shows that sensory axons will innervate other areas, even across sensory modalities, if there is a disruption of their normal target (Sur et al., 1990). There are simply not enough genes to permit a consideration of genetic control of behavior. Rather, clinical evidence indicates that cognitive functions are learned via the route of self-organization processes that assist the genetic blueprint. In this scenario, experience-dependent self-organization is an active dialogue between the brain and its environment.

O'Leary et al. (1992) suggested that the early cortex is devoid of area specificity and that a "proto cortex" is generated by the neuroepithelium that has generalized features but lacks a rigid regional specificity. The degree of plasticity associated with the final stage of cortical development (internal cortical microconnectivity) is critical because it will become the substrate for behavior.

Afferents greatly affect the regulation of intrinsic cortical connections and possibly contribute to synaptic weights and increased lateral inhibition. Therefore, epigenetic input can influence the final design of the neural system (Teyler and Fountain, 1987).

Lateralization as evidence of internal reorganization in the language area

Lateralization represents one possible way to alter the organization of a given area without creating an entirely new one. Laterality in the cortex of humans represents a behavioral and morphologic reorganization within the brain. Lateralization creates inequality of spatial arrangements in conjunction with physiologic alterations. When a cortical area in one hemisphere is larger than the other, it displays lateralization. Rosen et al. (1989) found that when laterality is present the combined size of both hemispheric areas yields a smaller total size than when there is no lateralization. Symmetrical brains have relatively larger amounts of callosal fibers, whereas asymmetric brains have a relative deficit of callosal connections (Galaburda et al., 1987). Weiskrantz (1977) suggested that the mechanism for cerebral dominance revolves around the nature of callosal connectivity. Laterality not only causes inequality of neuronal space between the hemispheres but also can alter the nature of connectivity simply on the basis of the dendritic tree lengths and patterns and the horizontal distance between cellular columns (Seldon, 1981a,b). Efferents on the right side spread to more columns, but left hemisphere temporal association areas columns collect information from more afferents (Seldon, 1981b). Scheibel (1984) noted that, during development, there is a greater increase in higher-order dendritic branches in the speech area on the left side than on the right side, which coincides with the beginnings of conceptualization and speech function. He noted that, in neonates, only the lower-order dendrites are present. Lateralization in the temporoparietal area of the temporal lobe in humans indicates a change in organization that relates, at least in part, to the evolution of language. Frost (1990) stated that initial lateralization may have been a consequence of handedness in conjunction with tool use, and that the neural reorganization served as a pre-adaptation for later development of language (Falk, 1980). Laterality of handedness and behaviors are present in extant primates (Sanford et al., 1984; Macneilage et al., 1987; Hopkins and Morris 1989; Hopkins et al., 1990; Dodson et al., 1992). Therefore, lateralization in the temporal lobe is not solely a function of language and handedness; it probably evolved much earlier than language.

In vitro computer imaging demonstrated that cell column morphology in human brains is markedly lateralized. Human laterality at the cell column level is seen predominantly in the left hemisphere and consists of more horizontal separation between cell columns and more non-neuronal spacing in the periphery. This pattern is not found in the chimpanzee, which has left–right equality nor in the rhesus monkey. The mean difference in the horizontal distance between columns of the two hemispheres in humans is 16% and ranges from 6 to 23%. The rhesus brains exhibit slight laterality on the right side and display a pattern that is different from the human pattern.

The shift in columnar morphology found in in vivo comparative histologic imaging studies from a monkey-like to a human pattern may be a result of the internal reorganization for language (Buxhoeveden et al., 1996). The implication is that this shift has been underway for a long time, though it is seemingly initiated by functions other than language. Evidence from fossil hominoids suggests the possibility that cerebral laterality extends as far back as the earliest human ancestors, the Australopithecines. Perhaps the more clearly defined examples of cerebral laterality in the speech areas is found in Neanderthals such as La Chappelle-Sux-Saints *Homo erectus* fossils and Australopithecus africanus (Le May, 1976).

There is less disputed evidence that early *Homo sapiens* was persistently right-handed. This is derived from sources such as art works of 5000 years ago (Coren and Porac, 1977). Microscopic analysis of wear patterns on Upper Paleolithic tools (about 35 000 years ago) indicate right-handedness. Tools from a few hundred thousand years ago (Middle Paleolithic) suggest the same (Keeley, 1977). Flakes manufactured by *Homo habilis* also suggest that the majority of users were right-handed.

Cases for bilateral symmetry (the absence of lateralization) are thought to be related to left-side dominance. In most studies, about 25% of human brains show little or no asymmetry in an area of the temporal lobe called the planum temporalis (Geschwind and Levitsky, 1968; Geschwind and Galaburda, 1985). Corbalis (1989) suggested that handedness is a response to bipedalism and the freeing of hands and subsequent tool use. In any case, there is no compelling reason to believe that the development of sophisticated language was present until around the time of the Upper Paleolithic "revolution", about 30 000 years ago. Recall that human language involves the use of symbolism, self-awareness, and belief systems, not just basic communication (Gazzaniga, 1989). The evidence that behavior was complex enough to mimic modern human behavior is only found in the Upper Paleolithic age with the advent of symbolism, art, adornment of jewelry, ceremonial burial, and much more.

Laterality per se is not specific to the anthropoid human and can be found elsewhere in the animal kingdom. The key to ascertaining the significance of lateralization is to find the peculiar form of lateralization utilized for a given area for a given species. Heilbroner and Holloway (1989) state that the left temporoparietal cortex, but not the right, started to change before the divergence of humans from the apes. Our research supports their view. It is even possible that the change began with the divergence of the apes from earlier Old World monkeys. Chimpanzees, which are perhaps the closest extant nonhuman relatives and which have some limited degree of linguistic ability, do not manifest a humanoid structural pattern for laterality. Yet, they also do not share the right-hemispheric emphasis that is present in rhesus monkeys.

As pointed out by Armstrong (1990), the presence of gross anatomic asymmetry in the posterior temporal regions is not a sufficient link to language because of the variations in human asymmetries and the presence of asymmetries in nonhuman primates. Most examinations of left Sylvian fissural length consistently reveal left-sided laterality in humans and apes (LeMay and Geschwind, 1975; LeMay, 1976) and more recently in monkeys (Heilbroner and Holloway, 1989). (Apes are genetically and anatomically much closer to humans than are monkeys. In fact, apes are taxonomically much closer to humans than they are to monkeys and it is incorrect to refer to an ape as a "monkey".) Asymmetrical left Sylvian fissural lengths in fossil hominoids must be interpreted with caution since they may reflect another aspect of laterality, i.e., handedness, instead of language. Hopkins (Hopkins and Morris, 1989; Hopkins et al., 1990) has pointed out that behavioral laterality can be found for many different functions within primates, and that individual species manifest varying degrees of laterality. Language is only one aspect of asymmetrical neuronal distribution. Laterality is a generalized trait of the primate nervous system. However, laterality in nonhuman primates does not necessarily imply humanoid qualities. Further studies on prosimians and other monkeys should shed more light on this topic, particularly the specific role played by language-area asymmetry. It has been proposed that lateralization and language are causal elements in schizophrenia (Crow et al., 1989; Crow, 1997). Evidence from MRI indicate certain morphologic findings for schizophrenia that appear to be consistent; an enlargement of the lateral ventricles, reduction in brain volume, possibly smaller left temporal lobe volume, and generalized decrease or absence of cortical asymmetry (Crow, 1997; Buckley, 1998). There is an interesting model that synthesizes the evolution of language with the advent of psychosis (especially schizophrenia). It is hypothesized that there is a genetic basis for psychosis and cerebral asymmetry that is located on the sex chromosomes (Laval

et al., 1998). It is argued that the independent development of each hemisphere is concomitant with both language and schizophrenia (Crow, 1997), thereby linking language, evolution, and schizophrenia.

The circuitry of the brain has undergone many changes at all levels from the callosal fibers that connect the two hemispheres, the interconnections between cortical and subcortical regions, to the microcircuitry of cell columns. Yet another indication of re-organization is the addition of new pathways. While a primary visual cortex may exist in two species, it may connect to 10 other areas in one species and to 15 in the other species. The trend in higher primate brains is to have far more intercommunication between sensory areas within their brains.

The unequal use of neurotransmitter pathways is another way that brain demonstrates lateralization. Asymmetry of neurotransmitters has also been documented in the mammalian brain in relation to motor and positional functions, especially with dopamine (Cabib, et al., 1995; Louilot and Choulli, 1997; Alonso, et al., 1997). A recent study seems to clearly support right hemisphere lateralization for dopamine. Dopaminergic neurons were found to be involved in affective perception, suggesting hemispheric roles for affective perception in normal and pathologic states (Besson and Louilot, 1995). Stress response may also be linked to asymmetrical dopamine systems (Carlson, et al., 1996; Sullivan and Gratton, 1998). Lateralization of noradrenaline (norepinephrine) in the olfactory bulbs of mice is also part of the generalized pattern of the asymmetrical distribution of neurotransmitters (Dluzen and Kreutzberg, 1996). Dopaminergic receptors are already lateralized in the fetal rat brain (Varlinskaya, et al., 1995). In humans, there is a growing body of evidence supporting early onset of laterality, including the asymmetrical distribution of metabolites in children (Hashimoto et al., 1995) and human growth hormones for handedness (Tan, 1995). Binding sites for serotonin-regulated gender differences, such as sexual behavior, aggression and impulse control, and serotonergic mental disorders were found to be sex-linked and asymmetrically distributed between hemispheres (Arato, et al., 1991). By comparison, other studies found no lateralization of serotonin ($5HT_2$) receptor binding sites in human cortex (Yates et al., 1991).

Conclusion: genes and the environment

This chapter reviewed the development of the human brain from conception to adult age and its evolution across time and species. The combination of ontogenetic and phylogenetic knowledge of the human brain can offer insights into the mechanisms that can lead to neurodevelopment disorders. In fact, the editors of the *Journal of the American Academy of Child and Adolescent Psychiatry* have initiated a 1998 series of invited columns that cover brain development in recognition of its critical importance in understanding childhood psychiatric disorders.

The examination of comparative structural and functional anatomy of the brain among species can help in the understanding of the phylogenetic role of the processes that orchestrate brain development. Not only do these processes support the concept of evolution by natural selection (e.g., influences of environment on neurogenesis), but they also help place into perspective behaviors called "maladaptive" that can be at the junction of evolutionary changes by being either obsolete or too precocious for the present time. For example, attention-deficit hyperactivity disorder represents a set of behaviors that may be adaptive in a different cultural milieu but are dysfunctional in our present society.

Disruption at any of the various steps of cortical development (neuronal migration, axonal formation, interneuronal connections) can result in disorders of higher brain functions, such as psychiatric disorders. Symptoms may appear only later in life when the higher cortical function is developmentally ready to be used (e.g., language, reading skills). Subtle disruptions of neuronal migration and synaptic formation have been proposed for disorders such as dyslexia and psychosis.

Genetic programs are the necessary (but not sufficient) factors that control brain development. Genes that contribute to the early events of brain development are being discovered, and it is possible that variants of these genes may be responsible for various developmental disorders. For example, one such gene, *LS1* on chromosome 17, was shown to regulate the early migration of neurons, and its defect leads to lissencephaly: disorders of brain formation in which the surface of the cortex appears smooth. How this genetic defect results in disturbances of neuronal migration is not fully understood. Mutant mouse strains, reared on the basis of abnormal behavior, have been useful in identifying molecular mechanisms underlying brain development. For example, the "reeler" gene, responsible for an abnormal laminar pattern of the cortex, was recently cloned.

Abnormality in the regulation of gene expression (e.g., how often, how much, how long, or at what developmental period a gene (DNA) is transcribed into a protein (RNA)) is another mechanism that can induce developmental disorders. This regulation is assumed by transcription factors. These transcription factors are proteins that bind to the

"promoter" region of the gene. The promoter region regulates the initiation of transcription. Disruption of the regulatory function of transcription has been linked to neuropsychiatric disorders such as Waardenburg syndrome, Prader–Willi syndrome, and fragile X syndrome. Many transcription factors are expressed in the brain. Often their patterns of expression respect boundaries of brain structures (e.g., *dlx-1* and *dlx-2* are expressed in the developing basal ganglia, *hox* in the hindbrain, engrailed genes in the cerebellum and midbrain; *emx* and *otx* in the cerebral cortex). Regionally limited brain abnormalities detected by functional neuroimaging studies can help the molecular geneticist to focus a search to specific genes that control the development of the identified regions. Defects in these genes can induce regionally specific abnormalities in given cell types, or in the "wiring" within the brain. Current theories propose that disruption in transcription factors plays a critical role in common psychiatric disorders.

Once the genetic program is in place (the necessary component to brain development), the environment contributes to the molding and consolidation of the developing brain. Indeed, environment influences the forming and strengthening of synaptic connections, which is mediated by growth factors. Recently, it was shown that early experiences can change cortical rearrangements and that these changes last into adulthood. Clearly, environmental events can significantly affect brain development during critical periods of maturation (e.g., windows of increased plasticity, increased vulnerability to insult, or opportunity for enrichment or treatment).

Brain maturation is a protracted process throughout childhood. Clearly, functional neuroimaging early in life has a better chance to clarify the trajectories of brain development and to help to trace back the normal and deviant maturational processes that underlie neuropsychiatric disorders. Genetic mechanisms need to be explored, and functional neuroimaging and molecular biology research conducted in synergy can optimize our understanding of the origin of brain disorders.

References

Alonso, S. J., Navarro, E., Santana, C. and Rodriquez, M. (1997). Motor lateralization, behavioral despair and dopaminergic brain asymmetry after prenatal stress. *Pharmacol. Biochem. Behav.*, **58**, 443–8.

Anderson, W. W. (1976). Endogenous bursting in Tritonia neurons at low temperature. *Brain Res.*, **103**, 407–11.

Armstrong, E. (1990). Evolution of the brain. In *The Human*

Nervous System, ed. E. Armstrong, pp. 1–16. New York: Academic Press.

Armstrong, E., Curtis, M., Buxhoeveden, D. P. et al. (1991). Cortical gyrification in the rhesus monkey: a test of the mechanical folding hypothesis. *Cereb. Cortex*, **1**, 426–32.

Arato, M., Frecska, E., Maccrimmon, D. J. et al. (1991). Serotonergic interhemispheric asymmetry: neurochemical and pharmaco-EEG evidence. *Prog. Neuropsychopharmacol. Biol. Psychiatry*, **15**, 759–64.

Arshavsky, Y. U., Berkinblit, M. B., Fukson, D. I., Gelfand, I. M. and Orlovsky, G. N. (1972). Recordings of neurons of the dorsal spinocerebellar tract during evoked locomotion. *Brain Res.*, **43**, 272–5.

Backton, J. and Kollok, S. (1989). Effect of forced unilateral nostril breathing on blink rates: relevance to hemispheric lateralization of dopamine. *Int. J. Neurosci.*, **46**, 53–9.

Barker, J. L. and Gainer, H. (1975). Studies on bursting pacemaker potential activity in Molluscan neurons I, II. *Brain Res.*, **84**, 461–77.

Barron, D. H. (1950). An experimental analysis of some factors involved in the development of the fissure pattern of the cerebral cortex. *J. Exp. Zool.*, **113**, 553–73.

Bentley, D. R. and Hoy, R. R. (1972). Genetic control of the neuronal network generating cricket (Teleogryllus gryllus) song patterns. *Animal Behav.*, **20**, 478–92.

Berman, A. J. and Berman, D. (1973). Fetal deafferentation: the ontogenesis of movement in the absence of peripheral sensory feedback. *Exp. Neurol.*, **38**, 170–6.

Besson, C. and Louilot, A. (1995). Asymmetrical involvement of mesolimbic dopaminergic neurons in affective perception. *Neuroscience*, **68**, 963–8.

Bockman, D. E. and Sohal, G. S. (1998). A new source of cells contributing to the developing gastrointestinal tract demonstrated in chick embryos. *Gastroenterology*, **114**, 878–82.

Bossom, J. S. and Ommaya, A. K. (1968). Visuo-motor adaptation (to prismatic transformation of the retinal image) in monkey with bilateral dorsal rhizotomy. *Brain*, **91**, 221–32.

Buckley, P. (1998). Structural brain imaging in schizophrenia. *Psychiatr. Clin. North Am.*, **21**, 77–92.

Bullock, T. H. (1961). The origins of patterned nervous discharge. *Behavior*, **17**, 125–35.

Buxhoeveden, D. P., Lefkowitz, W., Loats, P. and Armstrong, E. (1996). The linear organization of cell columns in human and nonhuman anthropoid Tpt cortex. *Anat. Embryol.*, **194**, 23–36.

Cabib, S., d'Amato, F., Neveu, P., Deleplanque, B., Le Moal, M. and Puglisi-Allegra, S. (1995). Paw preference and brain dopamine asymmetries. *Neuroscience*, **64**, 427–32.

Cambell, L. D., Dayton, D. H. and Sohal, G. S. (1986). Neural tube defects: a review of human and animal studies on the etiology of neural tube defects. *Teratology*, **34**, 171–87.

Campbell, L. R. and Sohal, G. S. (1990). The pattern of neural tube defects created by secondary reopening of the neural tube. *J. Child Neurol.*, **5**, 336–40.

Carlson, J. N., Visker, K. E., Keller, R. W. Jr and Glick, S. D. (1996). Left and right 6-hydroxydopamine lesions of the medial prefrontal cortex differentially alter subcortical dopamine utilization and the behavioral response to stress. *Brain Res.*, **711**, 1–9.

Carpenter, M. B. and Sutin, J . (1983). *Human Neuroanatomy*, 8th edn. Baltimore, MD: Williams and Wilkins.

Caviness, V. S., Kennedy, D. N., Bates, J. F. and Makris, N. (1997). The developing human brain: a morphometric profile. In *Developmental Neuroimaging: Mapping the Development of the Brain and Behavior*, eds. R. W. Thatcher, G. Reid Lyon, J. Rumsey and N. Krasnegor, pp. 3–14, San Diego, CA: Academic Press.

Chang, F. L., Steedman, J. G. and Lund, R. D. (1984). Embryonic cerebral cortex placed in the occipital region of newborn rats makes connections with host brain. *Brain Res.*, **315**, 164–6.

Chang, F., Steedman, J. G. and Lund, R. D. (1986). The lamination and connectivity of embryonic cerebral cortex transplanted into newborn rat. *J. Comp. Neurol.*, **244**, 401–11.

Chugani, H. T., Phelps, M. E. and Mazziotta, J. C. (1987). Positron emission tomography study of human brain functional development. *Ann. Neurol.*, **22**, 487–97.

Corbalis, M. C. (1989). Laterality and human evolution. *Psychol. Rev.*, **96**, 492–505.

Coren, S. and Porac, C. (1977). Fifty centuries of right handedness: the historical record. *Science*, **198**, 631–2.

Courchesne, E., Yeung-Courchesne, R., Press, G. A., Hesselink, J. R. and Jernigan, T. L. (1988). Hypoplasia of cerebrellar vermal lobes VI and VII in autism, *N. Engl. J. Med.*, **318**, 1349–54.

Crow, T. J. (1997). Schizophrenia as failure of hemispheric dominance for language. *Trends Neurosci.*, **20**, 339–43.

Crow, T. J., Ball, J., Bloom, S. R. et al. (1989). Schizophrenia as an anomaly of development of cerebral asymmetry. *Arch. Gen. Psychiatry*, **46**, 1145–50.

Das, S. K. and Ray, P. K. (1997). Ontogeny of neurotransmitter amino acids in human fetal brains. *Biochem. Mol. Biol. Int.*, **42**, 193–202.

Davis, W. J. (1969). The neuronal control of swimmeret beating in the lobster. *J. Exp. Biol.*, **50**, 99–117.

Davis, W. J. (1976). Organizational concepts in the central motor networks of vertebrates. In *The Neural Control of Locomotion*, vol. 18, eds. R. Herman and S. Grillner, New York: Plenum.

Davis, W. J. and Davis, W. S. (1973). Ontogeny of a simple locomotor system: role of the periphery in the development of central nervous circuitry. *Am. Zool.*, **32**, 1–30.

Dekaban, A. S. and Sadowsky, D. (1978). Changes in brain weights during the span of human life: relation of brain heights to body weights. *Ann. Neurol.*, **4**, 345–56.

Dluzen, D. E. and Kreutzberg, J. D. (1996). Norepinephrine is lateralized within the olfactory bulbs of male mice. *J. Neurochem.*, **66**, 1222–6.

Dodson, D. L., Stafford, D., Forsythe, C. Seltzer, C. P. and Ward, J. P. (1992). Laterality in quadrupedal and bipedal Prosimians: reach and whole-body turn in the mouse lemur (*Microcerbus murinus*) and the Galago (*Galago moholi*). *Am. J. Primatol.*, **26**, 191–202.

Dorovini-Zis, K. and Dolman, C. L. (1977). Gestational development of brain. *Arch. Pathol. Lab. Med.*, **101**, 192–5.

Dorsett, D. A., Willows, A. O. D. and Hoyle, G. (1973). The neuronal basis of behavior in *Tritonia*. IV. *J. Neurobiol.*, **4**, 287–300.

Emerit, M. B., Riad, M. and Hamon, M. (1992). Trophic effects of neurotransmitters during brain maturation. *Biol. Neonate*, **62**, 193–201.

Falk, D. (1980). A reanalysis of the South African Australopithecine natural endocasts. *Am. J. Phys. Anthropol.*, **53**, 525–39.

Favorov, O. V. and Kelly, G. (1994a). Minicolumnar organization within somatosensory cortical segregates: I. development of afferent connections. *Cereb. Cortex*, **4**, 408–27.

Favorov, O. V. and Kelly, G. (1994b). Minicolumnar organization within somatosensory cortical segregates: II. Emergent functional properties. *Cereb. Cortex*, **4**, 428–42.

Flechsig, P. (1876). *Die Leitungsbahnen im Gehirn und Ruckernmark des Menschen aufgrund entwicklungsgeschichtlicher Untersuchungen.* Leipzig: Engelmann.

Friede, R. L. (1989). *Developmental Neuropathology*, 2nd edn. Berlin: Springer-Verlag.

Frost, D. O. (1990). Sensory processing by novel, experimentally induced cross-modal circuits. *Ann. NY Acad. Sci.*, **608**, 92–112.

Galaburda, A. M. and Pandya, D. N. (1983). The intrinsic, architectonic and connectional organization of the superior temporal region of the rhesus monkey. *J. Comp. Neurol.*, **221**, 169.

Galaburda, A. M., Corsiglia, J., Rosen, G. D. and Sherman, G. F. (1987). Planum temporale asymmetry: reappraisal since Galaburda and Levitsky. *Neuropsychologia*, **25**, 853–68.

Gardner, C. P. (1976). The neuronal control of locomotion in the earthworm. *Biol. Rev.*, **51**, 25–52.

Gazzaniga, M. S. (1989). Organization of the human brain. *Science*, **245**, 947–52.

Geschwind, N. and Galaburda, A. M. (1985). Cerebral lateralization: biological mechanisms, associations, and pathology. I. *Arch. Neurol.*, **42**, 427–50.

Geschwind, N. and Levitsky, W. (1968). Human brain: left-right asymmetries in temporal speech region. *Science*, **161**, 186–7.

Giedd, J. N., Castellanos, F. X., Rajapakse, J. C., Vaituzis, A. C. and Rapoport, J. L. (1997). Sexual dimorphism of the developing human brain. *Prog. Neuropsychopharmacol. Biol. Psychiatry*, **21**, 1185–201.

Goffinet, A. M. (1984). The embryonic development of the cerebral cortex: what can we learn from the reptiles? In *Organizing Principles of Neural Development*, ed. S. C. Sharma. New York: Plenum.

Goldman, P. S. and Galkin, T. W. (1978). Prenatal removal of frontal association cortex in the fetal rhesus monkey: anatomical and functional consequences in postnatal life. *Brain Res.*, **152**, 451–85.

Grillner, S. (1985). Neurological basis of rhythmic motor acts in vertebrates. *Science*, **228**, 143–9.

Hamano, K., Iwasaki, N., Kawashima, K. and Takita, H. (1990). Volumetric quantification of brain volume in children using sequential CT scans. *Neuroradiology*, **32**, 300–3.

Hamburger, V., Wenger, E. and Oppenheim, R. (1966). Motility in the chick embryo in the absence of sensory input. *J. Exp. Zool.*, **102**, 133–60.

Hashimoto, T., Tayama, M., Miyazaki, M. et al. (1995). Developmental brain changes investigated with proton magnetic resonance spectroscopy. *Devel. Med. Child Neurol.*, **37**, 398–405.

Heilbroner, P. and Holloway, R. (1989). Anatomical brain asymmetries in monkeys: frontal, temporoparietal, and limbic cortex in Macaca. *Am. J. Phys. Anthropol.*, **80**, 203–11.

Hirano, S., Fuse, S. and Sohal, G. S. (1991). The effect of the floor plate on pattern and polarity in the developing central nervous system. *Science*, **251**, 310–13.

Hopkins, W. D. and Morris, R. D. (1989). Laterality for visual-spatial processing in two-language trained chimpanzees (*Pan troglodytes*). *Behav. Neurosci.*, **103**, 227–34.

Hopkins, W. D., Washburn, D. and Rumbaugh, D. (1990). Processing of form stimuli presented unilaterally in humans, chimpanzees (*Pan troglodytes*), and monkeys (*Macaca mulatta*). *Behav. Neurosci.*, **104**, 577–82.

Hubel, D. H. and Wiesel, T. N. (1972). Laminar and columnar distribution of genicular-cortical fibres in the macaque monkey. *J. Comp. Neurol.*, **158**, 421–50.

Hubel, D. H. and Wiesel, T. N. (1974). Sequence regularity and geometry of orientation columns in the monkey striate cortex. *J. Comp. Neurol.*, **158**, 267–94.

Iwasaka, N., Hamano, K., Okada, Y. et al. (1997). Volumetric quantification of brain development using MRI. *Neuroradiology*, **39**, 841–6.

Jacobson, M. (1991). *Developmental Neurobiology*, 3rd edn. New York: Plenum Press.

Jaeger, C. B. and Lund, R. D. (1981). Transplantation of embryonic occipital cortex to the brain of newborn rats. An autoradiographic study of transplant histogenesis. *Exp. Brain Res.*, **40**, 265–72.

Jerison, H. L. (1977). The theory of encephalization. *Ann. NY Acad. Sci.*, **299**, 146–60.

Johnston, M. V. (1995). Neurotransmitters and vulnerability of the developing brain. *Brain Dev.*, **17**, 301–6.

Kaas, J. (1987). The organization of the neocortex in mammal: implications for theories of brain function. *Annu. Rev. Psychol.*, **38**, 129–51.

Kandel, E. R., Schwartz, J. H., James, H. and Jessel, T. M. (1991). *Principles of Neural Science*, 3rd ed. Norwalk, CT: Appleton and Lange.

Kashin, S. M., Feldman, A. G. and Orlovsky, G. N. (1974). Locomotion of fish evoked by electrical stimulation of the brain. *Brain Res.*, **82**, 41–7.

Kato, T., Nishina, M., Matsiushita, K., Hori, E., Mito, T. and Takashima, S. (1997). Neuronal maturation and N-acetyl-L-aspartic acid development in human fetal and child brains. *Brain Dev.*, **19**, 131–3.

Keeley, L. H. (1977). The functions of paleolithic flint tools. *Sci. Am.*, **237**, 109–27.

Koester, S. E. and O'Leary, D. D. (1992). Functional classes of cortical projection neurons develop dendritic distinctions by class-specific sculpturing of an early common pattern. *J. Neurosci.*, **12**, 1382–93.

Kostovic, I. and Rakic, P. (1990). Developmental history of the transient subplate zone in the visual and somatosensory cortex of the macaque monkey and human brain. *J. Comp. Neurol.*, 297, 441–70.

Kreig, W. J. S. (1963). *Connections of the Cerebral Cortex.* Evanston II: Brain Brooks.

Landlesser, L. (1976). The development of neural circuits in the limb moving segments of the spinal cord. In *Neural Control of Locomotion,* ed. L. Landlesser. New York: Plenum Press.

Langworthy, O. R. (1933). Behavior patterns and myelination. *Contrib. Embryol.,* 24, 1–57.

Laval, S. H., Dann, J. C., Butler, R. J. et al. (1998). Evidence for linkage to psychosis and cerebral asymmetry (relative hand skill) on the X chromosome. *Am. J. Med. Genet.,* 81, 420–7.

Le Douarin, N. M. (1982). *The Neural Crest.* London: Cambridge University Press.

Leise, E. M. (1990). Modular constructs of nervous systems: a basic principle of design for vertebrates and invertebrates. *Brain Res. Rev.,* 15, 1–23.

LeMay, M. and Geschwind, N. (1975). Hemispheric differences in the brains of great apes. *Brain Behav. Evol.,* 11, 48–52.

LeMay, M. (1976). Morphological asymmetry in modern man, fossil man, and non-human primates. *Ann. NY Acad. Sci.,* 280, 349–66.

Lemire, R., Loeser, J., Leech, R. and Alvord, E. (1975). *Normal and Abnormal Development of the Human Nervous System.* New York: Harper Row.

Li, L. M., Cendes, F., Bastos, A. C., Andermann, F., Dubeau, F. and Arnold, D. L. (1998). Neuronal metabolic dysfunction in patients with cortical developmental malformations: a proton magnetic resonance spectroscopy imaging study. *Neurology,* 50, 755–9.

Louilot, A. and Choulli, M. K. (1997). Asymmetrical increases in dopamine turn-over in the nucleus accumbens and lack of changes in locomotor responses following unilateral dopaminergic depletions in the entorhinal cortex. *Brain Res.,* 778, 150–7.

Lucas Keene, M. F. and Hewer, E. E. (1931). Some observations on myelination in the human central nervous system. *J. Anat.,* 66, 1–13.

Lund, R. D. and Mustari, M. J. (1977). Development of the geniculorcortical pathway in rats. *J. Comp. Neurol.,* 173, 289–306.

Macneilage, P. F., Studdert-Kennedy, M. G. and Lindblom, B. (1987). Primate handedness reconsidered. *Behav. Brain Sci.,* 10, 247.

Mayeri, E. Koester, J. Kupperman, I., Liebeswar, G. and Kandel, E. R. (1974). Neural control of circulation in aplysia. *J. Neurophys.,* 37, 458–75.

Mountcastle, V. B. (1957). Modality and topographic properties of single neurons of cat's somatic sensory cortex. *J. Neurophysiol.,* 20, 408–34.

Mountcastle, V. B. (1978). An organizing principle for cerebral function: the unit module and the distributed system. In G. M. Edelman and V. B. Mountcastle. *The Mindful Brain: Cortical Organization and the Group-selective Theory of Higher Brain Function,* eds. G. M. Edelman and V. B. Mountcastle, pp. 7–51. Cambridge, MA: MIT Press.

Mountcastle, V. B. (1997). The columnar organization of the neocortex. *Brain,* 120, 701–22.

Nashner, L. M. (1981). Analysis of stance posture in humans. In *Handbook of Behavioral Neurobiology,* Vol. 5, eds. A. L. Towe and E. S. Luschci, pp. 527–65. New York: Plenum Press.

Nelson, J. S., Parisi, J. E. and Schochet, S. S. Jr (1993). *Principles and Practice of Neuropathology,* p. 24. St Louis, MO: Mosby.

Noback, C. R. and Demarest, R. J. (1981). *The Human Nervous System: Basic Principles of Neurobiology,* pp. 142–5. New York: McGraw-Hill.

Nottebohm, F. (1970). Ontogeny of bird song. *Science,* 167, 950–6.

Nottebohm, F. (1971). Vocalizations and breeding behavior of surgically deafened ring doves. (*Streptopelia risoria*). *Anim. Behav.,* 19, 313–27.

Nudo, R. J. and Masterson, R. B. (1990). Descending pathways to the spinal cord, IV: some factors related to the amount of cortex devoted to the cortical spinal tract. *J. Comp. Neurol.,* 296, 584–97.

O'Leary, D. D. M. and Stanfield, B. B. (1989). Selective elimation of axons extended by developing cortical neurons is dependent on regional locale: experiments utilizing fetal cortical transplants. *J. Neurosci.,* 9, 2230–46.

O'Leary, D. D., Schlaggar, B. L. and Stanfield, B. B. (1992). The specification of sensory cortex: lessons from cortical transplantation. *Exp. Neurol.,* 115, 121–6.

Oppenheim, R. W. (1991). Cell death during development of the nervous system. *Annu. Rev. Neurosci.,* 14, 453–501.

Pandya, D., Seltzer, B. and Barlos, H. (1988). Input–output organization of the primate cerebral cortex. In *Comparative Primate Biology,* vol. 4, *Neurosciences.* New York: Alan R. Liss.

Pearson, K. (1976). The control of walking. *Science,* 235, 72–86.

Perry, E. K., Piggott, M. A., Court, J. A., Johnson, M. and Perry, R. H. (1993). Transmitters in the developing and senescent human brain. *Ann. NY Acad. Sci.,* 695, 69–72.

Placzek, M., Tessier-Lavigne, M., Yamada, T., Jessell, T. M. and Dodd, J. (1990). Mesodermal control of neural cell identify: floor plate induction by the notochord. *Science,* 250, 985–8.

Pryse-Davies, J. and Beard, R. W. (1973). A necropsy study of brain swelling in the newborn with special reference to cerebellar herniation. *J. Pathol.,* 109, 51–73.

Rakic, P. (1976). Prenatal genesis of connections subserving ocular dominance in the rhesus monkey. *Nature,* 261, 467–71.

Rakic, P. (1978). Neuronal migration and contact guidance in primate telencephalon. *Postgrad. Med. J.,* 54, 25–40.

Rakic, P. (1988a). The specification of cerebral cortical areas: the radial unit hypothesis. *Science,* 242, 928–31.

Rakic, P. (1988b). Defects of neuronal migration and the pathogenesis of cortical malformations. *Prog. Brain Res.,* 73, 15–37.

Rakic, P. (1990). Principles of neural cell migration. *Experientia,* 46, 882–91.

Rakic, P., Suner, I. and Williams, R. W. (1991). A novel cytoarchitectonic area induced experimentally within the primate visual cortex. *Proc. Natl. Acad. Sci. USA,* 88, 2083–7.

Reiss, A. L., Abrams, M. T., Singer, H. S., Ross, J. L. and Denckla, M. B. (1996). Brain development, gender, and IQ in children. A volumetric imaging study. *Brain,* 119, 1763–74.

Richman, D. P., Stewart, R. M., Hutchinson, J. W. and Caviness, V. S. Jr (1975). Mechanical model of brain convolutional development. *Science,* 189, 18–21.

Rosen, G. D. Sherman, G. F. and Galaburda, A. M. (1989). Interhemispheric connections differ between symmetrical and asymmetrical brain regions. *Neuroscience*, **33**, 525–33.

Rumbaugh, D. M. (1977). *Language Learning by a chimpanzee: The LANA project*. New York: Academic Press.

Sanford, C., Gvin, K. and Ward, J. P. (1984). Posture and laterality in the bushbaby (*Galago senegalensis*). *Brain Behav. Evol.*, **25**, 217–24.

Scammon, R. E. (1932). The central nervous system. In *White House Conference on Child Health and Protection. Growth and Development of the Child*, section 1 (Medical Service), Part 2: *Anatomy and Physiology. Report of the Committee on Growth and Development*, pp. 176–90. London: Appleton.

Schoenwolf, G. C. and Smith, J. L. (1990). Mechanisms of neuralation: traditional viewpoint and recent advances. *Development*, 109, 243–70.

Scheibel, A. (1984). A dendritic correlate of human speech. In *Cerebral Dominance: The Biological Foundations*. eds. N. Geschwind and A. Galaburda. Cambridge, MA: Harvard University Press.

Seldon, H. L. (1981a). Structure of human auditory cortex. I. Cytoarchitectonics and dendritic distributions. *Brain Res.*, **229**, 277–94.

Seldon, H. L. (1981b). Structure of human auditory cortex. II. Axon distributions and morphological correlates of speech perception. *Brain Res.*, **229**, 295–310.

Sharma, K., Korade, Z. and Frank, E. (1995). Late-migrating neuroepithelial cells from the spinal cord differentiate into sensory ganglion cells and melanocytes. *Neuron*, **14**, 143–52.

Shik, M. L., Severen, F. V. and Orlovskii, G. N. (1966). Control of walking and running by means of electrical stimulation of the mid-brain. *Biofizyka*, **1**, 659–66.

Smart, I. H. M. and McSherry, G. M. (1986a). Gyrus formation in the cerebral cortex of the ferret. II. Description of the internal histological changes. *J. Anat.*, **147**, 27–43.

Smart, I. H. M. and McSherry, G. M. (1986b). Gyrus formation in the cerebral cortex of the ferret. I. Description of the external changes. *J. Anat.*, **146**, 141–52.

Smith, J. F. (1974). *Pediatric Neuropathology*, pp. 4–8, 10–14. New York: McGraw-Hill.

Sohal, G. S. (1992). The role of the target size in neuronal survival. *J. Neurobiol.*, **23**, 1124–30.

Sohal, G. S., Bockman, D. E., Ali, M. M. and Tsai, N. T. (1996). DiI labeling and homeobox gene islet-1 expression reveal the contribution of ventral neural tube cells to the formation of the avian trigeminal ganglion. *Int. J. Dev. Neurosci.*, **14**, 419–27.

Sohal, G. S., Ali, A. A. and Ali, M. M. (1998a). Ventral neural tube cells differentiate into craniofacial skeletal muscles. *Biochem. Biophys. Res. Commun.*, **252**: 675–8.

Sohal, G. S., Ali, M. M., Ali, A. A. and Bockman, D. E. (1999). Ventral neural tube cells differentiate into hepatocytes in the chick embryo. *Cell. Mol. Life Sci.*, **55**: 128–30.

Sohal, G. S., Ali, M. M. Galileo, D. S. and Ali, A. A. (1998c). Emigration of neuroepithelial cells from the hindbrain neural tube in the chick embryo. *Int. J. Dev. Neurosci.*, **16**, 477–81.

Strumwasser, F. (1975). Neuronal principles organizing periodic behaviors. In *Circadian Oscillations and Organization of the Nervous System*, ed. C. S. Pittendrigh. Cambridge, MA: MIT Press.

Sullivan, R. M. and Gratton, A. (1998). Relationships between stress-induced increases in medial prefrontal cortical dopamine and plasma corticosterone levels in rats: role of cerebral laterality. *Neuroscience*, **83**(1), 81–91.

Sur, M. Pallas, S. and Roe, A. (1990). Cross-modal plasticity in cortical development: differentiation and specification of sensory cortex. *Trends Neurosi.*, **13**, 227–33.

Szekely, G. Y., Czeh, G. and Voros, G. Y. (1969). The activity pattern of limb muscles in freely moving normal and deafferented newts. *Exp. Brain Res.*, **9**, 53–62.

Szentagothai, J. (1968). The modular architectonic principle of neural centers. *Rev. Physiol. Biochem. Pharmacol.*, **98**, 11–61.

Szentagothai, J. (1978). The neuron network of the cerebral cortex: a functional interpretation. The Ferrier Lecture 1977. *Proc. R. Soc. Lond. Ser. B*, **201**, 219–48.

Tan, U. (1995). Growth hormone limits brain/body development before birth in relation to sex, grasp-reflex asymmetry and familial sinistrality of human neonates. *Int. J. Neurosci.*, **82**, 105–11.

Taub, E. (1976). Motor behavior following deafferentation in the developing and motorically mature monkey. In *Neural Control of Locomotion*, eds. R. Herman and S. Griller. New York: Plenum Press.

Taub, E., Goldberg, I. and Taub, P. (1975). Deafferentation in monkeys: pointing at a target without visual feedback. *Exp. Neurol.*, **46**, 178–86.

Teyler, T. J. and Fountain, S. B. (1987). Neuronal plasticity in the mammalian brain: relevance to behavioral learning and memory. *Child Dev.*, **58**, 698–712.

Varlinskaya, E. I., Petrov, E. S., Robinson, S. R. and Smotherman, W. P. (1995). The asymmetrical development of the dopamine system in the fetal rat as indicated by lateralized administration of SKF-38393 and SCH-23390. *Pharmacol. Biochem. Behav.*, **50**, 359–67.

van der Knaap, M. S. and Valk, J. (1990). MR imaging of the various stages of normal myelination during the first year of life. *Neuroradiology*, **31**, 459–70.

Weiskrantz, L. (1977). On the role of cerebral commisures in animals. In *Structure and Function of Cerebral Commisures*, eds. I. Russel, M. van Hof and G. Berlucchi, pp. 475–478.

Weller, R. E. and Kaas, J. H. (1981). Retinotopic patterns of connections of area 17 with visual areas V-II and MT in macaque monkeys. *J. Comp. Neurol.*, **220**, 253–79.

Willis, J. A. (1974). The role of the electrogenic sodium pump in the modulation of pacemaker discharge of *Aplysia* neuron. *J. Cell Physiol.*, **84**, 463–72.

Wilmer, H. A. (1940). Changes in structural components of the human body from six lunar months to maturity. *Proc. Soc. Exp. Biol.*, **43**, 545–7.

Worthen, N. J., Gilbertson, V. and Lau, C. (1986). Cortical sulcal development seen on sonography: relationship to gestational parameters. *J. Ultrasound Med.*, **5**, 153–6.

Yakovlev, P. I. and Lecours, A. R. (1967). The myelogenic cycles of regional maturation of the brain. In *Regional Development of Brain in Early Life*, ed. A. Minowski, Davis, CA: Blackwells.

Yamada, T., Placzek, M., Tanaka, H., Dodd, J. and Jessell, T. M. (1991). Control of cell pattern in the developing nervous system: polarizing activity of the floor plate and notochord. *Cell*, **64**, 635–47.

Yates, M., Morris, C., Cheng, A. V., Ferrier, N. (1991). Laterality and 5HT$_2$ receptors in human brain. *Psychiatr. Res.*, **36**, 169–74.

Zeisel, S. H. (1997). Choline: essential for brain development and function. *Adv. Pediatr.*, **44**, 263–95.

8

Cognitive development from a neuropsychologic perspective

Daisy M. Pascualvaca and Gloria Morote

Introduction

The field of neuropsychology has made great advances in understanding how the adult brain is organized and how it functions. Relatively little is known, however, about the neural systems mediating normal cognitive development. At present, much of our understanding of brain–behavior relationships in children has been based primarily on adult models. Although valuable, these models have serious limitations when applied to children. Concepts such as critical periods, for example, refer exclusively to the developing organism. The immature brain differs from the mature brain in its neural organization. For example, while studies of laterality provide considerable data to suggest that hemisphere specialization begins early in life, the demarcation between cognitive functions that are differentially mediated by the two hemispheres is less clear cut in children than in adults (Luria, 1973). Concepts such as neural plasticity have been mostly applied to the developing brain, as the possibilities for neural re-organization and recovery of function following injury are remarkable in young organisms. Furthermore, the structure and function of the developing brain is profoundly responsive to and affected by experience. Adversity, whether through deprivation or through abusive environments, can have a deleterious and long-lasting impact on the brain's structural and functional organization (van der Kolk and Greenberg, 1987; Ito et al., 1993).

Recognition of the differences between the mature and the immature brain have led to the design of measures that are sensitive to developmental factors. Of all the techniques available neuroimaging provides a unique approach to the study of brain–behavior relationships in children. By allowing the investigator to observe the brain in vivo, neuroimaging now makes it possible to study the mechanisms that govern the development of cognition.

Studies using these powerful tools will challenge some, if not many, of our traditional concepts and offer invaluable contributions to the advancement of developmental neuroscience.

In this chapter, we will review the developmental trajectories of specific cognitive and neuropsychologic functions. Data from the cognitive, neuropsychologic and developmental literatures will be discussed. Although we will cover major developmental milestones and transitions, it is important to keep in mind that development is not a steady or linear process but rather is characterized by leaps, plateau, and even temporary regressions. As such, measurement of brain–behavior relationships in children requires an understanding of the developmental trajectories of various cognitive processes. In studying children, knowledge of these trajectories is critical to distinguish deviance from delay, because the performance of a normal 6-year-old may be indistinguishable from that of an adolescent with a developmental disability (see Fig. 8.1). Having an understanding of normal cognitive development is also critical to the selection of appropriate assessment instruments. This word of caution is important in developmental neuropsychology, where there has been a reliance on measures designed for adults whose brain–behavior relationships are more clearly understood than are those in children. Measures designed to capture deficits in adults with brain lesions may not be sensitive to the subtleties of deviations in normal development. Whenever possible, we will relate developmental trajectories to documented changes in neural tissue. It is important to note that despite the existence of a significant body of knowledge regarding both neurologic and cognitive development, mapping the correspondence between processes involved in brain maturation, such as myelination, and cognitive development remains a vast field of exploration. We will present Piaget's model, which has guided

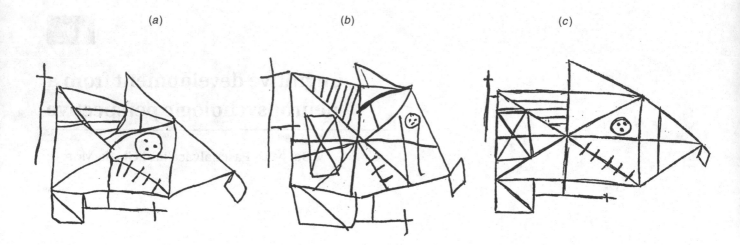

Fig. 8.1. Performance of a normal 6-year-old child (*a*), a 16-year-old-child with a nonverbal learning disability (*b*), and a normal 16-year-old child (*c*) on the Rey–Osterrieth Complex Figure Test.

much of the developmental research. The neuropsychologic findings will be related to Piagetian concepts, which, to this day, continue to influence our conceptualization of normal cognitive development.

Piaget's theory

Piaget (1952, 1954, 1976) proposed a comprehensive and ambitious theory of intellectual development. His observations regarding children's abilities to think, reason, and perceive their world have had a tremendous impact on our conceptualization of cognitive maturation. Piaget asserted throughout his work that cognitive changes are the result of qualitative changes in the way children understand their world. Children learn new concepts as they interact with their environment. At the same time, they adjust these concepts to incorporate changes in the environment. Cognitive development takes place as the child fits new information into his/her notion about the surroundings ("assimilation") and revises old concepts to fit the new information ("accommodation"). Piaget viewed intellectual development as reflecting a dynamic equilibrium between these two processes. Through assimilation and accommodation, the child forms "a schema," an organizing principle that is used to interpret the world.

Piaget conceptualized cognitive development as consisting of a sequence of stages, although it is important to emphasize that he envisaged a continuity of development over its entire course. Each stage derives logically and inevitably from the preceding one, with old schema incorporating new ones. He broadly summarized the stages of

cognitive development as the stage of sensorimotor intelligence (0–2 years), preoperational thought (2–7 years), concrete operations (7–11 years), and formal operations (11–15 years). The main characteristics of these stages are shown in Table 8.1.

Briefly, during the first 24 months of life, the infant learns about the environment by manipulating objects (e.g., through reaching, grasping, and pushing objects). Thinking independent of overt behavior is not yet developed. The child gradually begins to understand simple cause-and-effect relationships and, by the end of the sensorimotor stage, shows clear goal-directed behaviors. Over the next 5 years, during the preoperational stage, the child becomes increasingly able to conceptualize events and situations independent of actions. He/she continues to be egocentric, however, and his/her thoughts are still largely under the control of immediate experiences. By 7 years of age (in the concrete operations stage), the child begins to understand the viewpoint of others and makes logical decisions. He/she can also solve a variety of problems, although it is not until the next stage (the formal operations stage) that the child can apply logic to understand problems that are abstract. In the formal operations stage, there is a complete freeing of thought from direct experience and the adolescent shows hypothetical-deductive, as well as scientific-inductive, reasoning.

Piaget's model has generated much research and some of his findings have been challenged. Recent studies with infants and young children have consistently shown that mastery of many of the constructs he proposed are manifested much earlier. For example, Piaget proposed that object permanence (the recognition that objects exist even

Table 8.1. Piaget's stages of cognitive development

Stage	Age (years)	Characteristics
Sensorimotor	0–2	The child gains knowledge about objects by manipulating them Reflexive behaviors gradually evolve into intentional acts There is a rudimentary understanding of simple cause-and-effect relationships Object permanence develops
Preoperational	2–7	Development of internal representations of objects and events (symbols) Thought is egocentric in that the child fails to take others' point of view There is a tendency to fix attention on a limited aspect of a stimulus (centration) Thought is irreversible (unable to follow line of reasoning back)
Concrete operations	7–11	Emergence of logical operations (thought is no longer dominated by perceptions) Development of the ability to arrange objects according to a characteristic (seriation) Understanding of common characteristics among objects (classification) The child masters conservation (of number, area, mass, and volume) Reversibility of thought (ability to appreciate the invariant properties of objects) De-centering is attained (ability to consider all the salient features of a stimulus) The child can think logically but cannot apply logic to abstract problems
Formal operations	11–15+	Emergence of hypothetical-deductive reasoning Onset of scientific-inductive reasoning The child can understand abstractions from existing knowledge Evidence of logical, abstract, and systematic thinking

when not in view) is not mastered until approximately 9 months of age. Using a number of occlusion paradigms (e.g., a toy car rolling along a track that is partly hidden by a screen), Baillargeon (1995) has shown that infants as young as 2.5 months understand that the occluded object continues to exist. The difference in these timelines is likely to arise through the use of more refined measures that enable investigators to isolate specific cognitive processes involved in a particular task. For instance, Baillargeon (1995) suggested that the infant's failure to search for an object may not represent a lack of object permanence but may instead signal a difficulty in the ability to plan and search for objects. Despite such revisions, Piaget's model continues to provide a useful organizing framework within the developmental literature.

Development of specific cognitive functions

Attention

Piaget's description of the sensorimotor and preoperational stages provides some insight into the development of attention. Children in the preoperational stage (ages 2 to 7 years) are drawn by visual appearances and tend to focus on a single attribute, or the most compelling feature, of objects and situations. For example, when identifying geo-

metrical shapes, young children often confuse triangles, rectangles, and squares because they attend to only one feature of the shape (e.g., whether it has angles or not) (Wadsworth, 1984). By contrast, a child in the concrete operations stage (between the ages of 7 and 11) is able to attend to many more features when examining a shape (e.g., number of sides, lengths of sides) and, therefore, can identify it easily.

Neo-Piagetian theorists have found support for this developmental progression using problem-solving tasks. For example, Siegler (1981) found that 5-year-old children attend to and process only one salient dimension of the material. Nine-year-olds, in turn, will add a second, less-obvious dimension. By late childhood or early adolescence, children will take into account multiple features simultaneously. Similar developmental changes have been reported by investigators using a number of measures of attention such as vigilance tasks, speeded classification tasks, incidental learning tasks, selective listening tasks, and visual search tasks (for a review see Davies et al., 1984). These studies demonstrate that the ability to detect target information in the presence of distracting stimuli and to resist interference improves with age.

The improvement in processing efficiency and resistance to interference are, in part, responsible for an increase in short-term processing capacity observed during childhood (Cowan, 1997; Pressley and Schneider,

Table 8.2. Neuropsychologic models of attention and their proposed brain correlates

Model	Elements or processes	Brain regions
Mirsky (1987), Mirsky et al. (1991)	Focus–execute (scan information and execute response)	Inferior parietal, superior temporal, and striatal regions
	Sustain attention	Mesopontine reticular formation, midline and reticular thalamic nuclei
	Encode (retain and manipulate information)	Hippocampus and amygdala
	Shift	Dorsolateral prefrontal cortex
Posner and Petersen (1990)	Orienting to sensory stimuli	Posterior attention system
	Disengaging attention	Parietal lobe
	Moving attentional focus	Superior colliculus
	Engaging attention	Lateral pulvinar nucleus
	Detecting target events	Anterior attention system (cingulate gyrus and supplementary motor cortex)
	Maintaining an alert state	Noradrenaline (norepinephrine) innervation system particularly in the right hemisphere
Pribram and McGuinness (1975)	Arousal (orienting response)	Spinal cord through brainstem reticular formation
	Activation (readiness to respond)	Basal ganglia
	Effort (coordination of attention systems)	Hippocampus

1997). Short-term capacity refers to the amount of information that can be held in working memory at a given time and is frequently assessed by presenting subjects with sequences of simple stimuli of increasing length and asking them to repeat them immediately. Regardless of the specific type of material presented (e.g., digits or letters), there are clear developmental increases in the number of items children can recall with increasing age, and adult levels of performance typically are reached by 12 years of age (Dempster, 1981).

It is clear that the child's abilities to focus and modulate attentional focus are present as early as infancy (see review by Johnson, 1996) and become more efficient with age. However, little is known about how the different aspects of attention develop in normal children. Neuropsychologic models of attention propose that attention comprises different skills that are mediated by distinct brain regions (see Table 8.2 for a comparison of the main models of attention). Although the specific elements outlined in the models differ, most models include basic processes such as vigilance or arousal, selective attention or focusing, and the shifting of attention.

In developmental neuropsychology, these models have been applied almost exclusively to the study of children with conditions such as attention-deficit hyperactivity disorder (e.g., Barkley et al., 1992), autism (e.g., Courchesne et al., 1995; Pascualvaca et al., 1999), traumatic brain injury (e.g., Ewing-Cobbs et al., 1998), and spina bifida (Loss et al., 1998). These studies have noted attention problems in all the patient groups, although there appear to be some differences in the specific components that are impaired. For example, individuals with autism seem to have particular difficulties with shifting their focus of attention (Courchesne et al., 1995), whereas children who have sustained a traumatic brain injury show problems primarily in their ability to focus (Ewing-Cobbs et al., 1998).

Only a couple of studies have used these models to investigate the developmental trajectories of attention capacities in normal children. One of these studies was conducted by Rebok and colleagues (1997). Using Mirsky's model (Mirsky, 1987; Mirsky et al., 1991) as a conceptual framework, these investigators charted the developmental process of attentional capacities in an epidemiologic sample of children between 8 and 13 years of age. The results of this study indicate that the most rapid gains in attentional performance are seen between the ages of 8 and 10 years. For example, the percentage of omission errors on the Continuous Performance Test (CPT), a measure of sustained attention, declined by about half in this age range. Performance on the CPT leveled off between the ages of 10 and 13, except for the more difficult versions of this task (e.g., auditory CPT) on which performance continued to improve until adolescence. These developmental differences on the CPT are consistent with those reported by Greenberg and Waldman (1993) using a different version of this task. The developmental progression in sustained attention is consistent with maturation of the neural circuits that purportedly mediate this element of attention.

The ability to sustain attention, according to Mirsky, is associated with cellular activity in regions of the reticular activating system and other structures of the brainstem (Mirsky et al., 1991). Although these structures mature shortly after birth, the ascending projections from them to the cerebral cortex, which are also implicated in the regulation of sustained attention (Deutsch et al., 1987; Cohen et al., 1988), continue to develop well into adolescence (Rabinowicz, 1976; Hudspeth and Pribram, 1992).

Rebok and colleagues (1997) also found a marked improvement between ages 8 and 10 in the abilities to focus and to shift attentional focus. Changes in attentional performance seem to be less rapid after age 10, although there is some indication that attention continues to improve into adolescence. For example, reaction time scores in attention tasks continue to decrease across this time period (McKay et al., 1994). The continued improvement observed in the ability to focus, sustain, and shift attention suggests that the brain areas mediating these processes are not functionally mature in middle childhood.

There is also evidence to indicate that boys and girls show different developmental trajectories, with young girls being more efficient at focusing and sustaining attention. For example, 8-year-old girls make fewer commission errors on the CPT than do boys and take less time; they also make fewer errors on visual search tasks (Pascualvaca et al., 1997). The differences in favor of girls observed at 8 years of age decrease by 10 years and are imperceptible by adolescence (Rebok et al., 1997).

It is important to emphasize that adequate performance on traditional tests of attention depends on the integrity of many functional systems. Most neuropsychologic tests make extensive demands on the subjects and require the integrated activity of many brain regions (Cooley and Morris, 1990). The limitation of traditional tests can be overcome through the use of precise cognitive measures and brain imaging techniques. Brain imaging studies have elucidated the effects of specific variable factors, such as variations in the nature of the stimuli, mode of presentation, visual field of presentation, and type of response, on attentional performance (e.g., Posner et al., 1988; Pardo et al., 1991; Posner, 1993). These techniques will undoubtedly advance our understanding of the specific brain circuits involved in attention as well as of the development of these systems in normal children.

Executive functions

Attention and executive functions both refer to the ability to respond selectively to information. Consequently, the behavioral boundaries between these capacities are the subject of debate. Executive functions, however, encompass much more than attention. They incorporate many higher cognitive skills that are necessary to achieve a future goal (Luria, 1973). These include the ability to conceptualize situations flexibly, plan a course of action or goal, initiate the appropriate steps to accomplish this goal, and inhibit irrelevant or competing responses.

The behavioral descriptions of executive functions have been correlated with prefrontal cortical regions in nonhuman primates (e.g., Goldman-Rakic, 1987, 1988). The prefrontal cortex has intricate connections with the limbic system, caudate nucleus, superior colliculus, posterior association cortex, and motor regions within the frontal cortex. The richness of these connections implies a system that is capable of regulating complex behavior (Luria, 1973). At the present time, it is unclear whether specific executive functions are mediated by distinct regions within the prefrontal cortex or whether these functions are subserved by a common prefrontal region and distinguished by its unique sets of connections to other areas. Fuster (1985), for example, proposed that the abilities to resist interference, maintain set, and plan a response are localized in different parts of the prefrontal cortex. In contrast, Goldman-Rakic (1987) hypothesized that each of these component skills is mediated by different pathways that comprise the circuitry of the prefrontal cortex. For example, she proposed that the prefrontal–limbic connections may subserve the working memory component of executive functions, whereas the connections to the striatum, thalamus, and premotor cortex may mediate the selection and execution of specific responses.

The prefrontal cortex has traditionally been conceptualized as the slowest developing brain region based on the time course of its myelination (Rabinowicz, 1976; Hudspeth and Pribram, 1992). Given that this cortical area is late to mature, many investigators have suggested that executive functions are not fully operational until later in life, perhaps as late as adolescence. This assumption has been supported by the results of studies using clinical measures of executive functions, such as the Wisconsin Card Sorting Test (WCST). For example, Chelune and Baer (1986) administered the WCST to a group of children aged 6–12 years and found that there was a striking improvement in performance between 6 and 10 years of age (Fig. 8.2). Performance continued to improve, at a less accelerated rate, between 10 and 12 years of age, and it reached adult levels at about 12 years. These results have been interpreted as an indication that executive functions mature during early adolescence.

However, rudimentary types of executive function are observed in early childhood and even in infancy when

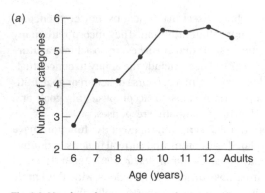
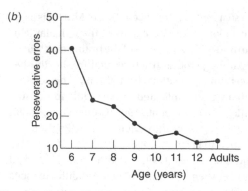

Fig. 8.2. Number of categories (*a*) and perseverative errors (*b*) on the Wisconsin Card Sorting Test by age (Chelune and Baer, 1986).

developmentally appropriate measures are used. One of these measures is the classic Piagetian object-permanence paradigm. This measure resembles the delayed-response inhibition task, which is sensitive to dorsolateral prefrontal functions in monkeys (Diamond and Goldman-Rakic, 1989). In the object-permanence task, a toy is hidden in one of two identical wells in front of the infant and, after a brief delay, the infant is allowed to reach for the toy. Once the infant reaches for the toy correctly, the toy is hidden in the other well in full view of the infant. Using this paradigm, Diamond (e.g., Diamond and Goldman-Rakic, 1989; Diamond, 1990) found that infants between 7 and 11 months made the classic "A not B" error; that is, they reached for the toy in the place where they had found it previously, rather than in the most recent hiding place. By 12 months of age, however, infants completed the task correctly without difficulty. Since this task requires the maintenance of a set over a brief delay (e.g., remembering where the toy was hidden) as well as the execution of an appropriate motor response while inhibiting an inappropriate response (i.e., reaching to the well that contained the toy in the previous trial), it is clear that rudimentary executive skills are present early in infancy.

Infants can not only maintain set and inhibit an inappropriate response but they can also withhold actions to obtain a reward. This ability, observed in children as young as 18 months of age, continues to improve during infancy and is associated with language competence (Vaughn et al., 1984). The association between language and inhibitory control is consistent with Luria's hypothesis (1959) that verbal mediation plays a role in the development of response inhibition.

Taken together, the consensus of recent findings indicates that the mastery of behaviors typically conceptualized as executive functions occurs at different ages, depending on the specific domains assessed. For example, using a number of executive tasks, Welsh et al. (1991) found

three stages of maturation: at ages 6, 10, and 12 years. Six-year-old children demonstrated simple planning and organized visual search, which included the ability to resist distraction and inhibit irrelevant responding. More developed impulse control and set maintenance and an increased ability to ignore distracting information were evident at 10 years of age. By 12 years of age, complex planning skills, verbal fluency, and motor sequencing reached adult levels. The specific functions mastered at each of these age levels and examples of tasks used to assess these functions are shown in Table 8.3. Using very different measures, a similar multistage progression was found by Passler et al. (1985) and by Becker, et al. (1987). These investigators outlined comparable stages of maturation, with the greatest period of development observed between 6 and 8 years of age.

It is important to note that, even though most studies have indicated complete mastery on tasks of executive functions by age 12, these functions are likely to continue maturing until late adolescence or adulthood. In fact, children of 12 years of age are not as flexible and efficient in their planning skills as are adults (Pea, 1982; Welsh et al., 1991). Adolescents are also likely to exhibit only incomplete mastery of tasks that require complex planning, organization, and inhibition of competing responses.

There are no consistent sex differences in the development of executive functions. Most studies have found either no differences between boys and girls (Welsh et al., 1991) or inconsistent differences only at the younger age groups (Passler et al., 1985). Girls are better at inhibiting motor movements (Macoby and Jacklin, 1974) and irrelevant responses (Pascualvaca et al., 1997) than boys, but it is not clear how these sex differences impact on their ability to plan and achieve a goal.

The developmental trajectory of executive functions parallels normal cognitive development. As discussed by Welsh and Pennington (1988), Piaget's theory of cognitive

Table 8.3. Developmental progression of behaviors associated with frontal lobe functioning

Age (years)	Processes	Name of instruments
6	Resistance to distraction	Visual Search Task
	Rudimentary response inhibition	Tower of Hanoi (3 rings)
	Simple strategic and planning	Speeded responding
10	Inhibition of irrelevant responding	Matching Familiar Figures Test
	Hypothesis generation	Wisconsin Card Sorting Test
	Organized search	
	Maintenance of set	
12	Verbal fluency efficiency	Verbal Fluency Test
	Goal setting (intermediate and final)	Tower of Hanoi (4 rings)
	Complex planning skills	Motor Planning
	Motor sequencing	

Source: From Welsh et al., 1991.

development resembles current concepts of executive functions and supports the premise that these functions are present during infancy. For instance, the concept of causality, which is mastered during the first year of life, involves rudimentary set maintenance, planning, and flexibility. Subsequent stages in Piaget's theory also provide examples of how executive functions change during cognitive development. Increased language competence during the preoperational stage (ages 2 to 7) allows greater verbal control, which, in turn, leads to improvement in the attainment of a goal. Subsequently, during the operational and formal operational stages, the child experiences a gradual distancing from the environmental stimuli and begins to reason logically about familiar situations (in the concrete operations stage, between the ages of 7 and 11), as well as about hypothetical events (during the formal operations stage, between 11 and 15 years). This gradual improvement in the ability to reason logically and understand hypothetical situations resembles the developmental progression of executive functions.

Memory

Contemporary views of memory posit that memory is not a unitary trait but rather comprises different skills (Table 8.4) that are mediated by distinct brain pathways (for a

review, see Schacter and Tulvin, 1994). At a general level, memory processes can be divided into short-term and long-term components. Short-term or working memory refers to the ability to represent information internally for brief periods of time (up to 20 s). Only a limited amount of information can be consciously processed while in short-term storage. In contrast, long-term memory contains virtually everything that the person has learned, including records of personal events, facts about the world, and information about how to do things.

The neural systems underlying short- and long-term memory processes also differ. Short-term capacity is mediated primarily by areas of the prefrontal cortex (Funahashi et al., 1993; Casey et al., 1995; Courtney et al., 1998; Ungerleider et al., 1998), whereas consolidation processes resulting in long-term memory is associated with the medial temporal region and neighboring structures (Bachevalier and Mishkin, 1984; Alvarez et al., 1994). Support for a distinction in the neural substrates subserving short- and long-term memory has been derived from the adult and developmental literature. However, there is evidence to suggest that the neurologic systems that support short- and long-term memory may change during the course of development. For example, compared with adults, normal children have shown a more diffuse pattern of activation on fMRI scans in the prefrontal cortex during working memory tasks (Casey et al., 1995). This finding may reflect an immature brain organization in children, particularly in areas that develop late. There is also some indication that the medial temporal region, which matures earlier than the prefrontal cortex, may mediate some aspects of short-term memory early in development (Hershey et al., 1998).

Short-term memory capacities can be further subdivided into verbal, visual (e.g., for objects, patterns, designs), and spatial systems (e.g., relationships among objects in space). Evidence for a dissociation of these systems has been found in cognitive (Baddeley, 1992), lesion (Levine et al., 1985), animal (Goldman-Rakic, 1987), positron emission tomographic (PET) (Jonides, et al., 1993; Courtney et al., 1996), and functional magnetic resonance imaging (fMRI) studies (D'Esposito et al., 1995). The evidence suggests that these memory systems are mediated by neighboring but distinct areas of the prefrontal cortex (e.g., Courtney et al., 1996). It is unclear, however, what specific role the prefrontal cortex plays in the working memory process.

Short-term memory improves dramatically during childhood and early adolescence, regardless of the specific type of material that children are asked to remember (e.g., verbal, visual, or spatial). For example, the number of unrelated words that children can recall doubles between 4 and 12 years, by which adult levels of performance are gener-

Table 8.4. Characteristics of different memory systems

Memory systems	Other terminology	Definition	Examples of tasks
Short-term memory	Working memory	Capacity to retain information for brief periods of time	Repetition of information (e.g., digits, letters, and words); immediate replication of spatial sequences; mental manipulation of stimuli for brief intervals
Episodic memory	Autobiographical memory	Recollection of past happenings	Remembering specific personal events; recalling significant events in the individual's experience
Semantic memory	Factual knowledge	Ability to remember novel information; acquisition and retention of factual material	Recalling stories, scenes, facts; answering questions of general knowledge
Declarative memory	Explicit memory	Includes memory for facts and events	Same as semantic memory
Nondeclarative memory	Implicit memory, procedural memory	Mastery of skills and habits unconsciously processed that facilitate performance	Priming tasks

ally achieved (Hulme et al., 1984). There is considerable debate as to whether these developmental changes reflect an increase in memory capacity itself (e.g., Pascual-Leone, 1970) or are secondary to improved processing strategies. The strategies that have received most support include a growth in the use of phonologic processes (e.g., internally generated phonologic or sound codes), an increase in lexical knowledge (e.g., a growth in vocabulary), and the emergence of rehearsal techniques (e.g., rehearsing items subvocally) (for a review see Gathercole, 1998). It is likely that the sharpening of these strategies also accounts for the improvement observed in visual working memory tasks. For example, preventing subvocal rehearsal disrupts visual pattern span (e.g., memory for geometric forms, shapes and objects) in 11-year-old children more dramatically than in 5-year-old children (Mills et al., 1996). Consequently, in addition to possible increases in the capacity to hold visual information in memory, the older children use a range of verbal strategies to retain information that are not accessible to the younger groups. Spatial memory tasks (i.e., those that tap memory for the locations of the objects in space) show a less dramatic developmental progression than visual memory tasks. The difference between these two developmental trajectories has been attributed to the greater difficulty in mediating spatial information verbally (Gathercole, 1998). Recent PET data in adults have provided support for this hypothesis. Specifically, Jonides et al. (1993) reported activation in language regions of the left hemisphere when adults were completing object memory tasks (i.e., recognition of novel geometric forms) that were not clearly observed on spatial memory tasks (e.g., dots in various location).

As with short-term memory, several systems have been hypothesized to subserve long-term memory in adults. For example, investigators have distinguished between episodic memory, or recollection of personal events and experiences, and semantic memory, or accumulated factual knowledge (e.g., Vargha-Khadem et al., 1997; Fernandez et al., 1998). The distinction between episodic and semantic memory has received relatively little attention in the developmental literature, in part because of the difficulty in assessing personal memories during the early years of life. Because of limitations in the assessment of memory functions in children, many investigators have conceptually organized memory into declarative and procedural systems, combining memories for facts and events into an integrated component. Declarative or explicit memory refers to the capacity for conscious recall of information and captures what the layman typically thinks of as memory. Procedural or implicit memory, by comparison, reflects expressed abilities (perceptual or motor) for which there is no conscious recollection. It includes the skills and habits that facilitate performance in novel tasks. For example, recall of a task is facilitated by prior exposure to a similar or identical task, even when the individual does not remember having had such exposure, a phenomenon known as priming. Studies in human adults and with animal models indicate that the declarative and procedural long-term memories are mediated by distinct brain pathways. Lesions of the medial temporal lobe, including the hippocampus, in nonhuman primates result in impairments in declarative memory, leaving performance on procedural or implicit memory tasks intact. Implicit memory is, in contrast, disrupted by lesions in areas of the striatum (e.g., Bachevalier, 1990). The results of animal studies also suggest that these memory systems emerge at different times in development, and that the system presumed to mediate declarative or explicit memory matures later in nonhuman primates (Bachevalier and Mishkin, 1984).

It is difficult to determine when these memory systems emerge in humans. The paucity of knowledge regarding developmental changes reflects limitations in the paradigms that can be used to assess memory in young children. Nonetheless, the available data suggest that tasks that measure implicit memory can be mastered by infants as young as 3½ months of age (for a review see Nelson, 1997). The early emergence of these functions is consistent with the early maturation of structures that comprise the striatum (caudate and putamen) (Hudspeth and Pribram, 1992). Infants between 6 and 12 months of age can also complete simple explicit memory tasks. However, more complex explicit memory tasks (or tasks with an explicit memory component), such as the delayed nonmatch-to-sample task, are not mastered until at least 18 months (Overman et al., 1992, 1993; Diamond, 1995), presumably because of their increased reliance on cortical structures (Malkova et al., 1995; Fernandez et al., 1998). The developmental trajectory of explicit memory continues throughout childhood, possibly reflecting further organization in the temporal lobe and neighboring cortical areas. In contrast, it is possible that less dramatic development occurs in implicit memory because the underlying neural system matures earlier in life.

It is clear that infants are capable of a rich repertoire of complex memories. By as early as 9 months of age, infants can recall specific events over delays of several weeks and even months (for reviews see Bauer, 1997; Rovee-Collier and Gerhardstein, 1997). The amount of information and type of material that children can remember increases steadily over the first few years of life. This development in memory capacities reflects several factors including (i) an improvement in the child's ability to encode more features of a stimulus, (ii) a decrease in the child's tendency to encode irrelevant information, (iii) an increase in the use of mnemonic strategies that promote learning, and (iv) an enhancement in metamemory or knowledge about memory.

In general, children's memories improve as their knowledge base expands (Pressley and Schneider, 1997). When children come to associate new information with a larger fund of knowledge, their memories become enriched. There are stronger connections among different types of material, which makes this material more accessible and easier to recall. As the knowledge base continues to grow, it facilitates the learning of new concepts that are related to concepts the child has already mastered.

During the school years, children also become increasingly adept at encoding the essential features of new stimuli and at registering fewer distracting events (Lane and Pearson, 1982). There is also a gradual improvement in the use of mnemonic strategies during childhood (for a review see Pressley and Schneider, 1997). Even 5-year-old children can use simple rehearsal strategies (e.g., rote repetition), but they do not rely on them consistently and may not derive as much benefit from their use. It is not until 8 years of age that children's use of rehearsal has a notable impact on their performance. Eight-year-old children rehearse single items spontaneously to learn new material, and, by 10 years of age, they can group items together and begin to organize information into categories. They can also plan specific strategies to facilitate their recall. Organizational strategies develop somewhat later than rehearsal techniques and are not seen consistently until approximately 10 years of age. With increasing age, mnemonic strategies also become more complex. For example, the use of elaboration becomes evident only in adolescence. These new techniques do not necessarily replace the old ones, but rather the older strategies continue to develop and become more efficient.

Another important aspect in the developmental progression of memory is a remarkable growth in children's knowledge about memory processes (metamemory, or the ability to make judgments and predictions about one's memory capacities). Young children are not aware of their memory capabilities (Kreutzer et al., 1975). For example, they tend to miscalculate the amount of time they require to learn a particular task and are not familiar with specific strategies that would facilitate their learning. During the school years, children gradually acquire knowledge about their memory capacities. For instance, they learn to allocate more time to material they have not yet mastered and are in a better position to appraise their readiness for tests. This knowledge clearly influences memory and learning, which, in turn, leads to enhanced metamemory (for a review see Schneider, 1997).

In addition to the processes that facilitate the encoding of new memories, there are also developmental differences in retrieval strategies, such as the use of categories and thematic cues to facilitate recall. The retrieval of memories grows steadily as other cognitive abilities mature. The difference between retrieval and recognition memories is a good example of how development in other cognitive systems influence recall. As shown in Fig. 8.3, 7-year-old children can recognize words in a list learning task as well as 16-year-olds, but they can spontaneously

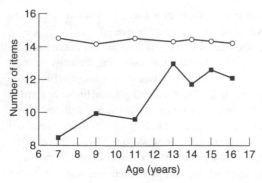

Fig. 8.3. Comparison of developmental changes in free and recognition recall. Free recall, ■; recognition recall, ○. (Material from the Rey Auditory Verbal Learning Test: A Handbook copyright (1996) by Western Psychological Services. Reprinted by permission of the publisher. Western Psychological Services. 12031 Wilshire Boulevard, Los Angeles, California 90025, USA. All rights reserved.)

retrieve fewer items. The difference between performance in recognition and free-recall tasks has been attributed to an increase in language competency. It may well be, however, that the difference between these two paradigms also reflects the concurrent maturation of executive functions. This is evident by the improvement in organized search strategies (Jetter et al., 1986) and decrease in susceptibility to interference and intrusion errors (Fiducia and O'Leary, 1990) observed during the school-age years.

Language

Many critical events in neural development take place during the years of language acquisition. Yet, little is known about the underlying neural correlates of language development. Studies of children who have sustained trauma early in life have shown that the developing language system can undergo striking changes in neural organization. For example, the studies of Woods and Teuber (1973), Milner (Milner et al., 1964; Rasmussen and Milner, 1977), Bates (Reilly et al., 1998), Feldman (Feldman et al., 1992), and Kohn and Dennis (1971) all indicate that lesions and even resection of the left hemisphere do not preclude the development of language. The findings of these studies also suggest that the two hemispheres can mediate many aspects of language early in life. The bilateral representation of language early in life may be a natural phenomenon of the developing system rather than a reaction to trauma (Bates, 1992). This hypothesis is supported by the results of recent evoked response potential (ERP) studies with normal children (Mills et al., 1994; Neville, 1995; Mills and

Neville, 1997), which indicate that lateralization of language increases during childhood. Although there are clear structural hemispheric differences in language areas even in the fetus (Chi et al., 1977), the results of recent ERP studies suggest that functional lateralization of language continues to develop over the first few months or years of life.

Language consists of six major components: the sound system (phonology), the content system (semantics), the rules of word formulation (morphology), the rules of sentence formation (syntax), the suprasegmental aspects of language (prosody), and the social use of language (pragmatics). The *phonologic* dimension reflects the ability to appreciate the distinct nature of individual speech sounds and sound patterns. *Semantics* refers to our knowledge of specific word meanings and understanding of relationships between words. *Morphology* describes the rules for combining morphemes (the smallest units of meaning) to form words and phrases. It also includes the use of inflection (as in the plural form) and derivation (creating new words by adding prefixes and suffixes). *Syntax* refers to the rules for joining words to make sentences. *Prosody* (also called the suprasegmental aspect of language) comprises vocal inflection, stress intonation, pausing, and other variables that contribute to the rhythmic aspects of language. Finally, *pragmatics* takes into account how variations in the intent of the speaker (e.g., goal or purpose) and the social milieu (e.g., speaker–listener relationship or situation) influence the linguistic output. Pragmatics includes the understanding and use of gestures as well as the social context in which language is used.

In the adult brain, these language dimensions are mediated by distinct neural systems. For example, after brain injury, understanding of words can be impaired while phonologic and syntactic processing remains intact (Allport and Funnell, 1981). Even different types of semantic knowledge can be selectively impaired by brain lesions (e.g., Warrington and Shallice, 1984). Recent neuroimaging studies have provided detailed information about the representation of specific linguistic processes in normal adults (e.g., Martin et al., 1995, 1996; Damasio et al., 1996) and differences in the functional organization of language between males and females (Shaywitz et al., 1995). Although comparable developmental studies are limited, the available evidence suggests that different dimensions of language can be dissociated in normal children (Neville, 1995), as well as in children with developmental language disorders (Korkman and Häkkinen-Rihu, 1994; Rapin and Allen, 1988). It is not known, however, how the neural systems that support specific language functions organize and become more refined during the course of normal development.

There are several principles of language development that are well documented. First, as noted above, language acquisition progresses at a remarkable pace during the first 3 years of life and coincides with rapid changes in neural development. Second, there are critical periods in the acquisition of language. Support for the concept of critical periods comes from different lines of investigation, including studies of children raised in grossly deprived environments (Curtiss, 1977), deaf isolates (Curtiss, 1989), and bilingual individuals (Johnson and Newport, 1989). Third, the emergence of language is an active process. Children generate their linguistic output and do not merely repeat what they have heard. Fourth, the course of language development is remarkably similar across individuals and cultures. Most children show a comparable progression in their acquisition of early language milestones.

The development of language begins well before the child speaks his first words (see Fig. 8.4 for a description of the early language milestones). During the third trimester of pregnancy, for example, the fetus reacts to the maternal voice (de Casper et al., 1994). Shortly after birth, infants show a consistent response to sounds (Locke, 1996, 1997) and to variations in vocal emotion (Caron et al., 1988). Auditory orienting responses appear several months later, at approximately 4 months of age, when the infant orients to the source of sound, responds to the human voice, and learns to recognize the caregiver's vocal characteristics. These early behaviors provide the rudimentary basis for language and social development and are vital to the acquisition of linguistic proficiency. Subsequent receptive milestones have not been clearly mapped, but it seems that at all levels of development, children are able to comprehend more language than they are able to speak.

Expressive milestones have been studied extensively. These milestones show a clear pattern of development (for reviews see Locke, 1997; Owens, 1992), beginning with cooing and the indiscriminate use of certain sounds (dada) during the first 4 months of life. These sounds give the infants a set of utterances that they can use in certain contexts and provides them with the opportunity to participate in social interactions. Babbling takes on speech-like characteristics and often overlaps with the emergence of the first few words between 10 and 12 months of age. Already by the end of the first year, babies use many single words to comment on their actions, the actions of others, and the environment around them. Most of the children's first words are labels for objects (e.g., dada, mama, and cookie), action words (e.g., eat, come, and go), and social

terms (e.g., bye and hi). Language explodes at around 2 years of age (Plunkett, 1993) when children also begin to show symbolic capacities in play and elaborate social behaviors. The most evident explosion is seen in the child's vocabulary. For example, at 2 years of age, most children have a vocabulary of at least 50 words and combine words into two-word phrases or utterances (e.g., want cookie). By 3 years of age, the child's vocabulary has increased to approximately 250 words, and he or she is using three-word phrases. These short phrases are devoid of articles, prepositions, and auxiliary verbs and are referred to as telegraphic speech because nonessential words are omitted. In English, where word order conveys meaning, 2- and 3-year-old children demonstrate the subject–action–object order as their first rule. By the end of the year, children begin to add grammatical inflections to their words (e.g., "-ed", resulting in "comed" for "came") and gradually expand the length of their sentences. They gradually begin to add elements to their speech, such as pronouns, prepositions, and grammatical morphemes, and elaborate the basic structure of the sentence to reflect more complex knowledge. Children possess perhaps as many as 400 words before they begin to apply the rules of linguistic morphology (Bates et al., 1994). By 4 years of age, the rapid development of language skills that characterize the first years of life is no longer seen.

By the time children enter school, at age 6 in the USA, they can use language to initiate conversation, maintain a topic, express feelings and emotions, and interact socially. They continue to refine their use of morphologic and syntactic rules and begin to view situations from the perspective of other people. By 8 years of age, children produce all phonemes correctly and exhibit the main characteristics of the adult grammar. Their language acquisition is not complete. In fact, language development continues through the school-age years and into adulthood (Johnson, 1996) in interaction with developing conceptual abilities, experience, and education. However, from this time on, additions to the linguistic system take the form of subtle refinements in the way language is used. The child becomes increasingly skilled at adapting his language to the specific situation and partner and shows an increased understanding of metaphoric language (e.g., feeling blue).

The association between language and cognitive development has been studied extensively since the early 1970s. Brown (1973), for example, noted strong parallels between the child's acquisition of language and Piaget's model of cognitive development. Specifically, Piaget emphasized the salience of objects and actions from the child's point of view, a salience that is supported by the first utterances. These utterances typically describe objects and actions

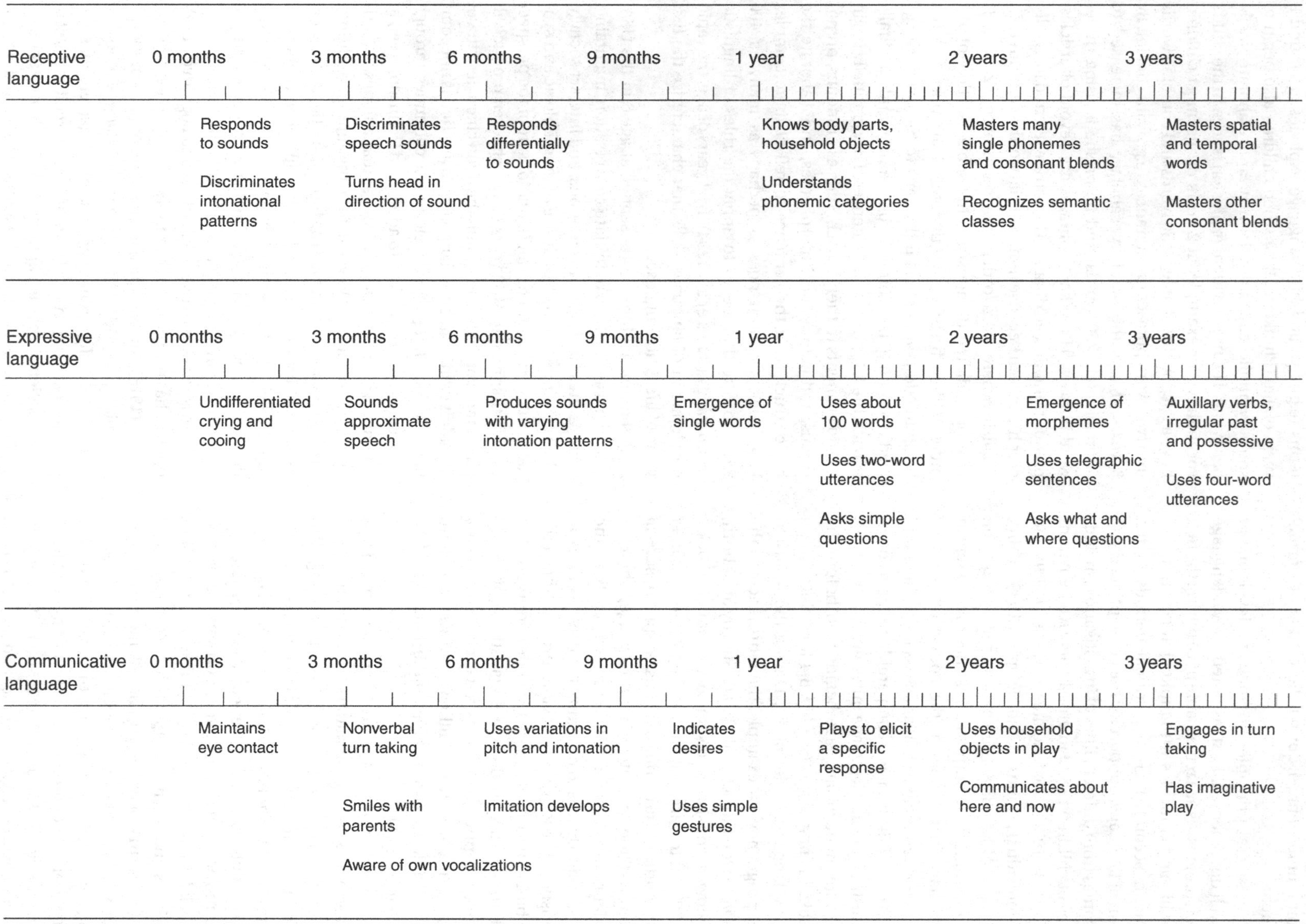

Receptive language

	0 months	3 months	6 months	9 months	1 year	2 years	3 years
	Responds to sounds	Discriminates speech sounds	Responds differentially to sounds		Knows body parts, household objects	Masters many single phonemes and consonant blends	Masters spatial and temporal words
	Discriminates intonational patterns	Turns head in direction of sound			Understands phonemic categories	Recognizes semantic classes	Masters other consonant blends

Expressive language

	0 months	3 months	6 months	9 months	1 year	2 years	3 years
	Undifferentiated crying and cooing	Sounds approximate speech	Produces sounds with varying intonation patterns		Emergence of single words	Uses about 100 words	Emergence of morphemes
						Uses two-word utterances	Uses telegraphic sentences
						Asks simple questions	Asks what and where questions
							Auxiliary verbs, irregular past and possessive
							Uses four-word utterances

Communicative language

	0 months	3 months	6 months	9 months	1 year	2 years	3 years
	Maintains eye contact	Nonverbal turn taking	Uses variations in pitch and intonation		Indicates desires	Plays to elicit a specific response	Engages in turn taking
		Smiles with parents	Imitation develops		Uses simple gestures	Uses household objects in play	Has imaginative play
		Aware of own vocalizations				Communicates about here and now	

Fig. 8.4. Early language milestones.

with which the child is familiar (e.g., want milk). However, contrary to Piaget's prediction, more advanced language milestones do not seem to follow specific cognitive competencies but rather emerge at the same time. Children use words to learn new concepts as well as to express ideas that they understand. Therefore, it seems that children in the sensorimotor period (birth to 2 years of age) draw upon concepts to master language, whereas children in more advanced stages use language to learn new concepts and to communicate what they know.

Visuospatial skills

This section provides a concise review of visual processing abilities. The organization of visual areas has been mapped extensively in primates and human adults (for reviews see Ungerleider and Mishkin, 1982; Ungerleider and Haxby, 1994; Courtney and Ungerleider, 1997). These studies reveal that visual cortical areas are organized into two functionally specialized pathways for object and spatial vision. The dorsal stream or "*where*" system provides information regarding the location of objects in space and the spatial relationship among objects. This pathway originates in area V1 and projects to the middle temporal area and to additional areas in the superior temporal and parietal cortex. The ventral stream or "*what*" system, in turn, recognizes the identity or nature of objects (e.g., color, pattern, and shape) regardless of spatial location and is mediated by the inferior temporal cortex. Regions in the occipitotemporal and occipitoparietal pathways are organized hierarchically. In other words, early processing areas within both pathways are dedicated to the detection of specific features (e.g., angles, edges), while areas involved in later processing subserve increasingly integrated and general perceptions (e.g., objects). This loss in specificity is accompanied by increasing selectivity for complex stimuli. For example, within the occipitotemporal pathway, neurons in V1 respond to contours and edges, whereas neurons in the inferior temporal cortex respond to global features such as faces.

An anomaly in the dorsal stream, particularly in the magnocellular visual system, which subserves transient processing may account for the difficulties in temporal processing hypothesized in developmental dyslexia (Eden et al., 1996). Disordered perceptions of spatial relationships (e.g., finger agnosia, visuospatial neglect, constructional apraxia) have been attributed to anomalies in the occipitotemporal pathway (Newcombe and Ratcliff, 1989). In addition, anomalies in areas of the ventral occipitotemporal cortex (e.g., collateral sulcus and lingual gyrus) can cause color-blindness (Damasio et al., 1980) and problems in visual discrimination. Specific areas within the central

occipitotemporal cortex are sensitive to the perception of faces (Desimone, 1991; Clark et al., 1996) and have been implicated in disorders of facial recognition (Damasio et al., 1982, 1990).

The occipitotemporal and occipitoparietal pathways show different developmental trajectories in nonhuman primates. Although both pathways are immature at birth, the occipitoparietal system matures at 2 months of age, approximately 1 month earlier than the occipitotemporal pathway (Distler et al., 1996). It is not known if the same finding applies to humans. The evidence suggests that these pathways are not fully mature at birth in human infants (for reviews see Cohen and Salapatek, 1975; Aslin et al., 1981). Neonates are sensitive to brightness and can discriminate between gross visual features but have difficulty identifying patterns and forms. Similarly, they can only detect gross movements in the visual field. At approximately 2 to 3 months of age, infants can track objects and discriminate simple forms. Between 2 and 12 months of age, the visual system matures rapidly and the infant becomes capable of making increasingly complex visual discriminations. The nature of their discriminations suggests that, in general, infants are attracted to high-contrast patterns and moving objects.

The infant's preference for movement and high-contrast features likely makes faces among the most interesting of visual stimuli. The study of facial recognition has received significant attention in recent years, not only because of the contribution of facial perception to the understanding of other perceptual abilities but also because of its role in the development of social competence. Studies of facial recognition have shown that, during the first weeks of life, infants recognize their mother's face. Facial recognition shows rapid qualitative changes during the first 7 months of life. In the early stages of development, infants rely on the external configuration of the mother's face (e.g., outer contour of the head and hairline) (Bushnell, 1982; Bushnell et al., 1989; Pascalis et al., 1995). Facial recognition becomes more refined in the first few months and, by the age of 5 months, infants are able to recognize the mother's face from its internal details (de Schonen and Mathivet, 1990). By 7 months of age, babies can recognize faces even when shown in different poses or from different vantage points (Fagan, 1976). Accuracy of facial recognition increases steadily during the first 5 years of life. By age 6, children can recognize faces as well as do adults but continue to have difficulty interpreting some facial expressions (Kolb et al., 1992). In fact, perception of facial expression continues to improve during childhood up until about 14 years of age. Kolb et al. (1992) argue that the neural substrates of facial recognition differ from those underlying the perception of facial expression, and that the latter ability reflects the integrity of the frontal lobes.

Motor and visuomotor

The development of motor functions is a remarkable process. In a matter of months, the crudely coordinated movements of the neonate are transformed into elegant and precise movements. Posture improves, coordination becomes more precise, and the infant begins to reach for and grasp objects. A review of motor development is beyond the scope of this chapter and only a cursory glance is presented here. Very briefly, motor development proceeds from general to specific. General movements are followed by refined actions and by subsequent integration of these movements. Motor development also progresses in cephalo–caudal and proximo–distal directions, with skilled manual movements appearing relatively late in development. Manipulatory dexterity shows greater precision with age. Skilled manual activities also become more automatic during childhood. For instance, increased speed in fine motor tasks such as repetitive and successive finger movements represent an important aspect of developmental progression (Denckla, 1973). Similarly, there is a marked increase in grip strength between the ages of 6 and 11 years. This increase is more dramatically seen in boys (3.6-fold) than in girls (2.6-fold) (Espenschade and Eckert, 1980).

In addition to improved motor coordination, strength and speed, there is a gradual decrease in extraneous movements during childhood. Extraneous motor movements are not unusual before the age of 7 when the child performs certain activities, but they become increasingly rare as the child develops. Similarly, motor impersistence, normal in younger children, constitutes an atypical feature in adolescents (Benton et al., 1983). Motor impersistence, the inability to maintain an action, is universal among 5-year-olds, decreases significantly between the ages of 5 and 7 and is relatively infrequent by age 10 (Benton et al., 1983). More complex motor behaviors such as inhibition of motor reactions are associated with executive functions and may not reach maturity until late adolescence.

Although visuospatial and visuomotor development have been covered separately in this chapter, integrative processes are equally important. A child's perceptual and motor functions can be well developed, but integration of visual perception with movements may continue to be problematic. Copying forms, for example, requires adequate interpretation of visual stimuli, execution of fine motor responses, and the integration of these processes.

Copying complex designs also engages other cognitive processes, including planning and organization of response patterns as well as shifting of attention between what is seen and what is being reproduced.

Summary and future directions

In this chapter, cognitive development has been discussed as comprising distinct functional systems that undergo a process of refinement with age. This process varies for the different cognitive functions and coincides with the maturation of intricate interactions among the various functional systems. For example, we have seen how the emergence of specific language competencies impact upon the refinement of executive functions and how these, in turn, affect the modulation of attentional capacities.

To date, the assessment of cognitive functions has been limited by the array of clinical tests available. These procedures do not tap isolated functions free from the interactive effects of other cognitive systems, and they may require skills that are beyond the child's developmental capabilities. Neuroimaging can overcome these limitations by providing an opportunity to localize the functional circuits that subserve performance on a task. By doing so, we can gain a better understanding of specific brain–behavior relationships in young children that have so far eluded us. Broadening the knowledge base of normal development from a neural perspective can also facilitate an understanding of aberrant development and consequent cognitive disorders.

Recent studies have already challenged traditional concepts of developmental trajectories. In some instances, they have shown that certain cognitive functions are present earlier than previously purported. For example, studies of infants (Casey and Richards, 1991) have shown that a rudimentary ability to sustain attention may be present far earlier than traditionally thought on the basis of clinical measures. At the same time, other studies have shown that cognitive functions may continue to undergo refinement and changes well into the adult years. The ceilings for maturation of various cognitive functions have been identified to be around the ages of 10 to 12 years, but this may simply reflect the limitations of neuropsychologic tests, which may not capture refinement at more advanced ages. Indeed, neuroimaging studies have shown that the brain continues to undergo striking reorganization even in adulthood (Courtney and Ungerleider, 1997). Therefore, functional neuroimaging holds great promise for mapping the brain maturational changes underlying neuropsychologic development in children and adolescents.

References

Allport, A. and Funnell, E. (1981). Components of the mental lexicon. *Philos. Trans. R. Soc. Lond.*, **295**, 397–410.

Alvarez, P., Zola-Morgan, S. and Squire, L. R. (1994). The animal model of human amnesia: long-term memory impaired and short-term memory intact. *Proc. Natl. Acad. Sci. USA*, **91**, 5637–41.

Aslin, R. N., Alberts, J. R. and Petersen, M. R. (eds.) (1981). *The Development of Perception: Psychophysiological Perspectives.* New York: Academic Press.

Bachevalier, J. (1990). Ontogenetic development of habit and memory formation in primates. In *Development and Neural Basis of Higher Cognitive Functions*, ed. A. Diamond, pp. 457–84. New York: New York Academy of Sciences Press.

Bachevalier, J. and Mishkin, M. (1984). An early and a late developing system for learning and retention in infant monkeys. *Behav. Neurosci.*, **98**, 770–8.

Baddeley, A. D. (1992). Working memory. *Science*, **255**, 556–9.

Baillargeon, R. (1995). Physical reasoning in infancy. In *The Cognitive Neurosciences*, ed. M. S. Gazzaniga, pp. 181–204. Cambridge, MA: MIT Press.

Barkley, R. A., Grodzinsky, G. M. and DuPaul, G. J. (1992). Frontal lobe functions in attention deficit disorder with and without hyperactivity: a review and research report. *J. Abnormal Child Psychol.*, **20**, 163–88.

Bates, E. A. (1992). Language development. *Curr. Opin. Neurobiol.*, **2**, 180–5.

Bates, E. A., Dale, P. S. and Thal, D. (1994). Individual differences and their implications for theories of language development. In *Handbook of Child Language*, eds. P. Fletcher and B. MacWhinney, pp. 96–151. Oxford: Blackwell.

Bauer, P. J. (1997). Development of memory in early childhood. In *The Development of Memory in Childhood*, ed. N. Cowan, pp. 83–111. Hove, UK: Psychology Press.

Becker, M. G., Isaac, W. and Hynd, G. (1987). Neuropsychological development of non-verbal behaviors attributed to 'frontal lobe' functioning. *Dev. Neuropsychol.*, **3**, 275–98.

Benton, A. L., de S. Hamsher, K., Varney, N. R. and Spreen, O. (1983). *Contribution to Neuropsychological Assessment.* New York: Oxford University Press.

Brown, R. (1973). *A First Language: The early stages.* Cambridge, MA: Harvard University Press.

Bushnell, I. W. (1982). Discrimination of faces by young infants. *J. Exp. Child Psychol.*, **33**, 298–308.

Bushnell, I. W., Sai, F. and Mullin, J. T. (1989). Neonatal recognition of the mother's face. *Br. J. Devel. Psychol.*, **7**, 3–15.

Caron, A. J., Caron, R. F. and MacLean, D. J. (1988). Infant discrimination of naturalistic emotional expressions: the role of face and voice. *Child Dev.*, **59**, 604–16.

Casey, B. J. and Richards, J. E. (1991). A refractory period for the heart rate response in infant visual attention. *Dev. Psychobiol.*, **24**, 327–40.

Casey, B. J., Cohen, J. D., Jezzard, P., et al. (1995). Activation of pre-frontal cortex in children during a nonspatial working memory task with functional MRI. *Neuroimage*, **2**, 221–9.

Chelune, G. J. and Baer, R. L. (1986). Developmental norms for the Wisconsin Card Sorting Test. *J. Clin. Exp. Neuropsychol.*, **8**, 219–28.

Chi, J. G., Dooling, E. C. and Gilles, F. H. (1977). Left–right asymmetries of the temporal speech areas in the human fetus. *Arch. Neurol.*, **34**, 346–8.

Clark, V. P., Keil, K., Maisog, J. M., Courtney, S., Ungerleider, L. G. and Haxby, J. V. (1996). Functional magnetic resonance imaging of human visual cortex during face matching: comparison with positron emission tomography. *Neuroimage*, **4**, 1–15.

Cohen, L. B. and Salapatek, P. (eds.) (1975). *Infant Perception: From Sensation to Cognition.* New York: Academic Press.

Cohen, R. M., Semple, W. E., Gross, M., Holcomb, H. H., Dowling, M. S. and Nordahl, T. E. (1988). Functional localization of sustained attention: comparison to sensory stimulation in the absence of instruction. *Neuropsychiatr. Neuropsychol. Behav. Neurol.*, **1**, 3–20.

Cooley, E. L. and Morris, R. D. (1990). Attention in children: a neuropsychologically based model for assessment. *Dev. Neuropsychol.*, **6**, 239–74.

Courchesne, E., Akshoomoff, N. A., Townsend, J. and Saitoh, O. (1995). A model system for the study of attention and the cerebellum: infantile autism. *Electroencephalogr. Clin. Neurophysiol.*, **44** (Suppl.), 315–25.

Courtney, S. M. and Ungerleider, L. G. (1997). What fMRI has taught us about human vision. *Curr. Opin. Neurobiol.*, **7**, 554–61.

Courtney, S. M., Ungerleider, L. G., Keil, K. and Haxby, J. V. (1996). Object and spatial working memory activate separate neural systems in human cortex. *Cerebr. Cortex*, **6**, 39–49.

Courtney, S. M., Petit, L., Maisog, J. M., Ungerleider, L. G. and Haxby, J. V. (1998). An area specialized for spatial working memory in human frontal cortex. *Science*, **279**, 1347–51.

Cowan, N. (1997). The development of working memory. In *The Development of Memory in Childhood*, ed. N. Cowan, pp. 163–9. Hove, UK: Psychology Press.

Curtiss, S. (1977). *Genie: A Psychological Study of a Modern Day "Wild Child".* New York: Academic Press.

Curtiss, S. (1989). The independence and task-specificity of language. In *Interaction in Human Development*, ed. A. Bornstein and J. Bruner, pp. 105–37. Hillsdale, NJ: Erlbaum.

Damasio, A. R., Yamada, T., Damasio, H., Corbett, J. and McKee, J. (1980). Central achromatopsia: Behavioral, anatomical and physiologic aspects. *Neurology*, **30**, 1064–71.

Damasio, A. R., Damasio, H. and van Hoesen, G. W. (1982). Prosopagnosia: anatomic basis and behavioral mechanisms. *Neurology*, **32**, 331–41.

Damasio, A. R., Tranel, D. and Damasio, H. (1990). Face agnosia and the neural substrates of memory. *Annu. Rev. Neurosci.*, **13**, 89–109.

Damasio, H., Grabowski, T. J., Tranel, D., Hichwa, R. D. and Damasio, A. R. (1996). A neural basis for lexical retrieval. *Nature*, **380**, 499–505.

Davies, D. R., Jones, D. M. and Taylor, A. (1984). Selective- and sustained-attention tasks: individual and group differences. In *Varieties of Attention*, eds. R. Parasuraman and D. R. Davies, pp. 395–446. Orlando, FL: Academic Press.

de Casper, A., Lecanuet, J. P., Busnel, M. C., Granier-Defere, C. and

Maugeais, R. (1994). Fetal reactions to recurrent maternal speech. *Infant Behav. Dev.*, **17**, 159–64.

D'Esposito, M., Detre, J. A., Alsop, D. C., Shin, R. K., Atlas, S. and Grossman, M. (1995). The neural basis of the central executive system of working memory. *Nature*, **378**, 279–81.

Dempster, F. N. (1981). Memory span: sources of individual and developmental differences. *Psychol. Bull.*, **89**, 63–100.

Denckla, M. D. (1973). Development of speed in normal children. *Dev. Med. and Child Neurol.*, **15**, 635–45.

de Schonen, S. and Mathivet, E. (1990). Hemispheric asymmetry in a face discrimination task in infants. *Child Dev.*, **61**, 1192–1205.

Desimone, R. (1991). Face-selective cells in the temporal cortex of monkeys. *J. Cogn. Neurosci.*, **3**, 1–8.

Deutsch, G., Papinicolaou, A. C., Bourbon, W. T. and Eisenberg, H. M. (1987). Cerebral blood flow evidence of right frontal activation in attention demanding tasks. *Int. J. Neurosci.*, **36**, 23–8.

Diamond, A. (1990). Rate of maturation of the hippocampus and the developmental progression of children performance on the delayed non-matching to sample and visual paired comparison tasks. *Anna. N. Y. Acad. Sci.*, **608**, 394–426.

Diamond, A. (1995). Evidence of robust recognition memory early in life even when assessed by reaching behavior. *J. Exp. Child Psychol.*, **59**, 419–74.

Diamond, A. and Goldman-Rakic, P. S. (1989). Comparison of human infants and rhesus monkeys on Piaget's AB task: evidence for dependence on dorsolateral prefrontal cortex. *Exp. Brain Res.*, **74**, 24–40.

Distler, C., Bachevalier, J., Kennedy, C., Mishkin, M. and Ungerleider, L. G. (1996). Functional development of the cortico-cortical pathway for motion analysis in the macaque monkey: a ^{14}C-2-deoxyglucose study. *Cereb. Cortex*, **6**, 184–95.

Eden, G. F., van Meter, J. W., Rumsey, J. M., Maisog, J. M., Woods, R. P. and Zeffiro, T. A. (1996). Abnormal processing of visual motion in dyslexia revealed by functional brain imaging. *Nature*, **382**, 66–9.

Espenschade, A. S. and Eckert, H. M. (1980). *Motor Development*, 2nd edn. Columbus, OH: Charles E. Merrill.

Ewing-Cobbs, L., Prasad, M., Fletcher, J. M., Levin, H. S., Miner, M. E. and Eisenberg, H. M. (1998). Attention after pediatric traumatic brain injury: a multidimensional assessment. *Child Neuropsychol.*, **4**, 35–48.

Fagan, J. F. (1976). Infants' recognition of invariant features of faces. *Child Dev.*, **47**, 627–38.

Feldman, H. M., Holland, A. L., Kemp, S. S. and Janosky, J. E. (1992). Language development after unilateral brain injury. *Brain Lang.*, **42**, 89–102.

Fernandez, G., Weyerts, H., Schrader-Bölsche, M. et al. (1998). Successful verbal encoding into episodic memory engages the posterior hippocampus: a parametrically analyzed functional magnetic resonance imaging study. *J. Neurosci.*, **18**, 1841–7.

Fiducia, D. and O'Leary, D. S. (1990). Development of a behavior attributed to the frontal lobes and the relationship to other cognitive functions. *Dev. Neuropsychol.*, **6**, 85–94.

Funahashi, S., Bruce, C. J. and Goldman-Rakic, P. S. (1993). Dorsolateral prefrontal lesions and oculomotor delayed-response performance. Evidence for mnemonic "scotomas". *J. Neurosci.*, **13**, 1479–97.

Fuster, J. M. (1985). The preferred cortex: mediator of cross-temporal contingencies. *Hum. Neurobiol.*, **4**, 169–79.

Gathercole, S. E. (1998). The development of memory. *J. Child Psychol. Psychiatr. Allied Disciplines*, **39**, 3–27.

Goldman-Rakic, P. S. (1987). Development of cortical circuitry and cognitive functions. *Child Dev.*, **58**, 601–22.

Goldman-Rakic, P. S. (1988). Topography of cognition: parallel distributed networks in primate association cortex. *Annu. Rev. Neurosci.*, **11**, 137–56.

Greenberg, L. M. and Waldman, I. D. (1993). Developmental normative data on the test of variables of attention (T.O.V.A.). *J. Child Psychol. Psychiatr. Allied Disciplines*, **34**, 1019–30.

Hershey, T., Craft, S., Glauser, T. A. and Hale. (1998). Short-term and long-term memory in early temporal lobe dysfunction. *Neuropsychology*, **12**, 52–64.

Hudspeth, W. J. and Pribram, K. H. (1992). Psychophysiological indices of cerebral maturation. *Int. J. Psychophysiol.*, **12**, 19–29.

Hulme, C., Muir, C., Thomson, N. and Lawrence, A. (1984). Speech rate and the development of short-term memory span. *J. Exp. Child Psychol.*, **38**, 241–53.

Ito, Y., Teicher, M. H., Glod, C. A., Harper, D., Magnus, E. and Gelbard, H. A. (1993). Increased prevalence of electrophysiological abnormalities in children with psychological, physical and sexual abuse. *J. Neuropsychiatr. Clin. Neurosci.*, **5**, 401–8.

Jetter, W., Poser, U., Freeman, R. B. and Markowitsch, J. H. (1986). A verbal long term memory deficit in frontal lobe damaged patients. *Cortex*, **22**, 229–42.

Johnson, B. A. (1996). *Language Disorders in Children*. Albany: Delmar.

Johnson, J. and Newport, E. (1989). Critical periods effects in second language learning. The influence of maturational state on the acquisition of English as a second language. *Cognit. Psychol.*, **21**, 60–99.

Johnson, M. (1995). The development of visual attention: a cognitive neuroscience perspective. In *The Cognitive Neurosciences*, ed. M. S. Gazzaniga, pp. 737–47. Cambridge, MA: MIT Press.

Jonides, J., Smith, E. E., Koeppe, R. A., Awh, E., Minoshima, S. and Mintun, M. A. (1993). Spatial working memory in humans as revealed by PET. *Nature*, **363**, 623–5.

Kohn, B. and Dennis, M. (1971). Patterns of hemispheric specialization after hemidecortication for infantile hemiplegia. In *Hemispheric Disconnection and Cerebral Function*, ed. M. Kinsbourne and W. L. Smith, pp. 34–47. Springfield, IL: Thomas.

Kolb, B., Wilson, B. and Taylor, I. (1992). Developmental changes in the recognition and comprehension of facial expression: implications for frontal lobe function. *Brain Cognit.*, **20**, 74–84.

Korkman, M. and Häkkinen-Rihu, P. (1994). A new classification of developmental language disorders (DLD). *Brain Lang.*, **47**, 96–116.

Kreutzer, M. A., Leonard, C. and Flavell, J. H. (1975). An interview study of children's knowledge about memory. *Monogr. Soc. Res. Child Dev.*, **40**, 1–60.

Lane, D. M. and Pearson, D. A. (1982). The development of selective attention. *Merrill-Palmer Quart.*, **28**, 317–27.

Levine, D. N., Warach, J. and Farah, M. J. (1985). Two visual systems in mental imagery: dissociation of "what" and "where" in imagery disorders due to bilateral posterior cerebral lesions. *Neurology*, 35, 1010–18.

Locke, J. L. (1996). Why do infants begin to talk? Language as an unintended consequence. *J. Child Lang.*, 23, 251–68.

Locke, J. L. (1997). Towards a biological science of language development. In *The Development of Language*, ed. M. Barrett, pp. 373–95. London: UCL Press.

Loss, N., Yeates, K. O. and Enrile, B. G. (1998). Attention in children with myelomeningocele. *Child Neuropsychol.*, 4, 7–20.

Luria, A. R. (1959). The directive function of speech in development and dissolution. *Word*, 15, 341–52.

Luria, A. R. (1973). *The Working Brain*. New York: Basic Books.

Macoby, E. E. and Jacklin, C. N. (1974). *The Psychology of Sex Differences*. Stanford: Stanford University Press.

Malkova, L., Mishkin, M. and Bachevalier, J. (1995). Long-term effects of selective neonatal temporal lobe lesions on learning and memory in monkeys. *Behav. Neurosci.*, 109, 212–26.

Martin, A., Haxby, J. V., Lalonde, F. M., Wiggs, C. L. and Ungerleider, L. G. (1995). Discrete cortical regions associated with knowledge of color and knowledge of action. *Science*, 270, 102–5.

Martin, A., Wiggs, C. L., Ungerleider, L. G. and Haxby, J. V. (1996). Neural correlates of category-specific knowledge. *Nature*, 379, 649–52.

McKay, K. E., Halperin, J. M., Schwartz, S. T. and Sharma, V. (1994). Developmental analysis of three aspects of information processing: sustained attention, selective attention, and response organization. *Dev. Neuropsychol.*, 10, 121–32.

Mills, C., Morgan, M. J., Milne, A. B. and Morris, D. M. (1996). Developmental and individual differences in visual memory span. *Curr. Psychol.*, 15, 53–67.

Mills, D. L. and Neville, H. J. (1997). Electrophysiological studies of language and language impairment. *Semin. Pediatr. Neurol.*, 4, 125–34.

Mills, D. M., Coffey, S. A. and Neville, H. J. (1994). Language acquisition and cerebral specialization in 20-month-old infants. *J. Cognit. Neurosci.*, 5, 326–42.

Milner, B., Branch, C. and Rasmussen, R. (1964). Observations on cerebral dominance: In *Disorders of Language*, ed. A. V. S. de Reuck and M. O'Connor, pp. 200–14. London: Churchill.

Mirsky, A. F. (1987). Behavioral and psychophysiological markers of disordered attention. *Environ. Health Perspect.*, 74, 191–9.

Mirsky, A. F., Anthony, B. J., Duncan, C. C., Ahearn, M. B. and Kellam, S. G. (1991). Analysis of the elements of attention: a neuropsychological approach. *Neuropsychol. Rev.*, 2, 109–45.

Nelson, C. A. (1997). The neurobiological basis of early memory development. In *The Development of Memory in Childhood*, ed. N. Cowan, pp. 41–82. Hove, UK: Psychology Press.

Neville, H. J. (1995). Developmental specificity in neurocognitive development in humans. In *The Cognitive Neurosciences*, ed. M. S. Gazzaniga, pp. 219–31. Cambridge, MA: MIT Press.

Newcombe, R. and Ratcliff, G. (1989). Disorders of visuospatial analysis. In *Handbook of Neuropsychology*, eds. F. Boller and F. Grafman, pp. 333–56. Amsterdam: Elsevier.

Overman, W. H., Bachevalier, J., Turner, M. and Peuster, A. (1992). Object recognition versus object discrimination: comparison between human infants and infant monkeys. *Behav. Neurosci.*, 106, 15–29.

Overman, W. H., Bachevalier, J., Sewell, F. and Drew, J. (1993). A comparison of children's performance on two recognition memory tasks: delayed nonmatch-to-sample vs. visual paired-comparison. *Dev. Psychobiol.*, 26, 345–57.

Owens, R. E. (1992). *Language Development: An Introduction*. Columbus: Merrill.

Pardo, J. V., Fox, P. T. and Raichle, M. E. (1991). Localization of a human system for sustained attention by positron emission tomography. *Nature*, 349, 61–4.

Pascalis, O., de Schonen, S., Morton, J., Deruelle, C. and Fabre-Grenet, M. (1995). Mother's face recognition in neonates: a replication and an extension. *Infant Behav. Dev.*, 18, 79–85.

Pascual-Leone, J. A. (1970). A mathematical model for the transition rule in Piaget's developmental stages. *Acta Psychol.*, 32, 301–45.

Pascualvaca, D. M., Anthony, B. J., Arnold, L. E. et al. (1997). Attention performance in an epidemiological sample of urban children: the role of sex and verbal intelligence. *Child Neuropsychol.*, 3, 13–27.

Pascualvaca, D. M., Fantie, B. D., Papageorgiou, M. and Mirsky, A. F. (1999). Attention capacities in children with autism: is there a general deficit in shifting focus? *J. Autism Dev. Dis. Disord.*, 28, 467–78.

Passler, M., Isaac, W. and Hynd, G. W. (1985). Neuropsychological development of behavior attributed to frontal lobe functioning in children. *Dev. Neuropsychol.*, 1, 349–70.

Pea, R. (1982). What is planning development the development of? In *Children's Planning Strategies*, eds. D. Forbes and M. T. Greenberg, pp. 5–28. San Francisco, CA: Jossey-Bass.

Piaget, J. (1952). *The Origins of Intelligence in Children*. New York: International University Press.

Piaget, J. (1954). *The Construction of Reality in the Child*. New York: Basic Books.

Piaget, J. (1976). *The Grasp of Consciousness*. Cambridge: Harvard University Press.

Plunkett, K. (1993). Lexical segmentation and vocabulary growth in early language acquisition. *J. Child Lang.*, 20, 43–60.

Posner, M. I. (1993). Seeing the mind. *Science*, 262, 673–74.

Posner, M. I. and Petersen, S. E. (1990). The attention system of the human brain. *Annu. Rev. Neurosci.*, 13, 25–42.

Posner, M. I., Petersen, S. E., Fox, P. T. and Raichle, M. E. (1988). Localization of cognitive operations in the human brain. *Science*, 240, 1627–31.

Pressley, M. and Schneider, W. (1997). *Introduction to Memory Development During Childhood and Adolescence*. New Jersey: Lawrence Erlbaum.

Pribram, K. H. and McGuinness, D. (1975). Arousal, activation, and effort in the control of attention. *Psychol. Rev.*, 82, 116–49.

Rabinowicz, T. (1976). Morphological features of the developing brain. In *Brain dysfunction in infantile febrile convulsions*, eds. M. A. B. Brazier and A. Coceani, pp. 1–23. New York: Raven Press.

Rapin, I. and Allen, D. A. (1988). Syndromes in developmental dysphasia and adult aphasia. In *Language, Communication, and the Brain*, ed. F. Plum. New York: Raven Press.

Rasmussen, T. and Milner, B. (1977). The role of early left-brain injury in determining lateralization of cerebral speech functions. *Ann. N. Y. Acad. Sci.*, **299**, 355–69.

Rebok, G. W., Smith, C. B., Pascualvaca, D. M., Mirsky, A. F., Anthony, B. J. and Kellam, S. G. (1997). Developmental changes in attentional performance in urban children from eight to thirteen years. *Child Neuropsychol.*, **3**, 28–46.

Reilly, J. S., Bates, E. A. and Marchman, V. A. (1998). Narrative discourse in children with early focal brain injury. *Brain Lang.*, **61**, 335–75.

Rovee-Collier, C. and Gerhardstein, P. (1997). The development of infant memory. In *The Development of Memory in Childhood*, ed. N. Cowan, pp. 5–39. Hove, UK: Psychology Press.

Schacter, D. L. and Tulving, E. (eds.) (1994). *Memory Systems.* Cambridge, MA: MIT Press.

Schneider, W. (1997). *Memory Development between Two and Twenty.* New Jersey: Lawrence Erlbaum.

Shaywitz, B. A., Shaywitz, S. E., Pugh, K. R. et al. (1995). Sex differences in the functional organization of the brain for language. *Nature*, **373**, 607–9.

Siegler, R. S. (1981). Developmental sequences within and between concepts. *Monogr. Soc. Res. Child Dev.*, **46**, (serial No. 189).

Ungerleider, L. G. and Haxby, J. V. (1994). What and where in the human brain. *Curr. Opin. Neurobiol.*, **4**, 157–65.

Ungerleider, L. G. and Mishkin, M. (1982). Two cortical visual systems. In *Analysis of Visual Behavior*, eds. D. J. Ingle, M. A. Goodale and R. J. W. Mansfield, pp. 549–86. Cambridge, MA: MIT Press.

Ungerleider, L. G., Courtney, S. M. and Haxby, J. V. (1998). A neural system for human working memory. *Proc. Natl. Acad. Sci. USA*, **95**, 883–90.

van der Kolk, B. A. and Greenberg, M. S. (1987). The psychobiology of the trauma response: hyperarousal, constriction, and addiction to the traumatic reexposure. In *Psychological Trauma*, ed. B. van der Kolk, pp. 63–87. Washington, DC: American Psychiatric Press.

Vargha-Khadem, F., Gadian, D. G., Watkins, K. E., Connelly, A., van Paesschen, W. and Mishkin, M. (1997). Differential effects of early hippocampal pathology on episodic and semantic memory. *Science*, **277**, 376–80.

Vaughn, B. E., Kopp, C. B. and Krakow, J. B. (1984). The emergence and constellation of self-control from eighteen to thirty months of age: normative trends and individual differences. *Child Dev.*, **55**, 990–1004.

Wadsworth, B. J. (1984). *Piaget's Theory of Cognitive and Affective Development*, 3rd edn. New York: Longman.

Warrington, E. K. and Shallice, T. (1984). Category specific semantic impairments. *Brain*, **107**, 829–53.

Welsh, M. C. and Pennington, B. F. (1988). Assessing frontal lobe function in children: views from developmental psychology. *Dev. Psychol.*, **4**, 199–230.

Welsh, M. C., Pennington, B. F. and Groisser, D. B. (1991). A normative-developmental study of executive function: a window of prefrontal function in children. *Dev. Neuropsychol.*, **7**, 131–49.

Western Psychological Services (1996). *Rey Auditory Verbal Learning Test.* Los Angeles, CA: Western Psychological Services.

Woods, B. T. and Teuber, H. L. (1973). Early onset of complementary specialization of cerebral hemispheres in man. *Trans. Am. Neurolog. Assoc.*, **98**, 113–17.

9

Cognitive and behavioral probes of developmental landmarks for use in functional neuroimaging

B. J. Casey, Kathleen M. Thomas, Tomihisa F. Welsh, Rona Livnat and Clayton H. Eccard

Introduction

Functional magnetic resonance imaging (fMRI) allows neuroscientists to examine the function of the human brain, especially the developing human brain, in a relatively noninvasive manner. Previous approaches were relatively indirect techniques such as scalp-recorded electroencephalography (EEG) and event-related brain potentials or brain imaging techniques that required exposure to ionizing radiation, for example positron emission tomography (PET), single photon emission computed tomography (SPECT), and X-ray computed tomography (CT). While these latter techniques may be used with pediatric patient populations when clinically warranted, the ethics of exposing children to unnecessary radiation for the advancement of science are still under debate (Casey and Cohen, 1996; Morton, 1996; Zametkin et al., 1996). With fMRI, developmental research is possible. This technique is described in detail in Chapter 3. In the current chapter age-appropriate behavioral paradigms and task designs for use with fMRI in the context of developmental studies are described.

The significance of studying functional brain changes in a developmental context becomes more apparent when we consider aspects of brain development in general (see Chapter 7). The brain continues to develop after birth and well into childhood. Huttenlocher (1990, 1997) has demonstrated that pruning and reorganization of some cortical regions are relatively protracted. While synaptic density reaches adult levels by approximately 5 months in the visual cortex, prefrontal cortex still shows a 10% greater synaptic density at 7 years than in adulthood. Similarly, PET studies of glucose metabolism suggest that maturation of local metabolic rates in prefrontal cortex closely parallel the time course of this overproduction and subsequent pruning of synapses (Chugani et al., 1987). A logical

conclusion from these findings is that cognitive processes such as memory and language, which rely heavily on the prefrontal, temporal, and association cortices, may function in a physiologically different manner in children than in adults. Whether this difference is qualitative or quantitative is yet to be determined.

To date, little is known regarding the neural bases of cognition in normally developing children, and the neural correlates of developmental disorders are even less well understood. Certain developmental disorders (e.g., attention-deficit hyperactivity disorder and obsessive-compulsive disorder) have shown abnormal brain metabolism in adult brain imaging studies (Swedo et al., 1989; Zametkin et al. 1990). Despite the significance of these findings, the study of childhood-onset disorders in adulthood, long after the appearance of the clinical symptoms, provides relatively limited information about the progression of the disorder with development. Noninvasive fMRI techniques provide a means of addressing the developmental physiologic course of a disorder in vivo. As a first step, the patterns detected by this technology for normal development must be established.

Paradigms for use in fMRI studies of children

There are few published studies using fMRI in children, although the number of studies reported at scientific meetings is increasing substantially. An important consideration in taking on this challenge is the development of appropriate cognitive and behavioral probes for children. Table 9.1 summarizes reported studies to date by type of behavioral paradigm; eight of these studies have been published to date, but many have been summarized previously (Thomas and Casey, 1999). Four general areas of research have been addressed. First, several neuroimaging studies

Table 9.1. Paradigms used to date in pediatric fMRI studies

| Paradigms | Study group | | | |
	Subjects	Age	Number	Citation
Sensorimotor tasks				
Passive visual stimulation	Sedated patients	6 weeks to 36 months	7	Born et al. (1996)[a]
	Unsedated normal	Adults	3	
	Sedated and unsedated patients	28 weeks' gestation to 36 months of age	30	Born et al. (1997)
	Congenital structural deformities of visual cortex	3 years	1	Hunter et al. (1998)
	Sedated	Older children	2	
	Unsedated			
	Sedated patients	4 days to 8 years	7	Joeri et al. (1996a)
	Unsedated healthy	Adults	10	
Tactile stimulation	Neurosurgery patients	22 months to 18 years	25	Kiriakopoulos et al. (1996)
	Neurosurgery patients, including children after a hemispherectomy involving the primary sensorimotor cortex	0–22 years	17 (14)	Graveline et al. (1998)
Unilateral and bilateral hand and finger movements	Patients including child with parietal tumor	8–14 years	7	Popp et al. (1996)
	Neurosurgery patients	22 months to 18 years	25	Kiriakopoulos et al. (1996)
Motor sequence task	Patients with affective disorders	9–11 years	6	Casey et al. (1997c)
	Normal volunteers	Adult	6	
Sensorimotor synchronization task	ADD boys	14 years (mean)	7	Rubia et al. (1998)
	Healthy boys	14 years (mean)	9	
Language tasks				
Verbal fluency and language task	Child with epilepsy and learning disability	9 years	1	Benson et al. (1996)[a]
Spelling and rhyming tasks	Children and adults with and without dyslexia		–	Dapretto et al. (1996)
Word generation	Complex partial epilepsy	9–17 years	7	Hertz-Pannier et al. (1995)
	Complex partial epilepsy	8–18 years	11	Hertz-Pannier et al. (1997)[a]
Phoneme deletion and discrimination	Dyslexic subjects and age-matched controls	13–19 years	20	Frost et al. (1997)[a]
Passive listening task	Sedated patient	15 months	1	Hirsch et al. (1997)
	Sedated patients	15 months	1	Hirsch et al. (1998)
		31 months	1	
		39 months	1	
Word generation and object naming	Normal volunteers	11–17 years	15	Bonello et al. (1998)
	Presurgical patients	6–16 years	20	Logan (1998)
Sentence comprehension and verb generation	Children with left hemisphere lesions	11–12 years	2	Booth et al. (1999)
	Healthy	Adults	4	
Living/nonliving word decisions	Normal volunteers	8–12 years	6	Vaidya et al. (1998)
Speech task, silent word generation, pair-judgement and naming tasks	Neurosurgery patients	22 months to 18 years	25	Kiriakopoulos et al. (1996)
	Patients with complex partial epilepsy, pre- and postsurgery	14 years (mean)	11	Hertz-Pannier et al. (1997)[a]

Table 9.1 (*cont.*)

Paradigms	Study group			
	Subjects	Age	Number	Citation
	Healthy and epileptic children and adults including presurgical epileptic patients	12–56 years	18	Kato et al. (1998)
	With and without reading disabilities	Adolescents	64	Vincent et al. (1998)
	Dyslexics	Adult	31	Pugh et al. (1998)
Spatial tasks				
Mental rotation	Children with left hemisphere lesions	11–12 years	2	Booth et al. (1999)
	Healthy	Adults	4	
Hierarchical spatial analysis of shape forms	Children, including 2 with lesions	10–15 years	7	Moses et al. (1997)
Memory and inhibition tasks				
Nonspatial working memory	Normal volunteers	9–11 years	6	Casey et al. (1995)[a]
		Adult	6	
Spatial working memory	Normal volunteers	8–10 years	6	Casey et al. (1997a)
	Normal volunteers	8–10 years	6	Orendi et al. (1997)
	Normal volunteers	8–12 years	7	Truwit et al. (1996)
	Normal volunteers	8–10 years	6	Thomas et al. (1999)[a]
Go-no-go task	Normal volunteers	7–12 years	9	Casey et al. (1997b)[a]
		Adults	9	
	Children with perinatal IVH	6–9 years	10	Casey et al. (1998b)
	Children with ADD, on and off medication		10	Vaidya et al. (1998)[a]
Go-no-go task (sinusoidal target probability)	Normal volunteers	7–11 years	9	Casey et al. (1998a)
		Adults	9	
Response selection task (incompatible SRT task)	Normal volunteers	7–11 years	10	Casey et al. (1997c)
	Normal volunteers	Adults	10	
Affect recognition tasks				
Affective face task	Normal volunteers	12–17 years	14	Baird et al. (1999)[a]
	Normal volunteers	Adults	10	

Notes:

[a]Journal article, not conference abstract.

ADD, attention deficit disorder; IVH, intraventricular hemorrhage; SRT, serial reaction time

have examined developing sensorimotor systems in infants and young children (Born et al., 1996, 1997; Joeri et al., 1996a,b; Popp et al., 1996). These studies have typically employed the use of sedation during the passive presentation of visual and auditory stimuli or required simple hand and finger movements of alert neurologic patients to map the sensorimotor cortex. Although these studies have been performed with the youngest children studied with fMRI to date, the majority of the studies used sedation and/or patient populations. In the studies using sedation, the interpretations of their data are limited because of the failure to include unsedated children or sedated adults as comparison groups. With studies using neurologic patients, the interpretations about the normal development of sensorimotor cortex based on mapping studies with neurosurgical patients is unclear. Second, a number of investigators (Hertz-Pannier et al., 1995, 1997; Benson et al., 1996; Dapretto et al., 1996; Kiriakopoulos et al., 1996; Frost et al., 1997; Hirsh et al., 1997; Logan, 1998; Vaidya et al., 1998) have begun to use fMRI to study language in children. These studies have investigated language function primarily in children with epilepsy, dyslexia, or early left hemisphere lesions, thereby limiting conclusions on the normal development of language. Nonetheless, these studies represent an important first step toward understanding the neural circuitry involved in language development. Third, the reorganization of the brain following early lateralized lesions has been a topic of much interest and the focus of at least two fMRI studies. These imaging studies were attempts to determine whether early left hemisphere lesions result in the reorganization of hemisphere-specialized functions (e.g., language) to the contralateral side. Booth et al. (1999) report preliminary 3 T fMRI data examining this question with regard to language. For the child in their sample with the largest early lesion, they observed regions of activation in the undamaged hemisphere that were homologous to the regions activated in healthy adults. These results may have implications for the plasticity of function following early brain lesions, specifically the relation between lesion size and location and subsequent cortical reorganization. Moses et al. (1997) report similar preliminary findings from a study of spatial analytic processing that showed activity in the contralateral hemisphere to that observed in normal developing children and adults. Finally, a number of neuroimaging studies have begun to address the functional development of the prefrontal cortex (Casey et al., 1995, 1997a,b,c, 1998a; Orendi et al., 1997; Truwit et al., 1996; Vaidya et al., 1998). These studies have addressed two cognitive processes that have been attributed to the prefrontal cortex: working memory and response inhibition. These studies will be described in greater detail later in this chapter.

Across the pediatric neuroimaging studies reviewed, two important issues emerged. First, in the process of developing cognitive and behavioral paradigms, it is important that the tasks be appropriate for children. Often tasks used with adults are modified or simplified for use with children. When taking this approach, investigators should ensure that the task is not too difficult or complex for children. Even simple tasks that require the subject to press more than one button can be difficult for young children because they are more likely to rely on visual input together with somatosensory feedback to position their fingers on the correct button. In the scanner environment, the child is lying down and typically cannot see her/his finger movements, which presents a problem for the child. Furthermore, when using a similar task with children and adults, task difficulty should be titrated across the different age ranges. Otherwise, differences in patterns of brain activity between groups may simply reflect differences in overall effort on the task rather than maturational changes in the behavior or the brain. Likewise, the lack of activity in certain brain regions of subjects performing poorly does not necessarily reflect the integrity of those brain regions, but rather a failure of the subject to recruit those areas. This issue is not specific to developmental research but applies to clinical research comparing patients with normal volunteers as well. Examples of how to titrate performance to a subject's individual ability include increasing task difficulty by degrading stimulus information, increasing the stimulus presentation rate, or increasing the memory load. Slowing the stimulus presentation rate or self-pacing tasks as a strategy for equating task performance between groups should be used with caution. Distinct patterns of brain activity have been observed as a function of varying stimulus presentation rate or self-pacing a task. For example, different brain regions were shown to be activated during the Stroop task (Stroop, 1935) when the stimulus presentation rate varied in a fixed-pace design (Bench et al., 1993) and similarly between subjects in a self-paced design (George et al., 1994). However, D'Esposito et al. (1997) argue that fixed-pace designs are sensitive to differences in both the duration and intensity of neural processing, whereas self-paced designs are less sensitive to differences in the duration of neural processing and more sensitive to differences in the intensity of local neural processing. For these reasons, when studying a patient or age group that is likely to show increased reaction times relative to controls, self-paced designs may be preferred.

Another concern that emerged when reviewing the current pediatric neuroimaging literature was the importance of developing appropriate comparison conditions within the behavioral paradigms. Most functional neuroimaging studies rely on subtractive methodology to identify active brain regions. Statistical subtractions are performed, comparing one condition with another. A well-recognized concern about subtractive methodology (Donders, 1969; Sergent et al., 1992) is whether it is possible to design conditions or tasks such that all of the "irrelevant" processes – those that are supposed to be subtracted out – are being performed in the same way or (in the case of neuroimaging studies) by the same anatomic structures in the control and experimental conditions. Failures to satisfy this assumption can produce misleading results. One approach to this problem is to analyze multiple subtraction pairings of conditions (e.g., Sergent, et al., 1992). For example, if a brain region shows activation in subtractions with two different control conditions (e.g., A – B and A – C), it is more likely to reflect processes related to condition A. This design can be further exploited by using a standard analysis of variance and comparing multiple conditions simultaneously (e.g., Sanders and Orrison, 1993).

Comparison conditions can be introduced by using extended periods of "on" versus "off" activations, commonly referred to as "blocked designs" or by using intermixed trial designs referred to as "event-related fMRI". Conventional blocked designs incorporate the use of experimental and control blocks that last several seconds or even minutes and have been used extensively with PET and SPECT studies of sensory and higher cortical function. Such block designs are a necessity when imaging hemodynamic responses that occur over periods of approximately 1 min but are not required for fMRI studies where activity can be observed within a few seconds. Event-related fMRI studies examine MR signal changes to brief stimulus events. For example, Savoy et al. (1995) showed that a clearly detectable signal change could be elicited with visual stimulation as brief as 34 ms in duration (see Rosen et al. (1998) for a review). These data suggest that it is possible to interpret transient changes in the MR signal analogous to electrophysiologic evoked potentials. Buckner and colleagues (Buckner et al., 1996; Dale and Buckner, 1997) were among the first to use event-related fMRI studies to demonstrate detectable changes related to single-task events. Since that time, a number of studies (Buckner et al., 1996; Konishi et al., 1997; Cohen et al., 1997; Courtney et al., 1997; Zarahn et al., 1998) have explored the use of event-related fMRI to separate sensorimotor activation temporally from cognitive-related activation (e.g., memory and inhibition). These issues, age-appropriate tasks, and appropriate task designs will be discussed within the context of a number of empirical studies.

Behavioral and cognitive paradigms of prefrontal cortical functioning

Given the prolonged physiologic development and reorganization of the frontal lobes, tasks believed to involve this region are ideal for investigating development. Two cognitive processes that have been attributed to the frontal lobe are working memory and response inhibition (Fuster, 1989). A number of normative pediatric fMRI studies have examined prefrontal cortical activity in children during working memory and response inhibition tasks (Casey et al., 1995, 1997b). In fact, the first published pediatric fMRI study examined prefrontal cortical activation in children performing a working memory task (Casey et al., 1995). One of the central themes of this chapter is the importance of examining the functional development of the frontal lobes and related circuitry. This is important for a number of reasons. First, as stated above, there is considerable development and reorganization of the frontal lobes

throughout childhood and adolescence. Second, the frontal lobes and related circuitry have been implicated in a number of developmental disorders.

One view of prefrontal function consistent with the approach that our laboratory has taken is that the prefrontal cortex supports representations of information (e.g., verbal, spatial, motor, emotional) against interference over time or from competing sources (Goldman-Rakic, 1987; Cohen and Servan-Schreiber, 1992). A number of classic developmental studies have demonstrated that these memory-related processes develop throughout childhood and adolescence (Flavell et al., 1966; Pascual-Leone, 1970; Case, 1972; Keating and Bobbitt, 1978).

In the current chapter we address the important themes of the development of age-appropriate behavioral paradigms and appropriate task designs in the context of four developmental fMRI studies. These empirical studies revolve around two central themes: maintenance of information in prefrontal cortex over time and suppression of competing responses in prefrontal cortex.

Maintenance of information in prefrontal cortex

The first published pediatric fMRI study examined prefrontal activation in children performing a working memory task (Casey et al., 1995). The purpose of this study, at the time, was to determine the feasibility of using fMRI to examine higher level cognitive processing in children. Six children between the ages of 9 and 11 years were scanned with fMRI while performing a working memory task used previously in adults (Cohen et al., 1994). The study included two task conditions: a memory condition and a comparison/control condition. The memory condition required children to observe sequences of letters and to respond whenever the current letter was the same as the letter occurring two trials back ("2-back memory task"). In the comparison condition, subjects monitored similar sequences of letters for any occurrence of a single, prespecified letter. Both the memory and comparison conditions required subjects to monitor sequences of letters presented visually one at a time, encode each letter, evaluate its identity, and respond to a target by pressing a button. The conditions differed in that the memory task required the subject to keep in mind both the identity and the order of the two previous letters, continuously updating this mental record over time. These latter cognitive operations are central to the concept of working memory (Baddeley, 1986) and consistent with our view of prefrontal involvement in the representation of information over time and against interference from competing sources.

Echo-planar images were acquired on a 1.5 T gradient

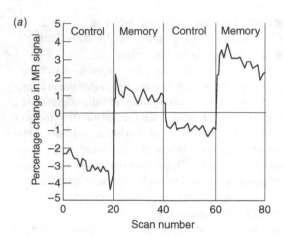 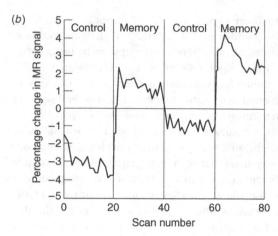

Fig. 9.1. Change in MR signal intensity as a function of the experimental manipulation (two-back memory task) for (*a*) the inferior frontal gyrus; (*b*) the middle frontal gyrus.

echo scanner using 5 inch(15 cm) surface coils while the children performed the memory and comparison conditions. Eight 5 mm coronal slices covering the frontal poles were acquired. Images were registered to a reference image to correct for movement using a modified version of Woods et al. (1992) three-dimensional automated image registration (AIR) algorithm. Movement did not correlate with the experimental manipulation but rather appeared to increase as a function of time on task and was minimal. The average movement across the entire study was less than 0.5 mm with 0.34 mm of movement in the x direction, and 0.47 mm in the y direction. Areas of significant activation were identified by performing pixel-wise t-tests comparing the memory and comparison conditions using a split-halves method, as follows. The first and second half of the data were analyzed separately and areas with significant values (e.g., 3.56, $p < 0.001$, one-tailed) in both comparisons were accepted as reliable regions of activity (the split-halves statistic approximates the p value of $< 0.001^2 = 0.000001$).

The results demonstrated reliable activity in the middle and inferior frontal gyri in five of the six children (Fig. 9.1). The graph depicts the change in MR signal intensity as a function of scans across time. The increases in activity nicely map onto the experimental manipulation. These results replicate an earlier fMRI study with adults showing inferior and middle frontal gyri activity using the same paradigm (Cohen et al., 1994) and a more recent event-related fMRI study of working memory (Cohen et al., 1997) showing dorsolateral activation during active maintenance of stimulus information. Table 9.2 illustrates the distribution of activity across frontal gyri for children and adults taken from the Casey et al. (1995) and Cohen et al. (1994) studies, respectively. Taken together, these two

Table 9.2. Distribution of prefrontal cortical activity in two fMRI studies defined by the number of active particles as a function of gyri

Frontal gyri	Number of active particles	
	Adults	Children
Superior frontal	4	3
Middle frontal	32	27
Inferior frontal	48	46
Anterior cingulate	4	9
Orbitofrontal	9	10

Sources: Adult data from the study of Cohen et al. (1994) and child data from that of Casey et al. (1995).

initial studies suggest a similar distribution of prefrontal cortical activity in children and adults during performance of a working memory task. However, the percentage change in signal observed for the children was on average two to three times that observed for the adults in the Cohen et al. (1994) study. Based on the behavioral data, the children had more difficulty with the task. On average, children performed at 70 to 75% accuracy in the Casey et al. (1995) study while adults performed at or above 90% accuracy in the Cohen et al. (1994) experiment. This study demonstrates the importance of collecting behavioral responses in the scanner but also raises concerns with regard to the interpretation of our findings given the behavioral differences. Are the differences maturational or strategic in nature or both?

A study that may help address this question is one by Braver et al. (1997) that examined prefrontal cortical activity as a function of increasing memory load in adults. They

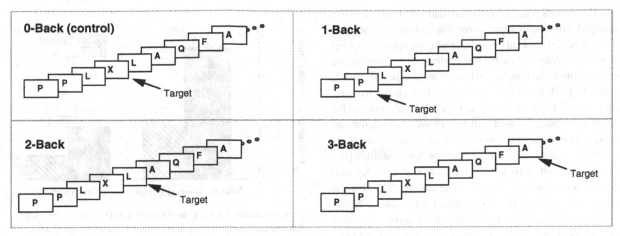

Fig. 9.2. Depiction of the *n*-back task. For the 0-back control condition, the target is the letter X. For the three memory load conditions, the target is any repeat of a letter presented one, two, or three trials back.

performed the same type of memory task but varied the memory load from 0 to 3, as demonstrated in Fig. 9.2. The subject monitored a sequential display of single letters and responded only when the current letter was the same as the letter *n* trials before it (e.g., if n = 2, then A–F–A or G–B–G, but not A–F–G–A or A–A). Subjects were practiced until they reached 90% accuracy on the highest memory load of three trials. The results revealed monotonic increases in percentage change in prefrontal cortex (Fig. 9.3). We mention this study because it is an elegant example of a task that may be especially well suited for developmental populations. This paradigm allows for the manipulation of memory load (number of trials back the subject must remember) by age and/or ability.

While our first study demonstrated the use of fMRI in pediatric populations, there was no direct comparison between children and adults since the child and adult studies were performed at different sites and with different scanning parameters. A similar working memory task was used to perform a more direct comparison of brain activation for children and adults. This study was an extension of a multisite collaboration with the primary goals of demonstrating the reproducibility of fMRI results across several sites in the USA and determining feasibility of using fMRI with pediatric populations.

Each participating group examined brain activity in both adults and children during performance of a spatial working memory task designed as an analog of the verbal working memory task. Instead of letters, colored dots were presented in one of four adjacent locations. The task was to press one of four buttons that corresponded to the location of the colored dot. In the memory condition, the task was to press the button that corresponded to the location of the

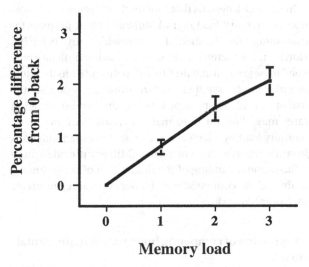

Fig. 9.3. Illustration of the monotonic increase in the MR signal intensity as a function of increasing memory load of zero, one, two, and three trials back for the dorsolateral prefrontal cortex.

dot *n*-trials back. While adults can perform the task at two and three trials back, typically children between the ages of 6 and 8 years can only perform the task at 1-back while older children (9–12 years) can do the task at 2-back. The number of trials back the subject had to remember was determined by individual ability. In the comparison or motor condition, the task was to press the button that corresponded to the location of the dot in the current trial (no memory load). Therefore, these conditions are identical except in the instructions to the subject and the memory demands.

As reported in Casey et al. (1998c), the results for adults were reproducible and reliable across all participating sites. The results from six children and eight adults at the Pittsburgh site demonstrated reliable activity in the right dorsolateral prefrontal cortex, right superior parietal cortex, and bilaterally in inferior parietal cortex during the memory condition relative to the motor condition (Fig. 9.4, p. 242). In part, these results suggest that spatial working memory tasks activate very similar cortical regions for school-age children and adults. However, despite an attempt to equate performance between age groups by varying memory load as a function of age, children performed less well than adults on both the memory and motor tasks. Adults performed near ceiling (99%) on the motor and memory tasks compared with the children, whose performance was significantly poorer (93% and 69%, respectively). Regional differences in activation (e.g., insular cortex and cingulate gyrus) between groups may reflect these performance differences.

In sum, task designs that inherently allow the manipulation of memory load or task difficulty yield promise for examining developmental progressions in behavior. However, the increment in memory load or difficulty may need to be gradual and fine-tuned to the individual subject in order to observe these progressions. For example, the use of degraded stimuli or varying stimulus presentation rates may allow for finer manipulations than increasing memory load by a factor of 1, 2 or 3. These manipulations in conjunction with event-related fMRI will provide a more refined understanding of the maturation of sensorimotor brain regions compared with higher cortical regions (e.g., prefrontal cortex).

Suppression of competing information in prefrontal cortex

Given the prevalence of inhibitory problems in children and related symptomatology in various developmental disorders (e.g., attention-deficit hyperactivity disorder, obsessive-compulsive disorder, Tourette's syndrome), the neural substrate of inhibitory control has received much attention. Consistent with the view put forth by Goldman-Rakic and others (Goldman-Rakic, 1987; Cohen and Servan-Schrieber, 1992), inhibitory control reflects the ability to support representations of information against interference from competing sources. Accordingly, when goals or task demands are well represented, then competing alternatives are suppressed. What prefrontal systems are involved in representing information against competing sources? Two examples of studies addressing this question are described below.

One classic paradigm for examining inhibition is the go-no-go task. At least one fMRI study using a go-no-go para-

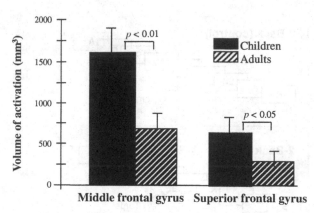

Fig. 9.5. Volume of activation of dorsolateral prefrontal cortex for children and adults during performance of a go-no-go task.

digm with healthy children has been published to date (Casey et al., 1997b). Nine children (7 to 12 years) and nine young adults (21 to 24 years) were scanned while performing a version of the go-no-go paradigm. The task required that the subject respond to all sequentially presented letters except X. Stimulus duration was 500 ms and the interstimulus interval was 1500 ms. The percentage of targets was maintained at 75% to build up a prepotent tendency to respond. Gradient-echo, echo-planar images (time to repetition (TR) 6000 ms, time to echo (TE) 40 ms, acquisition matrix 128 × 64) were acquired in eight 5 mm contiguous coronal slice locations during three task conditions: (i) inhibitory trials defined by the presence of 50% nontargets (i.e., Xs); (ii) control trials consisting of 100% targets (i.e., nonXs); and (iii) control trials consisting of 100% targets but with interstimulus intervals of 3500 ms, resulting in an equal number of motor responses as the inhibitory condition. The two comparison conditions thus controlled for stimulus parameters (number of stimuli and interstimulus interval) and response parameters (number of responses and inter-response interval), respectively.

An analysis of variance with a Bonferroni adjustment showed reliable activation in the anterior cingulate, inferior and middle frontal gyri, and orbitofrontal gyri for both the children and adults. In this investigation, the general location of activation in prefrontal cortex did not differ for children compared with adults, but the overall volume of prefrontal activation, particularly in dorsolateral prefrontal regions, was greater for children than adults (Fig. 9.5). This difference in the volume of dorsolateral prefrontal activity resulted from a lack of robust activity in these areas for the adults. Adults showed the most robust activity in more ventral regions of prefrontal cortex. Activity in the orbitofrontal and anterior cingulate cortex in children and adults correlated with behavioral performance on this response inhibition task such that greater activity in the orbitofrontal cortex was associated with the better performance, and greater activity in the anterior cingulate cortex with worse performance. It should be noted that those children with the best performance and the most orbitofrontal activity also had the most dorsolateral prefrontal activity. This observation suggests that children may be less selective in the portions of prefrontal cortex recruited in performance of the go-no-go task and/or rely on different strategies to perform the go-no-go task compared with adults. An event-related design may provide a clearer understanding of the neural mechanisms underlying response inhibition and their development. In a recent fMRI study by Konishi et al. (1997) using a go-no-go paradigm with a mixed trial design, right ventral prefrontal activation discriminated no-go from go trials in healthy adults. This finding is particularly interesting given that when we grouped our subjects (children and adults) by performance using a median split on the number of false alarms (i.e., responses to nontarget stimuli), we observed significant differences between groups only in ventral prefrontal cortex (Casey et al., 1996).

More recently we have begun to examine prefrontal activity related to the representation and suppression of information with emotional content. This work is based largely on Davidson's model of prefrontal asymmetries related to approach and avoidance behaviors (Davidson, 1994). Accordingly, appetitive or approach-related behavior is supported by the left prefrontal system, while negative or avoidance-related behaviors are presumably supported by the right prefrontal system. To examine this view of prefrontal asymmetries, we developed a task that we refer to as the "emotional n-back task". This task is a modified version of the working memory task described previously (Cohen et al., 1993; Casey et al., 1995) and includes emotionally evocative positive, negative, and neutral stimuli. The n-back task was superimposed onto backgrounds of emotionally evocative stimuli. Backgrounds of emotional and neutral content employed a subset of digitized slides from the International Affective Picture System (Lang et al., 1988) modified for use with children (McManis et al., 1995). This manipulation allowed us to assess the ability of a subject to suppress the representation of an emotional stimulus during maintenance of verbal information. The neutral background condition allows one to determine whether disruption in performance of the memory task is simply owing to distracting information in the background regardless of emotional type or whether it is a consequence of a specific type of interfering emotional response to the background. The control memory condition of 0-back (i.e., the detection of

a given letter) when superimposed on the different emotional backgrounds keeps subjects' vision fixated centrally and permits the examination of differences in patterns of brain activation as a function of emotional content irrespective of memory load (Fig. 9.6).

We had several predictions regarding the manipulations of memory and emotional content in this paradigm. First, we expected that the greatest disruption in performance of the memory condition would occur when the letters were superimposed on a withdrawal-related negative background and the least disruption would be observed when letters were superimposed on an approach-related positive background. These hypotheses were based on the assumption that the negative condition requires competing frontal systems (approach and withdrawal) to be activated simultaneously. In other words, representation and maintenance of verbal information (e.g., letters) is thought to be predominantly subserved by the left prefrontal cortex (Smith et al., 1996) or approach frontal system (Davidson, 1994) while representation of negative information is presumably subserved by the right prefrontal cortex or withdrawal/avoidant system. Therefore, when negative-related stimuli (e.g., a pointed gun, a wounded soldier, or a snarling dog) are presented, there is a conflict in the representation of behavioral goals. The negative-related stimuli are represented as an event to avoid whereas the letters are represented as events that are important to maintain (i.e., approach). For this reason, it was assumed that the negative stimulus information would be more disruptive because it required the representation of competing behavioral systems. When positive or approach-related stimuli are presented in conjunction with the task, the representation of behavioral goals are consistent so the subject's performance may even be primed or facilitated since a congruent behavioral system is activated.

Our behavioral data confirmed our hypothesis of worse memory performance during the presentation of negative information (81%) compared with performance during the presentation of positive (87%) and neutral information (84%), although these values did not reach significance for the small number of subjects (n = 10, p < 0.11).

The results from our initial imaging studies using this paradigm were promising with regard to our hypothesis of laterality of activity. For the first three subjects scanned during this task, all showed predominantly right prefrontal activity during the presentation of the negative backgrounds and predominantly left prefrontal activity during the presentation of the positive backgrounds. Figure 9.7 illustrates the pattern of activity for the two adult subjects. Similarly, the third subject, an 8-year-old child, showed a 3:1 ratio in right-to-left prefrontal activity during the presentation of

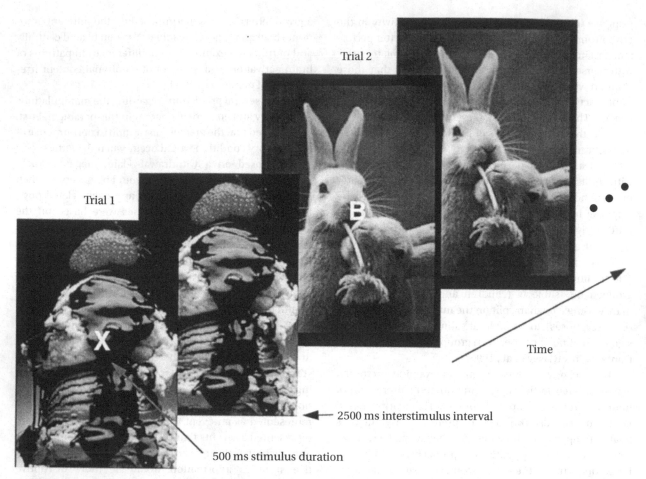

Fig. 9.6. Depiction of stimulus parameters for the emotional *n*-back task.

negative information and a 1:3 ratio in right-to-left prefrontal activity during the presentation of the negative backgrounds. However, the next three subjects scanned, either activated the hemispheres equally or showed the reverse pattern. Therefore, while the representation of emotional information is in part served by the prefrontal cortex in both children and adults, the laterality of this representation is less straightforward. Given this variability in pattern of activation across subjects, we have since moved to the presentation of face stimuli rather than pictures from the International Affective Picture System. Face stimuli allow for the control of picture complexity, size, familiarity, etc. across all conditions (e.g., positive, negative, and neutral).

Conclusions

In this chapter, a variety of paradigms have been described for use with developmental populations. These tasks, while limited primarily to the domain of prefrontal functioning, are quite broad with respect to the type of information processed (e.g., verbal, spatial, response, emotional). Across all four empirical studies described, similar locations of prefrontal activity were observed for school-aged children and adults. However, differences were observed in the magnitude of the patterns of activity, both in volume (Casey et al., 1997 a,b,c) and in percentage change (Cohen et al., 1994; Casey et al., 1995). These differences may be attributed to overall task difficulty. Even when attempts were made to titrate task difficulty across ages, young children performed less well than the adults. Many of these differences may be associated with differences in how quickly subjects mastered the tasks. Adults became more proficient in task performance (e.g., the spatial working memory task) as a function of time on-task in the scanner. The children, by comparison, did not increase their performance with time on task in the scanner. Some of the difficulty for children performing tasks in the scanner may

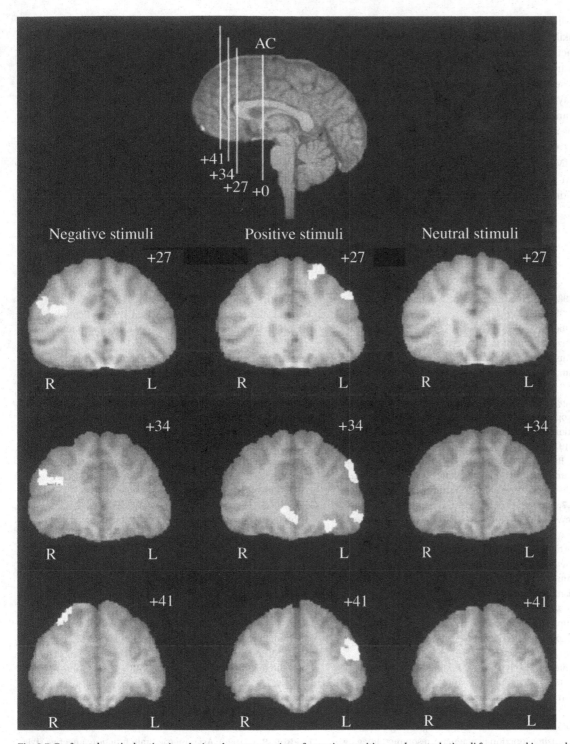

Fig. 9.7. Prefrontal cortical activation during the presentation of negative, positive, and neutral stimuli for coronal images located at +27, +34, and +41 mm anterior to the anterior commissure (AC) averaged across two young adults.

be the need to lie down, thus blocking a view of their hands. Their motor skills are not as sophisticated and so even with extended practice the children still benefit from visual feedback on where their hands and fingers are with respect to the response-recording device. Alternatively, children and adults may differ in the speed of acquiring new skills. These issues and others raised in the current chapter are just a few to be addressed as we continue to use functional neuroimaging with children. It is clear that innovative methods like fMRI will transform our current understanding of human brain development and hold significant implications for the study of developmental disorders.

References

Baddeley, A. (1986). Modularity, mass-action, and memory. *Q. J. Exp. Psychol.*, **38**, 527–33.

Baird, A. A., Gruber, S. A., Fein, D. A. et al. (1999). Functional magnetic resonance imaging of facial affect recognition in children and adolescents. *J. Am. Acad. Child Adolesc. Psychiatry*, **38**, 195–9.

Bench, C. J., Frith, C. D., Grasby, P. M. et al. (1993). Investigations of the functional anatomy of attention using the Stroop test. *Neuropsychologia*, **31**, 907–22.

Benson, R. R., Logan, W. J., Cosgrove, G. R. et al. (1996). Functional MRI localization of language in a 9-year-old child. *Can. J. Neurol. Sci.*, **23**, 213–19.

Bonello, C. M., Baird, A. A., Renshaw, P. F., Yurgelun-Todd, D. A. (1998). Structural and functional magnetic resonance imaging in the temporal lobes of children during word production. *Neuroimage*, **7**, S3.

Booth, J. R., MacWhinney, B., Thulborn, K. R. et al. (1999). Functional reorganization of activation patterns in children with brain lesions: whole brain fMRI imaging during three different cognitive tasks. *Progr. Neuropsychopharmacol. Biol. Psychiatry*, **23**, 669–82.

Born, P., Rostrup, E., Leth, H., Peitersen, B., Lou, H. C. (1996). Change of visually induced cortical activation patterns during development. *Lancet*, **347**, 543.

Born, P., Rostrup, E., Larsson, H. B. W., Leth, H., Miranda, M., Peitersen, B., Lou, H. C. (1997). Infant visual cortex function evaluated by fMRI. *Neuroimage*, **5**, S171.

Braver, T. S., Cohen, J. D., Nystrom, L. E., Jonides, J., Smith, E. E., Noll, D. C. (1997). A parametric study of prefrontal cortex involvement in human working memory. *Neuroimage*, **5**, 49–62.

Buckner, R. L., Bandettini, P. A., O'Craven, K. M. et al. (1996). Detection of cortical activation during averaged single trials of a cognitive task using functional magnetic resonance imaging. *Proc. Natl. Acad. Sci. USA*, **93**, 14878–83.

Case, R. (1972). Validation of a neo-Piagetian capacity construct. *J. Exp. Child. Psychol.*, **14**, 287–302.

Casey, B. J. and Cohen, J. D. (1996). In reply to: C. T. Morton, Is research in normal and ill children involving radiation exposure ethical? *Arch. Gen. Psychiatry*, **53**, 1059–60.

Casey, B. J., Cohen, J. D., Jezzard P. et al. (1995). Activation of prefrontal cortex in children during a nonspatial working memory task with functional MRI. *Neuroimage*, **2**, 221–9.

Casey, B. J., Trainor, R., Orendi, J., Schubert, A. (1996). A functional magnetic resonance imaging (fMRI) study of ventral prefrontal cortex mediation of response inhibition. *Proc. Soc. Neurosci.*, **22**, 1107.

Casey, B. J., Cohen, J. D., King, S. W. et al. (1997a). A developmental functional MRI study of cortical activation during a spatial working memory task. *Neuroimage*, **23**, S69.

Casey, B. J., Trainor R. J., Orendi, J. L., et al. (1997b). A developmental functional MRI study of prefrontal activation during performance of a go-no-go task. *J. Cogn. Neurosci.*, **9**, 835–47.

Casey, B. J., Badgaiyan, R. D., Franzen, P. L. et al. (1997c). Prefrontal activation as a function of response set. *Neuroimage*, **5**, S602.

Casey, B. J., Thomas, K. M., Welsh, T. F. et al. (1998a). A developmental fMRI study of prefrontal organization. *Neuroimage*, **7**, S512.

Casey, B. J., Thomas K. M., Welsh, T. F., Eccard, C. H., Livnat, R. and Pierri, J. N. (1998b). An fMRI study of response inhibition in children with striatal lesions. *Neuroimage*, **7**, S515.

Casey, B. J., Cohen, J. D., Davidson, R. et al. (1998c). Reproducibility of fMRI results across four institutions using a working memory task. *Neuroimage*, **8**, 249–61.

Chugani H. T., Phelps, M. E. and Mazziotta, J. C. (1987). Positron emission tomography study of human brain functional development. *Ann. Neurol.*, **22**, 487–97.

Cohen, J. D. and Servan-Schreiber, D. (1992). Context, cortex and dopamine: a connectionist approach to behavior and biology in schizophrenia. *Psychol. Rev.*, **99**, 47.

Cohen, J. D., Forman S. D., Casey, B. J. and Noll, D. C. (1993). Spiral-scan imaging of dorsolateral prefrontal cortex during a working memory task. In *Proceedings of the 12th Annual Meeting of the Society of Magnetic Resonance in Medicine*, p. 1413.

Cohen, J. D., Forman, S. D., Braver, T. S., Casey, B. J., Servan-Schreiber, D. and Noll, D. C. (1994). Activation of prefrontal cortex in a nonspatial working memory task with functional MRI. *Hum. Brain Map.*, **1**, 293–304.

Cohen, J. D., Perlstein, W. M., Braver, T. S. et al. (1997). Temporal dynamics of brain activation during a working memory task. *Nature*, **386**, 604–7.

Courtney, S. M., Ungerleider, L. G., Keil, K. and Haxby, J. V. (1997). Transient and sustained activity in a distributed neural system for human working memory. *Nature*, **386**, 608–11.

Dale, A. M. and Buckner, R. L. (1997). Selective arranging of rapidly presented individual trials using fMRI. *Hum. Brain Map.*, **5**, 329–40.

Dapretto, M., Bookheimer, S. Y., Cohen, M. S. and Wang, J. (1996). fMRI of language in dyslexic and normally developing children. *Neuroimage*, **3**, S434.

Davidson, R. J. (1994). Asymmetric brain function, affective style, and psychopathology: the role of early experience and plasticity. *Dev. Psychopathol.*, **6**, 741–58.

D'Esposito, M., Zarahn, E., Aguirre, G. K., Shin, R. K., Auerbach, P. and Detre, J. A. (1997). The effect of pacing of experimental stimuli on observed functional MRI activity. *Neuroimage*, **6**, 113–21.

Donders, F. C. (1969). On the speed of mental processes. In W. G. Koster (Original work published in 1868; reproduced in Attention and performance II (ed. and trans. W. G. Koster). *Acta Psychol.*, **30**, 412–31.

Flavell, J. H., Beach, D. R. and Chinsky, J. M. (1966). Spontaneous verbal rehearsal in a memory task as a function of age. *Child Dev.*, **37**, 283–99.

Frost, J. A., Binder, J. R., Newby, R. F. et al. (1997). Phonological processing in developmental dyslexia: an fMRI study. *Neuroimage*, **5**, S568.

Fuster, J. M. (1989). *The Prefrontal Cortex: Anatomy, Physiology and Neuropsychology of the Frontal Lobe*. New York: Raven Press.

George, M. S., Ketter, T. A., Parekh, P. I. et al. (1994). Regional brain activity when selecting a response despite interference. *Hum. Brain Map.*, **1**, 194–209.

Goldman-Rakic, P. S. (1987). Circuitry of primate prefrontal cortex and regulation of behavior by representational memory. In *Handbook of Physiology. The Nervous System. Higher Functions of the Brain*. Sect. 1, Vol. V, Part 1. eds. V. B. Mountcastle, F. Plum and S. R. Geiger, pp. 373–417. Bethesda, MD: American Physiological Society.

Graveline, C., Mikulis, D. J., Crawley, A. P. and Hwang, P. A. (1998). Regionalization evidence of sensorimotor plasticity pre and post hemispherectomy in children with epilepsy. fMRI and clinical studies. *Neuroimage*, **7**, S483.

Hertz-Pannier, L., Gaillard, W. D., Mott, S. et al. (1995). Functional MRI of language tasks: frontal diffuse activation patterns in children. *Hum. Brain Map.*, **1**(Suppl.), 231.

Hertz-Pannier, L., Gaillard, W. D., Mott, S. H. et al. (1997). Noninvasive assessment of language dominance in children and adolescents with functional MRI: a preliminary study. *Neurology*, **48**, 1003–12.

Hirsch, J., Kim, K. H. S., Souweidane, M. M. et al. (1997). fMRI reveals a developing language system in a 15-month old sedated infant. *Soc. Neurosci. Abst.*, **23**, 2227.

Hirsch, J., Kim, K. H. S., Souweidane, M. M. et al. (1998). Passive listening during fMRI reveals an extensive receptive language system in young and sedated children. *Neuroimage*, **7**, S513.

Hunter, J. V., Liu, G. T., Fletcher, D. W., Brown, L. W. and Haselgrove, J. C. (1998). Functional MRI in children with congenital structural abnormalities of the visual cortex. *Neuroimage*, **7**, S312.

Huttenlocher, P. R. (1990). Morphometric study of human cerebral cortex development. *Neuropsychologia*, **28**, 517–27.

Huttenlocher, P. R. (1997). Regional differences in synaptogenesis in human cerebral cortex. *J. Comp. Neurol.*, **387**, 167–78.

Joeri, P., Loenneker, T., Huisman, D., Ekatodramis, D., Rumpel, H. and Martin, E. (1996a). fMRI of the visual cortex in infants and children. *Neuroimage*, **3**, S279.

Joeri, P., Huisman, T., Loenneker, T., Ekatodramis, D., Rumpel, H. and Martin, E. (1996b). Reproducibility of fMRI and effects of pentobarbital sedation of cortical activation during visual stimulation. *Neuroimage*, **3**, S280.

Kato, T., Ohyu, J., Fukumizu, M. and Takashima, S. (1998). Assessment of language lateralization using functional near-infrared spectroscopy in bedside. *Neuroimage*, **7**, S207.

Keating, D. P. and Bobbitt, B. L. (1978). Individual and developmental differences in cognitive processing components of mental ability. *Child Dev.*, **49**, 155–67.

Kiriakopoulos, E. T., Wood, M. L. and Mikulis, D. J. (1996). fMRI in pediatric neurosurgical patients. *Neuroimage*, **3**, S490.

Konishi, S., Nakajima, K., Uchida, I., Sekihara, K. and Miyashita, Y. (1997). Temporally resolved no-go dominant brain activity in the prefrontal cortex revealed by functional magnetic resonance imaging. *Neuroimage*, **5**, S120.

Lang, P. J., Öhman, A. and Vaitl, D. (1988). *The International Affective Picture System*. [photographic slides] Gainesville, FL: The Center of Research in Psychophysiology, University of Florida.

Logan, W. J. (1998). Functional MRI language localization in children. In *Abstracts of the Society of Cognitive Neuroscience*, p. 127.

McManis, M. H., Bradley, M. M., Cuthbert, B. N. and Lang, P. J. (1995). Kids have feelings too: children's physiological responses to affective pictures. *Psychophysiology*, **32**, S53.

Morton, C. T. (1996). Is research in normal and ill children involving radiation exposure ethical? [Letter to the Editor] *Arch. Gen. Psychiatry*, **53**, 1059.

Moses, P., Martinez, A., Roe, K. et al. (1997). Functional MR imaging of children's spatial analysis of hierarchical forms. *Neuroimage*, **5**, S97.

Orendi, J. L., Irwin, W., Ward, R. T. et al. (1997). A fMRI study of cortical activity in children and adults during a spatial working memory task. *Neuroimage*, **5**, S603.

Pascual-Leone, J. A. (1970). A mathematical model for transition in Piaget's developmental stages. *Acta Psychol.*, **32**, 301–45.

Popp, C. A., Trudeau, J. D., Durden, D. et al. (1996). Functional MR imaging in children. *Neuroimage*, **3**, S594.

Pugh, K. R., Shaywitz, B. A., Shaywitz, S. E., et al. (1998). The relation between cortical activation profiles and regularity effects in reading: replications and extensions. *Neuroimage*, **7**, S216.

Rosen, B. R., Buckner, R. I. and Dale, A. M. (1998). Event-related functional MRI: past, present, and future. *Proc. Natl. Acad. Sci. USA*, **95**, 773–80.

Rubia, K., Overmeyer, S., Taylor, E. et al. (1998). Mesial hypofrontality in attention deficit hyperactivity disorder (ADHD) during motor timing: a study using fMRI. *Neuroimage*, **7**, S114.

Sanders, J. A. and Orrison, W. W. (1993). ANOVA tests for identification of FMRI activation. In *Proceedings of the 12th Annual Meeting of the Society of Magnetic Resonance in Medicine*, New York, p. 1376.

Savoy, R. L., Bandettini, P. A., O'Craven, K. M. et al. (1995). In *Proceedings of the 3rd Scientific Meeting of the Society for Magnetic Resonance*, vol. 2, p. 45.

Sergent, J., Zuck, E., Levesque, M. and MacDonald, B. (1992). Positron emission tomography study of letter and object processing: empirical findings and methodological considerations. *Cerebr. Cortex*, **80**, 68–80.

Smith, E. E., Jonides, J. and Koeppe, R. A. (1996). Dissociating verbal and spatial working memory using PET. *Cerebr. Cortex*, **6**, 11–20.

Swedo, S. E., Pietrini, P., Leonard, H. L. et al. (1989). Cerebral glucose metabolism in childhood-onset obsessive-compulsive disorder. *Arch. Gen. Psychiatry*, **49**, 690–4.

Thomas, K. M. and Casey, B. J. (1999). Functional MRI in pediatrics. In *Medical Radiology: Functional Magnetic Resonance Imaging*, eds. P. Bandettini and C. Moonen. New York: Springer-Verlag, in press.

Thomas, K. M., King, S. W., Franzen, P. L. et al. (1999). A developmental fMRI study of spatial working memory. *Neuroimage*, 10, 327–38.

Truwit, C. L., Le, T. H., Hu, X. et al. (1996). Functional MR imaging of working memory task activation in children: preliminary findings. *Neuroimage*, 3, S564.

Vaidya, C. J., Gabrieli, J. D. E., Rypma, B. et al. (1997). fMRI of frontal lobe function in children with attention deficit disorder on and off Ritalin. *Soc. Neurosci. Abst.*, 23, 859.

Vaidya, C. J., Austin, C., Kirkorian, C. et al. (1998). Selective effects of methylphenidate in attention deficit hyperactivity disorder: a functional magnetic resonance study. *Proc. Natl. Acad. Sci.* USA 95, 14494–9.

Vincent, D. J., Bryant, A. E., Worthington, W. C. et al. (1998). When can fMRI replace Wada for language localization? Two years experience. *Neuroimage*, 7, S147.

Woods, R. P., Cherry, S. R. and Mazziotta, J. C. (1992). Rapid automated algorithm for aligning and reslicing PET images. *J. Comp. Assist. Tomogr.*, 16, 620–33.

Zametkin, A. J., Nordahl, T. E., Gross, M. et al. (1990). Cerebral glucose metabolism in adults with hyperactivity of childhood onset. *N. Engl. J. Med.*, 323, 1361–6.

Zametkin, A. J., Schwartz, D. J., Ernst, M. and Cohen, R. M. (1996). In reply to: C. T. Morton, Is Research in normal and ill children involving radiation exposure ethical? *Arch. Gen. Psychiatry*, 53, 1060–1.

Zarahn, E., Aguirre, G. and D'Esposito, M. (1998). A trial-based experimental design for fMRI. *Neuroimage*, 6, 122–38.

Part 4

Psychiatric disorders

Functional neuroimaging methods have only recently begun to be applied to the study of child psychiatric disorders. As with many other areas of psychiatric research, scientific hypotheses tested in studies of children frequently have their roots, in part, in knowledge obtained in research on adults. The chapters in this section critically review the application of functional neuroimaging to the study of child psychiatric disorders, drawing on the background of adult neuroimaging research and our knowledge of childhood variations of adult-onset disorders. Theories of the neurobiology of child psychiatric disorders are discussed. Practical issues arising from imaging psychiatrically ill children, methods for addressing these issues, and related interpretative problems are explored. A wide variety of child psychiatric disorders are covered, ranging from those with early (solely childhood) onsets, such as autism, to those whose onset in childhood is rare, e.g., schizophrenia.

Chugani describes the full range of imaging studies of autism, a devastating and chronic disorder with an onset prior to age 3 years (Chapter 10). Jacobsen and Bertolino discuss their unique imaging studies of the rare form of schizophrenia with onset in childhood and the implications of their findings for developmental theories of schizophrenia (Chapter 11). Kowatch and his colleagues address childhood unipolar and bipolar depression, as well as neuroimaging paradigms developed to study the biology of mood and its disorders (Chapter 12). Rosenberg and his colleagues assess imaging research on the full spectrum of anxiety disorders, from phobias to panic and obsessive-compulsive disorder (Chapter 13) and Peterson critically evaluates the use of neuroimaging in defining the neural systems involved in Tourette's disorder (Chapter 14). Given the frequent comorbidity of child psychiatric disorders with specific developmental disorders, Wood and Flowers analyze the conceptual models underlying imaging studies of dyslexia and their relevance for the study of child psychiatric disorders (Chapter 15). Schweitzer and colleagues review the progress made in understanding the neuropathophysiology of attention-deficit hyperactivity disorder (ADHD) by means of functional neuroimaging, as well as the neurobehavioral probes worthy of use in future research on ADHD (Chapter 16) and, finally, Chowdhury and colleagues address the eating disorders of anorexia nervosa and bulimia nervosa, as well as those restricted to childhood (Chapter 17).

The reader will gain from this section knowledge of the latest research developments and pathophysiologic theories of specific child psychiatric disorders and glean from it information on the current status of brain imaging research in child psychiatry. Indeed, this comprehensive review covers practical challenges involved in scanning children, design issues arising from the heterogeneity of child psychiatry disorders, interpretative dilemmae posed by various imaging paradigms, advances in neurobiological knowledge gained through the use of neuroimaging, and the future potential of functional neuroimaging in child psychiatry. The identification of neural circuits underlying symptoms and vulnerabilities and of their specific disruptions in different disorders emerge as a goal worthy of pursuit given its implications for diagnosis and treatment.

10

Autism

Diane C. Chugani

Definition of autism

Autism is a developmental disorder defined by the presence of a triad of communication, social, and stereotypical behavioral characteristics with onset before 3 years of age. Previous estimates of the incidence of autism were 2–5 cases per 10 000 individuals (for review see Wing, 1993). Recent studies show a higher incidence of autism (approximately 1 in 1000), while the three to four times predominance of the disorder in males has remained constant (Bryson, 1996). Autism was first described by Kanner in 1943 in his landmark paper describing a group of children who showed language abnormalities, impairment in social interactions, and restricted interests and preoccupations. One year later, Asperger (1944) described a similar group of children. The term Asperger's syndrome is now used to describe high-functioning individuals with autistic features but relatively normal communication and cognitive skills (Gillberg, 1989; Volkmar et al., 1996).

Underlying the spectrum of autistic behaviors are undoubtedly multiple etiologies, only a small fraction of which have been so far identified. The reliance upon this behavioral definition is a consequence of a failure to identify biological markers for the majority of individuals with autistic behavior and is a source of difficulty in the design and reproducibility of functional imaging studies. The inexact nature of the diagnosis of autism and other pervasive developmental disorders is also the source of numerous practical problems for the families of autistic children in identifying appropriate medical, behavioral, and educational interventions necessary to promote optimal development of their children. In spite of the fact that there are various etiologies for autistic behavior, the possibility of a *common neurochemical mechanistic feature*, shared by multiple causes of autism, cannot be excluded. It is upon this premise that functional neuroimaging of groups of autistic subjects of unknown etiology are compared with nonautistic control groups in search of common biological substrates to define and understand autism better.

Clinical versus research criteria for the diagnosis of autism

The accurate diagnosis of autism and careful description of associated features of the subjects are essential criteria for obtaining meaningful functional imaging data and to allow comparison of results among groups (Table 10.1). The majority of the functional imaging studies published to date have utilized clinical diagnoses of autism based upon DSM-III-R (American Psychiatric Association, 1987), DSM-IV (American Psychiatric Association, 1994) or ICD-10 (World Health Organization, 1987) criteria. Various additional psychologic instruments, such as the Childhood Autism Rating Scales (CARS; Schopler et al., 1980), have also been employed. There has been a growing concensus in recent years that the Autism Diagnostic Interview-Revised (ADI-R; Lord et al., 1994) and the Autism Diagnostic Observation Scale (ADOS; Lord et al., 1989) developed by Lord and colleagues represent the gold standard for the diagnosis for autism for research purposes. These are excellent instruments with extensive validation for high-functioning autistic subjects over the age of 4 years (Lord et al., 1997). However, these instruments are overinclusive for lower-functioning individuals, who make up 75% of individuals with a clinical diagnosis of autism. The Prelinguistic Autism Diagnostic Observation Schedule (PL-DOS; DiLavore et al., 1995) was developed by the same group to address younger (less than the age of 6 years) children who have not yet developed phrase-level speech. The problem of stability of diagnosis of young autistic children (Lord and Schopler, 1989) can also be addressed by re-evaluating the children after several years (Lord, 1995).

Table 10.1. Summary of functional imaging studies in autistic subjects

Study	Subjects		Controls		Diagnostic criteria	Testing condition	Results
	Number (sex)	Age (years)	Number (sex)	Age (years)			
PET studies with 2-[18F]fluoro-2-deoxyglucose							
Rumsey et al. (1985)[a]	10M	18–36	15M	20–37	DSM-III	Rest, eyes covered	Global hypermetabolism
Horwitz et al. (1988)[a]	14M	18–39	14M	20–37	DSM-III	Rest, eyes covered	Fewer positive correlations between frontal and parietal cortices; lower correlations between thalamus, caudate nucleus, lenticular nucleui, and insula with frontal and parietal regions
de Volder et al. (1987)	11M, 7F	2–18	Normal Unilateral brain pathology Adults, 15	7, 14, 15 9, 12, 12.5 Mean 22	DSM-III	Sedated	Normal global and regional glucose metabolism
Herold et al. (1988)	16M	21–25	6M, 2F	22–53	DSM-III-R, ICD-10	Listening to music, eyes closed	No significant differences between groups in cerebral blood flow, oxygen consumption, and glucose metabolism
Heh et al. (1989)[a]	5M, 2F	19–36	7M, 1F	20–35	DSM-III, ICDS	Continuous performance task	No significant difference in cerebellar glucose metabolism
Buchsbaum et al. (1992)[a]	5M, 2F	19–36	13M	Mean 24	DSM-III, ICDS	Continuous performance task	Decreased glucose metabolism in right thalamus and putamen; less asymmetry in autistic group
Siegel et al. (1992)[a]	12M, 4F	17–38	19M, 7F	Mean 27	ICDS, DSM-III-R	Continuous performance task	Normal global glucose metabolism, decreased glucose metabolism in left putamen, increased metabolism in calcarine cortex, reversed asymmetry in rectal gyrus
Siegel et al. (1995)[a]	12M, 3F	17–38	13M, 7F	19–39	ICDS, DSM-III-R	Continuous performance task	Negative correlation of medial frontal glucose metabolism with attentional performance
Schifter et al. (1994)	9M, 4F	4–11	No control group	–	DSM-III-R	Rest, eyes open	Regional abnormalities of glucose metabolism by visual assessment in 4 of 13
Chugani et al. (1996)	14	10 months to 5 years	10	8 months to 5 years	DSM-IV	Rest	Bitemporal glucose hypometabolism, particularly in superior temporal gyrus and hippocampus
Haznedar et al. (1997)	5M, 2F	17–47	5M, 2F	20–47	ADI	Verbal learning test	Hypometabolism in right anterior cingulate gyrus
SPECT blood flow studies with ^{133}Xe							
Sherman et al. (1984)	7M	18–33	–	–	DSM-III	Rest, eyes open	Global hypoperfusion

Study	Subjects	Age	Comparison group	Comparison age	Diagnostic criteria	Condition	Findings
Zilbovicius et al. (1992)	12M, 9F	5–11	Nonautistic with slight language disorder: 10M, 4F	Mean 8.7	DSM-III-R	Sedated (controls not sedated)	No global or regional flow abnormalities in autistic group compared with language disorder group
Chiron et al. (1995)	14M, 4F	4–17	5M, 5F	4–16	ADI, ICD-10, DSM-III-R	Sedated (17 of 18); controls 2 of 10 sedated	Autistic group showed higher blood flow in right hemisphere compared to left; controls showed the reverse
Zilbovicius et al. (1995)	3M, 2F	3–4 and later at 6–7	5 / 7	3–4 / 6–12	DSM-III-R	Sedated	Longitudinal study showed bilateral hypoperfusion in frontal lobes at 3–4 years, but not at 6–7 years
SPECT blood flow studies with ^{99m}TC- HMPAO							
Ozbayrak et al. (1991)	1M, 22 y				Asperger's	Rest	Left occipital hypoperfusion
George et al. (1992)	4M	22–34	2M, 2F	25–32	DSM-III-R	Rest, eyes open	Global hypoperfusion; focally decreased flow in right lateral temporal and bilateral frontal lobes
McKelvey et al. (1995)	2M, 1F	14–17			Asperger's DSM-III-R, (Wing, 1981; Gillberg, 1989)	Rest, eyes open	Right hypoperfusion (diffuse in 1, temporal in 1, frontal and occcipital in 1; hypoperfusion of vermis and right cerebellum in 2
Mountz et al. (1995)	5M, 1F	9–21	5M, 2F	6–20	DSM-III-R, ASIEP, ABC	Rest, eyes open	Bilateral temporal and parietal hypoperfusion, with left hemisphere showing greater regional cerebral blood flow abnormalities than right
Functional mapping with $H_2\,^{15}O$ PET							
Happé et al. (1996)	5M	20–27	6M	24–65	Clinical diagnosis of Asperger's	"Theory of mind" task	Activation in Brodmann area 9 in autistic group and activation in area 8 in control group
Müller et al. (1999)[a]	4M, 1F	18–31	5M	23–30	DSM-IV, GARS	Language and auditory tasks	Reversed hemispheric dominance during verbal auditory stimulation; reduced cerebellar activation during nonverbal auditory perception
Müller et al. (1998)[a]	4M	18–31	5M	23–30	DSM-IV, GARS	Language and auditory tasks	Reduced activation in right dentate nucleus and left frontal area 46 and thalamus during expressive language task
Neurotransmitter function measured with PET							
Ernst et al. (1997)	8M, 6F	mean 13	7M, 3F	Mean 14	DSM-III-R	Sedated	[^{18}F]DOPA uptake reduced in medial prefrontal cortex
Chugani et al. (1997)	7M, 1F	4–11	4M, 1F	8–14	DSM IV, CARS, GARS	Sedated	Asymmetric α-[^{11}C]-methyltryptophan uptake in frontal cortex, thalamus and dentate nucleus of cerebellum

Table 10.1 (*cont.*)

Study	Subjects			Controls			Diagnostic criteria	Testing condition	Results
	Number (sex)	Age (years)		Number (sex)	Age (years)				
Chugani et al. (1999a)	Healthy autistic: 24M, 6F	2–15		Healthy siblings: 6M, 2F	2–14		ADI-R, DSM IV, CARS, GARS	Sedated; controls sedated	Whole-brain serotonin synthesis capacity showed different changes with age in autistic compared with nonautistic group
				Epilepsy: 9M, 7F	3 months to 14 years			Sedated (4/8)	
Metabolites measured with MRS									
Minshew et al. (1993)	11M	12–36		11M	12–36		DSM-III-R, ADI, ADOS	Not sedated	Decreased levels of phosphocreatine and esterified ends in dorsal prefrontal cortex
Hashimoto et al. (1997)	20M, 8F	2–12		16M, 9F	2–13		DSM-III-R	Sedated	No differences in *N*-acetylaspartate/choline ratio in voxel located in right parietal region; no lactate detected
Chugani et al. (1999b)	8M, 1F	3–12		Healthy siblings: 4M, 1F	8–14		DSM-IV, CARS, GARS	Sedated; controls not sedated	Lower *N*-acetylaspartate in cerebellum; lactate detected in frontal lobe in 1 autistic boy

Notes:

ABC, autistic behavior checklist; ASIEP, autistic symptom inventory educational profile; ADI, Autism Diagnostic Index; ADOS, Autism Diagnostic Observation Scale; CARS, Childhood Autism Rating Scale; DSM-III-R, *Diagnostic and Statistical Manual*, 3rd edn revised (American Psychiatric Association, 1987); GARS, Gilliam Autism Rating Scale; ICD-10, 10th draft of the *International Classification of Diseases* (World Health Organization, 1987); ICDS, interview for childhood disorders and schizophrenia.

[a] Indicates overlap in subject samples (different analyses of the same or overlapping sample).

Heterogeneity in etiology of autism

Autism may be a component feature of a number of disorders, such as fragile X syndrome (Payton et al., 1989; Piven et al., 1991), phenylketonuria (Friedman, 1969), tuberous sclerosis complex (Smalley et al., 1992), Rett syndrome (Hagberg, 1985), prenatal viral infection (reviewed in Lotspeich and Ciaranello, 1993), and several other conditions (reviewed in Ciaranello and Ciaranello, 1995). Manifestations vary according to developmental level and chronologic age, and there is marked heterogeneity of the behavioral characteristics among autistic individuals. Several studies have attempted to identify subtypes of symptom clusters. Classification systems of autistic subtypes generally are related to degree of severity and include intellectual functioning (Volkmar et al., 1987), social interactions (Wing and Gould, 1979), and behaviorally homogeneous subtypes (Sevin et al., 1995).

Functional imaging studies in autistic subjects

It is difficult to scan young children and to obtain appropriate age-matched controls; consequently, the majority of functional imaging studies of autistic subjects have employed adolescents and adults. In addition, the studies have overwhelmingly concentrated upon high-functioning autistic subjects since these individuals are able to cooperate with imaging procedures. This approach seriously limits our ability to probe the developmental changes in autistic brain. Moreover, adults with autism have an extended history of having undergone a variety of behavioral, sensory, dietary, herbal, and pharmacologic interventions. The effects of these treatments upon brain function are unknown and difficult to control. In addition, there may be chronic changes that occur with age in this disorder. Evidence for degenerative changes in cerebellar nuclei were suggested in older subjects in the neuropathology studies of Bauman and Kemper (1994).

Focal and global brain alterations in glucose metabolism

Increased global brain glucose metabolism in autism

The measurement of 2-deoxy-2-[^{18}F]-fluoro-D-glucose (FDG) with positron emission tomography (PET) has proved to be a valuable tool in identifying regional and global abnormalities in many neurologic conditions. The impact of this method toward the understanding of autism has been less clear. In the first study of glucose metabolism in autism, Rumsey et al. (1985) reported diffusely increased glucose metabolism by approximately 20% in a group of 10 autistic men compared with 15 healthy gender- and age-matched control subjects. The finding of globally increased glucose metabolism has not been replicated in subsequent FDG PET studies reported (de Volder et al., 1987; Herold et al., 1988; Siegel et al., 1992). However, there were methodologic differences in the subsequent studies; therefore, differences in global glucose metabolism in autistic adults cannot be discounted. For example, Herold et al. (1988) compared six male autistic subjects with six healthy males and two females. Similarly, Siegel et al. (1992) compared autistic adults (12 males, four females; 17–38 years) and normal controls (19 males, seven females; mean age 27 years) mixed for gender and found no difference in global glucose metabolism. Since there are gender differences in glucose metabolism on the same order of magnitude of those Rumsey et al. reported between autistic and normal men (Baxter et al., 1987), the inclusion of females in control groups could mask a true global increase in glucose metabolism. De Volder et al. (1987) reported no differences in global glucose metabolism in 18 autistic children (11 male, seven female aged 2–18 years) compared with a control group that comprised children (three normal children aged 7, 14, and 15 years; three children with unilateral pathology aged 9, 12, and 12.5 years) with various brain pathologies, as well as 15 adults (mean age 22 years). Few conclusions can be drawn from the de Volder study since glucose metabolism shows marked changes with age (Chugani et al., 1987; see below).

Regional brain glucose metabolism alterations in autism and related disorders

Horwitz et al. (1988) added four male autistic subjects to the series reported by Rumsey et al. (1985) and showed that the global brain glucose metabolic rate (CMRGlu) was 12% higher in the autistic group, a difference that was statistically significant. In addition, Horwitz et al. (1988) performed a correlation analysis that showed significantly fewer positive correlations between frontal and parietal cortices, with the most notable discrepancy found between the left and right inferior frontal regions. Furthermore, the thalamus and basal ganglia also showed less correlation with frontal and parietal cortices in the autistic group compared with the controls.

Focal abnormalities of glucose metabolism have been reported in a number of other studies in which global brain glucose metabolism was not addressed. Heh et al. (1989) studied glucose metabolism in the cerebellum based upon neuropathologic data showing fewer Purkinje and granule cells in the cerebellum (Bauman and Kemper, 1985; Ritvo et al., 1986) and vermal cerebellar hypoplasia measured by magnetic resonance imaging (MRI) (Courchesne et al., 1988). However, Heh et al. (1989), showed no significant difference in mean CMRGlu for cerebellar hemispheres or vermal lobes VI and VII in autistic subjects (five males and two females; 19–36 years) compared with control subjects (seven males, one female; 20–35 years). Schifter et al. (1994) studied a heterogeneous group of children (nine males, four females; 4–11 years) with autistic behavior coexisting with seizures, mental retardation, and neurologic abnormalities. Visual analysis of the FDG PET scans revealed that 5 of the 13 subjects had focal abnormalities located in different brain regions for each patient. Regions showing hypometabolism included right cerebellum and left temporal/parietal/occipital cortices; right parietal cortex, bilateral thalamus and left occipital cortex; right parietal and left temporal/parietal cortices; right parietal/occipital and left occipital cortices; and bilateral temporal lobes.

Buchsbaum et al. (1992) applied a visual continuous performance task, which was associated with greater right than left hemisphere metabolism in autistic subjects (five males, two females; 19–36 years) than in their normal control subjects (13 males; mean age 24 years). Siegel et al. (1992) studied 16 high-functioning autistic adults (12 males, four females; 17–38 years) and 26 normal controls (19 males, seven females; mean age 27 years) and reported that autistic subjects had a left greater than right anterior rectal gyrus asymmetry, as opposed to the normal right greater than left asymmetry in that region. The autistic group also showed low glucose metabolism in the left posterior putamen and high glucose metabolism in the right posterior calcarine cortex. The same group (Siegel et al., 1995) studied glucose metabolism in 15 adults with a history of infantile autism (12 males, three females; aged 17–38 years, mean 24 years; 15 of 16 subjects previously reported by Siegel et al. (1992)) and reported that autistic subjects showed abnormal thalamic glucose metabolism; correlations of task performance with pallidal metabolism suggested subcortical dysfunction during the attentional task in autism. Recently, Haznedar et al. (1997) performed MRI and glucose PET scans on seven high-functioning autistic patients (five males, two females; mean age 24.3 years) and seven sex- and age-matched normal adults. Right anterior cingulate was significantly smaller in relative volume and was metabolically less active in the autistic patients than in the normal subjects. However, these data were not corrected for partial volume effects (Hoffman et al., 1979), and the apparent decrease in glucose metabolism may be secondary to the reported volume decrease.

An association of autism in children with a history of infantile spasms has been long recognized (Riikonen and Amnell, 1981). Chugani et al. (1996b) reported that 18 children (seven males, 11 females; 10 months to 5 years of age) from a total of 110 children with a history of infantile spasms showed bilateral temporal lobe glucose hypometabolism on PET, with normal MRI scans. Long-term outcome data was obtained for 14 of the 18 children; 10 of the 14 children met DSM-IV criteria for autism. All 14 children had continued seizures and mental retardation. Two temporal lobe regions, superior temporal gyrus and hippocampus, showed significant hypometabolism compared with that in age-matched controls. These observations are relevant not only because histologic studies of brain tissue at autopsy from autistic subjects show abnormalities in hippocampus (Bauman and Kemper, 1994) but also because recent studies using volumetric MRI in patients with fragile X syndrome have found abnormalities in hippocampus (increased volume) and superior temporal gyrus (decreased volume) (Reiss and Freund, 1994).

Focal and global brain alterations in resting blood flow

A number of studies of autistic subjects measuring cerebral blood flow with single photon emission computed tomography (SPECT) can be found in the literature and report a variety of global and focal abnormalities. George et al. (1992) reported global hypoperfusion in the resting state in adult autistic men with seizures (four males; 22–34 years) compared with control subjects (two males, two females; 25–32 years). George et al. (1992) further observed pronounced hypoperfusion in the frontotemporal cortices, whereas McKelvey et al. (1995) localized most consistent hypoperfusion to the vermis and the right cerebellar hemisphere in three adolescent autistic subjects (two males, one female; 14–17 years). Mountz et al. (1995) also reported hypoperfusion in autistic subjects (five males, one female; 9–21 years) compared with the control group (five males, two females; 6–20 years) but localized it primarily to the left temporoparietal and the right anterior temporal region.

Zilbovicius et al. (1992) measured regional cerebral blood flow with SPECT and xenon-133 in 21 children (12 boys, nine girls; 5–11 years, mean 7.4) with autism according to DSM-III-R criteria. Five cortical brain areas including frontal, temporal, and sensory association cortices were examined. The group with autism showed no cortical regional abnormalities compared with an age-matched group of 14 nonautistic children with slight-to-moderate language disorders. While the autistic subjects in this study were sedated, the control group (those with language disorders) were not. Zilbovicius et al. (1995) also studied cerebral blood flow in preschool autistic children in a longitudinal study. Five autistic children (three males, two females) were studied at the age of 3–4 years and 3 years later and were compared with two age-matched comparison groups of nonautistic children (five children ages 3–4 years, and seven aged 6–12 years) with normal development. These investigators reported frontal hypoperfusion in the autistic children at ages 3–4 years, but not at the ages of 6–7; they concluded that these results indicated a delayed frontal maturation in childhood autism. Chiron et al. (1995) compared blood flow in 18 autistic children (14 males, four females; 4–14 years) with 10 control subjects (five males, five females; 4–16 years) and found blood flow was greater in the left hemisphere in control subjects but greater in the right in autistic patients. All but one of the autistic subjects was sedated with intrarectal pentobarbital (pentobarbitone) and, in some cases, intramuscular droperidol, while only two of the ten control subjects were sedated. While barbiturates have been reported to decrease cerebral metabolism in adults (Theodore et al., 1986), Chiron et al. (1992) used ^{133}Xe SPECT to show that cerebral blood flow changes induced by pentobarbital were not statistically significant in children.

Blood flow changes during the performance of tasks

In a functional mapping study using $H_2^{15}O$ PET, Happé et al. (1996) applied a "theory of mind" task that required attributing mental states to the characters of a narrative. The statistical parametric mapping analysis showed that the Asperger's group (five males, 20–27 years) showed a slightly different location of activation in inferior prefrontal cortex (Brodmann area 9 instead of 8) compared with the normal control group (six males; 24–65 years).

Müller et al. (1999) studied auditory perception and receptive and expressive language in five high-functioning autistic adults (four males, one female; 18–31 years) compared with five normal men (23–30 years) using an $H_2^{15}O$ activation paradigm. Scans were performed at rest, and while subjects listened to tones, listened to short sentences, repeated short sentences, and generated sentences. Analyses of peak activations revealed reduced or reversed dominance for language perception in temporal cortex, and reduced activation of auditory cortex and the cerebellum during acoustic stimulation in the autistic group. Data from the four autistic men and five normal men were reanalysed (Müller et al., 1998) to examine three predetermined regions of interest – dentate nucleus of the cerebellum, thalamus, and Brodmann area 46 – based upon serotonin (5-HT) synthesis studies showing abnormalities in these three regions in autistic boys (Chugani et al., 1997). The results of this study showed that the dorso-lateral prefrontal cortex (area 46) and thalamus in the left hemisphere and the right dentate nucleus showed less activation in the autistic men than in the control group for sentence generation. In contrast, with sentence repetition, increases in blood flow were significantly larger in left frontal cortex and right dentate nucleus in the autistic subjects than the control group. These data suggest that left frontal cortex, left thalamus, and right dentate nucleus showed atypical functional changes with language tasks in high-functioning autistic men.

Because of the small numbers of subjects, all of the functional mapping studies so far performed should be considered pilot studies. However, this is a promising approach for high-functioning subjects who are able to cooperate with the performance demands of this type of study.

Differences in brain metabolites

Magnetic resonance spectroscopy (MRS) is a technique that can be used to detect and quantify biochemicals in living brain using MRI technology. Phosphorus-31-MRS can be used to assess energy metabolism by quantifying steady-state levels of phosphocreatine, adenosine triphosphate (ATP), adenosine diphosphate (ADP), and inorganic orthophosphate (for reviews see Chapter 1 and Bottomley and Hardy, 1989). In addition, phospholipid metabolism can be assessed by the measurement of phosphomonoesters and phosphodiesters. Proton MRS (^{1}H MRS; for review see Moore, 1998) can be used to measure the levels of a number of brain metabolites, including N-acetylaspartate (NAA), which is a putative neuronal marker that is an indicator of neuronal function/viability, lactate, which is a metabolite of energy metabolism not normally detectable in brain but detected in some pathologic states (Jenkins et al., 1993), choline, creatine, and several neurotransmitters such as gamma-aminobutyric acid (GABA) and glutamate.

Using ^{31}P MRS to measure phosphorus metabolites in dorsal prefrontal cortex in 11 male autistic adolescents and adults (aged 12–36 years) and 11 age-, gender-, and socioeconomic-matched normal controls, Minshew et al. (1993) found decreased levels of phosphomonoesters, increased levels of phosphodiesters, and decreased levels of ATP. This group suggested that their results indicated decreased synthesis and/or increased breakdown of membrane phospholipids, with increased ATP consumption, perhaps related to abnormal dendritic integrity.

Hashimoto et al. (1997) performed ^{1}H MRS in occipital cortex in 28 patients with autism (20 males, eight females; 2–12 years), 28 age-matched patients with mental retardation (22 males, six females; 2–13 years) and 25 age-matched healthy children (16 males, nine females; 2–13 years). Peaks for NAA, choline, and creatine, but not lactate, were observed in each group. The NAA/choline ratio was lower in patients with mental retardation than in patients with autism and in controls, but there were no differences in the NAA/choline ratios between patients with autism and controls. Chugani et al. (1999b) performed ^{1}H MRS in nine autistic children (eight males, one female; 3–12 years, mean age 5.7 years) and five of their healthy nonautistic siblings (four males, one female; 6–14 years, mean age 9 years). Voxels of 8 ml were sampled in frontal cortex, temporal cortex, and cerebellum, and concentrations of NAA and lactate were measured using the cerebral water signal as an internal standard. Lactate, which is not normally detected in brain, was detected in one of the nine autistic children studied, but in none of the controls. These data are consistent with altered energy metabolism in some autistic children. NAA was significantly lower in cerebellum in the autistic group than in the sibling group, while mean NAA values for frontal lobe and temporal lobe did not significantly differ between the groups. The finding of lower NAA in cerebellum in the autistic group is consistent with neuropathology reports of decreased numbers of Purkinje cells and granule cells in cerebellar cortex from autistic individuals (Bauman and Kemper, 1994).

These promising preliminary MRS findings in autistic subjects suggest that further studies of autism with this technique are warranted. Studies reported so far used the single-voxel method and were limited in the regions of the brain that could be sampled in a scanning session. Newer spectroscopic imaging techniques now allow sampling of the entire brain within an acceptable scan acquisition time.

Focal and global brain alterations in neurotransmission

Studies investigating alterations in neurotransmitters, hormones, and their metabolites in the blood, cerebrospinal fluid (CSF), and urine of autistic patients have been numerous and have provided some evidence for the potential involvement of several neurotransmitters in autism (for review see Anderson, 1994). Furthermore, given there is evidence for dysfunction in widely distributed brain regions in autism (Minshew et al., 1997), the monoamine neurotransmitters are interesting candidates because of their widespread modulatory role in the brain. To this purpose, functional imaging has been used to examine the role for two monoamine transmitters, dopamine (Ernst et al., 1997) and serotonin (Chugani et al., 1997, 1999a), in autism.

Functional imaging evidence for dopaminergic dysfunction in autism

Ernst et al. (1997) studied 14 medication-free autistic children (eight males, six females; mean age 13 years) and 10 healthy children (seven males, three females; mean age 14 years) with ^{18}F fluorodopa (F-DOPA) using PET. F-DOPA is a precursor of dopamine, which is taken up, metabolized, and stored by dopaminergic terminals. Ernst and colleagues calculated the ratios of F-DOPA activity (as the region of interest/occipital cortex) measured between 90 and 120 min following tracer administration. Regions sampled were the caudate, putamen, midbrain, and lateral and medial anterior prefrontal regions (all regions rich in dopaminergic terminals), and occipital cortex (a region poor in dopaminergic terminals). They reported a 39% reduction of the F-DOPA ratio in the anterior medial prefrontal cortex/occipital cortex in the autistic group. There were no significant differences in any of the other regions measured. These authors suggested that decreased dopaminergic function in prefrontal cortex may contribute to the cognitive impairment seen in autism.

Functional imaging evidence for serotonergic dysfunction in autism

Although there is evidence for the potential involvement of several neurotransmitters in autism, the most consistent abnormal neurotransmitter findings involve serotonin. Schain and Freedman (1961) first reported increased blood serotonin in approximately one third of autistic patients. Studies of the serotonin metabolite 5-hydroxyindoleacetic acid (5-HIAA) in CSF have failed to demonstrate consistent abnormalities of central serotonergic tone (for review see Anderson et al., 1994). Pharmacologic treatments that decrease serotonergic neurotransmission, such as tryptophan depletion, have been reported to result in an exacerbation of symptoms in autistic subjects (McDougle et al., 1996a). Conversely, administration of serotonin-reuptake inhibitors appear to result in improvement of compulsive symptoms, repetitive movements, and social difficulties in autistic adults (Cook et al., 1992; Gordon et al., 1993; McDougle et al., 1996b). Finally, a role for serotonin in autism is also suggested by the recent finding that an inefficiently transcribed serotonin transporter polymorphism showed significantly higher incidence in autistic individuals and their families (Cook et al., 1997).

Chugani et al. (1997, 1999b) have applied α-[^{11}C]-methyl-L-tryptophan ([^{11}C]-AMT) as a PET tracer in autistic subjects. It is used to follow serotonin synthesis with PET (Diksic et al., 1990) because it is an analog of tryptophan, the precursor for serotonin synthesis. Following the administration of labeled or unlabeled AMT in rats, the synthesis of α-methylserotonin (AM-5HT) in brain has been demonstrated by high-pressure liquid chromatography (Missala and Sourkes, 1988; Diksic et al., 1990).

Synthesis of AM-5HT in brain has been localized to serotonergic neurons and nerve terminals by combined autoradiography detecting [3H]-AM-5HT and tryptophan hydroxylase immunocytochemistry at the electron microscopic level (Cohen et al., 1995). Furthermore, [3H]-AM-5HT present in nerve terminals could be released by K+-induced depolarization, suggesting that this tracer is stored within the releasable pool of serotonin (Cohen et al., 1995). Since AM-5HT, unlike serotonin, is not a substrate for the degradative enzyme monoamine oxidase (Missala and Sourkes, 1988), accumulation of AM-5HT occurs in serotonergic terminals. In addition, AMT, unlike tryptophan, is not incorporated into protein in significant amounts (Madras and Sourkes, 1965; Diksic et al., 1990). These properties of AMT make it a suitable tracer substance for the measurement with PET of serotonin synthesis in vivo in humans (Muzik et al., 1997; Nishizawa et al., 1997; Chugani et al., 1998).

Chugani et al. (1997) used [11C]-AMT and PET to study healthy, seizure-free children with autism (seven males, one female; 4–11 years) and their healthy nonautistic siblings (four males, one female; 8–14 years). All of the autistic subjects and three of the five siblings were sedated with pentobarbital or midazolam. Gross asymmetries of [11C]-AMT standard uptake value (SUV) in frontal cortex, thalamus, and cerebellum were visualized in seven autistic boys, but not in the one autistic girl studied nor in four of five siblings (Fig. 10.1a). Decreased [11C]-AMT accumulation was seen in the left frontal cortex and thalamus in five of seven autistic boys. This was accompanied by an elevated [11C]-AMT accumulation on the right in the cerebellum. The region of increased tracer accumulation in the cerebellum appeared to be in the dentate nucleus, based upon coregistration with the MRI. In the remaining two autistic boys, [11C]-AMT accumulation was decreased in the right frontal cortex and thalamus and elevated in the left dentate nucleus. No asymmetries were seen in the frontal cortex or thalamus of the sibling group (Fig. 10.1d); however, one sibling showed an increased [11C]-AMT accumulation in the right dentate nucleus. Interestingly, this boy had a history of calendar calculation and he ritualistically lined up his toys, behaviors commonly seen in autistic children. The overall difference in asymmetry scores between the autistic boys and their siblings was found to be statistically significant, and regional asymmetry scores in the frontal cortex and thalamus were also found to differ significantly. The specificity of these abnormalities in serotonin synthesis was apparent when comparing the

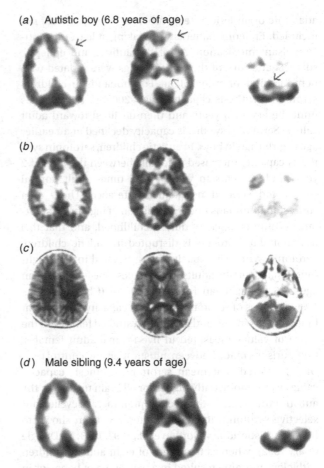

(a) Autistic boy (6.8 years of age)

(b)

(c)

(d) Male sibling (9.4 years of age)

Fig. 10.1. Scans for an autistic boy aged 6.8 years (a–c) and his brother aged 9.4 years (d). (a), (d) PET images using α-[11C]-methyltryptophan ([11C]-AMT); (b) PET image using [18F]-fluorodeoxyglucose scan; (c) MRI scan. Arrows denote decreased [11C]-AMT accumulation in left frontal cortex and left thalamus and increased [11C]-AMT accumulation in right dentate nucleus in the autistic child (left side of image is the right side of the brain).

[11C]-AMT scans with the FDG PET and MRI scans, both of which were normal by visual examination in the children studied (Fig. 10.1b,c).

Chugani et al. (1999a) also measured whole-brain serotonin synthesis capacity in autistic and nonautistic children at different ages using [11C]-AMT and PET. Global brain values for serotonin synthesis capacity were obtained for 30 healthy, seizure-free autistic children (24 males, six females; 2–15 years), eight of their healthy nonautistic siblings (six males, two females; 2–14 years), and 16 epileptic children without autism (nine males, seven females; 3 months to 13 years). Children in the epilepsy group had medically intractable seizures, but patients with multiple anatomic brain lesions (e.g., tuberous sclerosis) were not included. Epileptic patients were taking at least one anticonvulsant medication. All of the autistic and epileptic subjects and four of the eight siblings were sedated with pentobarbital or midazolam. For nonautistic children, serotonin synthesis capacity was >200% of adult values until the age of 5 years and then declined toward adult values. Serotonin synthesis capacity declined at an earlier age in girls than in boys. In autistic children, serotonin synthesis capacity increased gradually between the ages of 2 years and 15 years to values 1–1.5 times adult normal values and showed no gender difference. These data suggest that humans undergo a period of high brain serotonin synthesis capacity during childhood, and that this developmental process is disrupted in autistic children. Serotonin synthesis capacity was estimated in four high-functioning autistic adults (three males, one female; mean age 26.5 years; mean full scale IQ 70) (Chugani et al., 1996a). Values of serotonin synthesis capacity for different brain regions in one autistic woman studied fell within the range of values measured in five normal adult females. Comparisons made between autistic men and control men ($n=5$) showed that mean serotonin synthesis capacity values were significantly higher for all brain regions in the autistic group. Interestingly, clomipramine, a tricyclic nonselective serotonin-uptake inhibitor, has been shown to benefit autistic adults (Gordon et al., 1992, 1993; McDougle et al., 1992), whereas treatment of eight autistic children with clomipramine resulted in a worsening of behavior in six of the children, including increased tantrums, irritability, aggression, self-injury, and crying spells (Sanchez et al., 1996). Differences in response of autistic symptoms to serotonergic drugs between autistic adults and children would be expected in light of the findings with [11C]-AMT PET that young autistic children have lower serotonin synthesis than normal children, whereas autistic men have higher serotonin synthesis than normal men.

Intriguingly, manipulations of serotonin in animals during pre- and postnatal development can reproduce some of the pathologic findings in autistic brain reported by Bauman and colleagues (Bauman and Kemper, 1985, 1994). For example, Bauman and Kemper (1985) reported reduced neuronal cell size and increased cell number in the hippocampus of autistic brains. Treatment of pregnant rats with p-chlorophenylalanine to deplete serotonin resulted in a prolongation of the period of cell division in the pups in brain regions with dense serotonergic innervation, leading to increased neuronal cell numbers in hippocampus, superior colliculus, and several thalamic nuclei (Lauder and Krebs, 1978). Bauman and Kemper (1994) reported decreased complexity and extent of dendritic

arbors in the hippocampus of autistic brains. In the animal literature, Yan et al. (1997) have reported that depletion of serotonin with p-chlorophenylalanine or 5,7-dihydroxytryptamine in neonatal rat pups resulted in large decreases in the numbers of dendritic spines in the hippocampus.

The focal decreases in [11C]-AMT that were observed in the cortex and thalamus might be interpreted in light of developmental changes in serotonin mechanisms shown in animal studies. For example, it has been demonstrated recently that the serotonin transporter is transiently expressed by glutamatergic thalamocortical afferents (Lebrand et al., 1996; Bennett-Clarke et al., 1996) during the first 2 postnatal weeks in rats (note that a serotonin transporter polymorphism that is not efficiently transcribed shows a high incidence in the autistic individuals and their families (Cook et al., 1997)). During this period, these thalamocortical neurons take up and store serotonin, although they do not synthesize serotonin. While the role of serotonin in glutamatergic neurons with cell bodies located in the sensory nuclei of the thalamus is not yet known, there is evidence that the serotonin concentration must be neither too high nor too low during this period. Depletion of serotonin delays the development of the barrel fields of the rat somatosensory cortex (Blue et al., 1991; Osterheld-Haas and Hornung, 1996) and decreases the tangential arborization of the thalamocortical axons, resulting in reduced size of the barrel fields (Bennett-Clarke et al., 1994). Conversely, increased serotonin during this critical period results in increased tangential arborization of these axons and blurring of the boundaries of the cortical barrels (Cases et al., 1995, 1996). Developmental changes in serotonergic mechanisms have also been reported in the cerebellum. The $5HT_{1A}$ receptors are transiently expressed in cerebellum during brain development. In rat pups, there is high expression of the $5HT_{1A}$ receptor in the Purkinje cell layer between postnatal days 2 and 9, but there is no detectable $5HT_{1A}$ receptor in the cerebellum of adults (Miquel et al., 1994). These data suggest an important role for serotonin in Purkinje cells of the cerebellum during brain development. Bauman and her colleagues have also reported decreased numbers of Purkinje cells in the cerebellum (Bauman and Kemper, 1985) in autistic brains. These findings are particularly interesting in light of the focal increase in [11C]-AMT demonstrated in the dentate nucleus of the cerebellum (Chugani et al., 1997), since Purkinje cells project to the dentate nucleus. In sum, the frontal cortex, thalamus, and cerebellum may be particularly sensitive to changes in serotonin synthesis during development, and the abnormalities in these regions measured with [11C]-AMT PET may stem from develop-

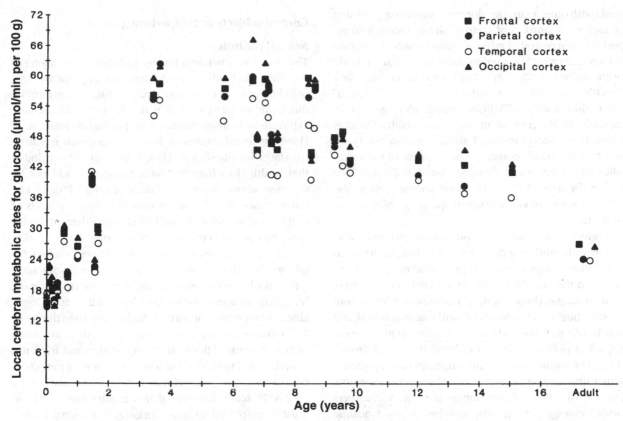

Fig. 10.2. Absolute values of local cerebral metabolic rates for glucose for cerebral cortex plotted as a function of age in 29 infants and children and seven young adults. In infants and children, points represent individual values; in adults, points are mean values from seven subjects, in which the size of the symbols equals the standard error of the mean. (Courtesy of Harry T. Chugani.)

mental alterations in serotonin synthesis. Focal alterations in [^{11}C]-AMT accumulation may represent either aberrant innervation by serotonergic terminals or altered function in anatomically normal pathways. Immunocytochemical studies in pathologic specimens are necessary in order to determine which is the case. Altered serotonergic neuromodulation of dentatothalamocortical synaptic activity could be one pathophysiologic mechanism underlying sensory dysfunction in autism.

Problems that need to be addressed in future studies of autism

Brain functional changes with development

Since autism is most commonly recognized in the second year of life, associated with regression in both social behavior and language in up to half of autistic children (Tuchman and Rapin, 1997), the study of young children soon after identification is more likely to yield important

information regarding the etiology of the disorder than the study of older autistic individuals, who are likely to have undergone various interventions. Furthermore, although autism is not a progressive disorder in the classical sense, the behavioral manifestations of autism do change with age, and, therefore, functional brain abnormalities also might change with age. Since functional imaging has demonstrated striking changes in brain glucose metabolism during the normal maturational process (Chugani et al., 1987), an evolution of brain regional values for other markers of brain function in autistic children compared with age-matched normal children may occur during development.

Quantitative analysis of local CMRGlu (lCMRGlu) shows that the brain follows a protracted glucose metabolic maturational course (Chugani et al., 1987). Neonatal lCMRGlu values, which are about 30% lower than adult rates, rapidly increase to exceed adult values by 2–3 years of age in the cerebral cortex and remain at these high levels until about 8–10 years, when lCMRGlu declines to reach adult rates by 16–18 years (Fig. 10.2). Correlation of these CMRGlu trends with other neurodevelopment events suggests that the ascending portion of rapid lCMRGlu increase corresponds to the period of rapid overproduction of synapses and nerve terminals known to occur in the human brain (Huttenlocher, 1979; 1990; Huttenlocher et al., 1982; Huttenlocher and de Courten, 1987). The "plateau" period, during which lCMRGlu exceeds adult values, corresponds to the period of increased cerebral energy demand as a result of transient exuberant connectivity relative to synaptic elimination. The segment of the metabolic maturational curve that corresponds to the lCMRGlu decline (between 10 and 16 years) corresponds to the period of selective elimination or "pruning" of excessive connectivity.

Developmental studies in nonhuman primates also demonstrate nonlinear developmental changes in neurotransmitter content and receptor binding (Goldman-Rakic and Brown, 1982; Lidow et al., 1991). For example, in the macaque, there is a steep rise in serotonin content in cortex beginning before birth and reaching a peak at 2 months of age, followed by a slow decline up to 3 years of age, when puberty occurs (Goldman-Rakic and Brown, 1982). The same group of investigators has reported a similar time course for expression of serotonin receptors (Lidow et al., 1991). These changes in serotonin markers parallel changes in synaptic number in the macaque cortex (Rakic et al., 1986; Bourgeois et al., 1994). Furthermore, these changes in synaptic number show a similar time course to that of the developmental changes in glucose metabolism in macaque and vervet monkeys (Jacobs et al., 1995).

In sum, it appears essential to include young children in functional imaging studies of autism to determine whether there are metabolic or neurochemical alterations during the process of brain development. The identification of specific neurochemical abnormalities during postnatal brain development in autism might lead to new strategies for intervention. Because of the dynamic nature of developing brain function, imaging studies in children need to take into account relatively large changes with age. While the use of age-matched control subjects will guard against drawing invalid conclusions that are artifacts of age differences between groups, this approach may decrease the sensitivity in detecting differences between groups owing to the introduction of age-generated variability. Muzik et al. (1999) have attempted to address this problem by devising a mathematical developmental function with identifiable parameters representing different stages of development, such as the CMRGlu value of the "plateau phase" and the age at which it begins to decline, that can be statistically compared among groups.

Control subjects or comparison groups

Normal controls

The most overwhelming barrier to functional imaging of disorders of childhood is obtaining an appropriate age-matched normal control group. The risks of performing functional imaging studies with PET or SPECT include exposure to ionizing radiation and sedation. Ernst et al. (1998) reviewed studies of low-level radiation exposure with large sample sizes and long follow-up and concluded that health risks from low-level radiation could not be detected above those of adverse events of daily life. Furthermore, they found no evidence that low levels of radiation were more harmful to children than to adults. Nonetheless, current recommendations for radiation dosimetry in children suggest a 10-fold lower dose limit for minors (less than 18 years of age) compared with adult doses (IRCP, 1988). Consequently, while the risks of most functional imaging studies to older children are acceptable, control studies of normal children less than the age of 6–8 years are more problematic. First, they are more difficult because of the need for cooperation and, in particular, the need to stay still in a scanner for long periods of time (for example, 30 min for an FDG scan and 90 min for a $[^{11}C]$-AMT scan). Because of this requirement, sedation must be employed for many imaging procedures, adding to the overall risk. However, several large studies indicate that this is a small risk, and that sedation of children can be done in a safe and highly efficacious manner in a hospital radiology department using a structured sedation program modeled after the guidelines of the American Academy of Pediatrics (Merola et al., 1995; Egelhoff et al., 1997). Second, very young children are not as capable of coping with the insertion of intravenous needles and the presence of a laboratory environment. Behavioral methods have been developed to address these issues for children. Acclimation techniques and strategies such as making the scanning environment more child-friendly (for example, using a facade to make the scanner look like a spaceship) have resulted in decreased stress to the children and increased cooperation, diminishing the need for sedation (Slifer et al., 1993, 1994; Rosenberg et al., 1997).

Siblings as a comparison group and the expanded phenotype of autism

Ethical guidelines recommend the study of children for comparison groups who may derive direct benefit from the study. Since there is considerable evidence that autism is genetically transmitted through family members carrying a milder phenotype (see below), the normal siblings of autistic children have served as control subjects. Older children with an autistic sibling are capable of understanding the psychologic, social, and economic impact of this genetic disorder on their family, as well as the value of their participation in the study. As a precaution against parental coercion, the child should be interviewed in the absence of the parents to ascertain the child's motivation (or lack of motivation) for participation in the study before obtaining the child's written assent.

Family and twin studies (reviewed in Piven and Folstein, 1994; Ciaranello and Ciaranello, 1995) have provided compelling evidence that genetic factors are important in the etiology of autism. The frequency of autism in subsequently born siblings is estimated at 6–8%, which is up to 200 times the risk in the general population (Bailey et al., 1996). Furthermore, three twin studies have detected pairwise concordance rates of approximately 65% in monozygotic and 0% in dizygotic pairs, producing a heritability estimate of over 90% (Folstein and Rutter, 1977; Steffenburg et al., 1989; Bailey et al., 1995). Epidemiologic, twin, and family studies have suggested that familial transmission of autism may involve a milder form of the disorder with an expanded autistic phenotype (Folstein and Rutter, 1988; Folstein and Piven, 1991; Landa et al., 1992). This phenotype is characterized by certain social personality characteristics, pragmatic language deficits, and a rigid style of behavior that are qualitatively similar to, but milder than, those features which define autism (Piven et al., 1994, 1997; Santangelo and Folstein, 1995). For example, Piven et al. (1994) found that parents and adult siblings often rated themselves as socially aloof, undemonstrative of emotion, unresponsive to the emotional cues of others, and untactful. Landa et al. (1990, 1991) detected marked deficits in the social use of language in the parents of autistic individuals compared with controls. Parents of autistic children were judged to provide too much detail and to give vague accounts, to be unable to give up their conversational turn, and to misinterpret statements frequently. High rates of anxiety and affective disorders have been reported in the family members of autistic individuals (reviewed in Piven and Folstein, 1994). Le Couteur et al. (1996) studied the behavioral phenotype in 28 monozygotic pairs and 20 dizygotic same-sex twin pairs in which one or both twins had autism. In the nonautistic twins, there was a high incidence of language delay and social deficits. Concordance for this broader phenotype was much greater in monozygotic than dizygotic twins, indicating a strong genetic component. Functional brain abnormalities underlying these behavioral deviances are also likely to be manifested in the siblings with the broader phenotype. However, the magnitude of these abnormalities are likely to be smaller, such that significant differences between autistic children and their siblings with a milder phenotype will be detectable.

Disease controls

Another approach for obtaining a comparison group is to employ a group of children with a different disorder but with otherwise normal development who might benefit from the study. This type of control does not constitute an ideal comparison group since their imaging studies will show abnormalities related to their disorder. If the abnormalities are limited to a certain brain region, the remainder of the brain might be used for comparison to the autistic group. Children with epilepsy, for example, have been shown to have focal increases in the uptake of the tracer $[^{11}C]$-AMT associated with epileptogenic cortex. Values for whole brain serotonin synthesis capacity have been calculated for children with epilepsy excluding the epileptogenic region for comparison of whole brain values in autistic children (Chugani et al., 1999a). It must be kept in mind when using this experimental approach, however, that adaptive changes can take place in other areas of the brain in response to the initial lesion.

Conclusions and future directions

Studies of glucose metabolism and blood flow have suggested a variety of global and focal brain abnormalities in autism. Newer more specific neurotransmitter probes, functional mapping, and MRS have begun to provide new clues to the biology of autism. However, data from the various imaging modalities have not yet converged to provide a unifying hypothesis of brain mechanisms. Brain regions implicated by functional imaging studies of autistic subjects are illustrated in part in Fig. 10.3. Frontal, medial prefrontal, temporal, and anterior cingulate cortical regions have been implicated with the various tracers. Abnormalities have also been reported in subcortical regions, such as basal ganglia, thalamus, and, cerebellum.

It is clear that functional imaging studies in young children, as well as new strategies for the assessment of developmental functional imaging data, are necessary to advance our understanding of autism. Furthermore, attention to the details of the design of future studies is essential. It is suggested that samples should not be merely gender matched, but that data from males and females should be analyzed separately because of gender differences in metabolic rates (Baxter et al., 1987), neurotransmitter synthesis (serotonergic gender differences reviewed in Chugani et al., 1998), and age of onset of

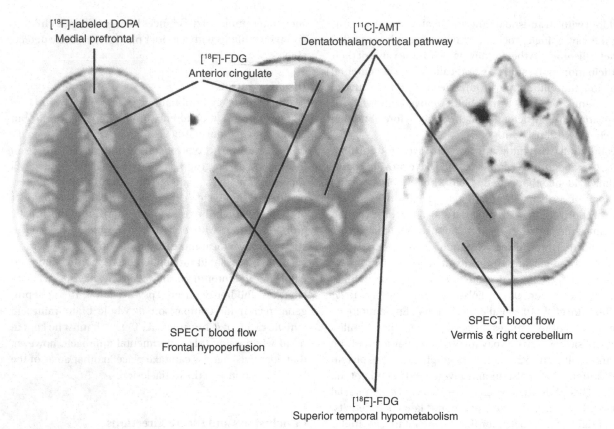

Fig. 10.3. Brain regions identified as abnormal in autistic subjects by various functional imaging modalities. Frontal, medial prefrontal, temporal, and anterior cingulate cortical regions have been implicated with the various functional tracers (AMT, α-methyltryptophan; FDG, fluorodeoxyglucose; DOPA, dihydroxyphenylalanine). Abnormalities have also been reported in subcortical regions such as the thalamus and cerebellum. A convergence of the data from the various imaging modalities to provide a unifying hypothesis of brain mechanisms responsible for autism has not yet emerged.

puberty (Tanner et al., 1976). In addition, the higher prevalence of autism in males suggests an effect of sex in this disorder. Likewise, maturational effects necessitate new mathematical approaches for analyzing cross-sectional data from subjects of different ages (for example see Muzik et al., 1999).

Alternatively, and perhaps ideally, longitudinal studies need to be undertaken to appreciate changes in functional brain activity with development more fully. Larger samples need to be examined. Although careful behavioral evaluation is essential to confirm the diagnosis, twin studies showing large differences in phenotype between identical twins suggest it is unlikely that behavioral methods will allow further refinement of subgroups of subjects with autism of differing etiologies. Genetic studies, however, may lead to the identification of new underlying etiologies, adding to the list of diseases associated with autism, and may aid in the subgrouping of subjects with more uniform neuroimaging abnormalities.

References

Anderson, G. M. (1994). Studies on the neurochemistry of autism. In *The Neurobiology of Autism*. eds. M. L. Bauman and T. L. Kemper, pp. 227–42. Baltimore: Johns Hopkins University Press.

American Psychiatric Association (1987). *Diagnostic and Statistical Manual III-Revised*. Washington, DC: American Psychiatric Association.

American Psychiatric Association (1994). *Diagnostic and Statistical Manual IV*, 4th edn. Washington, DC: American Psychiatric Association.

Asperger, H. (1994). Die "Autistischen Psychopathen" im Kindesalter. *Arch. Psychiatr. Nervenkr.*, **117**, 76–136.

Bailey, A., Le Couteur, A., Gottesman, I. and Bolton, P. (1995). Autism as a strongly genetic disorder: evidence from a British twin study. *Psychol. Med.*, **25**, 63–77.

Bailey, A., Phillips, W. and Rutter, M. (1996). Autism: towards an integration of clinical genetic, neuropsychological, and neurobiological perspectives. *J. Child Psychol. Psychiatry*, **37**, 89–126.

Bauman, M. and Kemper, T. L. (1985). Histoanatomic observations of the brain in early infantile autism. *Neurology*, **35**, 866–75.

Bauman, M. L. and Kemper, T. L. (1994). Neuroanatomic observations of the brain in autism. In *The Neurobiology of Autism*, eds. M. L. Bauman and T. L. Kemper, pp. 119–41. Baltimore: Johns Hopkins University Press.

Baxter, L. R., Mazziotta, J. C., Phelps, M. E. et al. (1987). Cerebral glucose metabolic rates in normal human females versus normal males. *Psychiatr. Res.*, **21**, 237–45.

Bennett-Clarke, C. A., Leslie, M. J., Lane, R. D. and Rhoades, R. W. (1994). Effect of serotonin depletion on vibrissae-related patterns in the rat's somatosensory cortex. *J. Neurosci.*, **14**, 7594–607.

Bennett-Clarke, C. A., Chiaia, N. L. and Rhoades, R. W. (1996). Thalamocortical afferents in rat transiently express high-affinity serotonin uptake sites. *Brain Res.*, **733**, 301–6.

Blue, M. E., Erzurumlu, R. S. and Jhaveri, S. (1991). A comparison of pattern formation by thalamocortical and serotonergic afferents in the rat barrel field cortex. *Cereb. Cortex*, **1**, 380–9.

Bottomley, P. A. and Hardy, C. J. (1989). Rapid, reliable in vivo assays of human phosphate metabolites by nuclear magnetic resonance. *Clin. Chem.*, **35**, 392–5.

Bourgeois, J.-P., Goldman-Rakic, P. S. and Rakic, P. (1994). Synaptogenesis in the prefrontal cortex of rhesus monkeys. *Cereb. Cortex*, **4**, 78–96.

Bryson, S. E. (1996). Brief report: epidemiology of autism. *J. Autism Dev. Disorders*, **26**, 165–7.

Buchsbaum, M. S., Siegel, B. V., Wu, J. C., Hazlett, E., Sicotte, N. and Haier, R. (1992). Brief report: attention performance in autism and regional brain metabolic rate assessed by positron emission tomography. *J. Autism Dev. Disorders*, **22**, 115–25.

Cases, O., Seif, I., Grimsby, J. et al. (1995). Aggressive behavior and altered amounts of brain serotonin and norepinephrine in mice lacking MAOA. *Science*, **268**, 1763–6.

Cases, O., Vitalis, T., Seif, I., de Maeyer, E., Sotelo, C. and Gaspar, P. (1996). Lack of barrels in the somatosensory cortex of monoamine oxidase A-deficient mice: role of a serotonin excess during the critical period. *Neuron*, **16**, 297–307.

Chiron, C., Raynaud, C., Maziere, B. et al. (1992). Changes in regional cerebral blood flow during brain maturation in children and adolescents. *J. Nucl. Med.*, **33**, 696–703.

Chiron, C., Leboyer, M., Leon, F., Jambaque, I., Nuttin, C. and Syrota, A. (1995). SPECT of the brain in childhood autism: evidence for a lack of normal hemispheric asymmetry. *Dev. Med. Child Neurol.*, **37**, 849–60.

Chugani, D. C., Muzik, O., Chakraborty, P. K., Mangner, T. J. and Chugani, H. T. (1996a). Brain serotonin synthesis measured with [^{11}C]-methyl-tryptophan positron emission tomography in normal and autistic adults. *Soc. Neurosci. Abst.*, **22**, 22.

Chugani, D. C., Muzik, O., Rothermel, R. et al. (1997). Altered serotonin synthesis in the dentatothalamo-cortical pathway in autistic boys. *Ann. Neurol.*, **14**, 666–9.

Chugani, D. C., Muzik, O., Chakraborty, P. K., Mangner, T. and Chugani, H. T. (1998). Human brain serotonin synthesis capacity measured in vivo with alpha-[C-11]methyl-L-tryptophan. *Synapse*, **28**, 33–43.

Chugani, D. C., Muzik, O., Behen, M., et al. (1999a). Developmental changes in brain serotonin synthesis capacity in autistic and non-autistic children. *Ann. Neurol.*, **45**, 287–95.

Chugani, D. C., Sundram, B. S., Behen, M., Lee, M.-L. and Moore, G. J. (1999b). Evidence of altered energy metabolism in autistic children. *Prog. Neuropsychopharmacol. Biol. Psychiatry*, **23**, 635–41.

Chugani, H. T., Phelps, M. E. and Mazziotta, J. C. (1987). Positron emission tomography study of human brain functional development. *Ann. Neurol.*, **22**, 487–97.

Chugani, H. T., da Silva, E. and Chugani, D. C. (1996b). Infantile spasms: III. Prognostic implications of bilateral hypometabolism on positron emission tomography. *Ann. Neurol.*, **39**, 643–9.

Ciaranello, A. L. and Ciaranello, R. D. (1995). The neurobiology of infantile autism. *Annu. Rev. Neurosci.*, **18**, 101–28.

Cohen, Z., Tsuiki, K., Takada, A., Beaudet, A., Diksic, M. and Hamel, E. (1995). In vivo-synthesis radioactively labeled α-methyl serotonin as a selective tracer for visualization of brain serotonin neurons. *Synapse*, **21**, 21–8.

Cook, E. H., Rowlett, R., Jaselskis, C. and Leventhal, B. L. (1992). Fluoxetine treatment of children and adults with autistic disorder and mental retardation. *J. Am. Acad. Child Adolesc. Psychiatry*, **31**, 739–45.

Cook, E. H., Courchesne, R., Lord, C. et al. (1997). Evidence of linkage between the serotonin transporter and autistic disorder. *Mol. Psychiatry*, **2**, 247–50.

Courchesne, E., Courchesne, R. Y., Press, G. A., Hesselink, J. R. and Jernigan, T. L. (1988). Hypoplasia of cerebellar vermal lobules VI and VII in autism. *N. Engl. J. Med.*, **813**, 1349–54.

de Volder, A., Bol, A., Michel, C., Congneau, M. and Goffinet, A. (1987). Brain glucose metabolism in children with the autistic syndrome: positron tomography analysis. *Brain Dev.*, **9**, 581–7.

Diksic, M., Nagahiro, S., Sourkes, T. L. and Yamamoto, Y. L. (1990). A new method to measure brain serotonin synthesis in vivo. I. Theory and basic data for a biological model. *J. Cereb. Blood Flow Metab.*, **9**, 1–12.

DiLavore, P. C., Lord, C. and Rutter, M. (1995). The pre-linguistic autism diagnostic observation schedule. *J. Autism Dev. Disorders*, **25**, 355–79.

Egelhoff, J. C., Ball, W. S. Jr, Koch, B. L. and Parks, T. D. (1997). Safety and efficacy of sedation in children using a structured sedation program. *Am. J. Roentgenol.*, **168**, 1259–62.

Ernst, M., Zametkin, A., Matochik, J., Pascualvaca, D. and Cohen, R. (1997). Low medial prefrontal dopaminergic activity in autistic children. *Lancet*, **350**, 638.

Ernst, M., Freed, M. E. and Zametkin, A. J. (1998). Health hazards of radiation exposure in the context of brain imaging research: special consideration for children. *J. Nucl. Med.*, **39**, 689–98.

Folstein, S. E. and Piven, J. (1991). Etiology of autism: genetic influences. *Pediatrics*, **87**, 767–73.

Folstein, S. E. and Rutter, M. L. (1977). Infantile autism: a genetic study of 21 twin pairs. *J. Child Psychol. Psychiatry*, **18**, 297–321.

Folstein, S. E. and Rutter, M. L. (1988). Autism: familial aggregation and genetic implications. *J. Autism Dev. Disorders*, **18**, 3–30.

Friedman, E. (1969). The "autistic syndrome" and phenylketonuria. *Schizophrenia*, **1**, 249–61.

George, M., Costa, D., Kouris, K., Ring, H. and Ell, P. (1992). Cerebral blood flow abnormalities in adults with infantile autism. *J. Nerv. Mental Dis.*, **180**, 413–17.

Gillberg, C. (1989). Asperger syndrome in 23 Swedish children. *Dev. Med. Child Neurol.*, **31**, 520–31.

Goldman-Rakic, P. S. and Brown, R. M. (1982). Postnatal development of monoamine content and synthesis in the cerebral cortex of rhesus monkeys. *Dev. Brain Res.*, **4**, 339–49.

Gordon, C. T., Rapoport, J. L., Hamburger, S. D., State, R. C. and Mannheim, G. B. (1992). Differential response of seven subjects with autistic disorder to clomipramine and desipramine. *Am. J. Psychiatry*, **149**, 363–6.

Gordon, C. T., State, R. C., Nelson, J. E., Hamburger, S. D. and Rapoport, J. L. (1993). A double-blind comparison of clomipramine, desipramine and placebo in the treatment of autistic disorder. *Arch. Gen. Psychiatry*, **50**, 441–7.

Hagberg, B. (1985). Retts syndrome: prevalence and impact on progressive severe mental retardation in girls. *Acta Paediatr. Scand.*, **74**, 405–8.

Happé, F., Ehlers, S., Fletcher, P. et al. (1996). "Theory of mind" in the brain. Evidence from a PET scan study of Asperger syndrome. *Neuroreport*, **8**, 197–201.

Hashimoto, T., Tayama, M., Miyazaki, M. et al. (1997). Differences in brain metabolites between patients with autism and mental retardation as detected by in vivo localized proton magnetic resonance spectroscopy. *J. Child Neurol.*, **12**, 91–6.

Haznedar, M., Buchsbaum, M., Metzger, M., Solimando, A., Spiegel-Cohen, J. and Hollander, E. (1997). Anterior cingulate gyrus volume and glucose metabolism in autistic disorder. *Am. J. Psychiatry*, **154**, 1047–50.

Heh, C. W. C., Smith, R., Wu, J. et al. (1989). Positron emission tomography of the cerebellum in autism. *Am. J. Psychiatry*, **146**, 242–5.

Herold, S., Frackowiak, R., Le Couteur, A., Rutter, M. and Howlin, P. (1988). Cerebral blood flow and metabolism of oxygen and glucose in young autistic adults. *Psychol. Med.*, **18**, 823–31.

Hoffman, E. J., Huang, S. C. and Phelps, M. E. (1979). Quantitation in positron emission computed tomography: 1. Effect of object size. *J. Comput. Assist. Tomogr.*, **3**, 299–308.

Horwitz, B., Rumsey, J., Grady, C. and Rapoport, S. (1988). The cerebral metabolic landscape in autism. Intercorrelations of regional glucose utilization. *Arch. Neurol.*, **45**, 749–55.

Huttenlocher, P. R. (1979). Synaptic density in human frontal cortex – developmental changes and effects of aging. *Brain Res.*, **163**, 195–205.

Huttenlocher, P. R. (1990). Morphometric study of human cerebral cortex development. *Neuropsychologia*, **28**, 517–27.

Huttenlocher, P. R. and de Courten, C. (1987). The development of synapses in the striate cortex of man. *Hum. Neurobiol.*, **6**, 1–9.

Huttenlocher, P. R., de Courten, C., Garey, L. J. and van der Loos, H. (1982). Synaptogenesis in human visual cortex: evidence for synapse elimination during normal development. *Neurosci. Lett.*, **33**, 247–52.

IRCP (1988). Radiation dose to patients from radiopharmaceutical. *Annals of the International Commission on Radiological Protection, Publication 53*, p. 15, New York: Pergamon Press.

Jacobs, B., Chugani, H. T., Allada, V. et al. (1995). Developmental changes in brain metabolism in sedated rhesus macaques and vervet monkeys revealed by positron emission tomography. *Cereb. Cortex*, **5**, 222–33.

Jenkins, B., Koroshetz, W., Beal, M. F. and Rosen, B. (1993). Evidence for an energy metabolism defect in Huntington's disease using localized proton spectroscopy. *Neurology*, **43**, 2685–95.

Kanner, L. (1943). Autistic disturbances of affective contact. *Nervous Child*, **2**, 217–50.

Killiany, R. J. and Moss, M. B. (1994). Memory function and autism. In *The Neurobiology of Autism*, eds. M. L. Bauman and T. L. Bauman, pp. 170–94. Baltimore: Johns Hopkins Press.

Landa, R., Piven, J., Wzorek, M. M. et al. (1990). Social language use in parents of autistic individuals. *Psychol. Med.*, **22**, 245–54.

Landa, R., Folstein, S. and Issacs, C. (1991). Spontaneous narrative-discourse performance of parents of autistic individuals. *J. Speech Hearing Res.*, **34**, 1339–45.

Landa, R., Piven, J., Wzorek, M. M., Gayle, J. O., Chase, G. A. and Folstein, S. E. (1992). Social language use in parents of autistic individuals. *Psychol. Med.*, **22**, 1245–54.

Lauder, J. M. and Krebs, H. (1978). Serotonin as a differentiation signal in early embryogenesis. *Dev. Neurosci.*, **1**, 15–30.

Lebrand, C., Cases, O., Adelbrecht, C. et al. (1996). Transient uptake and storage of serotonin in developing thalamic neurons. *Neuron*, **17**, 823–35.

Le Couteur, A., Bailey, A., Goode, S. et al. (1996). A broader phenotype of autism: the clinical spectrum in twins. *J. Child Psychol. Psychiatr. Allied Disciplines*, **37**, 785–801.

Lidow, M. S., Goldman-Rakic, P. S. and Rakic, P. (1991). Synchronized overproduction of neurotransmitter receptors in diverse regions of the primate cerebral cortex. *Proc. Natl. Acad. Sci. USA*, **88**, 10218–21.

Lord, C. (1995). Follow-up of two-year-olds referred for possible autism. *J. Child Psychol. Psychiatr. Allied Disciplines*, **36**, 1365–82.

Lord, C. and Schopler, E. (1989). The role of age at assessment, developmental level, and test in the stability of intelligence scores in young autistic children. *J. Autism Dev. Disorders*, **19**, 483–99.

Lord, C., Rutter, M., Goode, S. et al. (1989). Autism diagnostic observation schedule: a standardized observation of communicative and social behavior. *J. Autism Dev. Disorders*, **19**, 185–212.

Lord, C., Rutter, M. and LeCouteur, A. (1994). Autism diagnostic interview – revised: a revised version of diagnostic interview for caregivers of individuals with possible pervasive developmental disorders. *J. Autism Dev. Disorders*, **24**, 659–85.

Lord, C., Pickles, A., McLennan, J. et al. (1997). Diagnosing autism: analyses of data from the autism diagnostic interview. *J. Autism Dev. Disorders*, **27**, 501–17.

Lotspeich, L. J. and Ciaranello, R. D. (1993). The neurobiology and genetics of infantile autism. In *International Review of Neurobiology*, ed. R. Bradley, pp. 87–129. San Diego, CA: Academic Press.

Madras, B. K. and Sourkes, T. L. (1965). Metabolism of α-methyl-tryptophan. *Biochem. Pharmacol.*, **14**, 1499–506.

McDougle, C. J., Price, L. H., Volkmar, F. R. et al. (1992). Clomipramine in autism: preliminary evidence of efficacy. *J. Am. Acad. Child Adolesc. Psychiatry*, **31**, 746–50.

McDougle, C. J., Naylor, S. T., Cohen, D. J., Aghajanian, G. K., Heninger, G. R. and Price, L. H. (1996a). Effects of tryptophan depletion in drug-free adults with autistic disorder. *Arch. Gen. Psychiatry*, **53**, 993–1000.

McDougle, C. J., Naylor, S. T., Cohen, D. J., Volkmar, F. R., Heninger, G. R. and Price, L. H. (1996b). A double-blind, placebo-controlled study of fluvoxamine in adults with autistic disorder. *Arch. Gen. Psychiatry*, **53**, 1001–8.

McKelvey, J., Lambert, R., Mottron, L. and Shevell, M. (1995). Right-hemisphere dysfunction in Asperger's syndrome. *J. Child Neurol.*, **10**, 310–14.

Merola, C., Albarracin, C., Lebowitz, P., Bienkowski, R. S. and Barst, S. M. (1995). An audit of adverse events in children sedated with chloral hydrate or propofol during imaging studies. *Paediatr. Anaesth.*, **5**, 375–8.

Minshew, N., Goldstein, G., Dombrowski, S., Panchalingam, K. and Pettegrew, J. (1993). A preliminary ^{31}P MRS study of autism: evidence for undersynthesis and increased degradation of brain membranes. *Biol. Psychiatry*, **33**, 762–73.

Minshew, N. J. Goldstein, G. and Siegel, D. J. (1997). Neuropsychologic functioning in autism: profile of a complex information processing disorder. *J. Int. Neuropsychol. Soc.*, **3**, 303–16.

Miquel, M. C., Kia, H. K., Boni, C. et al. (1994). Postnatal development and localization of 5-HT$_{1A}$ receptor mRNA in rat forebrain and cerebellum. *Dev. Brain Res.*, **80**, 149–57.

Missala, K. and Sourkes, T. L. (1988). Functional cerebral activity of an analogue of serotonin formed in situ. *Neurochem. Int.*, **12**, 209–14.

Moore, G. J. (1998). Proton magnetic resonance spectroscopy in pediatric neuroradiology. *Pediatr. Radiol.*, **11**, 805–14.

Mountz, J., Tolbert, L., Lill, D., Katholi, C. and Liu, H. (1995). Functional deficits in autistic disorder: characterization by technetium-99m-HMPAO and SPECT. *J. Nucl. Med.*, **36**, 1156–62.

Müller, R. A., Chugani, D. C., Behen, M. E. et al. (1998). Impairment of dentato-thalamo-cortical pathway in autistic men: language activation data from positron emission tomography. *Neurosci. Lett.*, **245**, 1–4.

Müller, R. A., Behen, M. E., Rothermel, R. D. et al. (1999). Brain mapping of language and auditory perception in high-functioning autistic adults: a PET study. *J. Autism Dev. Disorders*, **29**, 19–31.

Muzik, O., Chugani, D. C., Chakraborty, P. K., Mangner, T. and Chugani, H. T. (1997). Analysis of [C-11]alpha-methyl-tryptophan kinetics for the estimation of serotonin synthesis rate in vivo. *J. Cereb. Blood Flow Metab.*, **17**, 659–69.

Muzik, O., Ager, J., Janisse, J., Shen, C., Chugani, D. C. and Chugani, H. T. (1999). A mathematical model for the analysis of cross-sectional brain glucose metabolism data in children. *Prog. NeuroPsychopharmacol. Biol. Psychiatry*, **23**, 589–600.

Nishizawa, S., Benkelfat, C., Young, S. N. et al. (1997). Differences between males and females in rates of serotonin synthesis in human brain. *Proc. Natl. Acad. Sci. USA*, **94**, 5308–13.

Osterheld-Haas, M. C. and Hornung, J. P. (1996). Laminar development of the mouse barrel cortex: effects of neurotoxins against monoamines. *Exp. Brain Res.*, **110**, 183–95.

Ozbayrak, K. R., Kapucu, O., Erdem, E. and Aras, T. (1991). Left occipital hypoperfusion in a case with Asperger syndrome. *Brain Dev.*, **13**, 454–6.

Payton, J. B., Steele, M. W., Wenger, S. L. and Minshew, N. J. (1989). The fragile X marker and autism in perspective. *J. Am. Acad. Child Adolesc. Psychiatry*, **28**, 417–21.

Piven, J. and Folstein, S. (1994). The genetics of autism. In *The Neurobiology of Autism*, eds. M. L. Bauman and T. L. Kemper, pp. 18–44. Baltimore: Johns Hopkins University Press.

Piven, J., Gayle, J., Landa, R., Wzorek, M. and Folstein, S. (1991). The prevalence of fragile X in a sample of autistic individuals diagnosed using a standardized interview. *J. Am. Acad. Child Adolesc. Psychiatry*, **30**, 825–30.

Piven, J., Wzorek, M., Landa, R. et al. (1994). Personality characteristics of the parents of autistic individuals. *Psychol. Med.*, **24**, 783–95.

Piven, J., Palmer, P., Jacobi, D., Childress, D. and Arndt, S. (1997). Broader autism phenotype: evidence from a family history of multiple-incidence autism families. *Am. J. Psychiatry*, **154**, 185–90.

Rakic, P., Bourgeois, J.-P., Eckenhoff, M. F., Zecevic, N. and Goldman-Rakic, P. S. (1986). Concurrent overproduction of synapses in diverse regions of the primate cerebral cortex. *Science*, **232**, 232–5.

Reiss, A. L., Lee, J. and Freund, L. (1994). Neuroanatomy of fragile X syndrome: the temporal lobe. *Neurology*, **44**, 1317–24.

Riikonen, R. and Amnell, G. (1981). Psychiatric disorders in children with earlier infantile spasms. *Dev. Med. Child Neurol.*, **23**, 747–60.

Ritvo, E. R., Freeman, B. J., Scheibel, A. B. et al. (1986). Lower Purkinje cell counts in the cerebella of four autistic subjects: initial findings of the UCLA–NSAC autopsy research report. *Am. J. Psychiatry*, **143**, 862–6.

Rosenberg, D. R., Sweeney, J. A., Gillen, J. S. et al. (1997). Magnetic resonance imaging of children without sedation: preparation with simulation. *J. Am. Acad. Child Adolesc. Psychiatry*, **36**, 853–9.

Rumsey, J., Duara, R., Grady, C. et al. (1985). Brain metabolism in autism. Resting cerebral glucose utilization rates as measured with positron emission tomography. *Arch. Gen. Psychiatry*, **42**, 448–55.

Sanchez, L. E., Campbell, M., Small, A. M., Cueva, J. E., Armenteros, J. L. and Adams, P. B. (1996). A pilot study of clomipramine in young autistic children. *J. Am. Acad. Child Adolesc. Psychiatry*, **35**, 537–44.

Santangelo, S. L. and Folstein, S. E. (1995). Social deficits in the families of autistic probands. *Am. J. Hum. Genetics*, **53**, 855.

Schain, R. J. and Freedman, D. X. (1961). Studies on 5-hydroxyindole metabolism in autism and other mentally retarded children. *J. Pediatr.*, **59**, 315–20.

Schifter, T., Hoffman, J., Hatten, H., Hanson, M., Coleman, R. and de Long, G. (1994). Neuroimaging in infantile autism. *J. Child Neurol.*, **9**, 155–61.

Schopler, E., Reichler, R. J., de Vellis, R. F. and Daly, K. (1980). Toward objective classification of childhood autism: childhood autism rating scale (CARS). *J. Autism Dev. Disorders*, **10**, 91–103.

Sevin, J. A., Matson, J. L., Coe, D., Love, S. R., Matese, M. J. and

Benavidez, D. A. (1995). Empirically derived subtypes of pervasive developmental disorders: a cluster analytic study. *J. Autism Dev. Disorders*, **25**, 561–78.

Sherman, M., Nass, R. and Shapiro, T. (1984). Regional cerebral blood flow in infantile autism. *J. Autism Dev. Disorders*, **4**, 438–40.

Siegel, B. V. Jr, Asarnow, R., Tanguay, P. et al. (1992). Regional cerebral glucose metabolism and attention in adults with a history of childhood autism. *J. Neuropsychiatry Clin. Neurosci.*, **4**, 406–14.

Siegel, B., Nuechterlein, K., Abel, L., Wu, J. and Buchsbaum, M. (1995). Glucose metabolic correlates of continuous performance test performance in adults with a history of infantile autism, schizophrenics, and controls. *Schizophr. Res.*, **17**, 85–94.

Slifer, K., Cataldo, M. F., Cataldo, M. D., Llorente, A. and Gerson, A. (1993). Behavior analysis of motion control for pediatric neuroimaging. *J. Appl. Behav. Anal.*, **26**, 469–70.

Slifer, K., Bucholts, J. and Cataldo, M. D. (1994). Behavioral training of motion control on young children undergoing radiation treatment without sedation. *J. Pediatr. Oncol. Nursing*, **11**, 55–63.

Smalley, S. L., Tanguay, P. E., Smith, M. and Gutierrez, G. (1992). Autism and tuberous sclerosis. *J. Autism Dev. Disorders*, **22**, 339–55.

Steffenburg, S., Gillberg, C., Hellgren, L. et al. (1989). A twin study of autism in Denmark, Finland, Iceland, Norway and Sweden. *J. Child Psychol. Psychiatr. Allied Disciplines*, **30**, 405–16.

Tanner, J. M., Whitehouse, R. H., Marubini, E. and Resele, L. F. (1976). The adolescent growth spurt of boys and girls of the Harpenden growth. *Ann. Hum. Biol.*, **3**, 109–26.

Theodore, W. H., di Chiro, G., Margolin, R., Fishbein, D., Porter, R.

J. and Brooks, R. A. (1986). Barbiturates reduce human cerebral glucose metabolism. *Neurology*, **36**, 60–4.

Tuchman, R. F. and Rapin, I. (1997). Regression in pervasive developmental disorders: seizures and epileptiform EEG correlates. *Pediatrics*, **99**, 560–6.

Volkmar, F. R., Sparrow, S. S., Goudreau, D., Cicchetti, D. V., Paul, R. and Cohen, D. J. (1987). Social deficits in autism: an operational approach using the Vineland adaptive behavior scales. *J. Am. Acad. Child Adolesc. Psychiatry*, **26**, 156–61.

Volkmar, F. R., Klin, A., Schultz, R. et al. (1996). Asperger's syndrome. *J. Am. Acad. Child Adolesc. Psychiatry*, **35**, 118–23.

Wing, L. (1981). Asperger's syndrome: a clinical account. *Psychol. Med.*, **11**, 115–29.

Wing, L. (1993). The definition and prevalence of autism. A review. *Eur. Child Adolesc. Psychiatry*, **2**, 61–74.

Wing, L. and Gould, J. (1979). Severe impairments of social interaction and associated abnormalities in children: epidemiology and classification. *J. Autism Dev. Disorders*, **9**, 11–29.

World Health Organization (1987). *International Classification of Diseases*, 10th Draft. New York: WHO.

Yan, W., Wilson, C. C. and Haring, J. H. (1997). Effects of neonatal serotonin depletion on the development of rat dentate granule cells. *Dev. Brain Res.*, **98**, 177–84.

Zilbovicius, M., Garreau, B., Tzourio, N. et al. (1992). Regional cerebral blood flow in childhood autism: a SPECT study. *Am. J. Psychiatry*, **149**, 924–30.

Zilbovicius, M., Garreau, B., Samson, Y. et al. (1995). Delayed maturation of the frontal cortex in childhood autism. *Am. J. Psychiatry*, **152**, 248–52.

11

Functional imaging in childhood-onsent schizophrenia

Leslie K. Jacobsen and Alessandro Bertolino

Introduction

This chapter will begin with a review of developmental theories of schizophrenia to provide a foundation for a discussion of functional brain imaging studies of childhood-onset schizophrenia. Two examples of such studies conducted with the National Institute of Mental Health (NIMH) childhood-onset schizophrenia sample are provided, followed by a discussion of future directions. Schizophrenia with onset during late adolescence or early adulthood is referred to as "adult-onset schizophrenia" whereas childhood-onset schizophrenia is usually defined as onset by the age of 12 years.

Etiology of schizophrenia

Since the 1970s, etiologic hypotheses about schizophrenia have shifted away from a view of the disorder as arising from pathologic processes occurring shortly prior to the onset of symptoms leading to diagnosis toward a neurodevelopmental conceptualization of the disorder. The neurodevelopmental hypothesis of schizophrenia asserts that schizophrenia results from an interaction between normal brain maturational events and a congenital brain lesion(s) (Weinberger, 1987). This shift in thinking is the result of cumulative evidence supporting the existence of brain morphologic and functional abnormalities in schizophrenia, together with the observation that disease onset typically occurs during late adolescence or early adulthood. Neurodevelopmental hypotheses argue that some brain abnormalities in people destined to develop schizophrenia may exist from birth, although symptoms of schizophrenia do not appear until affected brain areas and related circuitry mature (Murray and Lewis, 1987; Weinberger, 1987, 1995; Done et al., 1994; Jones et al., 1994; Murray, 1994).

One line of compelling evidence in support of the neurodevelopmental hypothesis of schizophrenia has come from animal studies. A large body of work in nonhuman primates by Patricia Goldman-Rakic and others has implicated the dorsolateral prefrontal cortex in working memory, a core aspect of cognition that is impaired in schizophrenia. In working memory tasks, information is presented and then must be recalled (Fuster and Alexander, 1971). A common paradigm used to test working memory in animals is the delayed response paradigm, wherein the animal is presented information (e.g., the location of a food pellet) that must be recalled after a delay interval. In humans, working memory is thought to provide a foundation for important higher cognitive functions, such as comprehension, thinking, and planning (Goldman-Rakic, 1994). Patients with schizophrenia perform poorly on tests of working memory, and this impairment may underlie a number of core symptoms of schizophrenia, including disorganization of thinking and behavior, an inability to modify strategies based upon experience, lack of initiative, and poverty of speech (Goldman-Rakic, 1991).

Adult monkeys with lesions of the dorsolateral prefrontal cortex perform at chance levels during tests of working memory. The perseverative errors that these animals frequently make, together with their distractibility and impulsivity, has led investigators to view them as a model for some dimensions of schizophrenia (Goldman-Rakic, 1991). In keeping with predictions from neurodevelopmental hypotheses, monkeys with dorsolateral prefrontal lesions created in infancy do not show deficits in performance on any task or in their behavior until 2 years of age (adolescence), at which point impairment appears and worsens with increasing age (Goldman, 1974). In contrast, lesions created in adolescent or adult monkeys are associated with immediate impairment in working memory performance. The delayed emergence of impairment in monkeys with lesions created in infancy is thought to reflect the late maturation of the dorsolateral prefrontal cortex and, consequently, the delayed integration of this cortical region into neural circuits subserving memory, particularly mesiotemporal–prefrontal cortical circuitry. In humans, the prefrontal brain area is the last to begin myelination and continues to myelinate throughout life (Yakovlev and Le Cours, 1964). Prior to maturation of this region, delayed response performance is mediated by other brain regions; consequently deficits related to dorsolateral prefrontal cortex lesions become apparent only once this region is mature and normally becomes more essential for working memory performance (Goldman, 1974; Goldman and Alexander, 1977).

Another animal model has been elaborated in rats (Lipska and Weinberger, 1995) in which neonatal hippocampal lesions are thought to interfere with the development of prefrontal cortex and with its integration into neural circuits. Such lesions produce a spectrum of changes in prefrontal function when the rats reach adulthood, resulting in abnormalities of cognition (Lipska et al., 1996), social behavior (Sams-Dodd et al., 1997), and gene expression (Lillrank et al., 1996). These animals become hyperresponsive to stress and to amphetamine challenge after puberty. Of particular relevance to childhood-onset schizophrenia is the observation that in certain strains of rats effects of hippocampal lesions emerge at an earlier age.

Adult-onset schizophrenia

Structural neuroimaging studies conducted in patients with onset of schizophrenia during late adolescence or early adulthood have produced a wealth of evidence in support of neurodevelopmental hypotheses of schizophrenia. The animal models described above predict that humans with schizophrenia will have smaller brain structures, particularly in frontal and temporal lobe regions, as the result of a neurodevelopmental lesion leading to failure of tissue development or to overly exuberant synaptic pruning during adolescence and/or early adulthood (Feinberg, 1982).

Consistent with this prediction, both autopsy studies and structural magnetic resonance imaging (MRI) studies in adult schizophrenia have demonstrated reduced medial temporal lobe volume, reduced frontal lobe volume, and enlarged lateral ventricles, as well as reduced midsagittal thalamic area and enlarged third ventricles (Andreasen et al., 1986, 1994a,b; Falkai and Bogerts, 1986; Jakob and Beckmann, 1989; Jeste and Lohr, 1989; Altshuler et al.,

1990; Bogerts et al., 1990a,b, 1993; Suddath et al., 1990; Arnold et al., 1991; Jernigan et al., 1991; Breier et al., 1992; Marsh et al., 1994; Zipursky et al., 1994; Flaum et al., 1995). Previous observations of basal ganglia enlargement now appear to reflect an effect of typical neuroleptic medications, as patients subsequently switched to atypical medication show normalization of basal ganglia volume (Chakos et al., 1995). Reduced total cerebral volume has also been observed, with recent autopsy work suggesting that this reduction is largely a result of decreased neuropil throughout the cortex, reflecting decreased synaptic density (Selemon et al., 1995). Consistent with this, in vivo brain MRI studies have found widespread reductions in cortical gray, but not white, matter, which are most prominent in frontal and temporal regions (Lim et al., 1996; Sullivan et al., 1998). Furthermore, the same pattern of gray matter reduction with white matter sparing has been observed in a sample of patients with congential rubella and schizophrenia-like symptoms, suggesting that this pattern of brain dysmorphology can result from a viral disturbance of early neurodevelopment (Lim et al., 1995).

Functional neuroimaging studies

Resting-state studies of cerebral glucose metabolism and blood flow in patients with adult-onset schizophrenia have yielded inconsistent findings (Chua and McKenna, 1995). Some have demonstrated reduced anterior-to-posterior ratios of metabolism in schizophrenia (Buchsbaum et al., 1984; DeLisi, et al., 1985); others have shown no group differences in frontal metabolism or blood flow (Wiesel et al., 1987; Ebmeier et al., 1995), and still others have shown increased frontal metabolism in schizophrenia (Szechtman et al., 1988).

Studies measuring glucose metabolism or blood flow during task performance have yielded more consistent findings. Hypofrontality has been demonstrated while schizophrenic adults performed the Wisconsin Card Sorting Test (Berman et al., 1992; Volz et al., 1997), the Tower of London (Andreasen et al., 1992), and the Continuous Performance Test (CPT) (Cohen et al., 1987; Siegel et al., 1993). Specific dysfunction of prefrontal-limbic neurocircuitry has been implicated in a study of monozygotic twins discordant for schizophrenia, which demonstrated that the schizophrenic twin's failure to activate prefrontal cortex during a working memory task was closely related to a reduction in left hippocampal volume (Weinberger et al., 1992). Hypofrontality has been particularly associated with deficit symptoms, which, along with poor performance on measures of frontal lobe functioning, is thought to result from the schizophrenic patients' inability to activate frontal regions (Andreasen et al., 1992; Siegel et al., 1993).

Proton magnetic resonance spectroscopy (^{1}H MRS) represents another in vivo imaging methodology that has been utilized to test the neurodevelopmental hypothesis of schizophrenia. This method permits in vivo measurement of some aspects of brain biochemistry. It detects signals arising from N-acetyl-containing moieties, mainly N-acetylaspartate (NAA). This compound is located within neurons (Urenjak et al., 1993), increases during development (Toft et al., 1994), and has been shown to be an intraneuronal marker sensitive to pharmacologic inhibition of mitochondrial energy metabolism and to a number of pathologic processes affecting the integrity of neurons (Arnold et al., 1990; de Stefano et al., 1995; Hugg et al., 1996, Cheng et al., 1997). Since neuronal number does not significantly increase after birth in humans or in monkeys, postnatal increases in NAA appear to reflect maturational processes. Proton MRS also detects signals arising from choline-containing compounds (Cho), such as glycerophosphocholine and phosphocholine (Miller, 1991; Barker et al., 1994), and from creatine plus phosphocreatine (Cre). Variation in the signal of Cho is associated with alterations in membrane turnover. Creatine and phosphocreatine buffer the ATP/ADP ratio. Previous single-voxel ^{1}H MRS studies of patients with adult-onset schizophrenia have reported reductions of NAA signal intensity or concentration in the mesial temporal lobes (Renshaw et al., 1995; Yurgelun-Todd et al., 1996), in the region of the hippocampus (Nasrallah et al., 1994; Maier et al., 1995), and in the frontal lobe (Buckley et al., 1994), but not without debate (Buckley et al., 1994; Fukuzako et al., 1995; Stanley et al., 1996; Bartha et al., 1997).

The use of ^{1}H MRS has evolved to permit imaging that maps signals acquired from a large number of small single-volume elements (Duyn et al., 1993). Using this technique, reductions in NAA levels in the hippocampal area and in the dorsolateral prefrontal cortex have been demonstrated in patients with adult-onset schizophrenia (Bertolino et al., 1996, 1998a,b; Deicken et al., 1997). These findings were independent of drug treatment and were consistent with developmental neuronal pathology (Bertolino et al., 1996, 1997, 1998a,b).

Proton MRS imaging has also been applied to an animal model of schizophrenia to test more directly the neurodevelopmental hypothesis of this disorder (Bertolino et al., 1997). In parallel to the rat model of schizophrenia of Lipska and colleagues (1993) described above, the mesial temporal lobe was ablated bilaterally in six monkeys within 3 weeks of birth and in six monkeys at 5 years of age (adult). Subsequent ^{1}H MRS imaging demonstrated

reduced NAA in the prefrontal cortex of animals who had undergone mesial temporal lobe ablation during infancy but not in animals undergoing this procedure as adults. These findings suggest that normal prefrontal cortical maturation is dependent upon neurons in this region receiving target feedback from mesiotemporal lobe neurons. This model also demonstrates that maldevelopment of prefrontal cortex and mesiotemporal–prefrontal cortical circuitry in schizophrenia could arise from early postnatal lesions of the mesiotemporal lobe (Bertolino et al., 1997).

Neuroreceptor imaging

Neurochemical brain imaging methodologies have permitted testing of the dopamine hypothesis of schizophrenia (Creese et al., 1976; Meltzer and Stahl, 1976). This hypothesis stemmed from the early observation that dopamimetic drugs, when taken in large quantities, can produce a schizophrenic-like psychosis. In addition, the antipsychotic potency of many neuroleptic drugs is correlated with the degree to which they bind to striatal dopamine receptors. More recent support for the involvement of dopamine in schizophrenia has come from observations of deterioration in performance on frontal lobe tasks (e.g., working memory tasks) in animals (Brozowski et al., 1979) and in humans (Stern and Langston, 1985) in whom dopaminergic afferents to frontal lobe have been lesioned. In a recent single photon emission computed tomography (SPECT) study using the dopamine D_2 receptor radioligand [^{123}I]-iodobenzamide ([^{123}I]-IBZM), patients with schizophrenia were found to have greater amphetamine-stimulated dopamine release than healthy controls, as measured by [^{123}I]-IBZM displacement, indicating increased dopamine transmission in schizophrenia (Laruelle et al., 1996; Abi-Dargham et al., 1998). More recently, the efficacy of atypical antipsychotic drugs, which have significant affinity for a wide range of receptor systems, has drawn attention to the role of other neurotransmitter systems in schizophrenia. These include serotonin (Abi-Dargham et al., 1997) and the gamma-aminobutyric acid (GABA) receptor complex (Benes et al., 1997).

While considerable evidence has accumulated in support of the neurodevelopmental hypothesis of schizophrenia, this hypothesis has its limitations (Weinberger, 1987). A major challenge to any neurobiologic hypothesis of schizophrenia is to account for atypical presentations of the disorder. Such cases test the boundaries of hypotheses based upon data collected from patients with more common disease manifestations and can result in a deeper understanding of disease mechanisms.

Childhood-onset schizophrenia

Phenomenology and neurobiology

The onset of schizophrenia in childhood, usually defined as onset by age 12, is extremely rare (Remschmidt et al., 1994) and therefore qualifies as an atypical presentation of schizophrenia. While no large-scale epidemiologic studies using rigorous diagnostic criteria have been conducted, it has been estimated that the prevalence of childhood-onset schizophrenia may be 50 times less than that of adult-onset schizophrenia (Karno and Norquist, 1989).

Because of the extreme rarity of childhood-onset schizophrenia, few systematic studies of phenomenology or neurobiology of this disorder have been conducted. Studies of phenomenology have demonstrated that, although it is rare, childhood-onset schizophrenia does occur and can be diagnosed using the same standard criteria used to diagnose adults with schizophrenia (American Psychiatric Association, 1994; Russell, 1994). Like other early-onset forms of multifactorial diseases (e.g. juvenile-onset diabetes mellitus, juvenile rheumatoid arthritis), childhood-onset schizophrenia is associated with greater disease severity and chronicity than adult-onset schizophrenia (Gordon et al., 1994).

Clinical studies have demonstrated prominent premorbid developmental delays in childhood-onset schizophrenia, especially in the areas of speech and language (Alaghband-Rad et al., 1995; Asarnow et al., 1995; Hollis, 1995). In addition, transient symptoms of pervasive developmental disorder, such as hand flapping and echolalia, are common in the prepsychotic period (Alaghband-Rad et al., 1995; Watkins et al., 1988; Russell et al., 1989). This is one area of phenomenologic distinction between childhood- and adult-onset schizophrenia, as symptoms of pervasive developmental disorder have not been reported in studies of the premorbid history of the latter (Done et al., 1994; Jones et al., 1994). The conspicuous prepsychotic developmental abnormalities seen in childhood-onset schizophrenia are consistent with a neurodevelopmental etiology, with the pattern suggesting that language-related brain areas, such as those in the temporal lobe, may be particularly affected.

Neurobiologic studies of childhood-onset schizophrenia are even fewer in number and have been conducted largely through the NIMH Childhood Onset Schizophrenia Project. This project has involved national recruitment of severely ill, treatment-refractory children and adolescents with well-documented onset of schizophrenia by age 12 (Gordon et al., 1994). Patients in this study undergo a period of drug-free washout to confirm diagnosis and to obtain baseline clinical ratings prior to initiation of atypical antipsychotic medication (Kumra et al., 1996, 1999). As a result a high degree of confidence in the accuracy of the diagnosis is possible with this sample. Furthermore, many of the neurobiologic studies of this sample have been conducted at the end of the medication-free phase to permit clear separation of medication effects from disease effects.

Neurobiologic studies of the NIMH childhood-onset schizophrenia sample have generally supported neurobiologic continuity between childhood- and adult-onset schizophrenia (Jacobsen and Rapoport, 1998). A pattern of abnormalities of eye tracking (Jacobsen et al., 1996), autonomic function (Zahn et al., 1997), and MRI brain morphology, (Jacobsen and Rapoport, 1998) similar to that found in adult-onset schizophrenia has been observed.

Structural brain imaging

Few systematic studies of brain morphology in pediatric schizophrenia have been conducted. One early axial computed tomography (CT) scan study by Schulz and colleagues (1983) of 15 adolescents with schizophrenia or schizophreniform disorder (mean age 16.5 ± 1.55 years; illness duration mean 13 months, range 5–24 months) demonstrated significant increases in ventricular volume in the schizophrenic group relative to both normal controls and a contrast group of borderline patients of similar ages, with greater increases in ventricular/brain ratio being related to poorer treatment response (Schulz et al., 1983). However, using MRI, this group later found no evidence of increased ventricular volume but instead found significantly smaller total brain volume in 17 schizophrenic patients aged 9–18 years (mean 14.3 years) when compared with 13 normal controls (mean age 14.9 years) (Friedman et al., 1996). After correction for group differences in total brain volume, there were no differences in hippocampal volume (Findling et al., 1996). Yeo and colleagues (1997) studied 20 children with schizophrenia spectrum disorders and 20 healthy children using structural MRI and found decreased amygdala and temporal cortex volumes, but normal hippocampal, ventricular, frontal and total brain volumes.

A recent analysis in which the brain morphology of 28 patients in the NIMH childhood-onset schizophrenia study was compared with that of 57 healthy controls matched for age, sex, and handedness and not differing in weight or height revealed significantly decreased (by 9.7%) total cerebral volume for the patients with schizophrenia (Jacobsen and Rapoport, 1998), as has been seen in adult-onset schizophrenia (Zipursky et al., 1991; Harvey et al.,

1993). Given these large group differences, all regional brain comparisons were conducted with analysis of covariance using total cerebral volume as the covariate. As has been observed in adult schizophrenia (Breier et al., 1992; Flaum et al., 1995), the lateral ventricles were increased in volume, and there was a trend for anterior frontal tissue volume (tissue anterior to the coronal plane intersecting the anterior-most point of the corpus callosum) to be decreased in size relative to that in healthy controls. The midsagittal thalamic area was also significantly decreased in patients with childhood-onset schizophrenia. A significant increase in the midsagittal area of the corpus callosum in patients with childhood-onset schizophrenia suggested that sparing of this white matter structure had occurred. In support of this notion, preliminary gray/white segmentation data suggest that the reduction in total cerebral volume in childhood-onset schizophrenia is primarily a consequence of a reduction in gray matter volume, with relative sparing of white matter (Giedd et al., 1996).

A longitudinal MRI brain imaging study of the NIMH childhood-onset schizophrenia sample has shown that, consistent with studies of adult schizophrenia, enlarged basal ganglia volumes on study entry normalize after patients are switched to atypical antipsychotic medication (Frazier et al., 1996). Perhaps most striking, however, has been the observation that the volumes of the lateral ventricles and temporal lobe structures are changing over time during adolescence in the sample more rapidly than in healthy matched controls. The rescanning of 16 patients with childhood-onset schizophrenia and 24 matched yoked controls 2 years following their initial scan indicated that ventricular volume increased more in children with schizophrenia than in healthy children (diagnosis × time F = 16.1; $p = 0.0003$) (Rapoport et al., 1997). In addition, midsagittal thalamic area decreased significantly in schizophrenic patients, but not in controls, over this time period (Rapoport et al., 1997). A rescan after 2 years in 10 patients with childhood-onset schizophrenia and 17 healthy yoked controls showed greater decreases in volumes over time of the right temporal lobe, bilateral superior temporal gyri, and left hippocampus in patients with childhood-onset schizophrenia (Jacobsen et al., 1998). Therefore, although medial temporal lobe structures were not found to be reduced in size in patients with childhood-onset schizophrenia upon their entry into the NIMH study (Jacobsen et al., 1996a), these structures may undergo abnormal developmental changes during adolescence leading to reduced size by early adulthood.

Functional brain imaging: cerebral glucose metabolism and blood flow

Very few functional brain imaging studies have been conducted in patients with childhood-onset schizophrenia. This fact stems not only from the rarity of this disorder but also from the demands that functional imaging studies place upon subjects. For all functional imaging modalities, it is important to remain still for the duration of the scan to avoid loss or distortion of data from movement artifact. For some modalities, functional imaging also requires performance of cognitive activation tasks, undergoing intravenous and/or arterial line placement, and being off of antipsychotic medication. Balancing these significant challenges is the important opportunity that functional neuroimaging methodologies provide for testing neurodevelopmental hypotheses of neuropsychiatric disorders.

To the best of our knowledge, only one brief report has appeared in the published literature to date in which cerebral blood flow (CBF) was examined in pediatric schizophrenia (Chabrol et al., 1986). This study compared 10 neuroleptic-naive adolescents with schizophrenia (mean age 16 ± 1.5, illness duration 1.6 ± 0.7 years) and 10 healthy sex- and age-matched controls using xenon-133 as tracer and demonstrated significant hypofrontality in the patients with schizophrenia. The state in which subjects were scanned was not specified.

The only study of cerebral glucose metabolism in childhood-onset schizophrenia has been conducted with a subset of the NIMH childhood-onset schizophrenia sample (Jacobsen et al., 1998). Of particular interest were comparisons between childhood- versus adult-onset schizophrenia. If early-onset schizophrenia is caused by a more pronounced lesion, then one would expect to see greater hypofrontality in patients with childhood-onset disease. To facilitate these comparisons, the methods previously applied to an adult-onset sample, who showed decreased frontal metabolism during the performance of an attentional task (Cohen et al., 1987), were adapted for use with the childhood sample. The adult study examined 16 patients (12 male, four female; mean age 28 ± 7 years) and 27 normal controls (15 male, 12 female; mean age 33 ± 12 years).

The childhood-onset schizophrenia study examined 16 patients (six girls, 10 boys), ages 12 to 18 years (mean ± SD 14.2 ± 1.7 years) with a mean age at onset of psychosis of 9.9 ± 1.8 years, using positron emission tomography (PET) and [18F]-fluorodeoxyglucose (FDG). As in the adult study (Cohen et al., 1987), patients discontinued their medications prior to scanning. Adult patients studied by Cohen were medication free for 13–73 days (mean 34 ± 18) prior to scanning. Childhood-onset patients were medication free for 9–32 days (mean 19.5 ± 5.9) prior to PET scanning. Patients were compared with 26 healthy control adolescents matched for age, gender, Tanner stage, and handedness. However, 19 of the normal control subjects had a sibling with attention-deficit hyperactivity disorder (ADHD), who had participated in a separate PET study (Ernst et al., 1994). PET scanning was performed using a method designed to minimize radiation exposure to subjects (Zametkin et al., 1993). As in the adult study, all subjects performed a computerized auditory CPT with eyes patched during FDG uptake (approximately 30 min).

Image analysis included both a region of interest (ROI) approach used previously to analyze data from the adult study and a newer pixel-based approach. For the ROI analysis, five slices most closely resembling anatomically defined templates were selected. Raw pixel values were converted into regional glucose metabolic rates (rCMRGlu, in 100 mg/min per g tissue) (Brooks, 1982) and these were then measured by an independent rater, blind to diagnosis, for 60 standard ROIs distributed within the five planes. Global CMRGlu was calculated by averaging values for glucose metabolism across all areas of the cortex sampled that were rich in gray matter. Regional CMRGlu values were normalized by dividing each subject's absolute CMRGlu for each ROI by his/her global CMRGlu.

For the pixel-based analysis, Statistical Parametric Mapping (SPM), version 1995 (Friston et al., 1991) was used. After transforming each image into a standard stereotactic space (Talairach and Tournoux, 1988), images were smoothed using a 10 mm × 10 mm × 6 mm Gaussian filter. Proportional scaling was used to control for intersubject differences in global CMRGlu. Between group comparisons were performed on a pixel-by-pixel basis, with the resulting value of t for each pixel being transformed to a Z score. Pixels corresponding to Z scores greater than or equal to 2.58 (or $p < 0.005$) were then subjected to a test of significance based on spatial extent (Friston et al., 1994). Spatially contiguous pixels (clusters) of a size corresponding to $p < 0.005$ were considered significant.

As in the adult study, results of the ROI-based analysis indicated that global CMRGlu in childhood-onset schizophrenia patients (14.13 ± 2.11 mg/min per 100 g) was comparable to that found in controls (14.01 ± 2.39 mg/min per 100 g). Also, similar to findings in the adult study, adolescents with childhood-onset schizophrenia had significantly lower metabolic rates than controls in their middle frontal gyrus (anterior frontal region of plane C) and superior frontal gyrus (anterior medial frontal region of plane E) (Fig. 11.1). The middle frontal gyral

region was identical to that identified as hypometabolic in the adult sample, while the other frontal region was one plane lower than that identified in the adult sample. Comparison of the effect sizes observed in the childhood- and the adult-onset samples failed to indicate more severe hypofrontality in early-onset schizophrenia. Within the early-onset schizophrenic group, metabolic rates of the brain regions showing hypofrontality was not significantly correlated with negative symptoms, as measured by the Scale for the Assessment of Negative Symptoms (SANS; Andreasen, 1983) total score, duration of illness, or total number of months that patients had received antipsychotic medication prior to study entry. (Comparable correlations were not reported for the adult study of Cohen et al. (1987).)

In addition to hypofrontality, adolescents with early-onset illness showed significantly higher metabolic rates in the region of the supramarginal gyrus (parietal region of plane B) and in the inferior frontal gyrus/insula (posterior frontal region of plane E) than did the controls. The hypermetabolism in the region of the inferior frontal gyrus/insula was similar to that seen in a subgroup of schizophrenic adults with poor CPT performance, whose "hits" (correct responses) were comparable to those of the childhood-onset sample, although they made fewer false alarm errors.

Because of technical failures during the childhood-onset study, performance data were available for only 13 schizophrenic and 20 control subjects, although all subjects performed the task. For the subgroups for whom CPT data were available, schizophrenic patients had significantly fewer CPT hits (correct button presses) and significantly more CPT false alarms (incorrect button presses) than did healthy controls. When the metabolic data were analyzed for the subgroups for whom performance data were available, all diagnostic differences were lost except for the posterior frontal region of plane E, where the patients had elevated metabolic rates.

Within the childhood-onset schizophrenic group, CPT false alarm rate was negatively correlated with CMRGlu for the right parietal (supramarginal) region on plane B ($r = 0.62$, $p < 0.05$) and the region of the right inferior frontal gyrus/insula ($r = 0.57$, $p < 0.05$). In controls, these same correlations were positive and significant for the right supramarginal region ($r = 0.73$, $p < 0.01$) and failed to reach significance for the inferior frontal gyrus/insula. Therefore, the hypermetabolic findings may reflect greater cognitive effort being expended by the patients in order to attend and perform, albeit poorly.

In contrast to the ROI-based analysis, the SPM analysis failed to reveal any regions of hypometabolism in schizo-

■ Schizophrenics < controls   ▨ Schizophrenics > controls

(a) 16 Childhood-onset schizophrenics, 26 matched controls

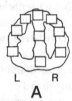 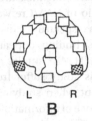 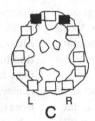 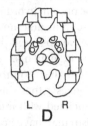 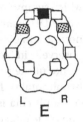

(b) 16 Later-onset schizophrenics, 27 matched controls

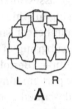 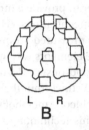 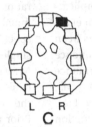 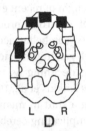 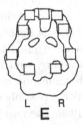

Fig. 11.1. Comparison of region-of-interest results of glucose metabolic studies of (a) 16 patients with childhood-onset schizophrenia studied by Jacobsen et al. (1997) and (b) 16 adult-onset schizophrenics studied by Cohen et al. (1987). Both childhood- and adult-onset patients demonstrated reductions in frontal metabolism, relative to age-matched controls, while performing a Continuous Performance Task. Only the childhood-onset group demonstrated biparietal hypermetabolism. Plane A is the most superior slice and lies 94 mm above the canthomeatal (CM) line; plane B is 84 mm and plane C is 67 mm above the CM line. Plane D contains the basal ganglia and thalamus and is 53 mm above the CM line. Plane E contains the lower frontal and temporal lobes and is 40 mm above the CM line. L, left, R, right.

phrenia but rather identified several hypermetabolic foci. The SPM method revealed increased metabolic rates in a region of the right pre/postcentral gyrus (Brodmann area 4/6), the left insula, the left inferior frontal gyrus (Brodmann area 47), and bilaterally in the cerebellum, a region not examined in the Cohen et al. (1987) study. The increase in bilateral cerebellar metabolic rate remained significant when the analysis was repeated after excluding the three schizophrenic subjects who had the most movement artifact, identified by visual inspection of PET scans prior to transforming them into standard stereotactic space. Subsequent ROI sampling of the left and right cerebellum from one slice (corresponding to level 0°12, atlas of Matsui and Hirano (1978) confirmed the bilateral hypermetabolism observed for this region.

Hypofrontality was demonstrated only when using the ROI-based approach, while cerebellar hypermetabolism was demonstrated with both data analytic approaches. While the pixel-based approach theoretically permits more refined localization, particularly when comparing different conditions within subjects, its accuracy may be compromised by deviations in brain anatomy associated with psychiatric disorder (schizophrenia, attention-deficit disorder) and/or with normal brain development, as well as by the need to interpolate to fill datapoints lying between the acquired slices. Because only the ROI-based analysis was used in the adult schizophrenia study, age-related comparisons are, of necessity, limited to this approach.

While the similarities in results for the childhood- and the adult-onset samples generated using the ROI-based analysis suggest a final common pathophysiology, the available data failed to suggest a straightforward relationship between the earlier onset of symptoms and the severity of neurodevelopmental lesion effects. An important limitation of this study, which may bear upon the relatively weak hypofrontality observed in the schizophrenic patients, was the inclusion of 19 siblings of subjects with ADHD as pediatric controls. Decreased frontal metabolism has been observed in both adults and adolescents with

ADHD (Zametkin et al., 1990; Ernst et al., 1994), albeit inconsistently (Ernst et al., 1997). While none of the controls in the present study met DSM criteria (American Psychiatric Association, 1994) for current or previous ADHD and all were older than the maximum age before which symptoms must be present in order to be diagnosed with ADHD, any decrease in frontal metabolism in these normal subjects would have obscured the hypofrontality observed in schizophrenic patients. Nonetheless, the failure of the pixel-based analysis to provide evidence of hypofrontality further suggests that this severe form of schizophrenia is not associated with more severe reductions in frontal metabolism than have been seen with PET in adult-onset schizophrenia.

The finding of cerebellar hypermetabolism in childhood-onset schizophrenia, seen with both data analytic approaches, is notable in light of recent evidence implicating the cerebellum in higher cortical processes (Kim et al., 1994). In healthy subjects, cerebellar activation has been demonstrated during verb generation and motor sequence learning, with activation declining as task performance became more automatic (Jenkins et al., 1994; Raichle et al., 1994), possibly reflecting a shift in mental strategy (Fiez, 1996). Previous reports implicating cerebellar dysfunction in schizophrenia include one report of decreased cerebellar metabolism in medicated adult patients studied at rest (Volkow et al., 1992) and one report of greater increases in cerebellar blood flow during cognitive task performance in schizophrenic adults (Steinberg at al., 1995). More recently, dysfunction of a prefrontal–thalamic–cerebellar network in schizophrenia was suggested by findings of reduced blood flow in these regions during practiced and novel memory tasks (Andreasen et al., 1996). These reports, together with observations from the present study, suggest that abnormal neural circuitry in schizophrenia involves the cerebellum, with the increase in cerebellar metabolism possibly resulting from failure of patients to shift to less effortful, more automatic strategies for performing the CPT.

Functional brain imaging: proton MRS

As with other functional imaging modalities, few previous ^{1}H MRS studies have been conducted in childhood-onset schizophrenia. Thomas and colleagues (1996) conducted a ^{1}H MRS study of 10 children with schizophrenia and 12 healthy controls in which ^{1}H spectra were measured in frontal gray matter bilaterally and in occipital gray matter. As has been observed in adult-onset schizophrenia (Bertolino et al., 1996, 1998a,b), the ratio of NAA/Cre was significantly lower in the frontal lobes of the schizophrenic children. There were no group differences in metabolite ratios in the occipital gray matter, suggesting some regional specificity for the frontal finding. Brooks and colleagues (1998) conducted a ^{1}H MRS study in children with schizophrenia spectrum symptoms (mean age 11 years) in which ^{1}H spectra were measured in the left frontal lobe. A decreased ratio of NAA/Cre was found for patients with schizophrenia spectrum disorder in this location. Although this finding appears to be consistent with findings from ^{1}H MRS studies of adult schizophrenia, the data from this study suffer from the lack of diagnostic clarity inherent when studying spectrum disorders and from the absence of information about metabolite ratios in other brain regions in these patients.

The above ^{1}H MRS studies of pediatric schizophrenia measured ^{1}H spectra from a small number of large voxels, precluding an adequate assessment of regional metabolite ratios. In order to provide a more thorough assessment of metabolite concentrations, ^{1}H MRS imaging in which ^{1}H spectra were measured from a large number of small single-volume elements was applied to a subgroup of the NIMH childhood-onset schizophrenia sample (Bertolino et al., 1998c) distinct from the subsample participating in the cerebral glucose metabolism study described above. Prior use of this technique to study patients with adult-onset schizophrenia demonstrated low levels of NAA in the hippocampal area and the dorsolateral prefrontal cortex, findings that were independent of treatment and consistent with developmental neuronal pathology (Bertolino et al., 1998a,b). Consequently, it was of major interest whether there were similarities in neurochemical patterns, as well as potential differences in the magnitude of any abnormalities, seen in childhood- versus adult-onset schizophrenia.

In this ^{1}H MRS imaging study, 14 children and adolescents (mean age $\pm$ SD 16.4 $\pm$ 1.7; 11 males) with childhood-onset schizophrenia and 14 healthy children and adolescents matched for sex and age (mean age 16.1 $\pm$ 2.1 years) were examined. All patients were on antipsychotic medication at the time of scanning. Exclusion criteria for both groups included a history of significant head injury, alcohol or drug abuse, and serious medical/neurologic illness. Multiple slice ^{1}H MRS imaging was performed on a conventional 1.5 T MR imaging system equipped with self-shielded gradients, using the method of Duyn et al. (1993) as modified by Bertolino and colleagues (1996, 1998a,b). The volume of brain to be included in the slices was chosen from a set of T_1-weighted 3 mm thick oblique axial images acquired in a plane parallel to the angle of the sylvian fissure, which maximized the cross-sectional profile of the hippocampus. Phase-encoding procedures were used to obtain a 32 × 32 array of spectra from volume elements in

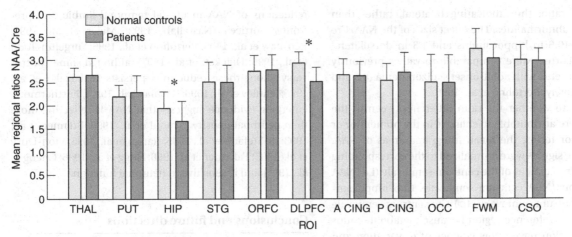

Fig. 11.2. Mean regional ratios of *N*-acetyl-containing compounds (NAA) to creatine plus phosphocreatine (Cre) for 14 patients with childhood-onset schizophrenia and 14 age- and sex-matched normal controls. Schizophrenic patients demonstrated regionally specific reductions in NAA/Cre ratios in the hippocampal regions and dorsolateral prefrontal cortex (*$p < 0.05$). THAL, thalamus; PUT, putamen; HIP, hippocampal area; STG, superior temporal gyrus; ORFC, orbitofrontal cortex; DLPFC, dorsolateral prefrontal cortex; A CING and P CING, anterior and posterior cingulate, respectively; OCC, occipital cortex; FWM, prefrontal white matter; CSO, centrum semiovale.

each selected slice. Each volume element (voxel) had nominal dimensions of 7.5 mm × 7.5 mm × 15 mm (0.84 ml). The ^{1}H MRS imaging sequence involved a spin-echo slice selection with repetition time (TR) of 2200 ms and echo time (TE) of 272 ms and included suppression of water and most of the signal arising from lipids in skull marrow and in surface tissues. The total length of the procedure was approximately 1 h. Foam padding was used to stabilize subjects' heads.

The raw ^{1}H MRS imaging data were processed by first locating the NAA, Cho, and Cre peaks for all voxels. Voxels in which these metabolite signals could not be identified (e.g., voxels located outside the head and on or near the skull's surface) were manually nulled. The signal strength in a range of 0.2 parts per million around the NAA, Cho, and Cre signal positions was integrated to produce four 32 × 32 arrays of metabolite signals corresponding to the four brain sections from which spectra were acquired. Obtaining absolute metabolite concentrations necessitates controlling for a number of additional variables, including field inhomogeneities, eddy current artifacts, and changes in metabolite T_1 and T_2 relaxation times owing to pathology, which would require significant additional scan time. Because total scan time had to be limited to what could be tolerated by this clinical population, metabolite signals were reported as ratios of the area under each peak: NAA/Cre, NAA/Cho and Cho/Cre.

A rater blind to diagnosis manually drew ROIs on the T_1-weighted coaxial MR images and then transferred them to the same location on the metabolite maps. These ROIs were drawn with reference to standard anatomic atlases (Talaraich and Tournoux 1988; Duvernoy and Cabanis, 1991) bilaterally in the hippocampal area, dorsolateral prefrontal cortex, superior temporal gyrus, orbitofrontal cortex, occipital cortex, anterior and posterior cingulate, centrum semiovale, prefrontal white matter, thalamus and putamen as described in Bertolino et al. (1996). Voxels that were contained within the anatomic ROI, but not present on the metabolite maps, were removed. Consequently, the final calculations were performed only on voxels containing ^{1}H spectra (approximately 700 voxels per study). A computer program calculated the average value of the area under each peak in all voxels within the ROIs on the metabolite maps.

A three-dimensional MRI dataset was also acquired to permit manual measurement of hippocampal and prefrontal lobe volumes to provide anatomic data to correlate with the ^{1}H MRS imaging data (Bertolino et al., 1996, 1998a). A physician also rated each patient at the time of scanning for positive and negative symptoms using the SAPS (Scale for the Assessment of Positive Symptoms), SANS, and BPRS (Brief Psychiatric Rating Scale).

As illustrated in Figs. 11.2 and 11.3 (p. 242), patients showed a significant bilateral reduction of NAA/Cre in the hippocampus ($p < 0.05$) and dorsolateral prefrontal cortex ($p < 0.04$) relative to their controls. There were no group differences for Cho/Cre for these regions. There was a trend for NAA/Cho to be reduced in the dorsolateral prefrontal cortex ($p < 0.06$). There was no main effect of hemisphere or interaction of diagnosis by hemisphere for any metabolite ratio, thus indicating bilateral, rather than lateralized, abnormalities. The effect sizes of the NAA/Cre reductions (0.6 in hippocampus and 1.3 in dorsolateral prefrontal cortex) were comparable to values previously found in patients with adult-onset schizophrenia (0.5 and 1.3, respectively; Bertolino et al., 1996).

To evaluate whether the ratio differences seen in the patients were attributable to changes in the numerator or denominator terms, the mean integrated areas of NAA, Cho and Cre signals were normalized to the corresponding mean integrated areas of the centrum semiovale (i.e., NAA hippocampus/NAA centrum semiovale, Cho hippocampus/Cho centrum semiovale, etc.) The centrum semiovale was used as a reference region because metabolite ratios from this region have a low coefficient of variation and because this region has not been implicated in the pathophysiology of schizophrenia (Bertolino et al., 1998b). Analysis of these normalized metabolite ratios showed a trend for NAA to be reduced bilaterally in the hippocampus ($p < 0.06$) and a reduction of NAA in the dorsolateral prefrontal cortex ($p < 0.1$). As in previous studies of patients with adult-onset schizophrenia (Bertolino et al., 1996, 1998a,b), no differences were found for Cho, which can be influenced by several physiologic, pharmacologic (Satlin et al., 1997), and pathologic processes, including neurodegenerative disease (Brenner et al., 1993; Gadian et al., 1994; Hetherington et al., 1995). Neither were differences found for Cre. The metabolite ratio differences observed between patients and healthy subjects in the childhood-onset schizophrenia study primarily reflected differences in NAA, a marker of neuronal integrity. The observation of reduced NAA in conjunction with normal Cho may imply the presence of neuronal damage unaccompanied by gliosis, such as might occur with a neurodevelopmental defect.

The NAA reductions were not found to be related to anatomic deviations nor to a number of clinical variables. Correlations between the volumes of the hippocampus and of the prefrontal lobe and the metabolite ratios in these regions were not significant (all r values were between 0.14 and 0.32). Correlations with symptoms, as measured by rating scales, and other clinical variables (age, age at onset of disease, current dose and years of treatment with neuroleptic drugs, and length of illness) failed to reveal significant relationships (all r values between 0.33 and 0.40). These findings suggest that the NAA reductions seen in schizophrenia are not related to progressive pathology, further reinforcing the likelihood that they reflect developmental neuropathology.

These MRS imaging findings are consistent with earlier findings in patients with adult-onset schizophrenia of reductions of NAA in mesial temporal limbic and prefrontal cortices (Nasrallah, 1993; Maier et al., 1995; Renshaw et al., 1995; Bertolino et al., 1996; Yurgelun-Todd et al., 1996; Deicken et al., 1997), although some controversy about these reductions persists (Fukuzako et al., 1995; Stanley et al., 1996; Bartha et al., 1997). Furthermore, emerging evidence suggests that NAA is reflecting more than neuronal density (Arnold et al., 1990; Brenner et al., 1993; de Stefano et al., 1995; Rango et al., 1995; Vion-Dury et al., 1995; Falconer et al. 1996; Hugg et al., 1996; Cheng et al., 1997) and is sensitive to neuronal function.

Conclusions and future directions

The functional imaging studies described in this chapter are among the first to be conducted in childhood-onset schizophrenia and provide valuable evidence that the underlying pathophysiology in this disorder is similar to that in adult-onset schizophrenia. Studies of regional CBF and glucose metabolism have provided evidence of task-related hypofrontality in early-onset disease, consistent with findings in adult schizophrenia. A comparison of glucose metabolism in childhood- and adult-onset schizophrenia using similar methods has revealed generally equivalent degrees of hypofrontality during the performance of an attentional task. MRS imaging findings in childhood-onset schizophrenia are consistent both for the extent and the localizaton of differences with earlier studies of patients with adult-onset schizophrenia that showed regionally specific reductions of NAA in mesial temporolimbic and prefrontal cortices suggestive of neuronal involvement in these areas. Overall, emerging neuroimaging findings support the hypothesis of a common pathophysiologic process specifically affecting mesial temporolimbic and prefrontal circuitries in patients with childhood- and adult-onset schizophrenia.

While these data suggest a similar pathophysiology for childhood- and adult-onset schizophrenia, the limited data available fail to suggest a straightforward relationship between the earlier onset of symptoms and the severity of effects of any neurodevelopmental lesion. Comparable effect sizes seen in both the PET study of CMRGlu and the MRS study fail to indicate greater brain-related abnormalities in early-onset schizophrenia. Limitations in statistical power, age differences in the childhood- and adult-onset samples, and/or differences in the control groups may have contributed to the failure to find such effects.

The failure to find more pronounced abnormalities in functional imaging studies of childhood-onset schizophrenia may seem inconsistent with the longitudinal structural MRI studies of the NIMH childhood-onset schizophrenia study described earlier in this chapter, which reported progressive reductions in the volume of temporal and mesial-temporal structures (including the hippocampus), the midsagittal thalamic area, and the whole brain, together with a progressive increase in the size of the ventricles (Rapoport et al., 1997; Jacobsen et al., 1998). However, patients in the MRS study were, on average, 2 years older than those participating in the PET study and those entering the longitudinal MRI study. The longitudinal MRI study of the NIMH sample has shown that the above-mentioned brain structures are changing more rapidly than is normal during the period from 14 to 16 years of age. If structural changes are associated with changes in function, the MRS study completed when adolescents with schizophrenia were, on average, 16.4 years old may have reflected such changes, leading to the observation of abnormalities similar to those seen in adult-onset schizophrenia. In contrast, the PET study, performed when patients were, on average, 14.2 years old, may have been conducted prior to the occurrence of these brain functional changes, thus resulting in a failure to observe more robust hypofrontality. Other factors possibly contributing to the minor inconsistency in findings from these two studies include the study of medicated patients in the MRS imaging study and unmedicated patients in the PET study and the use of siblings of patients with ADHD as normal controls in the FDG study. Finally, the two methods may be sensitive to different dimensions of pathology.

While the timing of brain-related changes in schizophrenia require further study, the findings discussed in this chapter suggest a window of progressive changes in brain morphology, and possibly physiology, that occur before the age of 16. Future functional brain imaging studies of patients with childhood-onset schizophrenia should focus on studying patients prior to and within this window. Ideally, future studies should employ longitudinal designs and include subjects between the ages of 7 and 18 years. Such data would provide invaluable information about the precise role of neurodevelopment in the symptoms and accompanying abnormalities of brain function observed in schizophrenia. The study of younger patients may elucidate the causes of the unusually early onset of illness.

Special challenges inherent in performing research with patients with childhood-onset schizophrenia include obtaining valid consent and assent, reducing movement during scanning, and significantly poorer performance of activation tasks than that achieved by healthy controls.

Minors participating in any research and their parents need to understand potential risks and discomforts associated with the research before providing assent and consent, respectively, for participation. Procedures, risks and discomforts should be described in simple language.

Patients with childhood-onset schizophrenia tend to move during scanning, which compromises image quality. The use of simulated scanning prior to data collection may improve the ability of these patients to remain still and, thus, enhance the quality of acquired data. To the best of our knowledge, there are no reports to date on the effectiveness of exposing psychotic children to a simulated scanning experience prior to their participating in an actual functional imaging experiment. However, Rosenberg and colleagues (1997) have demonstrated that simulated scanning prior to actual scanning reduces anxiety during actual scanning in children with obsessive-compulsive disorder.

The same factors that lead to increased movement during scanning on the part of patients with childhood-onset schizophrenia can also interfere with the performance of activation tasks, leading to significant group differences in task performance. As with studies of adults with schizophrenia, children and adolescents with schizophrenia may incorporate the experiment into their delusional system and/or be actively hallucinating during the experimental procedure, particularly if the study is performed during medication washout. While the presence of a parent or trusted adult during the procedure often helps, some patients may be unable to complete the study. The tradeoffs between maintaining patients on medication to optimize task performance and facilitate cooperation must be balanced against the introduction of potential artifacts resulting from psychotropic medications, with decisions depending, in part, on the specific hypotheses to be tested.

Despite the difficulties encountered in applying functional neuroimaging techniques to the study of childhood-onset schizophrenia, there is much to be gained from such an endeavor. Improvements in technology that decrease scanning time and increase the child friendliness of the scanning environment may help to overcome some of the limitations associated with severe psychotic illness. Further study, particularly employing longitudinal designs, may elucidate the developmental course of brain-related changes that contribute to early symptoms, both typical and atypical, and their evolution into adult-like schizophrenic illness. Such mapping of developmental brain changes may provide a window through which to view precursors to more typical adult-onset psychosis as well.

References

Abi-Dargham, A., Laruelle, M., Aghajanian, G. K., Charney, D. and Krystal, J. (1997). The role of serotonin in the pathophysiology and treatment of schizophrenia. *J. Neuropsychiatry Clin. Neurosci.*, **9**, 1–17.

Abi-Dargham, A., Gil, R., Krystal, J. et al. (1998). Increased striatal dopamine transmission in schizophrenia: confirmation in a second cohort. *Am. J. Psychiatry*, **155**, 761–7.

Alaghband-Rad, J., McKenna, K., Gordon, C. T. et al. (1995). Childhood-onset schizophrenia: the severity of premorbid course. *J. Am. Acad. Child Adolesc. Psychiatry*, **34**, 1273–83.

Altshuler, L. L., Casanova, M. F., Goldberg, T. E. and Kleinman, J. E. (1990). The hippocampus and parahippocampus in schizophrenic, suicide and control brains. *Arch. Gen. Psychiatry*, **47**, 1029–34.

American Psychiatric Association (1994). *Diagnostic and Statistical Manual of Mental Disorders*, 4th edn (DSM-IV). Washington, DC: American Psychiatric Association.

Andreasen, N. C. (1983). *Scale for the Assessment of Negative Symptoms (SANS)*. Iowa City, IA: The University of Iowa.

Andreasen N. C., Nasrallah H. A., Dunn, V. et al. (1986). Structural abnormalities in the frontal system in schizophrenia: a magnetic resonance imaging study. *Arch. Gen. Psychiatry*, **43**, 136–44.

Andreasen, N. C., Rezai, K., Alliger, R. et al. (1992). Hypofrontality in neuroleptic-naive patients and in patients with chronic schizophrenia: assessment with xenon 133 single-photon emission computed tomography and the Tower of London. *Arch. Gen. Psychiatry*, **49**, 943–58.

Andreasen N. C., Arndt, S., Swayze, V. et al. (1994a). Thalamic abnormalities in schizophrenia visualized through magnetic resonance image averaging. *Science*, **266**, 294–7.

Andreasen, N. C., Flashman, L., Flaum, M. et al. (1994b). Regional brain abnormalities in schizophrenia measured with magnetic resonance imaging. *J. Am. Med. Assoc.*, **272**, 1763–9.

Andreasen, N. C., O'Leary, D. S., Cizadlo, T., Arndt, S., Rezai, K., Ponto, L. L., Watkins, G. L. and Hichwa, R. D. (1996). Schizophrenia and cognitive dysmetria: a positron-emission tomography study of dysfunctional prefrontal-thalamic-cerebellar circuitry. *Proc. Natl. Acad. Sci. USA*, **93**, 9985–90.

Arnold D. L., Matthews, P. M., Francis, G. and Antel, J. (1990). Proton magnetic resonance spectroscopy of human brain in vivo in the evaluation of multiple sclerosis: assessment of the load of disease. *Magn. Reson. Med.*, **14**, 154–9.

Arnold, S. E., Hyman, B. T., van Hoesen, G. W. and Damasio, A. R. (1991). Some cytoarchitectural abnormalities of the entorhinal cortex in schizophrenia. *Arch. Gen. Psychiatry*, **48**, 625–32.

Asarnow, R. F., Brown, W. and Strandburg, R. (1995). Children with a schizophrenic disorder: neurobehavioral studies. *Eur. Arch. Psychiatry Clin. Neurosci.*, **245**, 70–9.

Barker, P. B., Breiter, S. N., Soher, B. J. et al. (1994). Quantitative proton spectroscopy of canine brain: in vivo and in vitro correlations. *Magn. Reson. Med.*, **32**, 157–63.

Bartha, R., Williamson, P. C., Drost, D. J. et al. (1997). Measurement of glutamate and glutamine in the medial prefrontal cortex of never treated schizophrenic patients and healthy controls by proton magnetic resonance spectroscopy. *Arch. Gen. Psychiatry*, **54**, 959–65.

Benes, F. M., Wickramasinghe, R., Vincent, S. L., Khan, Y. and Todtenkopf, M. (1997). Uncoupling of GABA(A) and benzodiazepine receptor binding activity in the hippocampal formation of schizophrenic brain. *Brain Res.*, **755**, 121–9.

Berman, K. F., Torrey, E. F., Daniel, D. G. and Weinberger, D. R. (1992). Regional cerebral blood flow in monozygotic twins discordant and concordant for schizophrenia. *Arch. Gen. Psychiatry*, **49**, 927–34.

Bertolino, A., Nawroz, S., Mattay V. S. et al. (1996). A specific pattern of neurochemical pathology in schizophrenia as assessed by multislice proton magnetic resonance spectroscopic imaging. *Am. J. Psychiatry*, **153**, 1554–63.

Bertolino, A., Saunders, R. C., Mattay, V. S., Bachevalier, J., Frank, J. A. and Weinberger, D. R. (1997). Proton magnetic resonance spectroscopic imaging in monkeys with mesial temporolimbic lesions. *Cereb. Cortex*, **7**, 740–8.

Bertolino, A., Callicott, J. H., Elman, et al. (1998a). Regionally specific neuronal pathology in untreated patients with schizophrenia: a proton magnetic resonance spectroscopic imaging study. *Biol. Psychiatry*, **43**, 641–8.

Bertolino, A., Callicott, J. H., Nawroz, S. et al. (1998b). Reproducibility of proton magnetic resonance spectroscopic imaging in patients with schizophrenia. *Neuropsychopharmacology*, **18**, 11–19.

Bogerts, B., Ashtari, M., Degreef, G., Alvir, J. M. J., Bilder, R. M. and Lieberman, J. A. (1990a). Reduced temporal limbic structure volumes on magnetic resonance images in first episode schizophrenia. *Psychiatry Res.* **35**, 1–13.

Bogerts, B., Falkai, P., Haupts, M. et al. (1990b). Post-mortem volume measurements of limbic system and basal ganglia structures in chronic schizophrenics: initial results from a new brain collection. *Schizophr. Res.*, **3**, 295–301.

Bogerts, B., Lieberman, J. A., Ashtari, M. et al. (1993). Hippocampus-amygdala volumes and psychopathology in chronic schizophrenia. *Biol. Psychiatry*, **33**, 236–46.

Breier, A., Buchanan, R. W., Elkashef, A., Munson, R. C., Kirkpatrick, B., Cellad, F. (1992). Brain morphology and schizophrenia. A magnetic resonance imaging study of limbic prefrontal cortex and caudate structures. *Arch. Gen. Psychiatry*, **49**, 921–6.

Brenner, R. E., Munro, P. M.G., Williams, S.C.R. et al. (1993). The proton NMR spectrum in acute EAE: the significance of the change in the Cho:Cre ratio, *Magn. Reson. Med.*, **29**, 737–45.

Brooks, R. A. (1982). Alternative formula for glucose utilization using labeled deoxyglucose. *J. Nucl. Med.*, **23**, 538–9.

Brooks, W. M., Hodde Vargas, J., Vargas, L. A., Yeo, R. A., Ford, C. C. and Hendren, R. L. (1998). Frontal lobe of children with schizophrenia spectrum disorders: a proton magnetic resonance spectroscopic study. *Biol. Psychiatry*, **43**, 263–9.

Brozowski, T. J., Brown, R. M., Rosvold, H. E. and Goldman, P. S. (1979). Cognitive deficit caused by regional depletion of dopamine in prefrontal cortex of rhesus monkey. *Science*, **205**, 929–32.

Buchsbaum, M. S., DeLisi, L. E., Holcomb, H. H. et al. (1984).

Anteroposterior gradients in cerebral glucose use in schizophrenia and affective disorders. *Arch. Gen. Psychiatry.* **41**, 1159–66.

Buckley, P. F., Moore, C., Long, H. et al. (1994). ¹H Magnetic resonance spectroscopy of the left temporal and frontal lobes in schizophrenia: clinical neurodevelopmental and cognitive correlates. *Biol. Psychiatry,* **36**, 792–800.

Chabrol, H., Guell, A., Bes, A. and Moron, P. (1986). Cerebral blood flow in schizophrenic adolescents. [Letter to the Editor] *Am. J. Psychiatry,* **143**, 130.

Chakos, M. H., Lieberman, J. A., Alvir, J., Bilder, R. and Ashtari, M. (1995). Caudate nuclei volumes in schizophrenic patients treated with typical antipsychotics or clozapine. *Lancet,* **345**, 456–7.

Cheng, L. L., Ma, M. J., Becerra, L. et al. (1997). Quantitative neuropathology by high resolution magic angle spinning proton magnetic resonance spectroscopy. *Proc. Natl. Acad. Sci. USA,* **94**, 6408–13.

Chua, S. E. and McKenna, P. J. (1995). Schizophrenia – a brain disease? A critical review of structural and functional cerebral abnormality in the disorder. *Br. J. Psychiatry,* **166**, 563–82.

Cohen, R. M., Semple, W. E., Gross, M. et al. (1987). Dysfunction in a prefrontal substrate of sustained attention in schizophrenia. *Life Sci.* **40**, 2031–9.

Creese, I., Burt, D. R. and Snyder, S. H. (1976). Dopamine receptor binding predicts clinical and pharmacological potencies of antischizophrenic drugs. *Science,* **192**, 481–3.

Deicken, R. F., Zhou, L., Corwin, F., Vinogradov, S. and Weiner, M. W. (1997). Decreased left frontal lobe N-Acetylaspartate in schizophrenia. *Am. J. Psychiatry,* **154**, 688–90.

DeLisi, L. E., Buchsbaum, M. S., Holcomb, H. H. et al. (1985). Clinical correlates of decreased anteroposterior metabolic gradients in positron emission tomography (PET) of schizophrenic patients. *Am. J. Psychiatry.* **142**, 78–81.

de Stefano, N., Matthews, P. M. and Arnold, D. L. (1995). Reversible decreases in N-acetylaspartate after acute brain injury. *Magn. Reson. Med.,* **34**, 721–7.

Done, D. J., Crow, T. L., Johnstone, E. C. and Sacker, A. (1994). Childhood antecedents of schizophrenia and affective illness: social adjustment at ages 7 and 11. *BMJ,* **309**, 599–703.

Duvernoy, H. M. and Cabanis, E. A. (1991). *The Human Brain Surface, Three-dimensional Sectional Anatomy, and MRI.* New York: Springer-Verlag.

Duyn, J. H., Gillen, J., Sobering, G., van Zijl, P. C. and Moonen C.T.W. (1993). Multisection proton MR spectroscopic imaging of the brain. *Radiology,* **188**, 277–82.

Ebmeier, K. P., Lawrie, S. M., Blackwood, D. H. R., Johnstone, E. C. and Goodwin, G. M. (1995). Hypofrontality revisited: a high resolution single photon emission computed tomography study in schizophrenia. *J. Neurol. Neurosurg. Psychiatry,* **58**, 452–6.

Ernst, M., Liebenauer, L. L., King, A. C., Fitzgerald, G. A., Cohen, R. M. and Zametkin, A. J. (1994). Reduced brain metabolism in hyperactive girls. *J. Am. Acad. Child Adolesc. Psychiatry,* **33**, 858–68.

Ernst, M., Cohen, R. M., Liebenauer, L. L., Jons, P. H. and Zametkin,

A. J. (1997). Cerebral glucose metabolism in adolescent girls with attention deficit/hyperactivity disorder. *J. Am. Acad. Child Adolesc. Psychiatry,* **36**, 1399–1406.

Falconer, J. C., Liu, S. J., Abbe, R. A. and Narayana, P. A. (1996). Time dependence of N-acetyl-aspartate, lactate, and pyruvate concentrations following spinal cord injury. *J. Neurochem.,* **66**, 717–22.

Falkai, P. and Bogerts, B. (1986). Cell loss in the hippocampus of schizophrenics. *Eur. Arch. Psychiatry Neurol. Sci.,* **236**, 154–61.

Feinberg, I. (1982). Schizophrenia: caused by a fault in programmed synaptic elimination during adolescence? *J. Psychiatr. Res.,* **17**, 319–34.

Fiez, J. A. (1996). Cerebellar contributions to cognition. *Neuron,* **16**, 13–15.

Findling, R. L., Friedman, L., Buck, J. et al. (1996). Hippocampal volume in adolescent schizophrenia. *Schizophr. Res.,* **18**, 185.

Flaum, M., Swayze, V. W., O'Leary, D. S. et al. (1995). Brain morphology in schizophrenia: effects of diagnosis, laterality and gender. *Am. J. Psychiatry,* **152**, 704–14.

Frazier, J. A., Giedd, J. N., Kaysen, D. et al. (1996). Brain magnetic resonance imaging rescan after two years of clozapine maintenance. *Am. J. Psychiatry,* **153**, 564–6.

Friedman, L., Findling, R. L., Buch, J. et al. (1996). Structural MRI and neuropsychological assessments in adolescent patients with either schizophrenia or affective disorders. *Schizophr. Res.,* **18**, 189–90.

Friston, K. J., Frith, C. D., Liddle, P. F. and Frackowiak, R. S. J. (1991). Comparing functional (PET) images: the assessment of significant change. *J. Cereb. Blood Flow Metab.,* **11**, 690–9.

Friston, K. J., Worsley, K. J., Frackowiak, R. S. J., Mazziotta, J. C. and Evans, A. C. (1994). Assessing the significance of focal activations using their spatial extent. *Hum. Brain Map.,* **1**, 210–20.

Fukuzako, H., Takeuchi, K., Hokazono, Y. et al. (1995). Proton magnetic resonance spectroscopy of the left medial temporal and frontal lobes in chronic schizophrenia: preliminary report. *Psychiatry Res. Neuroimaging,* **61**, 193–200.

Fuster, J. M. and Alexander, G. E. (1971). Neuron activity related to short term memory. *Science,* **173**, 652–4.

Gadian, D. G., Connelly, A., Duncan, J. S. et al. (1994). ¹H magnetic resonance spectroscopy in the investigation of intractable epilepsy. *Acta Neurol. Scand. Suppl.* **152**, 116–21.

Giedd, J. N., Castellanos, F. X., Rajapakse, J. C. et al. (1996). Quantitative analysis of gray matter volumes in childhood-onset schizophrenia and attention deficit/hyperactivity disorder. *Soc. Neurosci. Abst.,* **22**, 1166.

Goldman, P. S. (1974). An alternative to developmental plasticity: heterology of CNS structure in infants and adults. In *Plasticity and Recovery of Function in the Central Nervous System,* eds. D. G. Stein, J. J. Rosen and N. Butters, pp. 149–74. New York: Academic Press.

Goldman, P. S. and Alexander, G. E. (1977). Maturation of prefrontal cortex in the monkey revealed by local reversible cryogenic depression, *Nature,* **267**, 613–15.

Goldman-Rakic, P. S. (1987). Circuitry of primate prefrontal cortex and regulation of behavior by representational memory. In *Handbook of Physiology,* vol. 5, eds. V. B. Mountcastle, F. Plum and S. R. Geiger, pp. 373–417. Bethesda, MD: American Physiological Society.

Goldman-Rakic, P. S. (1991). Prefrontal cortical dysfunction in schizophrenia: the relevance of working memory. In *Psychopathology and the Brain*, eds. B. J. Carroll and J. E. Barrett, pp. 1–23. Hillsdale, NJ: Laurence Erlbaum.

Goldman-Rakic, P. S. (1994). Specification of higher cortical functions. In *Atypical Cognitive Deficits in Developmental Disorders: Implications for Brain Functions*, eds. S. H. and J. Grafman, pp. 3–17. Hillsdale NJ: Laurence Erlbaum.

Gordon, C. T., Frazier, J. A., McKenna, K. et al. (1994). Childhood-onset schizophrenia: an NIMH study in progress. *Schizophr. Bull.*, **20**, 697–712.

Harvey, I., Ron, M. A., Du Boulay, G., Wicks, D., Lewis, S. W. and Murray, R. M. (1993). Reduction of cortical volume in schizophrenia on magnetic resonance imaging. *Psychol. Med.*, **23**, 591–604.

Hetherington, H., Kuzniecky, R., Pan, J. et al. (1995). Proton nuclear magnetic resonance spectroscopic imaging of human temporal lobe epilepsy at 4.1 T. *Ann. Neurol.*, **38**, 396–404.

Hollis, C. (1995). Child and adolescent (juvenile onset) schizophrenia: a case control study of premorbid developmental impairments. *Br. J. Psychiatry*, **166**, 489–95.

Hugg, J. W., Kuzniecky, R. I., Gilliam, F. G., Morawetz, R. B. and Hetherington, H. P. (1996). Normalization of contralateral metabolic function following temporal lobectomy demonstrated by ^{1}H magnetic resonance spectroscopic imaging. *Ann. Neurol.*, **40**, 236–9.

Jacobsen, L. K. and Rapoport, J. L. (1998). Childhood onset schizophrenia; implications of clinical and neurobiological research. *J. Child Psychol. Psychiatr. Allied Disciplines*, **39**, 101–13.

Jacobsen, L. K., Giedd, J. N., Vaituzis, A. C. et al. (1996a). Temporal lobe morphology in childhood onset schizophrenia. *Am. J. Psychiatry*, **153**, 355–61.

Jacobsen, L. K., Hong, W. L., Hommer, D. W. et al. (1996b). Smooth pursuit eye movements in childhood onset schizophrenia: comparison with ADHD and normal controls. *Biol. Psychiatry*, **40**, 1144–54.

Jacobsen, L.K., Hamburger, S. D., van Horn, J. D. et al. (1997). Cerebral glucose metabolism in childhood onset schizophrenia. *Psychiatr. Res. Neuroimaging*, **75**, 131–44.

Jacobsen, L. K., Giedd, J. N., Castellanos, F. X. et al. (1998). Progressive reduction of temporal lobe structures in childhood onset schizophrenia. *Am. J. Psychiatry*, **155**, 678–85.

Jakob, H. and Beckmann, H. (1989). Prenatal developmental disturbances in the limbic allocortex in schizophrenics. *J. Neural Transmission*, **65**, 303–26.

Jenkins, I., Brooks, D., Nixon, P., Frackowiak, R. and Passingham, R. (1994). Motor sequence learning: a study with positron emission tomography. *J. Neurosci.*, **14**, 3775–90.

Jernigan, T. L., Zisook, S., Heaton, R. K., Moranvile, J. T., Hesselink, J. R. and Braff, D. L. (1991). Magnetic resonance imaging abnormalities in lenticular nuclei and cerebral cortex in schizophrenia. *Arch. Gen. Psychiatry.*, **48**, 881–90.

Jeste, D. V. and Lohr, J. B. (1989). Hippocampal pathologic findings in schizophrenia: a morphometric study. *Arch. Gen. Psychiatry.* **46**, 1019–24.

Jones, P., Rodgers, B., Murray, R. and Marmot, M. (1994). Child developmental risk factors for adult schizophrenia in the British 1946 birth cohort. *Lancet*, **344**, 1398–1402.

Karno, M. and Norquist, G. S. (1989). Schizophrenia: epidemiology. In *Comprehensive Textbook of Psychiatry*, 5th edn, eds. H. I. Kaplan and B. J. Sadock, pp. 699–705. Baltimore, MD: Williams and Wilkins.

Kim, S. G., Ugurbil, K. and Strick, P. L. (1994). Activation of a cerebellar output nucleus during cognitive processing. *Science*, **265**, 949–51.

Kumra, S., Frazier, J. A., Jacobsen, L. K. et al. (1996). Childhood-onset schizophrenia: a double-blind clozapine-haloperidol comparison. *Arch. Gen. Psychiatry*, **53**, 1090–7.

Kumra, S., Briguglio, C., Lenane, M. et al. (1999). Including children and adolescents with schizophrenia in medication-free research. *Am. J. Psychiatry*, **156**, 1065–8.

Laruelle, M., Abi-Dargham, A., van Dyck, C. H. et al. (1996). Single photon emission computerized tomography imaging of amphetamine-induced dopamine release in drug-free schizophrenic subjects. *Proc. Natl. Acad. Sci. USA*, **93**, 9235–40.

Lillrank, S. M., Lipska, B. K., Bachus, S. E., Wood, G. K. and Weinberger, D. R. (1996). Amphetamine induced c-*fos* mRNA expression is altered in rats with neonatal ventral hippocampal damage. *Synapse*, **23**, 292–301.

Lim, K. O., Beal, D. M., Harvey, R. L. et al. (1995). Brain dysmorphology in adults with congenital rubella plus schizohrenia-like symptoms. *Biol. Psychiatry*, **37**, 764–76.

Lim, K. O., Harris, D., Beal, M. et al. (1996). Gray matter deficits in young onset schizophrenia are independent of age of onset. *Biol. Psychiatry*, **40**, 4–13.

Lipska, B. K. and Weinberger, D. R. (1995). Genetic variation in vulnerability to the behavioral effects of neonatal hippocampal damage in the rat. *Proc. Natl. Acad. Sci.*, **92**, 8906–10.

Lipska, B. K., Jaskiw, G. E. and Weinberger, D. R. (1993). Post pubertal emergence of hyperresponsiveness to stress and amphetamines after neonatal excitotoxic hippocampal damage, a potential animal model of schizophrenia. *Neuropsychopharmacology*, **9**, 67–75.

Lipska, B., Moghaddam, B., Sams-Dodd, F. and Weinberger, D. R. (1996). Neonatal hippocampal damage in the rat models negative symptoms of schizophrenia. *Abstracts from the American College of Neuropsychopharmacology*, p. 126. Washington, DC: American College of Neuropsychopharmacology.

Maier, M., Ron, M. A., Barker, G. J. and Tofts, P. S. (1995). Proton magnetic resonance spectroscopy: an in vivo method of estimating hippocampal neuronal depletion in schizophrenia. *Psychol. Med.*, **25**, 1201–9.

Marsh, L., Suddath, R. Higgins, N. and Weinberger, D. R. (1994). Medial temporal lobe structures in schizophrenia: relationship of size to duration illness. *Schizophr. Res.*, **11**, 225–38.

Matsui, T. and Hirano, A. (1978). *An Atlas of the Human Brain for Computerized Tomography*. Tokyo: Igaku Shoin.

Meltzer, H. Y. and Stahl, S. M. (1976). The dopamine hypothesis of schizophrenia: a review. *Schizophr. Bull.*, **2**, 19–76.

Miller, B. L. (1991). A review of chemical issues in ¹H NMR spectroscopy: N-acetyl-L-aspartate, creatine and choline. *NMR Biomed.*, **4**, 47–52.

Murray, R. M. (1994). Neurodevelopmental schizophrenia: the rediscovery of dementia praecox. *Br. J. Psychiatry*, **165**, 6–12.

Murray, R. M. and Lewis, S. W. (1987). Is schizophrenia a neurodevelopmental disorder? *BMJ*, **295**, 681–82.

Nasrallah, H. (1993). Neurodevelopmental pathogenesis of schizophrenia. *Psychiatr. Clin. North Am.*, **16**, 269–80.

Nasrallah, H. A., Skinner, T. E., Schmalbrock, P. and Robitaille, P. M. (1994). Proton magnetic resonance spectroscopy of the hippocampal formation in schizophrenia: a pilot study. *Brit. J. Psychiatry*, **165**, 481–5.

Raichle, M. E., Fiez, J. A., Videen, T. O. et al. (1994). Practice related changes in human brain functional anatomy during nonmotor learning. *Cereb. Cortex*, **4**, 8–26.

Rango, M., Spagnoli, D., Tomei, G., Bamonti, F., Scarlato, G. and Zetta, L. (1995). Central nervous system transsynaptic effects of acute axonal injury: a ¹H magnetic resonance spectroscopy study. *Magn. Reson. Med.*, **33**, 595–600.

Rapoport, J. L., Giedd, J., Kumra, S. et al. (1997). Childhood onset schizophrenia: progressive ventricular change during adolescence. *Arch. Gen. Psychiatry*, **54**, 897–903.

Remschmidt, H. E., Schulz, E., Martin, M., Warnke, A. and Trott, G. (1994). Childhood-onset schizophrenia: history of the concept and recent studies. *Schizophr. Bull.*, **20**, 727–45.

Renshaw, P. F., Yurgelun-Todd, D. A., Tohen, M., Gruber, S. and Cohen, B. M. (1995). Temporal lobe proton magnetic resonance spectroscopy of patients with first-episode psychosis. *Am. J. Psychiatry*, **152**, 444–6.

Rosenberg, D. R., Sweeney, J. A., Gillen, J. S. et al. (1997). Magnetic resonance imaging of children without sedation: preparation with simulation. *J. Am. Acad. Child Adolesc. Psychiatry*, **36**, 853–9.

Russell, A. T. (1994). The clinical presentation of childhood onset schizophrenia. *Schizophr. Bull.*, **20**, 631–46.

Russell, A. T., Bott, L. and Sammons, C. (1989). The phenomenology of schizophrenia occurring in childhood. *J. Am. Acad. Child Adolesc. Psychiatry*, **28**, 399–407.

Sams-Dodd, F., Lipska, B. and Weinberger, D. R. (1997). Neonatal lesions of the rat ventral hippocampus result in hyperlocomotion and deficits in the social behavior in adulthood. *Psychopharmachology*, **132**, 303–10.

Satlin, A., Bodick, N., Offen, W. W. and Renshaw, P. F. (1997). Brain proton magnetic resonance spectroscopy (¹HMRS) in Alzheimer's disease: changes after treatment with xanomeline, an M1 selective cholinergic agonist. *Am. J. Psychiatry*, **154**, 1459–61.

Schulz, S. C., Koller, M.M., Kishore, P. R., Hamer, R. M., Gehl, J. J. and Friedel, R, O. (1983). Ventricular enlargement in teenage patients with schizophrenia spectrum disorder. *Am. J. Psychiatry*, **140**, 1592–5.

Selemon, L. D., Rajkowska, G. and Goldman-Rakic, P. S. (1995). Abnormally high neuronal density in the schizophrenic cortex. A morphometric analysis of prefrontal area 9 and occipital area 17. *Arch. Gen. Psychiatry*, **52**, 805–18.

Siegel, B. V., Buchsbaum, M. S., Bunney, W. E. et al. (1993). Cortical-striatal-thalamic circuits and brain glucose metabolic activity in 70 unmedicated male schizophrenic patients. *Am. J. Psychiatry*, **150**, 1325–36.

Stanley, J. A., Williamson, P. C., Drost, D. J. et al. (1996). An in vivo proton magnetic resonance spectroscopy study of schizophrenia patients. *Schizophr. Bull.*, **22**, 597–609.

Steinberg, J. L., Devous, M. D., Moeller, F. G. et al. (1995). Cerebellar blood flow in schizophrenic patients and normal control subjects. *Psychiatr. Res.*, **61**, 15–31.

Stern, Y. and Langston, J. W. (1985). Intellectual changes in patients with MPTP-induced parkinsonism. *Neurology*, **35**, 1506–9.

Suddath, R. L., Christison, G. W., Fuller Torrey, E., Casanova, M. F. and Weinberger, D. R. (1990). Anatomical abnormalities in the brains of monozygotic twins discordant for schizophrenia. *N. Engl. J. Med.*, **322**, 789–94.

Sullivan, E. V., Lim, K. O., Mathalon, D. et al. (1998). A profile of cortical gray matter volume deficits characteristic of schizophrenia. *Cereb. Cortex*, **8**, 117–24.

Szechtman, H., Nahmias, C., Garnett, E. S. et al. (1988). Effect on neuroleptics on altered cerebral glucose metabolism in schizophrenia. *Arch. Gen. Psychiatry*, **45**, 523–32.

Talairach, J. and Tournoux, P. (1988). *Coplanar Stereotaxic Atlas of the Human Brain.* New York: Thieme Medical.

Thomas, A. M., Ke, Y., Caplan, R. et al. (1996). Frontal lobe ¹HMR spectroscopy of children with schizophrenia. In *Proceedings of the 15th Annual Meeting of the Society of Magnetic Resonance in Medicine*, p. 1000.

Toft, P. B., Leth, H., Lou, H. C., Pryds, O. and Henriksen, O. (1994). Metabolite concentrations in the developing brain estimated with proton MR spectroscopy. *J. Magn. Reson. Imaging*, **4**, 647–80.

Urenjak, J., Williams, S. R., Gadian, D. G. and Noble, M. (1993). Proton nuclear magnetic resonance spectroscopy unambiguously identifies different neural cell types. *J. Neurosci.*, **13**, 981–9.

Vion-Dury, J., Salvan, A. M., Confort-Gouny, S., Dhiver, C. and Cozzone, P. (1995). Reversal of brain metabolic alterations with zidovudine detected by proton localised magnetic resonance spectroscopy. *Lancet*, **345**, 60–1.

Volkow, N. D., Levy, A., Brodie, J. D. et al. (1992). Low cerebellar metabolism in medicated patients with chronic schizophrenia. *Am. J. Psychiatry*, **149**, 686–8.

Volz, H. P., Gaser, C., Hager, F., Rzanny, R. et al. (1997). Brain activation during cognitive stimulation with the Wisconsin Card Sort Test – a functional MRI study in healthy volunteers and schizophrenics. *Psychiatr. Res.*, **75**, 145–57.

Watkins, J. M., Asarnow, R. F. and Tanguay, P. E. (1988). Symptom development in childhood onset schizophrenia. *J. Am. Acad. Child Adolesc. Psychiatry*, **6**, 865–78.

Weinberger, D. R. (1987). Implications of normal brain development for the pathogenesis of schizophrenia. *Arch. Gen. Psychiatry*, **44**, 660–9.

Weinberger, D. R. (1995). Schizophrenia: from neuropathology to neurodevelopment. *Lancet*, **346**, 552–7.

Weinberger, D. R., Berman, K. F., Suddath, R. and Torrey E. F. (1992). Evidence of dysfunction of a prefrontal-limbic network in schizophrenia: a magnetic resonance imaging and regional cerebral blood flow study of discordant monozygotic twins. *Am. J. Psychiatry*, **149**, 890–7.

Weisel, F. A., Wik, G., Sjogren, I., Blomqvist, G., Greitz, T. and Stone-Elander, S. (1987). Regional brain glucose metabolism in drug free schizophrenic patients and clinical correlates. *Acta Psychiatr. Scand.*, **76**, 628–41.

Yakovlev, P. I. and Le Cours, A. R. (1964). The myelogenetic cycles of regional maturation of the brain. In *Regional Development of the Brain in Early Life*, ed. A. Minkowski. Boston: Blackwell Scientific.

Yeo, R. A., Hodde-Vargas, J., Hendren, R. L. et al. (1997). Brain abnormalities in schizophrenia-spectrum children: implications for a neurodevelopmental perspective. *Psychiatry Res.*, **76**, 1–13.

Yurgelun-Todd, D. A., Renshaw, P. F., Gruber, S. A., Waternaux, C. M. and Cohen, B. M. (1996). Proton magnetic resonance spectroscopy of the temporal lobes in schizophrenics and normal controls. *Schizophr. Res.*, **19**, 55–9.

Zahn, T. P., Jacobsen, L. K., Gordon, C. T., McKenna, K., Frazier, J. A. and Rapoport, J. L. (1997). Autonomic nervous system markers of psychopathology in childhood onset schizophrenia. *Arch. Gen. Psychiatry*, **54**, 904–12.

Zametkin, A. J., Nordahl, T. E., Gross, M. et al. (1990). Cerebral glucose metabolism in adults with hyperactivity of childhood onset. *N. Engl. J. Med.*, **323**, 1361–6.

Zametkin, A. J., Liebenauer, L. L. Fitzgerald, G. A. et al. (1993). Brain metabolism in teenagers with attention-deficit hyperactivity disorder. *Arch. Gen. Psychiatry*, **50**, 333–40.

Zipursky, R. B., Lim, K. O. and Pfefferbaum, A. (1991). Brain size in schizophrenia. *Arch. Gen. Psychiatry*, **48**, 179–80.

Zipursky, R. B., Marsh, L., Lim, K. O. et al. (1994). Volumetric MRI assessment of temporal lobe structures in schizophrenia. *Biol. Psychiatry*, **35**, 501–16.

12

Pediatric mood disorders and neuroimaging

Robert A. Kowatch, Pablo A. Davanzo and
Graham J. Emslie

Introduction

Until recently, mood disorders were thought to have their onsets in adulthood and to be rare in children and adolescents. This view failed to take into account the possibility that the clinical presentations of mood disorders might differ with age. Research now has shown that mood disorders do occur in children and adolescents but present somewhat differently than in adults (Bowring and Kovacs, 1992; Birmaher et al., 1996). Recognition of this phenomenon has stimulated the use of neuroimaging techniques for research in these disorders; clinical applications have not been established.

This chapter will first present the clinical characteristics of these disorders in children and adolescents, briefly reviewing what is known about the neurobiology of these disorders; it will then present an overview of both adult and pediatric imaging studies of relevance to mood disorders.

Clinical aspects of mood disorders in children and adolescents

Child and adolescent mood disorders are complex in both their clinical presentations and neurobiology. These disorders commonly involve cognitive, affective, vegetative, and perceptual systems. The underlying neurobiology appears to involve multiple neurotransmitter and neuroendocrine systems. The developmental course and presentation vary, depending upon the age of the patient and what other disorders are comorbid. Bipolar disorders are particularly complex because often their initial presentation is a severe, sometimes psychotic, depression that later evolves into episodes of mania or hypomania. One of the hallmarks of pediatric bipolar disorders is mood lability and marked irritability.

The development of mood and its disorders occurs at much younger ages than was previously thought. Research suggests that children develop internal mood states between the ages of 12 and 18 months (Cicchetti et al., 1997) and can discriminate facial expressions when they are as young as 4 months of age (LaBarbera et al., 1976). Whereas psychoanalytic theory once taught that children could not experience depression before adolescence (Rie, 1966), it is now well established that mood disorders occur in childhood (see Epidemiology below). Children with a mood disorder are most often referred to clinicians because of their behavior. The most common referral patterns are (i) a child who is irritable, oppositional and negative, refusing to do work in school and having severe emotional outbursts at home and school; (ii) a child with unexplained physical complaints, such as headaches and stomach aches, whose degree of disability is in excess of any clear medical cause; (iii) the hyperactive, impulsive, motor-driven child, tearing up the world around – often with severe aggression, all along denying anything is wrong. None of these pictures fit the lay person's perception of the mood of a depressed child, and yet the first two are the typical presentations for depression and the third for bipolar disorder.

Epidemiology

Prevalence estimates of depressive disorders in children and adolescents range from 0.4 to 8.3% (Lewinsohn et al., 1986, 1993, 1994; Kashani et al., 1987a,b; Fleming and Offord, 1990; Burke et al., 1991; Shaffer et al., 1996) and are greater in adolescents than in children. These prevalence rates are only slightly lower than those for adults (Kessler et al., 1994), in whom the 12-month prevalence of major depressive disorder (MDD) is reported to be $10.3 \pm 0.8\%$ with females showing higher rates than males ($12.9 + 0.8\%$ females and

7.7 ± 0.8% males). In contrast, MDD in children appears to occur at approximately the same rate in girls and boys. The approximately 2:1 (female:male) ratio seen in adults emerges during adolescence (Emslie et al., 1990).

Bipolar disorders are equally as prevalent in children and adolescents as they are in adults, with an estimated prevalence of 1% (Kashani et al., 1987a,b; Lewinsohn et al., 1995). Bipolar disorders are also the most prevalent psychotic disorders in all age groups, including children and adolescents (Faedda et al., 1995). Wozniak et al. (1995) recently reported that of 262 children consecutively referred to a pediatric psychopharmacology clinic, 16% met DSM-III-R criteria for mania (American Psychological Association, 1989).

Signs and symptoms

Although the diagnostic criteria for MDD in children and adolescents are the same as those for adults, differences in symptomatic expression are substantial. Children tend to be more reactive to their environment and, therefore, may not consistently appear sad. Rather, their mood disturbance is most often expressed in variable days, consisting of normal moods and behavior interspersed with frequent periods of depressed feelings and irritability. Irritability is common in this age group, with irritable moods frequently resulting from sad feelings. Changes in social behavior may be manifested in adolescents by joining less socially desirable peer groups. Frequent complaints of boredom indicate loss of interest. School phobic reactions (fear of going to school) can also be symptomatic of depression. School refusal may constitute the primary problem for referral. With changes in appetite, children often become "picky" eaters, craving sweets or snack foods, and, in some instances, become voracious overeaters. Absence of usual weight gain, rather than weight loss, is common in the depressed child. Excessive weight gain is seen in some children and adolescents, but adolescents frequently lose weight. Depressed children often experience initial insomnia, not always objectively confirmed. Middle insomnia is not uncommon in small children (getting in bed with parents and siblings). Terminal insomnia is less common than in depressed adults. Psychomotor symptoms result in agitation and oppositional behavior, which often lead to a misdiagnosis of oppositional defiant disorder. Alternatively, some depressed children and adolescents complain of feeling slowed down, both in physical movement and thinking. Children with depression often present to pediatricians or general practitioners with vague somatic complaints including headaches, stomach aches, or other physical symptoms for which the physician can find no cause.

As with depression, while the DSM-IV criteria for bipolar disorders are the same for adults and children, there are developmental differences in symptom expression. For both children and adults, the essential feature of a bipolar I disorder is a clinical course characterized by one or more manic or mixed episodes. A child or adolescent who has had one or more episodes of major depression and at least one episode of hypomania, but no episodes of mania, is classified in DSM-IV as having a bipolar II disorder. Cyclothymia is a disorder of at least 1 year duration in which there are numerous periods of both hypomanic and depressive symptoms that do not meet criteria for mania or major depression. These symptoms may fluctuate within days, weeks, or months. The child or adolescent is not without symptoms for more than 2 months at a time.

Comorbidity

The diagnosis of a mood disorder is often obscured by the presence of other comorbid psychiatric diagnoses, as well as by general medical disorders. The most common comorbid diagnoses among bipolar adolescents are anxiety disorders, attention-deficit hyperactivity disorder (ADHD), conduct disorders, and substance abuse (Lewinsohn et al., 1995).

Natural course

The developmental course of mood disorders suggests a continuum of pathology from childhood to adulthood. Such developmental progression can be captured and utilized in brain imaging studies to further our understanding of the neural substrates of mood disorders. Similar to adults with depressive illness, depressed children and adolescents have a high rate of recurrence of their depression. Recurrence (i.e., a new episode of depression) has been reported in 54–72% of depressed children and adolescents followed for 3–8 years, with similar rates seen in inpatients (Garber et al., 1988; Emslie et al., 1997) and outpatients (Kovacs et al., 1984; McCauley et al., 1993; Rao et al., 1995).

Furthermore, early-onset depression often continues into adulthood. Kandal and Davies (1986) described poor adult outcomes in a large sample of adolescents (1004) identified as having depressive symptoms using a self-report scale. Similarly, in a retrospective, long-term follow-up study of 80 depressed and 80 nondepressed outpatient adolescents, Harrington et al. (1990) reported that depressed adolescents were more likely than nondepressed adolescents to have depression in adulthood; however, they note that most adult depressions are not preceded by adolescent depression.

The natural history of bipolar disorder in children and adolescents has received little study. McGlashen (1988) interviewed 62 adult patients who met DSM-III criteria for mania and divided them into two groups: 33 with adolescent onset of mania and 29 with adult onset of mania. He reported that among the adolescent-onset group, the mean age at which they first became symptomatic was 16 years. In comparing the course of the disorder, the adolescent-onset group had more hospitalizations, displayed more psychotic symptoms, and were more frequently misdiagnosed as having a schizoaffective disorder than the adult-onset group. Surprisingly, the adolescent-onset group had outcomes superior to those of the adult-onset group in terms of social relationships and their ability to work.

Strober et al. (1993) followed 58 adolescents who had been admitted to a psychiatric unit for a major depressive episode and found that during the 24-month follow-up period, mania occurred only in those patients who had a psychotic depression. In this psychotically depressed group, 28% went on to develop bipolar I disorder. In a similar follow-up study of depressed prepubertal children, Geller et al. (1994) reported that bipolarity was predicted by a family history of major mood disorders, major depressive disorder, or schizoaffective disorder. These studies show that bipolar disorders may first occur in childhood or adolescence, may sometimes present with schizophrenic-like symptoms, may be predicted by a past history of psychotic depression, and are associated with a family history of major mood disorders.

The neurobiology of mood disorders

Most neurotransmitter systems have been proposed as playing a role in mood disorders (Rush et al., 1998). Evidence from neuroanatomic, neurophysiologic, neurochemical, and behavioral studies in humans and animals also support the view that mood disorders are mediated by networks of interacting neural regions that are often widely spatially distributed (Mesulam, 1990; Sackeim et al., 1990; Soares and Mann, 1997b).

Neurotransmitter studies

Peripheral studies of neurotransmitters have primarily focused on norepinephrine, serotonin, and acetylcholine (Willner, 1985; Coyle, 1987; Gold et al., 1988; Zubenko et al., 1990). The interest in the bioamine hypothesis for depression originally arose from observations of depression caused by reserpine. Reserpine is an antihypertensive which depletes noradrenaline, dopamine, and serotonin and which can cause a depression, suggesting that depression, in part, results from a decrease in the availability of the mode of action of known antidepressant drugs, such as the specific serotonin-reuptake inhibitors, which increase serotonergic activity.

Although noradrenaline (norepinephrine) has been the most studied neurotransmitter in depression (Bunney and Davis, 1965; Schatzberg et al., 1982; Golden and Potter, 1986), results have been disappointing. Cerebrospinal fluid (CSF) concentrations of noradrenaline metabolite 3-methoxy-4-hydroxyphenylglycol have not clearly differed in adult patients with depression from those in controls, although Maas et al. (1968) reported decreased urinary excretion of the metabolite in bipolar patients in the depressed phase. Studies of children and adolescents are limited, although De Villiers et al. (1989) found no difference in noradrenergic function between depressed adolescents and controls.

Similarly, peripheral studies of serotonin (5-hydroxytryptamine) in adults with depression have not been helpful (Prange et al., 1974; van Pragg, 1977; Agren, 1980; Glennon, 1987), except for a subgroup of depressed patients. This subgroup, characterized by aggression, anxiety, impulsivity, and suicidality, showed low CSF 5-hydroxyindoleacetic acid, a product of serotonin metabolism. In children and adolescents, Ryan et al. (1992) reported abnormal neuroendocrine response to L-5-hydroxytryptophan in 37 prepubertal depressed children compared with 23 normal controls, suggesting a dysregulation of central serotonergic systems in childhood depression.

A theoretical framework characterizing the neurotransmitter systems involved in child and adolescent depression has been proposed by Rogeness et al. (1992), who adapted the model of Gray et al. (1981) for the neurobiology of anxiety disorders. Posited is an imbalance between a behavioral facilitory system (BFS) and a behavioral inhibitory system (BIS). The BFS is thought to be a primarily dopaminergic system, whereas the BIS is thought to involve noradrenergic and serotonergic systems. Rogeness et al. (1992) proposed that in child and adolescent major depression dopaminergic function (BFS) is depressed and noradrenergic and serotonergic (BIS) functions are elevated (Rogeness et al., 1992).

Neuroendocrine studies

Evidence implicating dysfunction of the hypothalamic–pituitary–adrenal axis, the hypothalamic–pituitary–thyroid axis, and the hypothalamic–pituitary–growth hormone axis has been reported in depression in adults. The neuroregulatory control of these axes involves many neurotransmitters including noradrenaline, acetylcholine, serotonin, and gamma-aminobutyric acid (GABA). Cortisol hypersecretion, present in adult depression, has not been identified in depressed children and adolescents (Puig-Antich et al., 1989; Kutcher et al., 1991), although depressed adolescents have shown a cortisol elevation at the approximate time of sleep onset (Dahl et al., 1989). However, nonsuppression of cortisol by dexamethasone has been found in many studies of depressed children and adolescents (Extein et al., 1982; Poznanski et al., 1982; Robbins et al., 1982; Doherty et al., 1986; Emslie et al., 1987). Inconsistent findings between studies may reflect differences in sampling, dosages, and the pharmacokinetics of dexamethasone (McCracken et al., 1988; Naylor et al., 1990).

Growth hormone releasing factor release is stimulated by noradrenergic, dopaminergic, and serotonergic neuronal input (Mendelson et al., 1978). Blunting of growth hormone release in response to hypoglycemia, desipramine, clonidine, and growth hormone releasing factor in depressed children and adolescents has been reported (Ryan et al., 1994). While these are among the most replicated results in this age group, the regulation of growth hormone by many neurotransmitters complicates their interpretation. Studies of thyroid axis abnormalities in children and adolescents are few. Kutcher et al. (1991) reported that nocturnal thyroid stimulating hormone values at 1.00 a.m. were elevated in 12 depressed adolescents, relative to normal controls, but there was no significant difference in the total amount secreted throughout the night.

Whereas several neurobiologic findings, like cortisol hypersecretion and reduced REM (rapid eye movement) latency, are present in mood disorders in adults, studies of pediatric patients are only suggestive of similar findings. Further research is needed to determine how these neurobiologic factors are involved in pediatric mood disorders. Functional neuroimaging studies are likely to be informative in this respect.

Neuroimaging studies

Most neuroimaging studies have been conducted in adults. Findings from these studies need to be compared with those in children to understand the developmental trajectory of neural abnormalities and their significance. This section will cover neuroimaging studies in adults, including activation studies using neurobehavioral probes, and the few imaging studies performed in children and adolescents.

Single-state studies of adults with mood disorders

Since 1972, more than 100 functional imaging studies using positron emission tomography (PET), single photon emission computed tomography (SPECT), or magnetic resonance spectroscopy (MRS) to study mood disorders in adults have been published. Most of these studies were completed with subjects scanned in a resting state. The results have been variable, likely because of differences in factors such as subject selection, diagnostic procedures, severity of illness, medication status, demographic characteristics, imaging techniques and analytic methods, and inadequate control over or variations in the state in which subjects were scanned. A thorough review of these studies is beyond the scope of this chapter, and the interested reader is referred to recent reviews by Drevets (1998), Mayberg (1997), and Soares and Mann (1997b).

The most replicated findings in well-designed PET and SPECT studies of cerebral blood flow and metabolism in depression, not confounded by medication effects (Drevets, 1998; Mayberg et al., 1994; Soares and Mann, 1997b), include (i) reductions in dorsolateral and dorsomedial prefrontal blood flow and glucose metabolism, with some, but not all, studies indicating that these abnormalities are reversed by antidepressant therapy; (ii) reduction in blood flow and glucose metabolism in the anterior cingulate gyrus in both unipolar and bipolar depression, which does not normalize following treatment, possibly because anatomic volumetric reductions may account, at least in part, for the apparent functional finding; (iii) increased blood flow and metabolism in the amygdala (left and possibly right) and medial thalamus in both unipolar and bipolar depression; and (iv) reduced blood flow and metabolism in the caudate in unipolar, but not bipolar, depression.

Abnormalities in the prefrontal cortex may be linked to neuropsychologic impairments in depression, and those in the anterior cingulate may reflect emotional processing and/or obsessive ruminations (Drevets, 1998). Drevets (1998) has highlighted the amygdala as the only structure in which blood flow and metabolism consistently show positive correlations with the severity of depression. Abnormal elevations of amygdala activity may be seen during sleep and in asymptomatic (remitted) subjects with familial depression who are not receiving treatment. Antidepressants that ameliorate symptoms and help to prevent relapse normalize amygdalar activity. Baseline amygdalar activity may predict relapse induced by a tryptophan-free diet (thought to deplete brain serotonin) in successfully treated, remitted patients, suggesting that it confers susceptibility to depression. Finally, resting-state amygdalar hypermetabolism at present appears to be unique to mood disorders.

Less consistent findings include reductions of blood flow and metabolism in the lateral temporal and parietal cortex, which may relate to neuropsychologic impairments associated with depression (Drevets, 1998; Soares and Mann, 1997b). Finally, increased blood flow has been reported in the cerebellar vermis in major depression, a finding that affects the interpretation of many SPECT studies which have normalized regional cerebral blood flow (rCBF) using the cerebellum as a reference (Drevets, 1998).

Alterations in blood flow and metabolism primarily reflect changes in synaptic activity (see Chapter 1). Regional brain differences may arise from increases or decreases in excitatory or inhibitory projections either within or distal to the region in which they are measured. The regions identified as abnormal by imaging studies agree with lesion studies in implicating neural circuits involving the frontal and temporal lobes and portions of the striatum, pallidum, and thalamus in the pathophysiology of depression (Drevets, 1998). Secondary depression, such as that seen in basal ganglia disorders (e.g., Huntington's or Parkinson's disease) or in other neuropsychiatric syndromes (e.g., obsessive-compulsive disorder), is likely to involve dysfunctional interactions between strucures within these same circuits, although the specific characteristics of these interactions are likely to differ.

Among the studies with the best control groups are two blood flow studies of adults with MDD. The first one used a two-dimensional probe ^{133}Xe method to study the resting rCBF patterns of a group of 41 depressed adults and 40 age- and gender-matched controls (Sackeim et al., 1990). This study, which carefully controlled for diagnosis, age, gender, handedness, and medication status, found that depressed subjects had both reduced global CBF and an abnormal topographic distribution of blood flow, with bilateral relative decreases in frontal, central, superior temporal, and anterior parietal regions compared with controls. These investigators postulated that blood flow decreases in these areas reflected dysfunction in a parallel distributed cortical network involving frontal and temporoparietal polymodal association areas. These polymodal association areas are thought to be directly involved in mood changes in depressed patients (Tucker, 1988).

The other study (Drevets et al., 1992) used PET to study rCBF in a homogenous sample of patients who met criteria for familial pure depressive disease (i.e., these subjects had primary MDD, as did a first-degree relative). Because neuroimaging changes may represent trait markers of the illness (Schlaepfer et al., 1997), state-dependent abnor-malities (Bench et al., 1995), or a combination of the two (Drevets, 1998), two patients groups – one symptomatic and one remitted – were compared with normal controls (10 per group). Symptomatic MDD subjects showed increased relative rCBF in the left prefrontal cortex, left amygdala, and left medial thalamus and decreased relative rCBF in the caudate bilaterally compared with normal controls. Remitted subjects also showed increased amygdalar activity, implicating this as a trait-related marker of depression. Remitted patients failed to show the increased left prefrontal rCBF seen in symptomatic subjects, suggesting that this finding is state related.

Drevets and Raichle (1992) postulate that two separate, but interconnected anatomic circuits are involved in adult MDD. One circuit involves the amygdala, the mediodorsal nucleus of the thalamus, and the ventrolateral and medial prefrontal cortex. This limbic–thalamo–cortical circuit, thought to act as an excitatory triangular circuit, is hypothesized to be overactive in symptomatic depression, as reflected in the increased rCBF in these areas. A second circuit, the limbic–striatal–pallidal–thalamic circuit, involves the striatum and the ventral pallidum and is connected to the first as a disinhibitory sideloop. Drevets and Raichle (1992) felt that their rCBF PET findings in this group of depressed and remitted subjects was compatible with a neural model of depression proposed by Swerdlow and Koob (1987), which hypothesized that underactivation of forebrain dopamine systems with a resultant enhancement of limbic–thalamo–cortical positive feedback leads to symptoms of MDD (Fig. 12.1).

Neuroreceptor imaging studies, reviewed by Soares and Mann (1997b), have provided evidence of alterations in the serotonergic system (e.g., a blunted metabolic response to serotonin release) in depressed patients, as well as possible alterations in the dopaminergic system (e.g., increased D_2 receptor binding and receptor density in the basal ganglia) of unipolar and bipolar patients.

Metabolic studies using ^{31}P and ^{1}H MRS, reviewed by Kato et al. (1998), suggest several abnormalities, including decreased phosphomonoester and phosphodiester levels in the frontal lobes and decreased phosphomonoesters in the temporal lobes, in patients with bipolar disorder in the euthymic state (Kato et al., 1998). The ^{31}P MRS studies have reported significant membrane phospholipid and energy metabolism abnormalities in the frontal and temporal lobes of adult bipolar patients (Kato et al., 1992, 1993; Deicken et al., 1995a,b; Moore et al., 1997). Several ^{1}H MRS studies reported significant choline abnormalities in the parietal lobes and basal ganglia of adult bipolar patients (Sharma et al., 1992; Stoll et al., 1992; Renshaw et al., 1997).

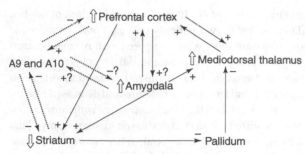

Fig. 12.1. Neuroanatomic circuits hypothesized to participate in the functional anatomy of unipolar major depression. Regions showing blood flow differences have adjacent open arrows, which indicate the direction of differences in flow in the depressives relative to controls. The regions' monosynaptic connections with each other are illustrated (solid arrows) with + indicating excitatory and − inhibitory projections, and with ? indicating where experimental evidence is limited. The portions of the prefrontal cortex affected involve primarily the ventrolateral and medial prefrontal cortex. The parts of the striatum under consideration are the ventromedial caudate and nucleus accumbens, which particularly project to the ventral pallidum. The major dopaminergic projections from the substantia nigra (A9) and the ventral tegmental area (A10) to these structures are illustrated with the dotted lines. (Reprinted with permission from Drevets et al. (1992). *Journal of Neuroscience*, 12, 3637.)

Structural neuroimaging studies of adults with mood disorders

The possibility exists that at least some trait-related abnormalities seen in mood disorders with functional neuroimaging may be attributable to anatomic deviations (Drevets, 1998). Structural imaging studies of adults with major depressive disorder and bipolar disorder have reported a variety of neuroanatomic abnormalities, the most consistent of which include an increased rate of subcortical white matter hyperintensities, increased ventricular size, decreased temporal lobe volume, decreased frontal lobe volume and changes in basal ganglia structures (Soares and Mann, 1997a). Recently, Drevets et al. (1997) have shown structural abnormalities in the subgenual prefrontal cortex of patients with both unipolar and bipolar disorder compared with normal controls. The subgenual prefrontal cortex consists of agranular cortex on the anterior cingulate gyrus ventral to the genu of the corpus callosum (corresponding to Brodmann areas 24 and 32). This area has extensive connections with the amygdala, hypothalamus, and brainstem monoaminergic nuclei (i.e., locus ceruleus, raphe). These structures have been associated with the regulation of emotion, autonomic function, sleep, appetite, and monoamine transmission. It has been postulated that a disruption of this neuronal pathway may

produce a disturbance in any or all of the functions associated with mood disorders (Drevets et al., 1997).

In bipolar disorder, many of the adult studies that acquired T_2-weighted magnetic resonance imaging (MRI) images have also reported finding white matter signal hyperintensities in the periventricular space of patients with bipolar I disease (Altshuler et al., 1995). These white matter signal hyperintensities could represent areas of astrogliosis, demyelination, encephalomalacia, or loss of axons (Bradley et al., 1984).

Neurobehavioral probes: recognition of facial expressions

The use of neurobehavioral probes in conjunction with functional imaging techniques may increase sensitivity and specificity in identifying the neural correlates of mood disorders. However, this involves a number of design challenges to insure valid experimental results (see Chapter 9). Sound task development may be conceptualized as involving the following stages (Gur et al., 1992): (i) selection of a unitary behavioral dimension for measurement; (ii) selection of tasks that tap into the chosen behavioral dimension and that have been validated within the constraints of experimental imaging paradigms; (iii) application of the chosen task with normal subjects to determine which brain areas are involved in the processing required by the neurobehavioral probe; and (iv) application of the neurobehavioral probe to well-characterized neuropsychiatric samples and matched normal control subjects.

Because impairments of social functioning in depressed adults have been hypothesized to stem, at least in part, from an inability to recognize facial expressions of emotion accurately (Persad and Polivy, 1993), several paradigms involving judgments of facial affect perception have been developed and implemented to investigate the functional neuroanatomy of depression. One such paradigm, the Ekman facial recognition paradigm, requires subjects to discriminate and name the emotions of 14 photographed facial expressions depicting seven primary human emotions: fear, anger, surprise, contempt or disgust, happiness, sadness, and indifference (Ekman and Oster, 1979). The Ekman photographs have been used in a variety of experiments to study the mechanisms of facial recognition and mood in brain-damaged, normal, and depressed subjects.

In 1994, Adolphs et al. studied S.M., a 30-year-old woman with Urbach–Wiethe disease using the Ekman facial recognition paradigm. Urbach–Wiethe disease is a rare, autosomal recessive condition that causes nearly complete bilateral destruction of the amygdala and in which affected individuals often show defective personal and social decision making (Hofer, 1973; Hofer et al., 1974). A T_1-weighted MRI of S.M.'s brain demonstrated extensive bilateral amygdala damage with sparing of the neocortex and hippocampus. When S.M. was tested with the Ekman facial recognition paradigm, her mood was rated as normal and she had normal visual–perceptual skills. Although S.M. was able to recognize familiar faces, she was unable to recognize the emotion of fear in any of the Ekman photographs. She was also unable to recognize similarities between expressions of different facial emotions. From these results, the authors concluded that the amygdala is necessary in humans both to recognize the emotion of fear and to recognize blends of multiple facial emotions.

These same authors expanded this study to three patients with damage to the left amygdala, three patients with damage to the right amygdala, 12 controls with brain damage but intact amygdalae, and seven normal subjects (Adolphs et al., 1995). In this experiment, which again used the Ekman facial recognition paradigm, subjects were asked to identify familiar faces, to draw pictures of facial expressions from memory, and to sort labels of emotions (e.g., happy, surprised, afraid) on the basis of the similarity and intensity of the emotion they denoted. Only bilateral, and not unilateral, damage to the amygdala impaired the processing of fearful facial emotions, while leaving the recognition of facial identity intact.

The Ekman facial photographs have proven less than ideal for neuroimaging studies because these photographs are asymmetrical, lit in varied ways, and contain both clothing and hair cues, thus introducing a number of potential confounds into studies of facial perception. To better control for such variables, the neuropsychiatry group at the University of Pennsylvania led by Ruben Gur and Roland Erwin created a more controlled set of facial photographs of professional actors and actresses portraying three emotions: happy, sad, or neutral (the PENN facial photographs). These photographs of faces are symmetrical, lighted in a standard way, and devoid of clothing or hair cues. In their first behavioral study using these photographs, Erwin et al. (1992) tested a group of young normal adults and reported a gender difference in the discrimination of facial emotions, with males being less sensitive than females to sad emotions in female faces, and females being more sensitive than males to all emotional expressions in male faces. Therefore, it appears that another factor – gender – also affects how facial emotions are perceived. Self-report mood ratings performed by the subjects during an emotion-discrimination task found that this task did not induce any changes in self-rated mood states.

Several behavioral studies have found that depressed adult subjects have difficulty recognizing facial emotional cues (Feinberg et al., 1986; Sweeney et al., 1989; Gaebel and Wolwer, 1992; Rubinow and Post, 1992). Various explanations have been offered for this deficit, including perceptual inaccuracies (Mandal and Bhattacharya, 1985) and slow processing of facial emotional cues (Cooley and Nowicki, 1989), but the source of this deficit is not yet fully understood. An alternative hypothesis proposed by Persad and Polivy (1993) was that the type of behavioral and emotional responses that facial cues elicit in depressed individuals lay at the core of their interactional difficulties.

Using a modified Ekman facial recognition paradigm, these investigators asked subjects to identify the emotion depicted in the Ekman photographs, identify what their behavioral response would be, explain their emotional reaction to the cue, and rate their degree of comfort with the cue (Persad and Polivy, 1993). Four groups of subjects were examined: 16 depressed college students enrolled in an introductory psychology course, 16 depressed psychiatric inpatients who met DSM-III criteria for major depression, 16 nondepressed college students also enrolled in an introductory psychology course, and 11 nondepressed psychiatric inpatients (two with anorexia, three with personality disorders, two with anxiety disorders, one with a pain disorder, and one with post-traumatic stress disorder). The depressed college student sample had a mean Beck Depression Inventory Score of 16, indicating mild depression, and the depressed inpatients a mean score of 37, indicating severe depression. Both depressed groups made more errors in facial recognition than did normal controls and nondepressed psychiatric inpatients, but neither of the depressed groups performed more poorly on any particular expression. Compared with the control groups, both depressed groups also reported more "freezing responses" (tensing up) toward the facial expressions, higher levels of fear ratings, and less comfort with their emotional reactions to the expressions of fear, anger, disgust, sadness, and indifference. Persad and Polivy concluded that depressed individuals have a generalized, nonspecific deficit in their perception of emotional cues, which includes problems at the level of facial recognition, behavioral reactions, and their own emotional reactions. Limitations of Persad and Polivy's study include their reliance on self-reports, the ecological validity (i.e., the relationship of responses to the Ekman paradigm versus real-life situations) of which is unknown. Nonetheless, these results suggest that the Ekman facial recognition paradigm not only involves the perceptual system but also stimulates behavioral and emotional responses that are affected in depression.

Gur et al. (1992) reported that depressed patients misinterpret neutral faces as sad and happy faces as neutral and that patients with more negative affect, as measured on the Positive and Negative Affect Scale, show less ability to discriminate neutral versus sad faces. This finding is in general agreement with the cognitive theory of depression by Beck (1971), which holds that cognitive dysfunctions are at the core of depressive illness. The data of Gur et al. suggest that not only is cognition impaired in depressive illness but also impaired are the perceptual processes involved in the discrimination of facial emotions.

Activation studies of facial recognition in normal adults and adolescents

The Ekman facial recognition paradigm described above and variations of it have been used in the study of emotion in functional imaging studies. Table 12.1 summarizes the various functional imaging studies that have used such neurobehavioral probes. This table reflects an evolution of the imaging modalities used and the types of neurobehavioral paradigm employed. The earliest studies used facial recognition tasks with PET or SPECT, while the later studies used paradigms involving film clips and autobiographical scripts with fMRI (discussed in a later section).

In an early ^{15}O PET study, Sergent et al. (1992) measured rCBF in seven normal adults, aged 22–31 years, during facial discrimination. Subjects were scanned during three visual tasks: discrimination of the gender of faces, identification of the faces of famous persons, and recognition of common objects. The gender discrimination task elicited activation (increased rCBF when subtracted from a grating control condition) in the right extrastriate cortex, while the face identification task additionally elicited activation of the fusiform gyrus and anterior temporal cortex of both hemispheres and the right parahippocampal gyrus. The object-recognition task increased rCBF in the left occipitotemporal cortex but failed to affect the right hemisphere regions activated during facial identification. In general, several cortical areas were involved in the processing of faces, but it appeared that the ventromedial region of the right anterior temporal lobe was uniquely activated during facial identification.

Using fMRI in conjunction with Ekman facial photographs, Breiter et al. (1996) measured activity in the amygdala of 18 normal men (mean age 26.5 years). In separate experiments, photographs of fearful versus neutral faces and happy versus neutral faces were presented. The amygdala was preferentially activated in response to fearful versus neutral faces, as well as in response to happy versus neutral faces, suggesting a possible generalized response to emotionally valenced stimuli. The fMRI measurements also indicated a rapid habituation of this neural response

in the healthy subjects. Similarly, using fMRI, Schneider et al. (1997) measured a significant increase in signal intensity in response to sad, as well as happy, facial expressions in the left amygdala in 12 right-handed normal subjects (seven males, five females) using the PENN facial photographs.

Finally, in a recent fMRI study of adolescents, Baird and colleagues (1999) studied 12 normal adolescents, ages 12–17 years (mean 13.9 years) using a facial discrimination paradigm that required the labeling of the emotional expressions of six different faces, all with fearful expressions. A significant increase in signal intensity in both amygdalae was seen in response to fearful facial expressions compared with the control task of viewing nonsense gray-scale images.

Neuroimaging using mood induction paradigms with normal adults

A number of functional imaging studies have used a variety of mood induction paradigms (see Table 12.1). Pardo et al. (1993) measured rCBF using ^{15}O PET in seven normal adult subjects (mean age of 24 years) scanned at rest and while they recalled or imagined a sad situation. Females activated areas in bilateral inferior and orbitofrontal cortex, while males activated the left and orbitofrontal cortex.

Similarly, George et al. (1995) used ^{15}O PET to study 11 normal female subjects (mean age 33 years) while they recalled specific happy, sad, or neutral life events. Compared to the resting condition in which subjects were told to close their eyes and concentrate on their sensory and emotional experience, transient sadness significantly increased rCBF bilaterally in the regions of the cingulate gyrus, right medial frontal gyrus, left dorsolateral prefrontal cortex, bilateral caudate, bilateral putamen, bilateral thalamus, bilateral fornix, left insula, and left midline cerebellum. In contrast, transient happiness resulted in no areas of significantly increased activity but rather was associated with significant and widespread reductions in cortical rCBF, especially in the right prefrontal and bilateral temporoparietal regions.

Using a cognitive task with ^{15}O PET to elicit affect, Schneider et al. (1996) imaged 12 normal subjects while they attempted to solve anagrams, some of which were designed to be unsolvable to induce learned helplessness, sadness, and anxiety. Compared with rest, both solvable and unsolvable anagram tasks increased activity in frontal and temporal regions. Dissociations seen in limbic structures suggested their involvement in the affective aspects of these tasks. The solvable task condition increased hippocampal rCBF and decreased

Table 12.1. Functional imaging studies and neurobehavioral probes

Study	Subjects (No.)	Age (mean ± SD or range, years)	Imaging modality spatial resolution; acquisition parameters	Probes	Control task	Results
Sergent et al. (1992)	Normal males (7)	22–31	PET H$_2^{15}$O; 5–6 mm	Facial gender categorization	Visual fixation	Face gender task: activation in the right extrastriate cortex
				Facial identity	Passive viewing of face	Face identity: activation of the fusiform gyrus and anterior temporal cortex of both hemispheres and the right parahippocampal gyrus
				Object recognition	Sine-wave gratings	Object recognition: increased rCBF in the left occipitotemporal cortex
Pardo et al. (1993)	Normal males (4) Normal females (3)	26 ± 7 24 ± 2	PET H$_2^{15}$O; 17 mm	Imagine or recall of a sad situation	Resting, eyes closed	Females: bilateral inferior and orbitofrontal cortices activation Males: left inferior and orbitofrontal cortices activation
Gur et al. (1994)	Normal males (21) Normal females (19)	26 ± 8 24 ± 6	^{133}Xe SPECT; 10 mm	Facial discrimination using PENN facial photographs, happy–neutral, sad–neutral age discrimination	Resting baseline	All three tasks produced right hemisphere activation Happy and sad discrimination produced right parietal activation Happy discrimination produced greater left frontal activation relative to sad discrimination
Schneider et al. (1994)	Normal males (5) Normal females (7)	22 ± 18	^{133}Xe SPECT; 10 mm	Mood induction using PENN facial photographs: happy, sad, sex discrimination	Resting baseline, eyes open	CBF increased during sad and happy inductions relative to sex discrimination and resting states Sad mood induction activated occipital temporal cortices
George et al. (1995)	Normal females (11)	33.3 ± 12.3	PET H$_2^{15}$O; 6.9 mm	Recall of sad and happy life events followed by PENN facial photographs	Resting baseline, eyes closed	Transient sadness increased rCBF in bilateral cingulate, medial prefrontal and mesial temporal cortices Transient happiness decreased rCBF in right prefrontal and bilateral temporoparietal cortices
Schneider et al. (1996)	Normal males (8) Normal females (4)	24.8 ± 4.5	PET H$_2^{15}$O; 6 mm; coregistered with T_2-weighted MRI	Unsolvable anagrams	Solvable anagrams and a resting baseline, eyes open, ears unoccluded	Both anagram tasks increased activity in frontal and temporal regions. The solvable task increased hippocampal activation and decreased mamillary bodies activity, while unsolvable anagrams increased CBF to the mamillary bodies and amygdala and decreased hippocampal activity

Table 12.1 (*cont.*)

Study	Subjects (No.)	Age (mean ± SD or range, years)	Imaging modality spatial resolution; acquisition parameters	Probes	Control task	Results
Breiter et al. (1996)	Normal males (18)	22–33; mean 26.5	Functional MRI 1.5 T; asymmetric spin-echo T_2^*-weighted, TR 3000/2000 ms, TE 50 ms, slice thickness 3.125 mm	Two experiments: Ekman fearful faces and Ekman happy faces	Ekman Neutral Faces	The amygdala was preferentially activated in response to fearful versus neutral faces and the amygdala also responded preferentially to happy versus neutral faces
Reiman et al. (1997)	Normal females (12)	23.3 ± 3.2	PET $H_2^{15}O$; 10 mm	Emotion-generating film clips of happiness, sadness, and disgust; recall of autobiographical scripts	Neutral film clips and neutral autobiographical scripts	Film- and recall-generated emotion increased activity in the medial prefrontal cortex and thalamus Film-generated emotion was associated with increases in activity bilaterally in the occipitotemporoparietal cortex, lateral cerebellum, hypothalamus, and in a region that included the anterior temporal cortex, amygdala, and hippocampal formation Recall-generated sadness was associated with increases in activity in the vicinity of the anterior insular cortex
Lane et al. (1997)	Normal females (12)	23.3 ± 3.2	PET $H_2^{15}O$; 10 mm	Film clips of happiness, sadness, and disgust and recall of autobiographical scripts of the same three emotions	Three neutral film clips and three neutral autobiographical scripts	Happiness, sadness, and disgust increased activity in the thalamus and medial prefrontal cortex; these three emotions were also associated with activation of anterior and posterior temporal structures, primarily when induced by film Recalled sadness was associated with increased activation in the anterior insula Happiness was distinguished from sadness by greater activity in the vicinity of ventral mesial frontal cortex
Schneider et al. (1997)	Normal males (7) Normal females (5)	29.7 ± 4.3	Functional MRI 1.5 T; T_2^*-weighted FLASH, TR 240 ms, TE 60 ms, slice thickness 4 mm	Mood induction using PENN facial photographs: happy, sad	Resting baseline, eyes open	A significant increase in signal intensity was found during sad as well as happy mood induction in the left amygdala

Study	Subjects (n)	Mean age	Imaging method	Task	Findings
Elliott et al. (1997)	Depressed adults (6) Normal controls (6)	Mean 34.7	PET $H_2^{15}O$	Easy and hard Tower of London tasks	Depressed subjects, compared with their controls, failed to show significant activation in the cingulate and striatum and also failed to show the normal augmentation of activation in the caudate nucleus, anterior cingulate, and right prefrontal cortex that was associated with increasing task difficulty
Beauregard et al. (1998)	Depressed males (3) Depressed females (4) Normal males (3) Normal females (4)	Mean 42 Mean 42 Mean 45 Mean 45	Functional MRI: 1.5 T; echo-planar, TE 54 ms, slice thickness 5 mm	Color film clip to elicit transient sadness A neutral film clip of house renovation	Transient sadness elicited significant activation in both groups of subjects in the medial and inferior prefrontal cortices, the middle temporal cortex, the cerebellum, and the right caudate. While viewing the sad film clip, the depressed subjects showed significantly greater activations in the left medial prefrontal cortex and in the right cingulate than did the control group
Baird et al. (1999)	Normal males (5) Normal females (7)	Mean 13.9	Functional MRI: 1.5 T echo planar, TE 40 ms, slice thickness 3 mm	Three unique nonsense gray-scale images Facial discrimination and labeling of fearful expressions	A significant increase in signal intensity was found in both amygdalae in response to recognition of fearful facial expressions

Notes: CBF, cerebral blood flow; rCBF, regional cerebral blood flow; TE, time to echo; TR, time to repetition.

mamillary body rCBF, whereas unsolvable anagrams increased mamillary body and amygdalar CBF and decreased hippocampal rCBF.

To explore the neural bases of externally versus internally generated human emotion, Reiman et al. (1997) measured rCBF using PET in 12 healthy normal females while they watched short film clips with either emotionally laden or neutral content. Tasks alternated between emotion-generating and control film and recall tasks. Both film- and recall-generated emotion significantly increased activity in the medial prefrontal cortex and thalamus. Film-generated emotion increased rCBF bilaterally in the occipitotemporoparietal cortex, lateral cerebellum, and hypothalamus. Recall-generated sadness was associated with increases in the anterior insular cortex.

Activation studies of adult mood disorders

Using a Tower of London task to study frontal lobe function, Elliott et al. (1997) used PET to measure rCBF in five patients with unipolar depression (mean Hamilton score 23.8) and controls matched for age, gender, and educational levels. Unlike controls, depressed subjects failed to show significant activation in the cingulate and striatum and failed to show the normal augmentation of activation in the caudate nucleus, anterior cingulate, and right prefrontal cortex that was associated with increasing task difficulty, suggesting impaired function of these regions in depression.

Blunted activation of the left cingulate in depression has also been demonstrated using a Stroop task with ^{15}O PET. George et al. (1997) studied 11 mood-disordered adults (nine men, two women; six unipolar, three biopolar II, and two bipolar I) and an equal number of age- and sex-matched controls. A control task involved color naming, a standard Stroop task required subjects to name the colors of ink in which incongruent color names appeared (e.g., "red" printed in blue ink), and a sad Stroop task required the naming of the colors of ink in which emotional words (e.g., grief, misery, sad, bleak) appeared. Depressed subjects were able to activate the left dorsolateral prefrontal cortex, a region commonly hypoactive at rest in depression and hypoactive during the control task in this study. In contrast, activation seen during the interference task (i.e., naming of incongruent colors) was reduced in the left mid-cingulate, as well as in left insula and right superior temporal gyrus. No significant group differences were seen during the sad Stroop test.

Using fMRI, Beauregard et al. (1998) studied seven adults (four women and three men) with major depression (mean age 42 years) and age- and gender-matched controls.

Subjects were imaged while watching a color film clip designed to elicit sadness and while watching a neutral film clip. Transient sadness elicited significant activation in both groups in the medial and inferior prefrontal cortices, the middle temporal cortex, the cerebellum, and the right caudate, suggesting the participation of circuits involving these regions in this emotion. However, relative to controls, depressed subjects showed significantly greater activation while viewing the sad film clip in the left medial prefrontal cortex and right cingulate.

Neuroimaging of pediatric mood disorders

Studies of children and adolescents with mood disorders are just emerging. There have been a few structural studies of children and adolescents with mood disorders, the interpretation of which must be integrated with the changes that are known to occur with brain maturation (Chugani et al., 1987; Chugani and Phelps, 1991; Chiron et al., 1992). This limits direct comparisons with studies of adults. Structural imaging studies of children and adolescents with mood disorders using MRI have begun to implicate the frontal and temporal lobes and basal ganglia.

Hendren et al. (1991) reported clinically abnormal MRI scans in two of three children hospitalized for MDD. The first was a 13-year-old male whose MRI showed abnormally asymmetrical lateral ventricles (right larger than the left), suggesting right-sided ventricular enlargement and decreases in surrounding brain tissue. The second subject was a 12-year-old male whose MRI showed a small area of abnormal signal intensity in the area of the left anterior basal ganglia or medial temporal lobe.

In a volumetric MRI study, Steingard et al. (1996) compared 65 children and adolescents (mean age 13 years) who were hospitalized for either MDD or dysthymia with 18 hospitalized psychiatric controls (mean age 10.7 years) without a depressive disorder: 11 with conduct disorder/oppositional defiant disorder, two with ADHD, three with post-traumatic stress disorder, and two with an adjustment disorder. Volumetric analyses were used to measure frontal lobe volumes, lateral ventricular volumes, and total cerebral volumes for all subjects. To correct for differences in absolute cerebral volume associated with different body and head size, the ratios of frontal lobe and lateral ventricular volumes to total cerebral volume were used to compare differences between the two groups; a multivariate analysis was used to control for the effects of age, gender, and diagnosis. The depressed group had reduced frontal lobe volumes (significantly smaller frontal lobe to total cerebral volume ratio) and increased ventricular volumes (significantly larger ventricular to total cerebral volume ratio), but normal total cerebral volumes relative to their nondepressed psychiatric controls. The reduction in frontal lobe volume resembles that reported in depressed adults with MDD, suggesting some continuity of deviations in brain anatomy.

In the first anatomic MRI study of pediatric bipolar patients, Botteron et al. (1995) compared T_1- and T_2-weighted MRI scans from eight manic children and adolescents and five age-, but not gender-matched normal subjects. They reported increased rates of subcortical white matter signal hyperintensities, abnormal temporal horn asymmetries, and ventricular abnormalities in four of the bipolar patients, and only one of the normal controls by clinical interpretation. Areas of hyperintensity on MRI usually are caused by increased water content and have been associated with ischemia, inflammation, and demyelination. While the significance of these hyperintensities in children and adolescents with bipolar disorders is uncertain at this time, these findings are consistent with those of MRI studies of adults with bipolar I disorders, which frequently find white matter signal hyperintensities in the periventricular space (Altshuler et al., 1995).

Using ^{1}H MRS, Steingard et al. (1998) studied 14 adolescents with MDD (mean age 15.6 years) and 26 normal controls (mean age 14.3 years). Depressed adolescents showed an increase in the ratio of choline to creatine in the orbitofrontal cortex relative to controls, but normal N-acetylaspartate to creatine ratios. These findings are similar to findings in adult MDD (Charles et al., 1994) and suggest alterations in cholinergic neurotransmission in the orbitofrontal cortex.

In a recent SPECT study with ^{99m}Tc-labeled hexamethylpropyleneamine oxime (HMPAO), Kowatch et al. (1999) compared the rCBF in a resting condition of a group of seven adolescents (mean age 15.5 years; range 13–18 years) with symptomatic MDD (DSM-III-R criteria) to those of seven age- and gender-matched normal controls. Previously, the authors have obtained SPECT brain scans on depressed children and adolescents who were inpatients, and visual analysis of these studies suggested abnormalities (relative bilateral hypoperfusion) of the frontal cortex and mesial temporal lobes (Kowatch et al., 1993). This controlled study used a voxel-based T-image analysis to compare the rCBF patterns of a group of adolescents with MDD with those of control adolescents. After normalizing regional to whole brain counts, higher relative rCBF was found in the right mesial temporal cortex, the right superior–anterior temporal lobe, and the left inferolateral temporal lobe in the depressed group relative to controls. Decreased relative rCBF in the depressed group

compared with the control group was localized to the left parietal lobe, the anterior thalamus, and the right caudate. The most spatially extensive area of abnormally low rCBF was in the left superior parietal cortex. Some of these differences are shown in Figs. 12.2 and 12.3.

These preliminary findings suggest that portions of the right and left temporal lobes, the left parietal lobe, the anterior thalamus, and the right caudate may be involved in adolescent MDD. Parietal lobe rCBF abnormalities in MDD adults have been reported in a number of SPECT studies (Sackeim et al., 1990; Austin et al., 1992; Philpot et al., 1993; Lesser et al., 1994). Mesulam (1985) noted that, in monkeys, the superior parietal lobe receives projections from the primary somatosensory cortex and is designated as the unimodal somatosensory association area. Although lesions of the left parietal cortex area in humans are associated with deficits in motor planning (de Renzi et al., 1983), the role of the left superior parietal cortex in MDD has yet to be elucidated. The authors also found high levels of relative rCBF in the right mesial temporal cortex, the right superior anterior temporal lobe, and the left inferolateral temporal lobe. The temporal lobes are central to the limbic–thalamic–cortical circuit believed to contribute to the regulation of mood (Ketter et al., 1996; Mayberg 1997). In addition, the majority of adult SPECT studies have reported decreases in temporal lobe rCBF (Soares and Mann, 1997b). Although the above studies implicate the temporal lobes in the pathophysiology of MDD in both adults and adolescents, the direction of the abnormality (low in adult MDD and high in adolescent MDD) is inconsistent. These findings raise the possibility of developmental differences in the neurobiology of adolescent versus adult MDD. Finally, adolescents with MDD show rCBF abnormalities implicating the limbic–thalamic–cortical circuit and portions of the basal ganglia, consistent with rCBF findings in adults with MDD.

Conclusions and future directions

Functional imaging studies have the potential to provide valuable information about the neurobiologic basis of child and adolescent mood disorders and their development into adult mood disorders. Significant progress in this type of research is expected from improvements in functional imaging technologies, the development of normative data bases, and the use of multimodal imaging methods. The goals of brain imaging research will be to delineate the neural circuits underlying mood disorders, the neurobiologic differences among specific mood disorders and etiological subgroups, and the biology of

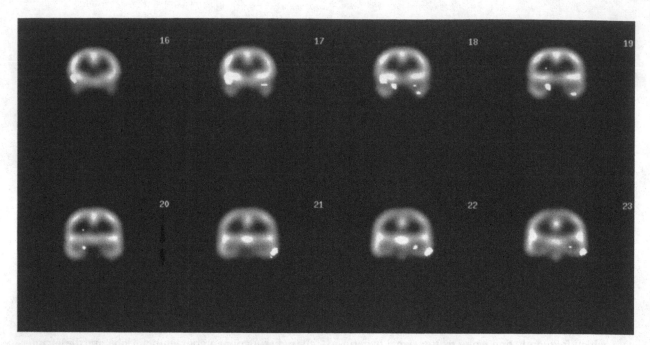

Fig. 12.2. SPECT T images of coronal brain slices illustrating relative increases in rCBF in seven adolescents with major depression, relative to normal controls ($p < 0.01$). Slices 16–20 illustrate increases in the right mesial and lateral temporal lobe and slices 21–23 illustrate the increases in the left lateral temporal lobe. These T images have been overlaid on the normal adolescent model brain in which the individual brain slices have been averaged together in a 3:1 ratio.

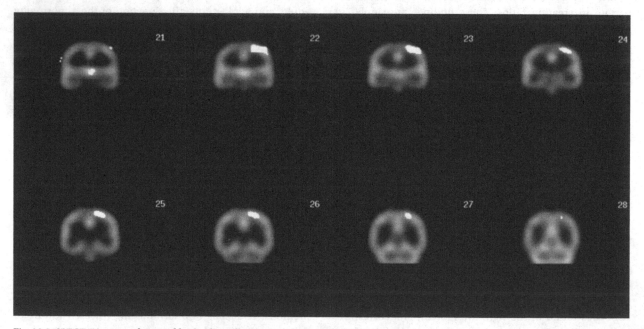

Fig. 12.3. SPECT T images of coronal brain slices illustrating relative decreases in rCBF in seven adolescents with major depression, relative to normal controls ($p < 0.01$). Slice 21 illustrates the thalamic decreases and slices 22–27 illustrate the left parietal decreases.

transient mood states and ongoing trait vulnerabilities, and, ultimately, to contribute to the development of focused and rational treatments, both pharmacologic and behavioral.

To achieve these aims, specific behavioral subtyping (i.e., the study of homogeneous diagnostic groups) is needed. Longitudinal designs of specific diagnostic subgroups will be particularly helpful in elucidating state-versus trait-related brain abnormalities, correlates of depressive and manic phases of bipolar illness, and the impact of developmental influences on brain physiology. Age and gender, as well as other maturational variables such as sexual maturity (Tanner stage), will need to be considered when designing and interpreting functional neuroimaging studies in children and adolescents with mood disorders. Studies of integrated neural activity will predominantly utilize fMRI because of its lack of ionizing radiation and its excellent temporal resolution. Behavioral paradigms that target specific affective and mood-related cognitive processes and that take into consideration age and gender effects should prove useful. Such paradigms can be developed to examine the neural correlates of behavioral aspects of mood disorders (e.g. effects on the perception of facial affect), as well as to evaluate the responsiveness of certain neural structures, such as the amygdala or other limbic structures. The ability to link abnormalities in integrated neural activity with abnormalities of brain neurochemistry may fuel the development of rational therapies for addressing pathophysiology.

Functional imaging studies should be complemented by controlled, quantitative, and, preferably, longitudinal structural imaging studies. Quantitative image analysis techniques, as well as improved characterization of qualitative abnormalities such as white matter hyperintensities (their extent, number, and localization), are needed for use in well-controlled studies of specific subgroups. Where volumetric differences are identified, appropriate adjustments are required in functional image data analysis to avoid partial volume artifacts introduced by such anatomic differences.

Acknowledgements

Support from the National Institute of Mental Health (NIMH), Bethesda, MD (grant K07-MH01057 to R.A.K.) is gratefully acknowledged. We appreciate the administrative support of Kenneth Z. Altshuler M.D., Stanton Sharp Distinguished Chair, Professor and Chairman, Department of Psychiatry.

References

Adolphs, R., Tranel, D., Damasio, H. and Damasio, A. (1994). Impaired recognition of emotion in facial expressions following bilateral damage to the human amygdala. *Nature*, 372, 669–72.

Adolphs, R., Tranel, D., Damasio, H. and Damasio, A. R. (1995). Fear and the human amygdala. *J. Neurosci.*, 15, 5879–91.

Agren, H. (1980). Symptom patterns in unipolar and biopolar depression correlating with monoamine metabolites in crebrospinal fluid, I. General patterns. *Psychiatry Res.*, 3, 211–23.

Altshuler, L. L., Curran, J. G., Hauser, P., Mintz, J., Denicoff, K. and Post, R. (1995). T_2 hyperintensities in bipolar disorder: magnetic resonance imaging comparison and literature meta-analysis. *Am. J. Psychiatry*, 152, 1139–44.

American Psychological Association (1989). *Diagnostic and Statistical Manual of Mental Disorders*, 3rd edn. Washington, DC: American Psychiatric Association.

Austin, M. P., Dougall, N., Ross, M. et al. (1992). Single proton emission tomography with ^{99m}Tc-exametazime in major depression and the pattern of brain activity underlying the psychotic/neurotic continuum. *J. Affect. Disord.*, 26, 31–43.

Baird, A., Gruber, S., Fein, D. et al. (1999). Functional magnetic resonance imaging of facial affect recognition in children and adolescents. *J. Am. Acad. Child Adolesc. Psychiatry*, 38, 195–9.

Beauregard, M., Leroux, J. M., Bergman, S. et al. (1998). The functional neuroanatomy of major depression: an fMRI study using an emotional activation paradigm. *Neuroreport*, 9, 3253–8.

Beck, A. T. (1971). Cognition, affect, and psychopathology. *Arch. Gen. Psychiatry*, 24, 495–500.

Bench, C. J., Frackowiak, R. S. and Dolan, R. J. (1995). Changes in regional cerebral blood flow on recovery from depression. *Psychol. Med.*, 25, 247–61.

Birmaher, B., Ryan, N. D., Williamson, D. E., Brent, D. A. Kaufman, J., Dahl, R. E., Perel, J. and Nelson, B. (1996). Childhood and adolescent depression: a review of the past 10 years. Part I. *J. Am. Acad. Child Adolesc. Psychiatry*, 35, 1427–39.

Botteron, K. N., Vannier, M. W., Geller, B., Todd, R. D. and Lee, B. C. P. (1995). Preliminary study of magnetic resonance imaging characteristics in 8- to 16-year olds with mania. *J. Am. Acad. Child Adolesc. Psychiatry*, 34, 742–9.

Bowring, M. A. and Kovacs, M. (1992). Difficulties in diagnosing manic disorders among children and adolescents. *J. Am. Acad. Child Adolesc. Psychiatry*, 31, 611–14.

Bradley, W. G., Waluch, V., Brant-Zawadzki, M., Yardley, R. A. and Wycoff, R. R. (1984). Patchy, perivascular white matter lesions in the elderly: a common observation during NMR imaging. *Noninvasive Med. Imaging*, 1, 35–41.

Breiter, H. C., Etcoff, N. L., Whalen, P. J. et al. (1996). Response and habituation of the human amygdala during visual processing of facial expression. *Neuron*, 17, 875–87.

Bunney, W. E., Jr and Davis, J. M. (1965). Norepinephrine in depressive reactions: a review. *Arch. Gen. Psychiatry*, 13, 483–94.

Burke, K. C., Burke, J. D., Rae, D. S. and Regier, D. A. (1991). Comparing age at onset of major depression and other psychiatric disorders by birth cohorts in five US community populations. *Arch. Gen. Psychiatry*, **48**, 789–95.

Charles, H. C., Lazeyras, F., Krishnan, K. R., Boyko, O. B., Payne, M. and Moore, D. (1994). Brain choline in depression: in vivo detection of potential pharmacodynamic effects of antidepressant therapy using hydrogen localized spectroscopy. *Prog. Neuropsychopharmacol. Biol. Psychiatry*, **18**, 1121–7.

Chiron, C., Raynaud, C., Maziere, B. et al. (1992). Changes in regional cerebral blood flow during brain maturation in children and adolescents. *J. Nucl. Med.*, **33**, 696–703.

Chugani, H. T. and Phelps, M. E. (1991). Imaging human brain development with positron emission tomography. *J. Nucl. Med.*, **32**, 23–6.

Chugani, H. T., Phelps, M. E. and Mazziotta, J. C. (1987). Positron emission tomography study of human brain functional development. *Ann. Neurol.*, **22**, 487–97.

Cicchetti, D., Rogosch, F. A., Toth, S. L. and Spagnola, M. (1997). Affect, cognition, and the emergence of self-knowledge in the toddler offspring of depressed mothers. *J. Exp. Child Psychol.*, **67**, 338–62.

Cooley, E. L. and Nowicki, S. Jr (1989). Discrimination of facial expressions of emotion by depressed subjects. *Genet. Soc. Gen. Psychol. Monogr.*, **115**, 449–65.

Coyle, J. T. (1987). Biochemical development of the brain: neurotransmitters and child psychiatry. In *Psychiatric Pharmacosciences of Children and Adolescents*, ed. C. Popper, pp. 3–26. Washington, DC: American Psychiatric Press.

Dahl, R., Puig-Antich, J., Ryan, N. et al. (1989). Cortisol secretion in adolescents with major depressive disorder. *Acta Scand.*, **80**, 18–26.

Deicken, R. F., Fein, G. and Weiner, M. W. (1995a). Abnormal frontal lobe phosphorous metabolism in bipolar disorder. *Am. J. Psychiatry*, **152**, 915–18.

Deicken, R. F., Weiner, M. W. and Fein, G. (1995b). Decreased temporal lobe phosphomonoesters in bipolar disorder. *J. Affect. Disord.*, **33**, 195–9.

de Renzi, E., Faglioni, P., Lodesani, M. and Vecchi, A. (1983). Performance of left brain-damaged patients on imitation of single movements and motor sequences. Frontal and parietal-injured patients compared. *Cortex*, **19**, 333–43.

De Villiers, A. S., Russell, V. A., Carstens, M. E. et al. (1989). Noradrenergic function and hypothalamic–pituitary–adrenal axis activity in adolescents with major depressive disorder. *Psychiatry Res.*, **27**, 101–9.

Doherty, M. B., Madansky, D., Kraft, J. et al. (1986). Cortisol dynamics and test performance of the dexamethasone suppression test in 97 psychiatrically hospitalized children aged 3–16 years. *J. Am. Acad. Child Psychiatry*, **25**, 400–8.

Drevets, W. C. (1998). Functional neuroimaging studies of depression: the anatomy of melancholia. *Annu. Rev. Med.*, **49**, 341–61.

Drevets, W. C. and Raichle, M. E. (1992). Neuroanatomical circuits in depression: implications for treatment mechanisms. *Psychopharmacol. Bull.*, **28**, 261–74.

Drevets, W. C., Videen, T. O., Price, J. L., Peskorn, S. H., Carmichael, S. T. and Raichle, M. E. (1992). A functional anatomical study of unipolar depression. *J. Neurosci.*, **12**, 3628–41.

Drevets, W. C., Price, J. L., Simpson, J. R., Jr et al. (1997). Subgenual prefrontal cortex abnormalities in mood disorders. *Nature*, **386**, 824–7.

Ekman, P. and Oster, H. (1979). Facial expressions of emotion. *Annu. Rev. Psychol.*, **30**, 527–54.

Elliott, R., Baker, S. C., Rogers, R. D. et al. (1997). Prefrontal dysfunction in depressed patients performing a complex planning task: a study using positron emission tomography. *Psychol. Med.*, **27**, 931–42.

Emslie, G. J., Weinberg, W. A., Rush, A. J., Weissenburger, J. and Parkin-Feigenbaum, L. (1987). Depression and dexamethasone suppression testing in children and adolescents. *J. Child Neurol.*, **2**, 31–7.

Emslie, G. J., Weinberg, W. A., Rush, A. J., Adams, R. M. and Rintelmann, J. W. (1990). Depressive symptoms by self report in adolescence: phase I of the development of a questionnaire for depression by self-report. *J. Child Neurol.*, **3**, 114–21.

Emslie, G. J., Rush, A. J., Weinberg, W. A., Gullion, C. M., Rintelmann, J. W. and Hughes, C. W. (1997). Recurrence of major depressive disorder in hospitalized children and adolescents. *J. Am. Acad. Child Adolesc. Psychiatry*, **36**, 785–92.

Erwin, R. J., Gur, R. C., Gur, R. E., Skolnick, B., Mawhinney-Hee, M., Smailis, J. (1992). Facial emotion discrimination: I. Task construction and behavioral findings in normal subjects. *Psychiatry Res.*, **42**, 231–40.

Extein, I., Rosenberg, G., Pottash, A., Gold, M. (1982). The dexamethasone suppression test in depressed adolescents. *Am. J. Psychiatry*, **139**, 1617–19.

Faedda, G. L., Baldessarini, R. J., Suppes, T., Tondo, L., Becker, I. and Lipschitz, D. S. (1995). Pediatric-onset bipolar disorder: a neglected clinical and public health problem. *Harvard Rev. Psychiatry*, **3**, 171–95.

Feinberg, T. E., Rifkin, A., Schaffer, C. and Walker, E. (1986). Facial discrimination and emotional recognition in schizophrenia and affective disorders. *Arch. Gen. Psychiatry*, **43**, 276–79.

Fleming, J. E. and Offord, D. R. (1990). Epidemiology of childhood depressive disorders: a critical review. *J. Am. Acad. Child Adolesc. Psychiatry*, **29**, 571–80.

Gaebel, W. and Wolwer, W. (1992). Facial expression and emotional face recognition in schizophrenia and depression. *Eur. Arch. Psychiatr. Clin. Neurosci.*, **242**, 46–52.

Garber, J., Kriss, M. R., Koch, M. and Lindholm, L. (1988). Recurrent depression in adolescents: a follow-up study. *J. Am. Acad. Child. Adolesc. Psychiatry*, **27**, 49–54.

Geller, B., Fox, L. W. and Clark, K. A. (1994). Rate and predictors of prepubertal bipolarity during follow-up of 6- to 12-year-old depressed children. *J. Am. Acad. Child Adolesc. Psychiatry*, **33**, 461–8.

Geller, B., Sun, K., Zimerman, B., Luby, J. and Frazier, J. (1995). Complex and rapid-cycling in bipolar children and adolescents: a preliminary study. *J. Affect. Disord.*, **34**, 259–68.

George, M. S., Ketter, T. A., Parekh, P. I., Horwitz, B., Herscovitch, P. and Prost, R. M. (1995). Brain activity during transient sadness and happiness in healthy women. *Am. J. Psychiatry*, **152**, 341–51.

George, M. S., Ketter, T. A., Parekh, P. I. et al. (1997). Blunted left cingulate activation in mood disorder subjects during a response interference task (the Stroop). *J. Neuropsychiatry Clin. Neurosci.*, **9**, 55–63.

Glennon, R. A. (1987). Central serotonin receptors as targets for drug research. *J. Med. Chem.*, **30**, 1–12.

Gold, P. W., Goodwin, F. K. and Chrousos, G. P. (1988). Clinical and biochemical manifestations of depression: relation to the neurobiology of stress. *N. Engl. J. Med.*, **319**, 348–53.

Golden, R. M. and Potter, W. Z. (1986). Neurochemical and neuroendocrine dysregulation in affective disorders. *Psychiatr. Clin. North Am.*, **9**, 313–27.

Gray, J. A., Davis, N., Feldon, J., Nicholas, J., Rawlins, P. and Owen, S. R. (1981). Animal models of anxiety. *Prog. Neuropsychopharmacol.*, **5**, 143–57.

Gur, R. C., Erwin, R. J. and Gur, R. E. (1992). Neurobehavioral probes for physiologic neuroimaging studies. *Arch. Gen. Psychiatry*, **49**, 409–14.

Gur, R. C., Ragland, J. D., Resnick, S. M. and Skolnick, B. E. (1994). Lateralized increases in cerebral blood flow during performance of verbal and spatial tasks: relationship with performance level. *Brain and Cognit.*, **24**, 244–58.

Harrington, R., Fudge, H., Rutter, M. and Hill, J. (1990). Adult outcomes of childhood and adolescent depression. *Arch. Gen. Psychiatry*, **47**, 465–73.

Hendren, R. L., Hodde-Vargas, J. E., Vargas, L. A., Orrison, W. W. and Dell, L. (1991). Magnetic resonance imaging of severely disturbed children – a preliminary study. *J. Am. Acad. Child Adolesc. Psychiatry*, **30**, 466–70.

Hofer, P. A. (1973). Urbach–Wiethe disease (lipoglycoproteinosis; lipoid proteinosis; hyalinosis cutis et mucosae). A review. *Acta Derm. Venereol.*, **53**(Suppl.), 1–52.

Hofer, P. A., Larsson, P. A., Goller, H., Laurell, H. and Lorentzon, R. (1974). A clinical and histopathological study of twenty-seven cases of Urbach–Wiethe disease. Dermatologic, gastroenterologic, neurophysiologic, ophthalmologic and roentgendiagnostic aspects, as well as the results of some clinico-chemical and histochemical examinations. *Acta Pathol. Microbiol. Scand., Pathol.*, (Suppl.) **245**, 1–87.

Kandal, D. B. and Davies, M. (1986). Adult sequela of adolescent depressive symptoms, *Arch. Gen. Psychiatry*, **43**, 255–62.

Kashani, J. H., Beck, N. C., Hoeper, E. et al. (1987a). Psychiatric disorders in a community sample of adolescents. *Am. J. Psychiatry*, **144**, 584–9.

Kashani, J. H., Carlson, G. A., Beck, N. C. et al. (1987b). Depression, depressive symptoms, and depressed mood among a community sample of adolescents. *Am. J. Psychiatry*, **144**, 931–4.

Kato, T., Takahashi, S., Shiori, T. and Inubushi, T. (1992). Brain phosphorous metabolism in depressive disorders detected by phosphorus-31 magnetic resonance spectroscopy. *J. Affect. Disord.*, **26**, 223–30.

Kato, T., Takahashi, S., Shiori, T. and Inubushi, T. (1993). Alterations in brain phosphorous metabolism in bipolar disorder detected in vivo ^{31}P and ^{7}Li magnetic resonance spectroscopy. *J. Affect. Disord.*, **27**, 53–9.

Kato, T., Inubushi, T. and Kato, N. (1998). Magnetic resonance spectroscopy in affective disorders. *J. Neuropsychiatr. Clin. Neurosci.*, **10**, 133–47.

Kessler, R. C., McGonagle, K. A., Nelson, C. B., Hughes, M., Swartz, M. and Blazer, D. G. (1994). Sex and depression in the national comorbidity survey. II. Cohort effects. *J. Affect. Disord.*, **30**, 15–26.

Ketter, T. George, M., Kimbrell, T., Benson, B. and Post, R. (1996). Functional brain imaging, limbic function, and affective disorders. *Neuroscientist*, **2**, 55–65.

Kovacs, M., Feinberg, T. L. and Crouse-Novak, M. A. (1984). Depressive disorders in childhood. II. A longitudinal study of the risk for a subsequent major depression. *Arch. Gen. Psychiatry*, **41**, 643–9.

Kowatch, R. A., Devous, M. D. S., Grannemann, B. G., Emslie, G. D., Trivedi, M. H. and Weinberg, W. A. (1993). A preliminary report of regional cerebral blood flow in depressed adolescents. In *Proceedings of a Meeting of the American Academy of Child and Adolescent Psychiatry*, San Antonio, Texas, p. 34.

Kowatch, R. A., Devous, M. D. S., Harvey, D. C. et al. (1999). A SPECT HMPAO study of regional cerebral blood flow in depressed adolescents and normal controls. *Prog. Neuropsychopharm. Biol. Psychiatry*, **23**, 643–56.

Kutcher, S., Malkin, D., Silverberg, J. et al. (1991). Nocturnal cortisol, thyroid stimulating hormone, and growth hormone secretory profiles in depressed adolescents. *J. Am Acad. Child Adolesc. Psychiatry*, **30**, 407–14.

LaBarbera, J. D., Izard, C. E., Vietze, P. and Parisi, S. A. (1976). Four- and six-month-old infants' visual responses to joy, anger, and neutral expressions. *Child Dev.*, **47**, 535–8.

Lane, R. D., Reiman, E. M., Ahern, G. L., Schwartz, G. E. and Davidson, R. J. (1997). Neuroanatomical correlates of happiness, sadness, and disgust. *Am. J. Psychiatry*, **154**, 926–33.

Lesser, I. M., Mena, I., Boone, K. B., Miller, B. L., Mehringer, C. M. and Wohl, M. (1994). Reduction of cerebral blood flow in older depressed patients. *Arch. Gen. Psychiatry*, **51**, 677–86.

Lewinsohn, P. M., Duncan, E. M., Stanton, A. K. and Hantzine, M. (1986). Age at onset for first unipolar depression. *J. Abnorm. Psychol.*, **95**, 387–3.

Lewinsohn, P. M. Hops, H., Roberts, R. E., Seeley, J. R. and Andrews, J. A. (1993). Adolescent psychopathology: I. Prevalence and incidence of depression and other DSM-III-R disorders in high school students. *J. Abnorm. Psychol.*, **102**, 133–44.

Lewinsohn, P. M., Clarke, G. N., Seeley, J. R. and Rhodes, P. (1994). Major depression in community adolescents: age at onset, episode duration, and time to recurrence. *J. Am. Acad. Child Adolesc. Psychiatry*, **33**, 809–18.

Lewinsohn, P. M., Klein, D. N. and Seeley, J. R. (1995). Bipolar disorder in a community sample of older adolescents: presence, phenomenology, comorbidity, and course. *J. Am. Acad. Child Adolesc. Psychiatry*, **34**, 454–63.

Maas, J. W. Fawcett, J. and Dekirmenjian, H. (1968). 3-Methoxy-4-hydroxyphenylglycol (MHPG) excretion in depressed states: a pilot study. *Arch Gen. Psychiatry*, **19**, 129–34.

Mandal, M. K and Bhattacharya, B. B. (1985). Recognition of facial affect in depression. *Percept. Motor Skills*, **61**, 13–14.

Mayberg, H. S. (1997). Limbic-cortical dysregulation: a proposed model of depression. *J. Neuropsychiatr. Clin. Neurosci.*, **9**, 471–81.

Mayberg, H. S., Lewis, P. J., Regenold, W. and Wagner, H. N. Jr (1994).

Paralimbic hypertension in unipolar depression. *J. Nucl. Med.*, **35**, 929–34.

McCauley, E., Myers, K., Mitchell, J., Calderon, R., Schloredt, K. and Treder, R. (1993). Depression in young people: initial presentation and clinical course. *J. Am. Acad. Child Adolesc. Psychiatry*, **32**, 714–22.

McCracken, J. T., Rubin, R. T. and Poland, R. E. (1988). Neuroendocrine aspects of primary endogenous depression. VI: Receiver operating characteristic analysis of the cortisol suppression index versus the dexamethasone suppression test in patients and matched controls. *Psychiatry Res.*, **26**, 69–78.

McGlashen, T. H. (1988). Adolescent versus adult onset of mania. *Am. J. Psychiatry*, **145**, 221–3.

Mendelson, W. B. Sitaram, N., Wyatt, R. J., Gillin, J. C. and Jacobs, L. S. (1978). Methoscopolamine inhibition of sleep related growth hormone secretion. Evidence for a cholinergic secretory mechanism. *J. Clin. Invest.*, **61**, 1683–90.

Mesulam, M. (1985). *Principles of Behavioral Neurology*. Philadelphia, PA: Davis.

Mesulam, M. M. (1990). Large-scale neurocognitive networks and distributed processing for attention, language, and memory. *Ann. Neurol.*, **28**, 597–613.

Moore, C. M., Christensen, J. D., Lafer, B., Fava, M. and Renshaw, P. F. (1997). Lower levels of nucleoside triphosphate in the basal ganglia of depressed subjects: a phosphorous-31 magnetic resonance spectroscopy study. *Am. J. Psychiatry*, **154**, 116–18.

Naylor, M. W., Greden, J. F. and Alessi, N. E. (1990). Plasma dexamethasone levels in children given the dexamethasone suppression test. *Biol. Psychiatry*, **27**, 592–600.

Pardo, J. V., Pardo, P. J. and Raichle, M. E. (1993). Neural correlates of self-induced dysphoria. *Am. J. Psychiatry*, **150**, 713–19.

Persad, S. M. and Polivy, J. (1993). Differences between depressed and nondepressed individuals in the recognition of and response to facial emotional cues. *J. Abnorm. Psychol.*, **102**, 358–68.

Philpot, M. P., Banerjee, S., Needham-Bennett, H., Costa, D. C. and Ell, P. J. (1993). ⁹⁹ᵐTc-HMPAO single photon emission tomography in late life depression: a pilot study of regional cerebral blood flow at rest and during a verbal fluency task. *J. Affect. Disord.*, **28**, 233–40.

Poznanski, E. O., Carroll, V. J., Benegas, M. E., Cook, S. C. and Grossman, J. A. (1982). The dexamethasone suppression test in prepubertal depressed children. *Am. J. Psychiatry*, **139**, 321–4.

Prange, A. J. Jr, Wilson, I. C., Lynn, C. W., Alltop, L. B. and Stikeleather, R. A. (1974). L-Tryptophan in mania: contribution to a permissive hypothesis of affective disorders. *Arch. Gen. Psychiatry*, **30**, 56–62.

Puig-Antich, J., Dahl, R., Ryan, N. et al. (1989). Cortisol secretion in prepubertal children with major depressive disorder. *Arch. Gen. Psychiatry*, **46**, 801–9.

Rao, U., Ryan, N. D., Birmaher, B. et al. (1995). Unipolar depression in adolescents: clinical outcome in adulthood. *J. Am. Acad. Child Adolesc. Psychiatry*, **34**, 566–78.

Reiman, E. M., Lane, R. D., Ahern, G. L. et al. (1997). Neuroanatomical correlates of externally and internally generated human emotion. *Am. J. Psychiatry*, **154**, 918–25.

Renshaw, P. F., Lafer, B., Babb, S. M. et al. (1997). Basal ganglia

choline levels in depression and response to fluoxetine treatment: an in vivo proton magnetic resonance spectroscopy study. *Biol. Psychiatry*, **41**, 837–43.

Rie, H. E. (1966). Depression in childhood. A survey of some pertinent contributions. *J. Am. Acad. Child Psychiatry*, **5**, 653–85.

Robbins, D. R., Alessi, N. E., Yanchyshyn, G. W. and Colfer, M. (1982). Preliminary report on the dexamethasone suppression test in adolescents. *Am. J. Psychiatry*, **139**, 942–3.

Rogeness, G. A., Javors, M. A. and Pliszka, S. R. (1992). Neurochemistry and child and adolescent psychiatry. *J. Am. Acad. Child Adolesc. Psychiatry*, **31**, 765–81.

Rubinow, D. R. and Post, R. M. (1992). Impaired recognition of affect in facial expression in depressed patients. *Biol. Psychiatry*, **31**, 947–53.

Rush, A., Stewart, R., Garver, D. and Waller, D. (1998). Neurobiological bases for psychiatric disorders. In *Comprehensive Neurology*, eds. R. Rosenberg and D. Pleasure, pp. 887–919. New York: Wiley.

Ryan, N. D., Birmaher, B., Perel, J. M. et al. (1992). Neuroendocrine response to L-5-hydroxytryptophan challenge in prepubertal major depression. Depressed vs. normal children. *Arch. Gen. Psychiatry*, **49**, 843–51.

Ryan, N. D., Dahl, R. E., Birmaher, B. et al. (1994). Stimulatory tests of growth hormone secretion in prepubertal major depression: depressed versus normal children. *J. Am. Acad. Child Adolesc. Psychiatry*, **33**, 824–33.

Sackeim, H. A., Prohovnik, I., Moeller, J. R. et al. (1990). Regional cerebral blood flow in mood disorders. I. Comparison of major depressives and normal controls at rest. *Arch. Gen. Psychiatry*, **47**, 60–70.

Schatzberg, A. F., Orsulak, P. J., Rosenbaum, A. J. et al. (1982). Toward a biochemical classification of depressive disorders, V: heterogeneity of unipolar depression. *Am. J. Psychiatry*, **139**, 471–5.

Schlaepfer, T. E., Pearlson, G. D., Wong, D. F., Marenco, S. and Dannals, R. F. (1997). PET study of competition between intravenous cocaine and [¹¹C] raclopride at dopamine receptors in human subjects. *Am. J. Psychiatry*, **154**, 1209–13.

Schneider, F., Gur, R. C., Jaggi, J. L. and Gur, R. E. (1994). Differential effects of mood on cortical cerebral blood flow: a 133-xenon clearance study. *Psychiatry Res.*, **52**, 215–36.

Schneider, F., Gur, R. E., Alavi, A. et al. (1996). Cerebral blood flow changes in limbic regions induced by unsolvable anagram tasks. *Am. J. Psychiatry*, **153**, 206–12.

Schneider, F., Grodd, W., Weiss, U. et al. (1997). Functional MRI reveals left amygdala activation during emotion. *Psychiatry Res.*, **76**, 75–82.

Sergent, J., Ohta, S. and Macdonald, B. (1992). Functional neuroanatomy of face and object processing: a positron emission tomography study. *Brain*, **115**, 15–36.

Shaffer, D., Fisher, P., Dulcan, M. K. et al. (1996). The NIMH diagnostic interview schedule for children version 2.3 (DISC-2.3): description, acceptability, prevalence rates, and performance in the MECA study. Methods for the epidemiology of child and adolescent mental disorders study. *J. Am. Acad. Child Adolesc. Psychiatry*, **35**, 865–77.

Sharma, R., Venkatasubramanian, P. N., Barany, M. and Davis, J. M. (1992). Proton magnetic resonance spectroscopy of the brain in schizophrenic and affective patients. *Schizophr. Res.*, **8**, 43–9.

Soares, J. C. and Mann, J. J. (1997a). The anatomy of mood disorders – review of structural neuroimaging studies. *Biol. Psychiatry*, **41**, 86–106.

Soares, J. C. and Mann, J. J. (1997b). The functional neuroanatomy of mood disorders. *J. Psychiatr. Res.*, **31**, 393–432.

Steingard, R. J., Renshaw, P. F., Yurgelun-Todd, D. et al. (1996). Structural abnormalities in brain magnetic resonance images of depressed children. *J. Am. Acad. Child Adolesc. Psychiatry*, **35**, 307–11.

Steingard, R., Renshaw, P., Yurgelun-Todd, D. and Wald, L. (1998). Proton MRS studies of the orbitofrontal cortex of depressed adolescents. *Biol. Psychiatry*, **43**, 28S.

Stoll, A. L., Renshaw, P. F., Sachs, G. S. et al. (1992). The human brain resonance of choline-containing compounds is similar in patients receiving lithium treatment and controls: an in vivo proton magnetic resonance spectroscopy study. *Biol. Psychiatry*, **32**, 944–9.

Strober, M., Lampert, C., Schmidt, S. and Morrell, W. (1993). The course of major depressive disorder in adolescents. I. Recovery and risk of manic switching in a follow-up of psychotic and non-psychotic subtypes. *J. Am. Acad. Child Adolesc. Psychiatry*, **32**, 34–42.

Sweeney, J. A., Wetzler, S., Stokes, P. and Kocsis, J. (1989). Cognitive functioning in depression. *J. Clin. Psychol.*, **45**, 836–42.

Swerdlow, N. and Koob, G. (1987). Dopamine, schizophrenia, mania, and depression: toward a unified hypothesis of cortico-striato-pallido-thalamic function. *Behav. Brain Sci.*, **10**, 197–245.

Tucker, D. (1988). *Neuropsychological Mechanisms of Affective Self-regulation*, pp. 1–22. Washington, DC: American Psychiatric Press.

van Praag, H. M. (1977). *Depression and Schizophrenia: A Contribution on Their Chemical Pathologies.* New York: Spectrum.

Willner, P. (1985). *Depression: A Psychobiological Synthesis.* New York: Wiley.

Wozniak, J., Biederman, J., Kiely, K. et al. (1995). Mania-like symptoms suggestive of childhood-onset bipolar disorder in clinically referred children. *J. Am. Acad. Child Adolesc. Psychiatry*, **34**, 867–76.

Zubenko, G. S. Moossy, J. and Kopp, U. (1990). Neurochemical correlates of major depression in primary dementia. *Arch. Neurol.*, **47**, 209–14.

13

Neuroimaging of childhood-onset anxiety disorders

David R. Rosenberg, Lori Anne D. Paulson,
Frank P. MacMaster and Gregory J. Moore

Introduction

The emergence of newer, noninvasive approaches to brain research since the 1980s, for example magnetic resonance spectroscopy (MRS) and functional magnetic resonance imaging (fMRI), has provided findings of critical relevance to childhood-onset anxiety disorders. These techniques are particularly well suited for studying pediatric populations where radiation exposure limits the use of positron emission tomography (PET) and single photon emission computed tomography (SPECT). This chapter will discuss the use of these techniques in childhood-onset anxiety disorders.

For many years, investigations in adult psychiatric disorders have been extended to child populations with the intent of verifying the finding in children in a "top-down" fashion. In the process, the developmental focus was often lost. Recent investigations have kept the developmental focus at the forefront, while applying a systems neuroscience approach to childhood-onset neuropsychiatric disorders, including pediatric anxiety. Understanding the underlying neutral substrate of childhood-onset anxiety disorders requires knowledge of the normal functional development of the brain. Recent investigations have begun to refine and map systematically the developmental trajectory of brain functions in normal children and to apply this knowledge to the study of childhood-onset neuropsychiatric disorders (Casey et al., 1995, 1997b; Rosenberg et al., 1997a,b; Rosenberg and Keshavan, 1998). The techniques of fMRI and MRS provide in vivo noninvasive approaches for studying neural circuitry in childhood anxiety disorders. Moreover, these techniques permit delineation of critical developmental "windows" of abnormality in brain anatomy and function in pediatric anxiety disorders.

Implementing a neuroscience approach to develop-mental systems in the study of childhood-onset anxiety disorders offers several critical advantages. Anxiety disorders frequently emerge during childhood even though they are not always diagnosed at their time of onset. In contrast to other neuropsychiatric disorders such as depression, the presentation of many anxiety disorders in children is quite similar to their presentation in adulthood, suggesting that the risk for certain core anxiety symptoms emerges during early childhood development. Studies of anxiety disorders during childhood near the time of onset can, therefore, minimize potential confounds of illness chronicity and treatment effects and begin to clarify the contributions of neurodevelopmental abnormalities to the pathogenesis of anxiety disorders.

A developmental approach to examining brain circuits can best explain the frequent childhood and adolescent onset of anxiety, as well as the modification of its presentation with age. Because fMRI and MRS are noninvasive and without radiation risks, repeated studies can be performed to elucidate the longitudinal course of anxiety as well as the impact of psychotropic medication, cognitive behavioral therapy, and illness duration on brain function and chemistry.

This chapter will review brain imaging studies in various childhood-onset anxiety disorders, including obsessive-compulsive disorder (OCD), generalized anxiety disorder (GAD), panic disorder, specific phobia, social phobia, and post-traumatic stress disorder (PTSD), as well as suggest directions for future investigation. Not all anxiety disorders have been examined by neuroimaging techniques. For example, to our knowledge there are no published neuroimaging studies in patients with separation anxiety disorder, despite its high prevalence (Benjamin et al., 1990) and early age of onset (Keller et al., 1992). OCD is the most investigated anxiety disorder and will occupy the largest place in this review. Finally, it is important to note that many fMRI and MRS studies have examined only a limited number of brain regions. Therefore, brain regions that are not mentioned either show no abnormalities or have not been analyzed.

One major concern in the study of anxiety disorders is the potential confound of "normative" anxiety that arises from participating in a medical procedure. Indeed, differences in brain activity have been shown as a function of anxiety state using both [^{18}F]-fluorodeoxyglucose (FDG) PET and the ^{133}Xe inhalation technique (Gur et al., 1987). Consequently, we discuss initially techniques of simulation training to reduce anxiety in subjects prior to functional neuroimaging data collection.

Simulation training for anxiety reduction

As with any medical procedure, brain imaging studies elicit anxiety in participants, particularly in children. To minimize levels of anxiety during MRI scanning, Rosenberg et al. (1997d) trained pediatric subjects in a simulation scanner that mimicked the actual MRI scanning environment. The simulation MRI scanner was equipped with a genuine scanner patient tube, 55 cm in diameter (kindly supplied by General Electric), a sound system, gurney bed, mirrors, and an airflow apparatus located in the bore of the scanner. The training process involved a graded exposure behavioral program. Parents and their children first toured the MRI center, where they were encouraged to ask questions and observe MRI studies in progress. Subjects then entered the simulation scanning room and were gradually introduced to the scanning procedure. Subjects were asked to lie down on the moveable patient table and were given ear plugs. Once the radio frequency coil was placed over the subject's head, rhythmic sounds of the MR procedure were played over a high-fidelity audio system. During the entire simulation procedure, all children had their pulse, blood pressure, and respiration continuously monitored. The Subjective Units of Discomfort Scale (SUDS), which measures distress on a scale of 0 to 100 (0 being no distress and 100 being overwhelming distress), was also administered (Wolpe et al., 1973). After the MRI simulation, children under the age of 12 received stickers and treats as rewards.

Rosenberg et al. (1997d) examined the efficacy of simulation scanning in 16 healthy pediatric subjects who were 7–17 years of age and in 16 age- and sex-matched, severely anxious children with OCD. Both healthy controls and OCD children exhibited a significant decrease in both subjective and objective anxiety as a result of the preliminary simulation scanning. Moreover, when levels

of anxiety of pediatric control subjects, who were not trained in the simulation scanner, were compared with control subjects trained in the simulation scanner, the pretrained group experienced significantly less subjective and objective distress during MRI data acquisition. None of the subjects who had been trained in the simulation scanner suffered a claustrophobic reaction in the actual scanner, whereas 10% of pediatric subjects ($n = 10$) not trained in the simulation scanner had a claustrophobic reaction necessitating discontinuation of the MRI procedure. This reduced anxiety resulted in improved comfort and cooperation during data collection, reduced head motion artifact, and increased signal-to-noise ratios (SNR). Parents and their children found the simulation experience reassuring and were grateful for the opportunity to "practice" and become comfortable with the MRI scanner. More striking were the results that occurred in patients with OCD, who began with higher levels of anxiety and demonstrated a more dramatic decrease in anxiety levels.

Simulation scanning may reduce the need for sedation for completion of MRI studies in children. This is important because sedation may introduce confounds when interpreting functional neuroimaging data. The simulation scanner also reduces the costs of scanning since the children are less apprehensive and require less time to settle down. The simulation scanning process typically takes 15–30 min in most children; however, it may take longer when children require extra reassurance (Rosenberg et al., 1997d). It should be noted, however, that constructing an actual simulation scanner is expensive; typical costs for scanner construction, equipment, and scanner time lie in the range of US $10 000–15 000. Because of these high costs, some groups have adopted alternative strategies for desensitizing children, such as presenting videotapes that demonstrate the procedures, utilizing a working scanner when it is not in use for data collection, or constructing less-expensive simulation scanners. MRI studies can also be greatly facilitated in those institutions that have an MRI center located in a children's hospital. An environment designed to make the appearance of a hospital less intimidating can further help children habituate to the actual scanning process.

Another potential confound is pharmacologically induced anxiety. For example, stimulants like caffeine may have anxiogenic effects. In fact, Moore et al. (1999) used ^{1}H MRS to demonstrate that intravenous caffeine induced changes in lactate concentration in the anterior cingulate and insular cortices in healthy volunteers. Therefore, it is important to control the amount of caffeine (caffeine-containing sodas, chocolate) consumed by children.

Obsessive-compulsive disorder

Since the late 1980s, there has been an increasing recognition of OCD as a severe, highly prevalent, and chronically disabling disorder characterized by repetitive, ritualistic thoughts, ideas, impulses, and behaviors over which individuals have little control. Characteristic obsessions and compulsions include pathologic doubting, fear of germs, need for symmetry, checking, washing, hoarding, and religious scrupulosity. The lifetime prevalence of OCD is 2–3% (Flament et al., 1988; Valleni-Basile et al., 1994; Hanna, 1995), and as many as 80% of all patients have a disease onset in children and adolescence (Pauls et al., 1995). The mean age of onset of OCD in referred children and adolescents ranges from 9 years (Riddle et al., 1990) to 10.7 years of age (Last and Strauss, 1989).

Neurobiologic studies have begun to clarify the pathophysiology of OCD. Converging lines of evidence support basal ganglia–frontal cortical pathway dysfunction as a basis for OCD (Modell et al., 1989; Wise and Rapoport, 1989; Baxter et al., 1992; Insel, 1992) (Fig. 13.1, p. 242). Brain structures related to fear (i.e., amygdala, hippocampus) act in concert with the frontal thalamic loop, which is implicated in OCD (Fig. 13.2, p. 242). Increased rates of OCD symptoms in basal ganglia disorders such as Tourette's syndrome, Sydenham's chorea, and postencephalitic parkinsonism (von Economo, 1931; Pitman et al., 1987) and the fact that psychosurgical lesions of ventral prefrontal cortex (anterior cingulum) can decrease OCD symptoms (Jenike et al., 1991) provide indirect support for this hypothesis. More direct evidence comes from functional neuroimaging studies in adult patients with childhood onset of OCD. These studies have demonstrated increased metabolic activity in ventral prefrontal cortex and the head of the caudate nucleus (Benkelfat et al., 1990; Hoehn-Saric et al., 1991; Baxter et al., 1992; Swedo et al., 1992a,b; Rauch et al., 1994; Breiter and Rauch, 1996; Schwartz et al., 1996). However, despite the high prevalence and frequent childhood onset, there have been few studies of children with this disorder. The neuroimaging findings in OCD will be discussed in terms of the structures affected, the networks identified by activation tasks, and the changes detected in neurotransmitters.

Structures implicated in obsessive-compulsive disorder

Basal ganglia and ventricular size

In two early studies using computed tomographic (CT) scans. Behar et al, (1984) found significantly larger ventric-

ular brain ratios in 16 adolescents with OCD (13 males, three females) relative to age- and sex-matched control subjects, whereas Luxenberg et al. (1988) found significantly smaller caudate volumes in late adolescent and young adult male patients with OCD compared with controls. Caudate abnormalities were most pronounced in younger patients with OCD (J. Rapoport, personal communication). Using MRI, Rosenberg et al. (1997c) examined striatal volumes in 19 nondepressed, treatment-naive pediatric patients with OCD, ages 8–17 years, and 19 age- and sex-matched controls. The patients with OCD had significantly smaller striatal volumes than the controls, and their striatal volumes negatively correlated with OCD symptom severity. Striatal volumes, however, did not correlate with duration of illness, age of onset of illness, age of child, or intracranial volume. Children with OCD also had increased third ventricular volumes relative to age- and sex-matched controls. Consistent with these findings, Giedd et al. (1995) also found selective anatomic basal ganglia abnormalities in 24 pediatric patients with Sydenham's chorea and OCD compared with 48 matched controls. The sizes of the caudate, putamen, and globus pallidus were larger in the Sydenham's chorea group compared with controls; no size differences were found in total cerebral, prefrontal, midfrontal, or thalamic volumes.

Frontal cortex and corpus callosum

Consistent with a prior study in adult patients with OCD (Robinson et al., 1995), Rosenberg and colleagues (1997c) did not find any significant differences in MRI measurements of total prefrontal cortical gray or white matter volumes between 19 pediatric patients with OCD, aged 7–17 years and 19 age- and sex-matched controls. However, prior functional neuroimaging studies in adult patients with OCD had found abnormally high glucose metabolic activity in ventral prefrontal cortex (Baxter, 1992). Morphometric measurement of the total prefrontal cortex may not be sensitive enough to detect subtle case–control differences in structures such as ventral prefrontal cortex. Indeed, subsequent studies of the regional morphology of the corpus callosum are consistent with ventral prefrontal deviance (Rosenberg et al., 1997b). Specifically, abnormalities in the genu of the corpus callosum were identified. Fibers that connect the ventral prefrontal cortex and the striatum cross between the cerebral hemispheres at this point (Seltzer and Pandya, 1986). Patients with OCD who were between the ages of 7.2–17.7 years were found to have larger genu sizes than age- and sex-matched controls. The increased genu sizes correlated positively with OCD symptom severity but not with illness duration. Increased genu size of the corpus callosum in

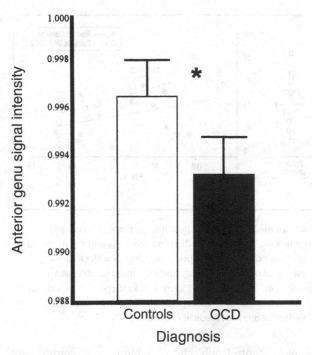

Fig. 13.3. Anterior genu signal intensity in patients with obsessive-compulsive disorder (OCD) and controls ($*F_{(1,37)} = 5.47$; $p = 0.025$). (Created by Frank P. MacMaster.)

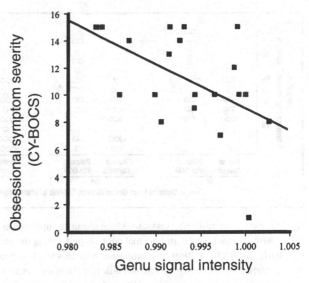

Fig. 13.4. Genu signal intensity in relation to symptom severity ($r = 0.55$; $p = 0.01$) as measured by the Children's Yale–Brown Obsessive Compulsive Scale (CY-BOCS). (Created by Frank P. MacMaster.)

patients with OCD could be the result of increased myelinization of fibers in that area relative to that in controls. In fact, the normal age-related increase in the total corpus callosum area (Giedd et al., 1996; Rajapakse et al., 1996) was absent in patients with OCD. Earlier myelinization could result in increased corpus callosum size in these patients. However, no significant difference in corpus callosum area between adult patients with OCD and controls has been observed (Jenike et al., 1996), consistent with the hypothesis that myelinization of axons may be more gradual in healthy children than in those with OCD, only catching up toward the end of adolescence or in early adulthood. It is also possible that these findings may reflect a greater number of synaptic connections or less pruning in young patients with OCD, resulting in increased axonal density.

The following findings support the hypothesis of enhanced myelinization of corpus callosum fibers in OCD. MacMaster et al. (1999) compared regional corpus callosum signal intensity from midsagittal MRI in 21 treatment-naive patients with OCD, 7.2–17.2 years of age, and 21 case-matched healthy controls. Although controversial, the measure of MRI signal brightness, or signal intensity (SI), is believed to reflect myelination (van der Knapp and Valk, 1989; Laissy et al., 1993; Belmonte et al., 1995).

MacMaster et al. (1999) found lower SI in the anterior genu region of the corpus callosum connecting the ventral prefrontal cortex and the striatum in OCD compared with controls (Fig. 13.3). The lower was the genu SI, the more severe were the OCD symptoms (Fig. 13.4). No correlation was detected between illness duration and genu SI. MacMaster and colleagues (1999) hypothesized that a deficit in myelination occurring in patients with OCD may result in abnormal signal transmission and function of ventral prefrontal–striatal circuitry.

Anterior cingulate

More recently, Rosenberg and Keshavan (1998) reported increased ventral prefrontal cortex and anterior cingulate volumes in 21 treatment-naive pediatric patients with OCD relative to age- and sex-matched controls. Increased volumes were associated with increased OCD symptom severity, but not with illness duration. No anatomic abnormalities were observed in posterior cingulate cortex, dorsolateral prefrontal cortex, or temporal cortex. Moreover, an age-related increase in anterior cingulate volumes in healthy pediatric controls was not observed in these pediatric patients. Increased anterior cingulate volumes, particularly in younger patients with OCD, were consistent with prior observations of increased genu size of the corpus callosum (Rosenberg et al., 1997b). Larger anterior cingulate volumes tended to be associated with smaller striatal volumes in pediatric patients with OCD,

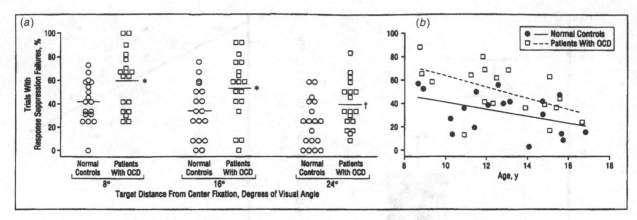

Fig. 13.5. Response inhibition tasks. (*a*) Mean response suppression failures for medication-naive pediatric patients with obsessive-compulsive disorder (OCD) and normal controls performing the antisaccadic task. Lines through distributions represent the mean value. (*$p = 0.01$; $^+p = 0.02$). (*b*) Response suppression failures as a function of age for medication-naive pediatric patients with OCD and normal controls performing the antisaccadic task. Note the marked inverse correlation between age and total number of response suppression errors in patients with OCD and a trend for such an effect in controls. (Adapted from Figure 2, Rosenberg, D. R., Averbach, D. H., O'Hearn, K. M. et al. (1997a). Reprinted from Oculomotor response inhibition abnormalities in pediatric obsessive compulsive disorder, *Archives of General Psychiatry*, 1997, 54(9), 831–8, copyright 1995–1997. American Medical Association.)

(Rosenberg et al., 1997c; Rosenberg and Keshavan, 1998). This neuroanatomic dysplasia in OCD might represent an increase in pruning and/or a decrease in neural tissue in the striatum, whereas the increased ventral prefrontal cortical volumes might represent a delay in pruning and/or an excess of neural brain elements. The increased volume observed in the anterior cingulate in OCD may be indicative of a delay in the normal pruning processes that occur during this period, further implicating a putative developmental abnormality.

Cognitive/behavioral activation tasks

Another strategy used to examine neural networks in OCD involves the use of functional neuroimaging in conjunction with activation tasks. This neurocognitive/behavioral approach has the advantage of exploiting the richness of neuropsychologic research, which develops theoretical models and provides a priori hypotheses. Such experimental paradigms require the development and testing of activation tasks appropriate for the model to be tested and for use with brain imaging technologies.

Response inhibition tasks

Based on the theory that OCD may represent the expression of abnormal inhibitory processes, tasks of inhibition have been sought for use in brain imaging studies. Along these lines, Rosenberg et al. (1997a) measured three core prefrontal functions in treatment-naive pediatric patients with OCD (aged 7 to 18 years) and age- and sex-matched

healthy control subjects: (i) inhibition of contextually inappropriate responses, (ii) delayed responses involving working memory (requiring a response to new situations on the basis of stored information without benefit of sensory cue information), and (iii) the ability to prepare a response in advance of its initiation. The Antisaccadic Response Suppression Task was used to test these functions. In this task, subjects fixate their eyes on a central target (such as a red dot), then look the same distance, but in the opposite direction of targets presented to the left or right of the center fixation (8, 16, or 24 degrees). Therefore, if a target appeared to the left, subjects need to shift their eyes 8° to the right. This test requires the suppression of a powerful reflexive response to look toward novel peripheral targets and the ability to drive the eyes volitionally away from a target when no cue exists in the periphery. The inability of subjects to drive their eyes away from and in the opposite direction of the peripheral target is classified as a response suppression failure. A selective deficit in neurobehavioral response inhibition was observed in patients with OCD, particularly in younger patients, compared with age- and sex-matched controls (Fig. 13.5); these patients showed no deficits on measures of delayed response and preparatory set. Controls began to master neurobehavioral response inhibitions tasks approximately 5 years earlier than did patients with OCD; as a result, comparable performance was observed between 16-year-old patients with OCD and 11-year-old healthy control subjects. In addition, response inhibition failures correlated significantly with striatal and ventral prefrontal cortical volumetric MRI measures (Rosenberg and Keshavan, 1998), suggesting a developmental neurobiologic model for relating anatomic findings with clinical and behavioral OCD symptoms.

Ventral prefrontal–striatal circuits appear to play a crucial role in mediating responses suppression (Rosvold and Mishkin, 1961; Luria, 1966; Goldman and Rosvold, 1970; Iversen and Mishkin, 1970; Goodglass and Kaplan, 1972; Passingham, 1972; Rosenkilde, 1979; Stuss and Benson, 1983; Diamond, 1990; Cummings, 1993; Sweeney et al., 1996), whereas dorsal prefrontal cortex has been shown to mediate delayed response and preparatory set functions (Goldman and Rosvold, 1970; Funahashi et al., 1989). Consistent with this, functional neuroimaging studies in healthy volunteers have reported functional activation of ventral prefrontal cortico–striatal circuitry in tasks of inhibition such as the antisaccadic oculomotor response inhibition task (Sweeney et al., 1996) and the go-no-go task (Casey et al., 1997). Consequently, dysplasia in ventral prefrontal–striatal circuits might give rise to OCD by disrupting a neurocognitive function that mediates ongoing purposive behaviors. The localization of a neuro-anatomic abnormality that correlates with deficits in neurobehavioral tasks known to be subserved by this brain region provides an ideal focus for functional neuroimaging using fMRI. The fMRI technique can monitor in vivo the spatial localization and time course of functional abnormalities. Such studies are now being conducted in our laboratory.

Symptom provocation

Another type of behavioral activation paradigm used to study OCD is that designed to provoke symptoms. Using fMRI, Breiter et al. (1996) studied 10 adult patients with OCD and five normal control subjects during control and experimental conditions designed to induce OCD symptoms. The subjects were asked to hold a neutral stimulus object, with the knowledge that a feared stimulus object would be introduced half-way through the scan. The feared stimulus objects included blindly faked versions of (i) tissue soaked in toilet water, (ii) plastic bags from contaminated waste barrels, and (iii) tissue with nose effluvium. Increased activation of the ventral prefrontal–striatal circuits was found in patients with OCD but not in healthy controls. Abnormal activation was also observed in these patients in temporolimbic regions, i.e., the hippocampus. Adapting the technique designed and developed by Rauch and colleagues (1994) and Breiter and associates (1996), Rosenberg and Thulborn have initiated similar studies in pediatric patients with OCD with comparable findings (unpublished data).

Conclusion

Findings from activation studies appear promising. Thus far, they support neurocognitive and neurofunctional theories of OCD. The challenge of neuroimaging research is to further the understanding of mechanisms underlying the hypothesized processes in order to provide clues on how to modify these processes and develop focused, rational, and effective therapeutic interventions. In this regard, the elucidation of the role of neurochemical substrates in the dysfunction of the neural circuits involved in OCD is critical.

Neurochemical substrates

Serotonin

Pharmacologic treatment studies have suggested a critical role for serotonin in OCD. Serotonin reuptake inhibitors (e.g., fluvoxamine, sertraline) are effective in treating OCD, whereas dopamine and noradrenaline reuptake inhibitors (e.g., amitriptyline, desipramine) are less effective (Pigott, 1996). Other studies have found the serotonin transporter protein (5HTPR) capacity, as indexed in platelets by ^{3}H-paroxetine, to be decreased in pediatric patients with OCD (Sallee et al., 1996). Researchers have also found the brain regions with the greatest binding of the potent selective serotonin reuptake inhibitor (SSRI) citalopram to be the caudate nucleus and nucleus accumbens (Insel, 1992). Moreover, the ventral prefrontal cortex and the striatum are densely innervated by serotonin-containing neurons (Smith and Parent, 1986). Finally, animal studies have shown that a sustained administration of SSRI to guinea pigs increases serotonin release by desensitizing terminal serotonin autoreceptors in the orbital prefrontal cortex. Findings such as these have spawned the "serotonin hypothesis of OCD", which postulates that OCD is mediated by serotoninergic alterations in ventral prefrontal–striatal circuits.

Studies investigating alterations of neurotransmitters in blood and the serotonin metabolite 5-hydroxyindoleacetic acid (5-HIAA) in cerebrospinal fluid (CSF) of patients with OCD have found positive correlations between drug-induced decreases in platelet serotonin concentrations (Flament et al., 1985) and CSF 5-HIAA levels (Thoren et al., 1980) in adult patients with OCD; however, other studies have failed to detect such a relationship (Pandey et al., 1993). Studies of platelet serotonin and CSF, however, provide a poor index of brain function and chemistry.

Recently, Rosenberg et al. (1998) compared seven children with OCD (aged 8 to 13 years) with seven age-matched controls using PET and α-[^{11}C]-methyl-L-tryptophan ([^{11}C]-AMT), an analog of tryptophan and a tracer for serotonin synthesis (Diksic et al., 1991). Tryptophan is converted to serotonin by tryptophan hydroxylase, the rate-limiting enzyme in serotonin synthesis. Preliminary data indicated a reduction in serotonin synthesis in the caudate nucleus of treatment-naive, pediatric patients with OCD, relative to controls (Fig. 13.6, p. 242). Five children were scanned twice: before and after a 3-week treatment with the SSRI paroxetine. Treatment response was associated with increased serotonin synthesis in the caudate nucleus in three children (Fig. 13.6, p. 242).

Because PET scanning involves exposure to ionizing radiation, the study of healthy children as controls is problematic. The risk–value attached to radiation exposure at the doses used in brain imaging studies is difficult to address because of the emotional impact at the mention of radiation. In fact, health hazards associated with low-level radiation have not been detected in any of the large studies conducted to date. Despite the lack of evidence of excess risk of low-level radiation exposure above the expected risks of daily life, most Institutional Review Boards (IRBs) consider low-level radiation exposure to be above minimal risk. In the aforementioned study (Rosenberg et al., 1998), comparison subjects for the patients with OCD included developmentally normal siblings of patients with OCD or autism. The IRB of the Children's Hospital of Michigan at Wayne State University School of Medicine, where the study was performed, did not allow the study of healthy children without a first-degree relative with a significant neuropsychiatric disorder. On the one hand, the use of siblings of affected patients as comparison groups may not be ideal because they may carry a genetically determined brain abnormality predisposing them to the disorder, but without expression of the symptoms. Indeed, the IRB approved these protocols in siblings because of their increased risk for developing neuropsychiatric disorders. For example, if brain serotonergic abnormalities are found to constitute a pathophysiologic mechanism in OCD, then it is possible that their high-risk siblings may also have serotonergic abnormalities. On the other hand, the use of siblings as a comparison group can reduce intersubject variability, increasing the chance to detect differences related to diagnostic status.

Glutamatergic neurotransmitter

MRS permits investigators to monitor directly and noninvasively brain chemistry without radiation exposure (see Chapter 4). Proton MRS can identify compounds that include the neuronal marker N-acetylaspartate (NAA) (Birken and Oldendorf, 1989), glutamate/glutamine, gamma-aminobutyric acid (GABA) (Glx), creatine/phosphocreatine (Cr), choline compounds (Cho), and *myo*-inositol (myo-I).

The ability to measure Glx concentrations by MRS may be especially relevant, because glutamatergic–serotonin modulation may be involved in the pathogenesis of OCD (Rosenberg and Keshavan, 1998). Indeed, glutamate plays a critical role in the striatum (Becquet et al., 1990), which receives dense glutamatergic projections from the prefrontal cortex (Taber and Fibiger, 1993, 1994). The caudate nucleus, in particular, receives a very large glutamatergic innervation from the cerebral cortex such that if the frontal cortex or the hemicortex is ablated, there is a marked reduction of glutamate concentrations in the rat caudate nucleus (Kim et al., 1977). In addition, Becquet et al. (1990) have demonstrated a potent presynaptic inhibitory glutamatergic control of serotonin release, possibly via GABA interneurons, in the cat caudate nucleus.

Preliminary MRS studies have shown elevated glutamatergic concentrations in the caudate nucleus of pediatric patients with OCD compared with controls (Rosenberg et al., 1998). Following 12 weeks of SSRI treatment, the level of glutamatergic concentrations in the caudate nucleus decreased in patients with OCD (Moore et al., 1998) (Fig. 13.7). This reduction was associated with a reduction in OCD symptom severity (Fig. 13.8).

Using ^{1}H MRS, Ebert et al. (1997) demonstrated reduced NAA levels, suggestive of neuronal dysfunction, in the striatum and anterior cingulate of 12 patients with OCD that correlated with symptom severity, but not with illness duration. No abnormalities were observed in the parietal cortex. A reduction of NAA levels in the ventral prefrontal cortex and striatum may be indicative of underlying metabolic abnormalities in OCD (Ebert et al., 1997). These results demonstrate how ^{1}H MRS can be used for the in vivo monitoring of brain chemistry and the impact of psychotropic medication on brain neurochemistry, as it relates to the medication's therapeutic effect. Moreover, this technology involves no radiation risks or blood sampling, both of which are best avoided in pediatric research studies. It should be noted, however, that considerable development and refinement of methods is necessary before determination of the precise meaning of the MRS signals is possible.

Summary

To date, functional neuroimaging has most consistently identified the caudate nucleus, ventral prefrontal cortex, and anterior cingulate as neural substrates of OCD. These regions have shown abnormal serotonergic and/or glutamatergic function. These findings evidence the great potential of brain imaging for unraveling the mechanisms

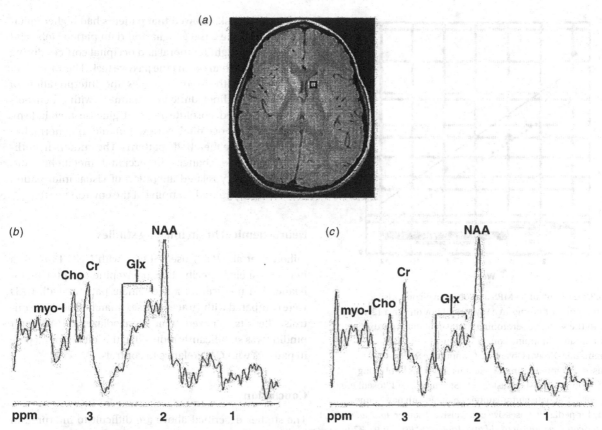

Fig. 13.7. MRS studies on a 9-year-old boy with obsessive-compulsive disorder. (*a*) Proton MRS of a 0.7 ml volume of interest centered in the left caudate, as shown by the box on the T_1-weighted MR image.(*b*) Spectrum obtained at baseline in the treatment-naive state. (*c*) Spectrum obtained after a 12-week trial of the selective serotonin reuptake inhibitor paroxetine. NAA, *N*-acetylaspartate; Glx, glutamate/glutamine; Cr, creatine/phosphocreatine; Cho, choline-containing compounds; myo-I, myoinositol. (Permission granted from the Williams & Wilkins Publishing House; Moore, G. J., MacMaster, F. P., Stewart, C., and Rosenberg, D. R. (1998). Caudate glutamatergic changes with paroxetine therapy for pediatric obsessive compulsive disorder, *Journal of the American Academy of Child and Adolescent Psychiatry*, 27(6), 663–7.)

underlying OCD. Functional networks, as well as neurobiochemical systems, need to be examined in a systematic fashion. This work needs to be interactive with genetic research, which requires the identification of homogeneous phenotypes (which brain imaging may provide) but which can also define subgroups to be studied using neuroimaging.

Generalized anxiety disorder

Epidemiologic catchment area studies have found a high lifetime prevalence rate of 3.7% for GAD (called overanxious disorder in DSM-III-R) in 5596 nonreferred children aged 14–17 years (Whitaker et al., 1990), a prevalence of 2.4% in 1869 children 12–16 years (Bowen et al., 1990), and 2.9% for 792 11 year olds (Anderson et al.,

1987). In a pediatric primary care setting, a sample of 300 children aged 7–11 years demonstrated a 15.4% prevalence of anxiety disorders, with simple phobia, separation anxiety disorder, and GAD being the most prevalent (Benjamin et al., 1990). The prevalence of GAD in this population was 4.6%. Median age of onset of GAD was found to be 10 years (Keller et al., 1992). To date, there have been only three published brain imaging studies in adults with GAD, and none in children or adolescents with GAD.

Benzodiazepine cerebral effects

Wu et al. (1991) utilized PET to measure brain glucose metabolism in 18 patients with GAD and 15 healthy control subjects. Measurements in patients with GAD were taken at three different times: baseline, pretreatment (or baseline

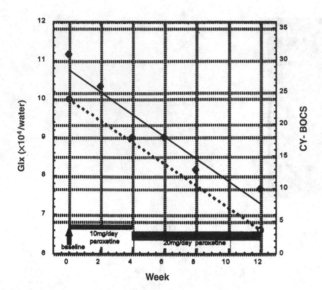

Fig. 13.8. Summary of ¹H MRS and obsessive-compulsive symptomatology findings in a 9-year-old boy during a 12-week trial with the selective serotonin reuptake inhibitor paroxetine. Glx, glutamate/glutamine concentrations (- - -); CY-BOCS, Children's Yale–Brown Obsessive Compulsive Scale (—). (Permission granted from the Williams & Wilkins Publishing House; Moore, G. J., MacMaster, F. P., Stewart, C. and Rosenberg, D. R. (1998). Caudate glutamatergic changes with paroxetine therapy for pediatric obsessive compulsive disorder, *Journal of the American Academy of Child and Adolescent Psychiatry*, 27(6), 663–7.)

2), and following a 21-day double-blind treatment with clorazepate (8) or placebo (10). During the first baseline, subjects (GAD and controls) were required only to observe the degraded stimulus of a continuous performance task (CPT) (passive task). In the pretreatment and post-treatment studies, subjects actively had to identify target stimuli during a CPT (active, vigilance task) before and after receiving either a benzodiazepine (clorazepate) or placebo for 21 days. The use of two different cognitive tasks during baseline permitted the identification of the regions of the brain involved in attention, determined through comparisons of activity during the passive versus active tasks. Attention is likely to activate regions involved in anxiety, which is characterized by a heightened state of vigilance. The identified regions were then targeted in the assessment of treatment effects.

During the passive visual task, patients with GAD showed lower basal ganglia (particularly putamen and globus pallidus) metabolic rates and higher glucose metabolism in occipital cortex, right posterior temporal cortex, and the right precentral frontal gyrus relative to controls. Comparison of the two baseline studies (active

task, passive task) showed that patients had higher metabolic rates in the basal ganglia and right parietal lobe and lower rates in right temporal and occipital cortices during the active task than during the passive task. The absence of comparison with controls makes the interpretation of these latter findings difficult. Treatment with a benzodiazepine reduced absolute rates of glucose metabolism, particularly in occipital cortex, but did not normalize regional glucose metabolic patterns. The authors hypothesized that the changes in occipital metabolic rates reflected anxiety-related alteration of visual information processing (increased scanning of the environment).

Neurochemical brain imaging studies

Tiihonen et al. (1997) used SPECT with NNC 13-8241, a new ¹²³I-labeled specific benzodiazepine receptor radioligand. Ten medication-naive female patients with GAD were compared with 10 age- and sex-matched healthy controls. Results showed that benzodiazepine receptor binding was significantly reduced in the left temporal pole in patients with GAD relative to controls.

Conclusions

The studies described above are difficult to interpret, in part because of the complex designs that involve the interaction of various factors such as the use of different conditions and pharmacologic intervention. Issues of primary versus secondary effects of the biochemical changes, as well as of the changes in symptoms, are difficult to sort out in pharmacologic studies and require the use of careful study designs. The serotonin receptor SPECT study is of great interest but, like most brain imaging studies, suffers from low statistical power because of the small sample size; it requires replication.

It is clear that abnormalities in integrated brain activity, indexed by measurements of glucose metabolism, need to be characterized neurobiochemically. An interesting proposition is that benzodiazepine receptor dysfunction may be secondary to GABAergic abnormalities (Allen et al., 1995). The ¹H MRS technique at high magnetic fields (4 T and higher) may provide a means with which to examine this hypothesis (Rothman et al., 1993; Keltner et al., 1997).

Panic disorder

As described in DSM-IV (American Psychiatric Association, 1994), the diagnosis of panic disorder can be made with or without agoraphobia (fear of crowds and being unable to escape from places where panic attacks may occur). Panic disorder is characterized by recurrent panic attacks or the fear of developing a panic attack. A panic attack is characterized by feelings of impending doom and/or fear of dying, with typical physical and psychologic symptoms. Retrospective studies of adults with panic disorder indicate that panic disorder typically begins in adolescence or early adulthood (Moreau and Follett, 1993) and is uncommon before puberty (Black and Robbins, 1990; Klein et al., 1992). The peak age of onset of panic disorders is 15 to 19 years (von Korff et al., 1985). In a study of 754 pubertal sixth- and seventh-grade girls in the USA, 5.3% of the girls reported a history of having had at least one panic attack (Hayward et al., 1992). Interestingly, panic attacks increased significantly during sexual maturation, with rates of 8% for females at Tanner stage 5 (sexually mature) and 0% for the 94 girls at Tanner stages 1 or 2 (sexually immature). This increased frequency of panic attacks with sexual maturation could not be explained by differences in chronologic age (Bernstein et al., 1996). This suggests the influence of sexual steroid hormones on the induction of panic attacks.

Pollack et al. (1996) found that over 54% of 194 adults with panic disorder had a history of childhood anxiety disorders, and patients with a history of childhood anxiety disorders had significantly more comorbid mood disorders during adulthood. Furthermore, over 60% of adults with panic disorder who had a history of childhood anxiety disorder had been diagnosed with two or more anxiety disorders during childhood. The comorbidity among anxiety and mood disorders must be considered in designing brain imaging studies. Neuroimaging studies in adults with panic disorder have begun to delineate the neurobiology of this disorder (Sallee and Greenwald, 1995; Goddard and Charney, 1997).

Structural abnormalities

To identify more homogeneous subtypes of panic disorder, Dantendorfer et al. (1996) divided a sample of 120 patients with panic disorder (53 males, 67 females) into two groups: one with nonepileptic electroencephalographic (EEG) abnormalities (35) and one without EEG abnormalities (85). Twenty eight patients with EEG abnormalities were able to complete an MRI successfully. These 28 subjects were sex- and age-matched with 28 patients with GAD without EEG abnormalities and with 28 healthy subjects, all with normal EEG. The EEG was evaluated clinically by a psychiatrist. Although EEG abnormalities were more frequent in patients with panic disorder than rates reported for healthy subjects, their role in panic disorder is unclear,

and the choice of this discriminating factor not well justified. Subjects were compared on structural MRI, read clinically by three experienced neurologists who were blind to all subject information. MRI abnormalities were present in over 60% of the patient group with abnormal EEG, 17.9% of the patient group with normal EEG readings, and 3.6% of the controls. Patients with panic disorder had significantly more septohippocampal abnormalities than controls, which included smaller right hippocampi and the presence of a cavum septum pellucidum. The implication of hippocampal abnormalities is consistent with functional neuroimaging findings.

Functional neuroimaging

Utilizing PET and $H_2{}^{15}O$ with 16 patients with panic disorder and 25 control subjects, Reiman et al. (1986) reported that those patients who were most susceptible to lactate-induced panic attacks (eight) had abnormally high global brain oxygen metabolism and deviant asymmetries of parahippocampal regional cerebral blood flow (rCBF) and oxygen metabolism.

Using PET and FDG during the performance of an auditory discrimination attention task, Nordahl et al. (1990) compared 12 patients with panic disorder (five males, seven females) with 30 healthy volunteers (16 males, 14 females). Similar to Reiman's results (1986), the patient group showed abnormal hippocampal asymmetry. However, global brain glucose metabolism was not altered. In addition, regional glucose metabolism was abnormally low in the left inferior parietal lobe and anterior cingulate cortex and abnormally high in the orbitofrontal cortex.

More recently, Dager et al. (1995) used ^1H MRS to compare the effects of hyperventilation on brain lactate in seven patients with panic disorder (four males, three females) and seven healthy comparison subjects (five males, two females). Hyperventilation normally increases brain lactate concentrations. This study was stimulated by previous observations of abnormally large increases in brain lactate in patients with panic disorder during lactate administration (Dager et al., 1994). Prior to hyperventilation, these patients had brain lactate levels similar to those of controls, but they demonstrated a significantly greater increase in brain lactate than controls in response to the same degree of hyperventilation (Dager et al., 1995). Blood levels of lactate measured before and after hyperventilation did not differ significantly between the patients and the healthy controls, underscoring the importance of direct evaluation of the brain regions of interest as opposed to relying on peripheral indices of brain function and chemistry. Here again, the mechanism of increased lactate production in the activation state in individuals with panic disorder remains unclear.

Conclusion

The brain regions implicated in panic disorder by the above studies are consistent with the brain networks subserving fear and anxiety. Structural asymmetries, such as those reported in the hippocampal/parahippocampal regions, may be chance findings as a result of the high variability and small differences of left–right measures or may reflect developmental processes that contribute to brain lateralization. The functional significance of these findings needs to be further explored.

Specific (simple) phobias

As defined by DSM-IV (American Psychiatric Association, 1994), specific phobia, previously referred to as simple phobia, consists of fear and anxiety associated with specific objects (e.g., snakes) or situations (thunder and lightning), which result in significant impairment. Adults with specific phobias recognize their symptoms to be excessive and unreasonable, while children may be unable to do so (Bernstein et al., 1996). When exposed to the phobic stimulus, children with specific phobia experience feelings of dread, intense anxiety, physiologic symptoms, and marked fear (Silverman and Rabian, 1993). Anderson et al. (1987) studied a sample of 792 nonreferred 11-year-old children and found that specific phobias occurred in 2.4% of this sample. Assessment of 300 children aged 7 to 11 years in a pediatric primary care setting demonstrated specific phobia to be the most prevalent anxiety disorder in this population, with a prevalence rate of 9.2% (Benjamin et al., 1990). To date, there have been no published brain imaging studies in pediatric patients with specific phobia.

The only imaging study of specific phobia is that of Rauch et al. (1995), who used PET with $H_2^{15}O$ in a within-subject symptom provocation design. Seven adults (one male, six females) with simple phobia were assessed during both neutral and individually tailored procedures designed to provoke their particular phobias. Comparison of phobic versus neutral conditions demonstrated significantly increased rCBF in the anterior cingulate, insular, anterior temporal, somatosensory, and posterior medial orbitofrontal cortices and the thalamus. The authors speculated that the somatosensory activation induced by symptom provocation might be caused by tactile imagery (such as the imagery of touching a box containing the feared animal).

Social phobia social anxiety disorder

Social phobia is characterized by intense and excessive fear of social and/or performance situations such as public speaking, eating in front of others, or using public restrooms (American Psychiatric Association, 1994). Patients with social phobia recognize their symptoms to be excessive and unreasonable, and the symptoms go beyond appropriate nervousness. Social phobia most often emerges during early to middle adolescence (Schneir et al., 1992; Strauss and Last, 1993). Equal numbers of males and females are affected (Bernstein et al., 1996). Patients with social phobia and those with DSM-III-R avoidant disorder share many of the same characteristics (Last et al., 1992; Bernstein et al., 1996). The critical distinguishing factor is that avoidant disorder has an earlier age of onset than does social phobia (Francis et al., 1992), which suggests that avoidant disorder and social phobia may lie on the same neurodevelopmental continuum (Bernstein et al., 1996). Therefore, avoidant disorder has been subsumed under social phobia in DSM-IV. Black and Uhde (1995) recently described selective mutism as a social phobic condition as well. Patients with selective mutism do not talk in specific social settings (e.g., in a class) but do speak in other situations (e.g., at home) (American Psychiatric Association, 1994). In fact, Black and Uhde's (1995) comprehensive analysis of 30 patients with selective mutism demonstrated that 90% of patients with selective mutism met criteria for social phobia on the basis of their inability to speak in certain situations. Only three published studies of neuroimaging in social phobia exist, none of which includes children.

Using morphometric MRI, Potts et al. (1994) studied 22 patients (36 ± 8 years of age; 13 males, nine females) with social phobia and 22 age- and sex-matched controls and found no significant differences between case–control pairs in total cerebral, striatal, or thalamic volumes. However, patients with social phobia exhibited a significantly greater age-related decrease in putamen volumes than did controls, but the change in volume did not correlate with severity of illness.

Using ^{1}H MRS, Davidson et al., (1993) studied 20 patients (aged 35.7 ± 6.7 years; 11 males, nine females) with social phobia and 20 age- and sex-matched healthy comparison subjects. Compared with controls, at baseline, social phobics had significantly lower MRS signals of various markers of neuronal viability in the thalamus and caudate nucleus (Cho and Cr SNR values) and also diffusely in cortical and subcortical areas (NAA). Severity of social phobic symptoms correlated inversely with MRS signals (Cho, Cr, and NAA SNR values) in subcortical regions. After treatment with clonazepam, the SNR values for Cho and Cr increased in some, but not all, social phobic patients compared with their pretreatment states. These exploratory findings suggest the presence of diffuse neuronal abnormality. However, the exact nature of this neuronal abnormality cannot be specified given the uncertain functional significance of the MRS signals.

A subsequent repeat ^{1}H MRS study in 19 social phobic patients (aged 42.0 ± 11.6 years; five males, 14 females) and 10 controls (aged 37.8 ± 10.5 years; six males, four females) showed significantly lower MRS signals of neuronal viability (NAA/Cr) associated with greater MRS signal related to serotonin function (myo-I/NAA) in the cerebral gray matter (Tupler et al., 1997). The effect of an 8-week treatment with the benzodiazepine clonazepam did not alter any of the MRS measures.

Here again, while data are too scant to implicate specific neuronal networks in social phobia, they suggest the presence of detectable abnormalities.

Post-traumatic stress disorder

PTSD follows exposure to a traumatic event or situation that would be stressful to anyone. However, the difference between a normal response and that in PTSD is that the stressor is re-experienced repeatedly despite constant efforts to avoid stimuli that remind or re-expose the individual to the trauma. To meet DSM-IV criteria (American Psychiatric Association, 1994), symptoms must persist for at least 1 month and the disorder must result in significant impairment and emotional distress. Although the classic image of a person suffering from PTSD is "shell shock" from battle or war, this syndrome is not uncommonly seen in children and adolescents exposed to severe trauma, e.g., kidnapping, rape, physical/sexual abuse, or natural disasters (Terr, 1996).

Structural imaging studies

Anatomic MRI studies of adult patients with PTSD have demonstrated subtle structural brain abnormalities including an increased incidence of a small cleft in the callosal-septal interface and a cavum of the septum pellucidum (Krishnan et al., 1988; Myslobodsky et al., 1995; Canive et al., 1997). Five of ten male patients with PTSD aged 33 ± 7.3 years had this latter abnormality compared with only 3 of 21 healthy male comparison subjects aged 31 ± 6.7 years (Myslobodsky et al., 1995). A cavum of the septum pellucidum is likely to be a neurodevelopmental deviance that may reflect an abnormality of cell migration,

myelinization stages, pruning, or a combination of all three. Such a neurodevelopmental anomaly may be a potential marker of susceptibility to the development of PTSD. It may represent an epiphenomenon of the actual mechanisms that confer vulnerability to PTSD.

One model of PTSD involves the hypothesis that stress-related rises in cortisol levels have adverse effects on hippocampal function. When nonhuman primates are exposed to stressful situations, cortisol levels increase and produce neurotoxic effects on the hippocampus (Sapolsky et al., 1990), a structure known to subserve the consolidation of memory. Its role in memory may be particularly relevant in PTSD, a disorder characterized by unwanted and often distorted memories of the traumatic event.

Bremner et al. (1995) used volumetric MRI to compare hippocampal volumes in 26 Vietnam veterans with PTSD with 22 comparison subjects without PTSD but matched for age, sex, race, educational and socioeconomic status, and history of alcohol use. Patients with PTSD had significantly smaller right hippocampal volumes than comparison subjects, without volumetric differences in the basal ganglia or the temporal lobe as a whole. A similar MRI study (Gurvits et al., 1996) compared seven Vietnam veterans with chronic combat-induced PTSD with seven without PTSD and eight healthy comparison subjects. Here again, patients with PTSD had significantly smaller left and right hippocampal volumes than both the veterans without PTSD and the normal controls (Fig. 13.9). No significant differences were detected for total brain volume, ventricular volume, ventricular-to-brain ratio, or amygdalar volumes. Scores on the Combat Exposure Scale correlated with hippocampal volume, suggesting that stress associated with the traumatic event may have had neurotoxic effects on the hippocampus (Gurvits et al., 1996). Alternatively, decreased hippocampal volume may be a neurodevelopmental abnormality that confers vulnerability to PTSD.

Recently, Bremner et al. (1997) used volumetric MRI in adult patients with PTSD secondary to childhood physical and sexual abuse. Seventeen adult patients with PTSD who had been sexually and physically abused were compared with 17 controls matched for age, sex, race, handedness, education, height, weight and alcohol abuse. The patients with PTSD had significantly reduced left hippocampal volumes compared with controls, but no volumetric abnormalities of the amygdala, temporal lobe, or the basal ganglia.

Functional neuroimaging study

Using PET and H$_2$^{15}O, Rauch et al. (1996) conducted a study of eight adult patients with PTSD (aged 41.1 ± 3.7 years;

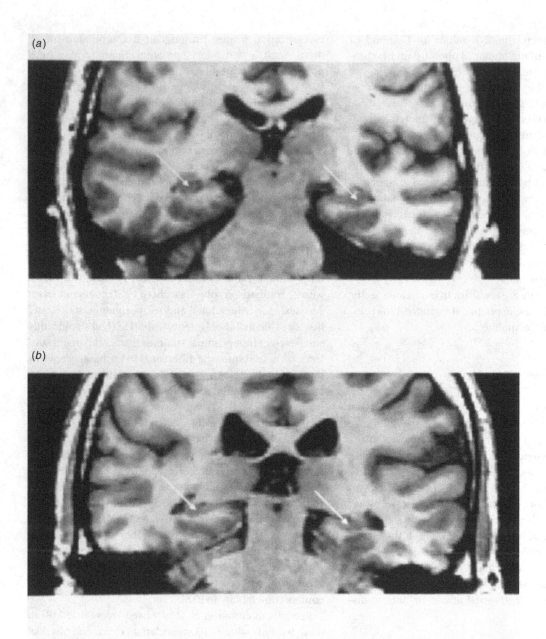

Fig. 13.9. MRI in (*a*) a veteran without post-traumatic stress disorder (PTSD) and (*b*) a veteran with PTSD. (Reprinted by permission of Elsevier Science from Magnetic resonance imaging study of hippocampal volume in chronic combat-related posttraumatic stress disorder, by Gurvits, T., *Biological Psychiatry*, 40(11), 1091–1099, Copyright 1996 by the Society of Biological Psychiatry.)

two males, six females) during exposure to an "active" script (intended to evoke PTSD symptoms) and to a neutral control script. Compared with the neutral condition, the active condition showed increased rCBF in right limbic, paralimbic, and visual cortex, and decreased rCBF in left inferior frontal and middle temporal cortices. These results provide additional evidence that limbic and paralimbic systems contribute to the expression of PTSD symptoms.

The authors hypothesized that increased rCBF in the visual cortex may reflect the patient's visual re-experience of the traumatic event.

Summary

The structural imaging findings suggest that functional dysfunction in the hippocampus is associated with PTSD.

Future functional brain imaging studies will need to examine this hypothesis carefully and to correct functional data for potential differences in size (correcting for partial volume effect, see Chapters 1 and 2).

Neuroimaging and diagnostic specificity

In reviewing studies exploring the neural substrates of anxiety disorders, it is tempting to ponder the scientific grounds for grouping various maladaptive behaviors under the common umbrella of anxiety disorders. While too few data exist with which to address this issue, the possibility that a modified taxonomy of psychiatric disorders might emerge is intriguing, as well as provocative. Relevant to this issue are two studies that have constrasted different anxiety disorders to identify both common and distinct functional neuroanatomic substrates.

Rauch et al. (1997) combined data from 23 adults with OCD (eight), simple phobia (seven), and PTSD (eight) who participated in $H_2^{15}O$ PET studies using a symptom provocation paradigm. Symptom provocation activated the right inferior frontal and posterior medial orbitofrontal cortices and bilaterally the insular cortex, lenticulate nuclei, and brainstem in all three disorders. A significant correlation was observed between severity of anxiety and rCBF in the brainstem. These findings suggested that paralimbic dysfunction might be common to the pathogenesis of these three anxiety disorders. However, it is unclear whether this shared activation pattern merely reflects the normal pathway of anxiety or a specific pathway involved in maladaptive behaviors that characterize these anxiety disorders. The study of anxiety in healthy controls will be critical for answering this question.

Lucey and colleagues (1997) compared rCBF across three different anxiety disorders: OCD (15), panic disorder with agoraphobia (15), and PTSD (16) using SPECT with ^{99m}Tc-labeled hexamethyl-propyleneamine oxime ([^{99m}TC]-HMPAO). They observed significant differences between patients with OCD, PTSD, and panic disorder, and healthy comparison subjects. Specifically, patients with OCD and PTSD exhibited abnormally low rCBF in bilateral superior frontal cortices and in the right caudate nucleus. In addition, global CBF was correlated with the severity of anxiety, and left and right caudate rCBF were correlated inversely with PTSD symptom severity. The authors hypothesized that some of the common findings in OCD and PTSD may reflect similarities in symptoms, with both disorders involving repetitive, ritualistic behaviors and intrusive thoughts.

Based on the above findings of common regional brain activation during symptom provocation across anxiety dis-

orders, it is possible that the dysfunction is rather temporal (not detected using the temporal resolution of the order of 8 min, which is the minimal scan interval time in PET blood flow studies) than at the spatial level (same regions activated). Anxiety disorders may result from an inability of functional systems that mediate "normal" anxiety to habituate. This hypothesis can best be tested in fMRI studies, which afford better temporal resolution (scans can be repeated at a faster pace than in PET studies).

Conclusion and future directions

In summary, the literature on neuroimaging studies of childhood-onset anxiety disorders is remarkable by its paucity in children, but also in adults. Neuroimaging tools are just beginning to be utilized for unraveling the neural mechanisms underlying neuropsychiatric disorders; yet they promise to provide unprecedented information.

Developmental neurobiologic models for pediatric anxiety disorders are of importance because they will guide future research. Current neurobiologic models have been generated for adult anxiety disorders, and there is a need to include in these models the contribution of brain development and maturation to allow better understanding of the origin of these disorders. As briefly mentioned in this chapter, the taxonomy of anxiety disorders is likely to be modified as we understand their pathogenesis better. Currently, there is some emphasis in identifying homogeneous phenotypes of psychiatric disorders to help in the search for vulnerability or even causal genes. Synergistic advances in clinical (behavioral and psychopharmacologic), genetic, and neuroimaging research are expected to provide the basis for a new generation of focused, rational, and effective preventive and therapeutic interventions.

The rapid advances in noninvasive brain imaging offer an unprecedented opportunity to test model-generated hypotheses in pediatric anxiety disorders. Precise, quantitative, high-resolution MRI studies are crucial to detect any underlying anatomic abnormalities. Moreover, since volumetric abnormalities have already been observed in certain anxiety disorders, such measures can help to guide fMRI and MRS studies. If volumetric differences exist between patients with anxiety disorders and controls, precise mesurement is mandatory for the interpretation of any putative functional, metabolic, or neurochemical abnormalities. This is especially critical when studying pediatric populations where developmental maturation is ongoing. Keshavan (1997) has discussed neural network dysplasias with differential brain maturational abnormalitites in neurodevelopmental disorders such as OCD. Longitudinal studies, as well as studies of unaffected, first-degree relatives at increased risk for developing anxiety disorders, are needed to clarify whether the regions already implicated by structural and functional imaging studies of affected adults, such as ventral prefrontal–striatal regions in OCD or hippocampal/parahippocampal regions in panic disorders and PTSD, are degenerative, developmental, or some combination of both.

References

Allen, A. J., Leonard, H. and Swedo, S. E. (1995). Current knowledge of medications for the treatment of childhood anxiety disorders. *J. Am. Acad. Child Adolesc. Psychiatry*, **34**, 976–86.

American Psychiatric Association (1994). *DSM-IV: Diagnostic and Statistical Manual of Mental Disorders*, 4th edn. Washington, DC: American Psychiatric Press.

Anderson, J. C., Williams, S., McGee, R. and Silva, P. A. (1987). DSM-III disorders in preadolescent children: prevalence in a large sample from the general population. *Arch. Gen. Psychiatry*, **44**, 69–76.

Baxter, L. R. (1992). Neuroimaging studies of obsessive-compulsive disorders. *Psychiatr. Clin. North Am.*, **15**, 871–84.

Baxter, L. R., Schwartz, J. M. and Bergman, K. S. (1992). Caudate glucose metabolic rate changes with both drug and behavior therapy for obsessive-compulsive disorder. *Arch. Gen. Psychiatry*, **49**, 681–9.

Becquet, D., Faudon, M. and Hery, F. (1990). In Vivo evidence for an inhibitory glutamatergic control of serotonin release in the cat caudate nucleus: involvement of GABA neurons. *Brain Res.*, **519**, 82–88.

Behar, D., Rapoport, J. L., Berg, C. J. et al. (1984). Computerized tomography and neuropsychological test measures in adolescents with obsessive-compulsive disorder. *Am. J. Psychiatry*, **141**, 363–9.

Belmonte, M., Egaas, B., Townsend, J. and Courchesne, E. (1995). NMR intensity of corpus callosum differs with age but not with diagnosis of autism. *Neuroreport*, **6**, 1253–6.

Benjamin, R. S., Costello, E. J. and Warren, M. (1990). Anxiety disorders in a pediatric sample. *J. Anxiety Disord.*, **4**, 293–316.

Benkelfat, C., Nordahl, T. E., Semple, W. E., King, C., Murphy, D. L. and Cohen, R. M. (1990). Local cerebral glucose metabolic activity in obsessive-compulsive disorder: Patients treated with clomipramine. *Arch. Gen. Psychiatry*, **47**, 840–848.

Bernstein, G. A., Borchardt, C. M. and Perwien, A. R. (1996). Anxiety disorders in children and adolescents: a review of the past 10 years. *J. Am. Acad. Child Adolesc. Psychiatry*, **35**, 1110–19.

Birken, D. L. and Oldendorf, W. H. (1989). *N*-Acetyl-L-aspartic acid: a literature review of a compound prominent in ¹H-NMR spectroscopic studies of brain. *Neurosci. Biobehav. Rev.*, **13**, 23–31.

Black, B. and Robbins, D. R. (1990). Case study: panic disorder in children and adolescents. *J. Am. Acad. Child Adolesc. Psychiatry*, **29**, 36–44.

Black, B. and Uhde, T. W. (1995). Psychiatric characteristics of children with selective mutism: a pilot study. *J. Am. Acad. Child Adolesc. Psychiatry*, **34**, 847–56.

Bowen, R. C., Offord, D. R. and Boyle, M. H. (1990). The prevalence of overanxious disorder and separation anxiety disorder: results from the Ontario Child Health Study. *J. Am. Acad. Child Adolesc. Psychiatry*, **29**, 753–8.

Breiter, H. C. and Rauch, S. L. (1996). Functional MRI and the study of OCD: from symptom provocation to cognitive-behavioral probes of cortico-striatal systems and the amygdala. *Neuroimaging*, **4**, S127–38.

Breiter, H. C., Rauch, S. L., Kwong, K. K. et al. (1996). Functional magnetic resonance imaging of symptom provocation in obsessive compulsive disorder. *Arch. Gen. Psychiatry*, **53**, 595–606.

Bremner, J. D., Randall, P., Scott, T. M. et al. (1995). MRI-based measurement of hippocampal volume in patients with combat-related posttraumatic stress disorder. *Am. J. Psychiatry*, **152**, 973–81.

Bremner, J. D., Randall, P., Vermetten, E. et al. (1997). Magnetic resonance imaging-based measurement of hippocampal volume in posttraumatic stress disorder related to childhood physical and sexual abuse – A preliminary report. *Biol. Psychiatry*, **41**, 23–32.

Canive, J. M., Lewine, J. D., Orrison, W. W. J. et al. (1997). MRI reveals gross structural abnormalities in PTSD. *Ann. N. Y. Acad. Sci.*, **821**, 512–15.

Casey, B. J., Cohen, J. D., Jezzard, P. et al. (1995). Activation of prefrontal cortex in children during a non-spatial working memory task with functional MRI. *Neuroimaging*, **2**, 221–9.

Casey, B. J., Trainor, R. J., Orendi, J. L. et al. (1997). A developmental functional MRI study of prefrontal activation during performance of a go-no-go task. *J. Cognit. Neurosci.*, **9**, 835–47.

Cummings, J. L. (1993). Frontal-subcortical circuits and human behavior. *Arch. Neurol.*, **50**, 873–80.

Dager, S. R., Marro, K. L., Richards, T. L. and Metzger, G. D. (1994). Preliminary application of magnetic resonance spectroscopy to investigate lactate-induced panic. *Am. J. Psychiatry*, **151**, 57–63.

Dager, S. R., Strauss, W. L., Marro, K. I. et al. (1995). Proton magnetic resonance spectroscopy investigation of hyperventilation in subjects with panic disorder and comparison subjects. *Am. J. Psychiatry*, **152**, 666–72.

Dantendorfer, K., Prayer, D., Kramer, J. et al. (1996). High frequency EEG and MRI brain abnormalities in panic disorder. *Psychiatr. Res.*, **68**, 41–53.

Davidson, J. R., Krishnan, K. R., Charles, H. C. et al. (1993). Magnetic resonance spectroscopy in social phobia: preliminary findings. *J. Clin. Psychiatry*, **54**(Suppl.), 19–25.

Diamond, A. (1990). Developmental progression in human infants and infant monkeys, and the neural bases of inhibitory control of reaching. In *The Development and Neural Bases of Higher Cognitive Functions*, ed. A. Diamond, pp. 267–317. New York: Academy of Science Press.

Diksic, M., Nagahiro, S., Chaly, T., Sourkes, T. L., Yamamoto, Y. L.

and Feindel, W. (1991). Serotonin synthesis rate measured in living dog brain by positron emission tomography. *J. Neurochem.*, **56**, 153–62.

Ebert, D., Speck, O., Konig, A., Berger, M., Hennig, J. and Hohagen, F. (1997). 1-H-Magnetic resonance spectroscopy in obsessive-compulsive disorder: evidence for neuronal loss in the cingulate gyrus and the right striatum. *Psychiatr. Res.*, **74**, 173–6.

Flament, M. F., Rapoport, J. L., Berg, C. J. et al. (1985). Clomipramine treatment of childhood obsessive compulsive disorder: A double-blind controlled study. *Arch. Gen. Psychiatry*, **42**, 977–83.

Flament, M. F., Whitaker, A. and Rapoport, J. L. (1988). Obsessive compulsive disorder in adolescence: an epidemiological study. *J. Am. Acad. Child Adolesc. Psychiatry*, **27**, 764–71.

Francis, G., Last, C. G. and Strauss, C. C. (1992). Avoidant disorder and social phobia in children and adolescents. *J. Am. Acad. Child Adolesc. Psychiatry*, **31**, 1086–9.

Funahashi, S., Bruce, C. J. and Goldman-Rakic, P. S. (1989). Mnemonic coding of visual space in the monkey's dorsolateral prefrontal cortex. *J. Neurophysiol.*, **61**, 331–49.

Giedd, J. N., Rapoport, J. L., Kruesi, M. J. P. et al. (1995). Sydenham's chorea: magnetic-resonance-imaging of the basal ganglia. *Neurology*, **45**, 2199–202.

Giedd, J. N., Vaituzis, A. C., Hamburger, S. D. et al. (1996). Quantitative MRI of the temporal lobe, amygdala, and hippocampus in normal human development: ages 4–18 years. *J. Compar. Neurol.*, **366**, 223–30.

Goddard, A. W. and Charney, D. S. (1997). Toward an integrated neurobiology of panic disorder. *J. Clin. Psychiatry*, **58**(Suppl. 2), 4–11.

Goldman, P. S. and Rosvold, H. E. (1970). Localization of function within the dorsolateral prefrontal cortex of the rhesus monkey. *Exp. Neurol.*, **27**, 291–304.

Goodglass, H. and Kaplan, E. (1972). *An Assessment of Aphasia and Related Disorders*. Philadelphia, PA: Lea and Fibiger.

Gur, R. C., Gur, R. E., Resnick, S. M., Skolnick, B. E., Alavi, A. and Reivich, M. (1987). The effect of anxiety on cortical cerebral blood flow and metabolism. *J. Cereb. Blood Flow Metab.*, **7**, 173–7.

Gurvits, T. V., Shenton, M. E., Hokama, H. et al. (1996). Magnetic resonance imaging study of hippocampal volume in chronic combat-related posttraumatic stress disorder. *Biol. Psychiatry*, **40**, 1091–9.

Hanna, G. L. (1995). Demographic and clinical features of obsessive-compulsive disorder in children and adolescents. *J. Am. Acad. Child Adolesc. Psychiatry*, **34**, 19–27.

Hayward, C., Killen, J. D., Hammer, L. D. et al. (1992). Pubertal stage and panic attack history in sixth- and seventh-grade girls. *Am. J. Psychiatry*, **149**, 1239–43.

Hoehn-Saric, R., Pearslon, G., Harris, G. Machlin, S. and Camargo, E. (1991). Effects of fluoxetine on regional cerebral blood flow in obsessive-compulsive patients. *Am. J. Psychiatry*, **148**, 1243–5.

Insel, T. R. (1992). Toward a neuroanatomy of obsessive-compulsive disorder. *Arch. Gen. Psychiatry*, **49**, 739–44.

Iversen, S. D. and Mishkin, M. (1970). Perseverative interference in monkeys following selective lesions of the inferior prefrontal convexity. *Exp. Brain Res.*, **11**, 376–86.

Jenike, M. A., Baer, L., Ballantine, T. et al. (1991). Cingulotomy for refractory obsessive-compulsive disorder: a long-term follow-up of 33 patients. *Arch. Gen. Psychiatry*, **48**, 548–55.

Jenike, M. A., Breiter, H. C., Baer, L. et al. (1996). Cerebral structural abnormalities in obsessive-compulsive disorder: a quantitative morphometric magnetic resonance imaging study. *Arch. Gen Psychiatry*, **53**, 625–32.

Keller, M. B., Lavori, P. W., Wunder, J., Beardslee, W. R., Schwarts, C. E. and Roth, J. (1992). Chronic course of anxiety disorders in children and adolescents. *J. Am. Acad. Child Adolesc. Psychiatry*, **31**, 595–9.

Keltner, J. R., Wald, L. L., Frederick, B. B. and Renshaw, P. F. (1997). In vivo detection of GABA in human brain using a localized double-quantum filter technique. *Magn. Reson. Med.*, **37**, 366–71.

Keshavan, M. S. (1997). Neurodevelopment and schizophrenia: Quo vadis? In *Neurodevelopmental Models of Psychopathology*, eds. M. S. Keshavan and R. Murray, pp. 267–770. London: Cambridge University Press.

Kim, J. S., Hassler, R., Haug, P. and Paik, K. S. (1977). Effect of frontal cortex ablation on striatal glutamic acid level in rat. *Brain Res.*, **132**, 370–4.

Klein, D. F., Mannuzza, S., Chapman, T. and Fyer, A. J. (1992). Child panic revisited. *J. Am. Acad. Child Adolesc. Psychiatry*, **31**, 112–14.

Krishnan, K. R., Ellinwood, E. H. J. and Goli, V. (1988). Structural brain changes revealed by MRI. *Am. J. Psychiatry*, **145**, 1316.

Laissy, J. P., Partrux, B., Duchateau, C. et al. (1993). Midsagittal MR measurement of the corpus callosum in healthy subjects and diseased patients: a prospective survey. *Am. J. Neuroradiol.*, **14**, 145–54.

Last, C. G. and Strauss, C. C. (1989). Obsessive-compulsive disorder in childhood. *J. Anxiety Disord.*, **3**, 295–302.

Last, C. G., Perrin, S., Hersen, M. and Kazdin, A. E. (1992). DSM-III-R anxiety disorders in children: sociodemographic and clinical characteristics. *J. Am. Acad. Child Adolesc. Psychiatry*, **31**, 1070–76.

Lucey, J. V., Costa, D. C., Adshead, G. et al. (1997). Brain blood flow in anxiety disorders. OCD, panic disorder with agoraphobia and post-traumatic stress disorder on 99mTcHMPAO single photon emission tomography (SPET). *Br. J. Psychiatry*, **171**, 346–50.

Luria, A. R. (1966). *Higher Cortical Function in Man*, 2nd edn. New York: Basic Books.

Luxenberg, J. S., Swedo, S. E., Flament, M. F., Friedland, R. P., Rapoport, J. and Rapoport, S. I. (1988). Neuroanatomical abnormalities in obsessive-compulsive disorder determined with quantitative X-ray computed tomography. *Am. J. Psychiatry*, **145**, 1089–93.

MacMaster, F. P., Dick, E. L., Keshavan, M. S. and Rosenberg, D. R. (1999). Corpus callosal signal intensity in treatment-naive pediatric obsessive compulsive disorder. *Progr. Neuropsychopharmacol. Biol. Psychiatry*, **23**, 601–12.

Modell, J. G., Mountz, J. M., Curtis, G. C. and Greden, J. F. (1989). Neurophysiologic dysfunction in basal ganglia/limbic striatal and thalamocortical circuits as a pathogenetic mechanism of obsessive-compulsive disorder. *J. Neuropsychiatry*, **1**, 27–36.

Moore, G. J., MacMaster, F. P., Stewart, C. and Rosenberg, D. R. (1998). Caudate glutamatergic changes with paroxetine therapy for pediatric obsessive compulsive disorder. *J. Am. Acad. Child Adolesc Psychiatry*, **27**, 663–7.

Moore, G. J., Tancer, M. E. and Uhde, T. W. (1999). Dynamic proton MRS in an intravenous caffeine model of anxiety reveals focal increases in lactate. *Depression Anxiety*, in press.

Moreau, D. and Follett, C. (1993). Panic disorder in children and adolescents. *Child Adolesc. Psychiatr. Clin. North Am.*, **2**, 581–602.

Myslobodsky, M. S., Glicksohn, J., Singer, J. et al. (1995). Changes of brain anatomy in patients with posttraumatic stress disorder: a pilot magnetic resonance imaging study. *Psychiatr. Res.*, **58**, 259–64.

Nordahl, T. E., Semple, W. E., Gross, M. et al. (1990). Cerebral glucose metabolic differences in patients with panic disorder. *Neuropsychopharmacology*, **3**, 261–72.

Pandey, S. C., Kim, S. W., Davis, J. M. and Pandey, G. N. (1993). Platelet serotonin-2 receptors in obsessive-compulsive disorder. *Biol. Psychiatry*, **33**, 367–72.

Passingham, R. E. (1972). Visual discrimination learning after selective prefrontal ablations in monkeys. *Neuropsychologia*, **10**, 27–39.

Pauls, D. L., Alsobrook, J. P., Goodman, W., Rasmussen, S. and Leckman, J. F. (1995). A family study of obsessive-compulsive disorder. *Am. J. Psychiatry*, **152**, 76–84.

Pigott, T. A. (1996). OCD: where the serotonin selectivity story begins. *J. Clin. Psychiatry*, **57**, 11–20.

Pitman, R. E., Green, R. C., Jenike, M. A. and Mesulam, M. M. (1987). Clinical comparison of Tourette's disorder and obsessive-compulsive disorder. *Am. J. Psychiatry*, **144**, 1166–71.

Pollack, M. H., Otto, M. W., Sabatino, S. et al. (1996). Relationship of childhood anxiety to adult panic disorder: correlates and influence on course. *Am. J. Psychiatry*, **153**, 376–81.

Potts, N. L., Davidson, J. R., Krishnan, K. R. and Doraiswamy, P. M. (1994). Magnetic resonance imaging in social phobia. *Psychiatr. Res.*, **52**, 35–42.

Rajapakse, J. C., Giedd, J. N., Rumsey, J. M., Vaituzis, A. C., Hamburger, S. D. and Rapoport, J. L. (1996). Regional MRI measurements of the corpus callosum: a methodological and developmental study. *Brain Dev.*, **18**, 379–88.

Rauch, S. L., Jenike, M. A., Alpert, N. M. et al. (1994). Regional cerebral blood flow measured during symptom provocation in obsessive-compulsive disorder using oxygen 15-labeled carbon dioxide and positron emission tomography. *Arch. Gen. Psychiatry*, **51**, 62–70.

Rauch, S. L., Savage, C. R., Alpert, N. M. et al. (1995). A positron emission tomographic study of simple phobic symptom provocation. *Arch. Gen. Psychiatry*, **52**, 20–8.

Rauch, S. L., van der Kolk, B. A., Fisler, R. E. et al. (1996). A symptom provocation study of posttraumatic stress disorder using positron emission tomography and script-driven imagery. *Arch. Gen. Psychiatry*, **53**, 380–7.

Rauch, S. L., Savage, C. R., Alpert, N. M., Fischman, A. J. and Jenike, M. A. (1997). The functional neuroanatomy of anxiety: a study of three disorders using positron emission tomography and symptom provocation. *Biol. Psychiatry*, **42**, 446–52.

Reiman, E. M., Raichle, M. E., Robins, E. et al. (1986). The application of positron emission tomography to the study of panic disorder. *Am. J. Psychiatry*, **143**, 469–77.

Riddle, M. A., Schahill, L. and King, R. (1990). Obsessive compulsive disorder in children and adolescents: phenomenology and family history. *J. Am. Acad. Child Adolesc. Psychiatry*, **29**, 766–72.

Robinson, D., Wu, H., Munne, R. A. et al. (1995). Reduced caudate nucleus volume in obsessive-compulsive disorder. *Arch. Gen Psychiatry*, **52**, 393–8.

Rosenberg, D. R. and Keshavan, M. S. (1998). Toward a neurodevelopment model of obsessive compulsive disorder. *Biol. Psychiatry*, **43**, 623–40.

Rosenberg, D. R., Averbach, D. H., O'Hearn, K. M., Seymour, A. B., Birmaher, B. and Sweeney, J. A. (1997a). Oculomotor response inhibition abnormalities in pediatric obsessive compulsive disorder. *Arch. Gen. Psychiatry*, **54**, 831–8.

Rosenberg, D. R., Keshavan, M. S., Dick, E. L. et al. (1997b). Corpus callosal morphology in treatment naive pediatric obsessive compulsive disorder. *Prog. NeuroPsychopharmacol. Biol. Psychiatry*, **21**, 1269–83.

Rosenberg, D. R., Keshavan, M. S., O'Hearn, K. M. et al. (1997c). Fronto-striatal measurement of treatment-naive pediatric obsessive compulsive disorder. *Arch. Gen. Psychiatry*, **54**, 824–30.

Rosenberg, D. R., Sweeney, J. A., Gillen, J. S. et al. (1997d). Simulation for desensitization of children requiring MRI. *J. Am. Acad. Child Adolesc. Psychiatry*, **36**, 853–9.

Rosenberg, D. R., MacMaster, F. P., Parrish, J. K. et al. (1998). 1-H MRS measurement of caudate glutamatergic changes associated with paroxetine therapy for pediatric obsessive compulsive disorder. In *Proceedings of the 6th Scientific Meeting of the International Society for Magnetic Resonance in Medicine*, p. 1808.

Rosenkilde, C. E. (1979). Functional heterogeneity of the prefrontal cortex in the monkey: a review. *Behav. Neural Biol.*, **25**, 301–45.

Rosvold, H. E. and Mishkin, M. (1961). Non-sensory effects of frontal lesions on discrimination learning and performance. In *Brain Mechanisms and Learning*, ed. J. F. Delafresnaye, pp. 555–76. Oxford: Blackwell.

Rothman, D. L. Petroff, O. A. C., Behar, K. L. and Mattson, R. H. (1993). Localized 1H NMR measurements of GABA levels in the human brain in vivo. *Proc. Natl. Acad. Sci. USA*, **90**, 5662–6.

Sallee, R. and Greenwald, J. (1995). Neurobiology. In *Anxiety Disorders in Children and Adolescents*, ed. J. S. March, pp. 3–34. New York: Guiliford.

Sallee, F. R., Richman, H., Beach, K., Sethuraman, G. and Nesbitt, L. (1996). Platelet serotonin transporter in children and adolescents with obsessive-compulsive disorder or Tourette's syndrome. *J. Am. Acad. Child Adolesc. Psychiatry*, **35**, 1647–56.

Sapolsky, R. M., Uno, H., Rebert, C. S. and Finch, C. E. (1990). Hippocampal damage associated with prolonged glucocoticoid exposure in primates. *J. Neurosci.*, **10**, 2897–902.

Schneir, F. R., Johnson, J., Hornig, C. D., Liebowitz, M. R. and Weissman, M. M. (1992). Social phobia: comorbidity in an epidemiologic sample. *Arch. Gen. Psychiatry*, **49**, 282–8.

Schwartz, J. M., Stoessel, P. W., Baxter, L. R., Martin, K. M. and Phelps, M. E. (1996). Systematic changes in cerebral glucose metabolic rate after successful behavior modification treatment of obsessive-compulsive disorder. *Arch. Gen. Psychiatry*, **53**, 109–13.

Seltzer, B. and Pandya, D. N. (1986). The topography of commissural fibers. In *Two Hemispheres, One Brain. Functions of the Corpus Callosum*, eds. H. H. F. Lepore and M. Ptito, pp. 47–73. New York: Liss.

Silverman, W. K. and Rabian, B. (1993). Simple phobias. *Child Adolesc. Psychiatr. Clin. North Am.*, **2**, 603–22.

Smith, Y. and Parent, A. (1986). Differential connections of caudate nucleus and putamen in the squirrel monkey (*Saimiri sciureus*). *Neuroscience*, **18**, 347–71.

Strauss, C. C. and Last, C. G. (1993). Social and simple phobias in children. *J. Anxiety Disord.*, **7**, 141–52.

Stuss, D. T. and Benson, D. F. (1983). Frontal lobe lesions and behavior. In *Localization in Neuropsychology*, ed. A. Kertesz, pp. 429–49. New York: Academic Press.

Swedo, S. E., Leonard, H. L. and Rapoport, J. L. (1992a). Childhood-onset obsessive compulsive disorder. *Psychiatr. Clin. North Am.*, **15**, 767–73.

Swedo, S. E., Pietrini, P. and Leonard, H. L. (1992b). Cerebral glucose metabolism in childhood-onset obsessive-compulsive disorder: Revisualization during pharmacotherapy. *Arch. Gen. Psychiatry*, **49**, 690–4.

Sweeney, J. A., Mintun, M. A., Kwee, S. et al. (1996). A positron emission tomography study of voluntary saccadic eye movements and spatial working memory. *J. Neurophysiol.* **75**, 454–68.

Taber, M. T. and Fibiger, H. C. (1993). Electrical stimulation of the medial prefrontal cortex increases dopamine release in the striatum. *Neuropsychopharmacology*, **9**, 271–5.

Taber, M. T. and Fibiger, H. C. (1994). Cortical regulation of acetylcholine release in rat striatum. *Brain Res.*, **639**, 354–6.

Terr, L. C. (1996). *Child and Adolescent Psychiatry: A Comprehensive Textbook*, 2nd edn. Baltimore: Williams and Wilkins.

Thoren, P., Asberg, M., Cronholm, B., Jornestedt, L. and Traskman, L. (1980). Clomipramine treatment of obsessive compulsive disorder: I. A controlled clinical trial. *Arch. Gen. Psychiatry*, **37**, 1281–5.

Tiihonen, J., Kuikka, J., Rasanen, P. et al. (1997). Cerebral benzodiazepine receptor binding and distribution in generalized anxiety disorder: a fractal analysis. *Mol. Psychiatry*, **2**, 463–71.

Tupler, L. A., Davidson, J. R., Smith, R. D., Lazeyras, F., Charles, H. C. and Krishnan, K. R. (1997). A repeat proton magnetic resonance spectroscopy study in social phobia. *Biol. Psychiatry*, **42**, 419–24.

Valleni-Basile, L. A., Garrison, C. Z., Jackson, K. L. et al. (1994). Frequency of obsessive-compulsive disorder in a community sample of young adolescents. *J. Am. Acad. Child Adolesc. Psychiatry*, **33**, 782–91.

van der Knapp, M. S. and Valk, J. (1989). The reflection of histology in MR imaging of Pelizaeus–Merzbacher disease. *Am. J. Neuroradiol.*, **10**, 99–103.

von Economo, C. (1931). *Encephalitis Lethargica: Its Sequelae and Treatment*. London: Oxford University Press.

von Korff, M. R. Eaton, W. W. and Keyl, P. M. (1985). The epidemiology of panic attacks and panic disorder. Results of three community surveys. *Am. J. Epidemiol.* **122**, 970–81.

Whitaker, A., Johnson, J., Shaffer, D. et al. (1990). Uncommon troubles in young people: prevalence estimates of selected psychiatric disorders in a non-referred adolescent population. *Arch. Gen Psychiatry*, **47**, 487–96.

Wise, S. and Rapoport, J. L. (1989). Obsessive-compulsive disorder: is it basal ganglia dysfunction? In *Obsessive-Compulsive Disorder in Children and Adolescents*, ed. J. L. Rapoport, pp. 327–47. Washington, DC: American Psychiatric Press.

Wolpe, J., Brady, J. P., Serber, M., Agras, W. S. and Liberman, R. P. (1973). The current status of systematic desensitization. *Am. J. Psychiatry*, **130**, 961–5.

Wu, J. C., Buchsbaum, M. S., Hershey, T. G., Hazlett, E., Sicotte, N. and Johnson, J. C. (1991). PET in generalized anxiety disorder. *Biol. Psychiatry*, **29**, 1181–99.

14

Tourette's syndrome: what are we really imaging?

Bradley S. Peterson and Prakash Thomas

Introduction

This chapter will discuss and integrate the numerous conflicting findings produced by a wide variety of functional imaging studies in Tourette's syndrome (TS) performed by different investigators under different experimental protocols over a large number of years. We hope in our analysis to identify the neural systems that seem to be most strongly implicated in the pathophysiology of this disorder. We also hope in our analysis to enliven the typically static interpretation of brain images by emphasizing the dynamic interplay of pathophysiology and adaptation, not only in the people who have this particular illness but also in the many others who have difficulty controlling a wide array of unwanted impulses. This dynamic interplay of pathophysiology and adaptation presents important difficulties for the interpretation of existing TS functional imaging studies that will affect the design of the next generation of studies in TS and other developmental neuropsychiatric disorders.

Phenomenology

Simple and complex tics

The tics of TS are rapid, purposeless jerks of brief duration that most commonly affect musculature of the face, head, neck, shoulders, and vocal apparatus. They less commonly affect the torso and extremities. These rapid and brief movements are referred to as "simple" motor or phonic tics, and they are the kind of tics most frequently seen in patients with TS. With increasing age, individuals who have TS become particularly adept at the temporary inhibition of their tics, although tics cannot be inhibited indefinitely. Less commonly seen in TS are slower, semi-purposeful movements of longer duration, which are referred to as "complex" tics. These include movements such as tapping, touching, rubbing, uttering of words or phrases, and coprolalia.

Highly complex tics can be exceptionally difficult to distinguish from compulsive behaviors and stereotypies. Tics are commonly preceded by a persistent, intrusive awareness of an urge to tic or to move the body part in which the tic will occur, and this urge is relieved, if only momentarily, immediately upon performing the tic behavior (Leckman et al., 1993). This premonitory urge and the patient's preoccupation with it can be difficult to distinguish from the obsessional urges that typically precede compulsive behaviors.

Genetic basis

Family genetic and twin studies have provided compelling evidence that TS has strong genetic determinants (Price et al., 1985; Pauls et al., 1986, 1991). These genetic determinants, once they are identified and characterized, will offer the opportunity of studying the neuroanatomic and functional basis of involuntary urges and their behavioral counterparts in a relatively homogeneous disorder. The study of similar urges and behaviors can then inform the study of disorders that are more heterogeneous, though etiologically related to TS.

Although the vertical transmission of the putative TS vulnerability genes does not seem to involve the X-chromosome, males are between 4 and 10 times more likely than females to be affected with TS (Burd et al., 1986; Comings et al., 1990; Nomoto and Machiyama, 1990; Apter et al., 1993). These sex-specific prevalence differences must have a neural correlate, and functional imaging studies must ultimately account for them. In addition, because the male preponderance of TS easily can lead to

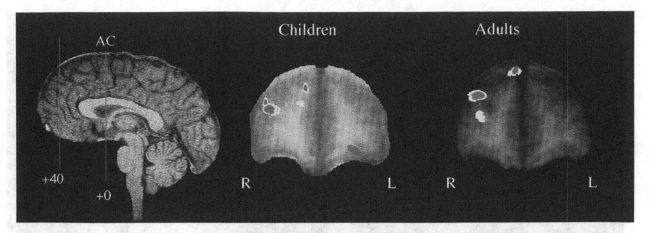

Fig. 9.4. Dorsolateral prefrontal cortical activity for children ($n=6$) and adults ($n=8$) during performance of a spatial working memory task. AC, anterior commissure.

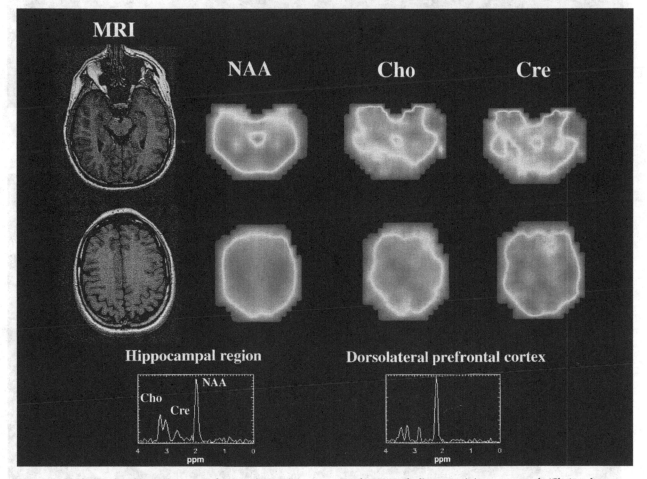

Fig. 11.3. Metabolite signal intensity maps of *N*-acetyl-containing compounds (NAA), choline-containing compounds (Cho) and creatine/phosphocreatine (Cre) with coaxial MRI for a patient with childhood-onset schizophrenia. The upper slabs are taken at the level of the hippocampal region and the lower slabs at the level of the dorsolateral prefrontal cortex. The left side of the brain is on the right of the figure, and vice versa. Color images are scaled to the highest value of each metabolite signal intensity for each ^{1}H MRS imaging slice, so that the *pattern* of regional distribution of metabolite signal intensities within the same slice can be compared between subjects, although the color intensity from the same anatomic location cannot be compared between subjects. The spectra shown are representative of the hippocampus and dorsolateral prefrontal cortex.

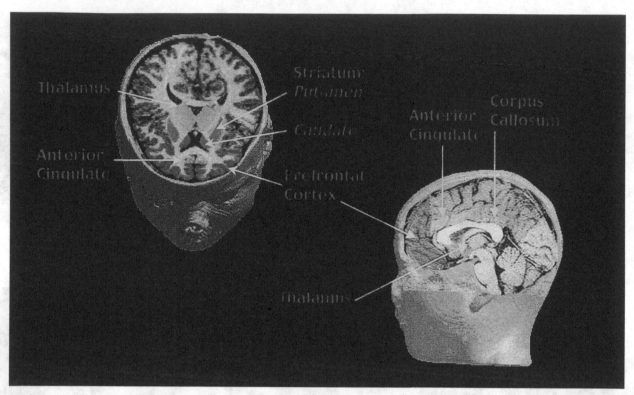

Fig. 13.1. Research has shown that certain brain structures are involved in the neurobiology of obsessive-compulsive disorder. (Created by Frank P. MacMaster.)

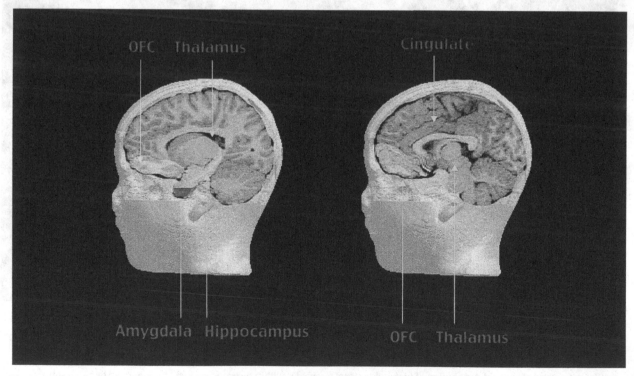

Fig. 13.2. Structures such as the thalamus, cingulate, amygdala, hippocampus and the orbital frontal cortex (OFC) are activated in the emotion fear. (Created by Frank P. MacMaster.)

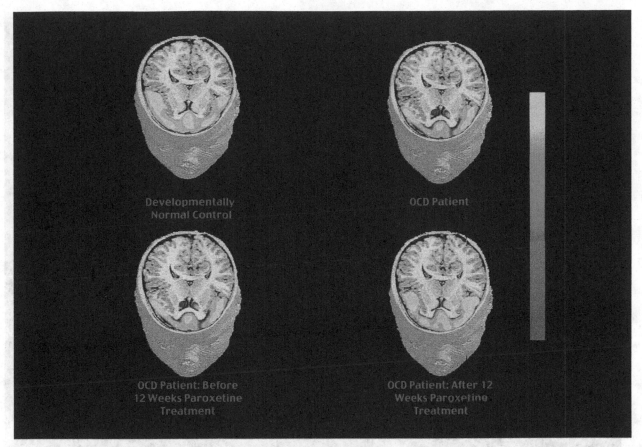

Fig. 13.6. Positron emission tomography with α-[^{11}C]-methyl-L-tryptophan showing serotonin synthesis levels in the ventral–striatal brain areas of a developmentally normal control, a patient with obsessive-compulsive disorder (OCD), and a patient before and after drug treatment with paroxetine. Higher serotonin synthesis levels correspond to the areas highlighted in yellow, while low serotonin synthesis levels correspond to areas in blue. (Created by the laboratory of Dr David Rosenberg.)

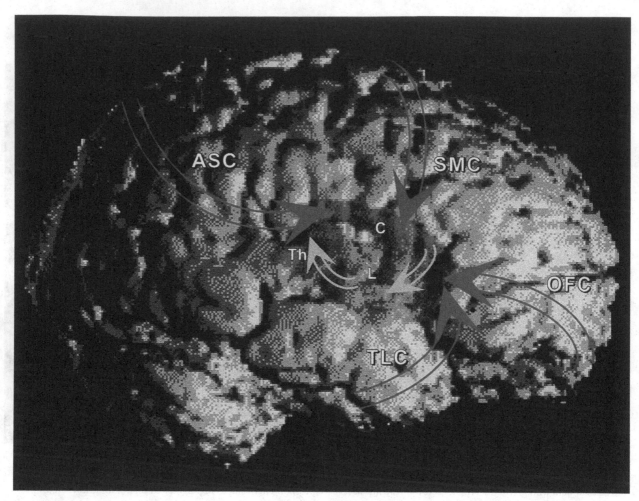

Fig. 14.1. Cortico–striato–thalamo–cortical (CSTC) circuits. White, cerebral cortex; red, caudate nucleus (labeled "C"); green, lenticular nucleus (labeled "L"); purple, thalamus (labeled "Th"); ASC, association cortex; SMC, sensorimotor cortex; OFC, orbitofrontal cortex; TLC, temporolimbic cortex. See Fig. 14.3*a* for a more detailed schematic drawing of connectivity in CSTC circuits. Here excitatory cortico–striatal projections are represented with red arrows. Projections from OFC and TLC are primarily to ventral striatum, whereas those from SMC and ASC are primarily to dorsal striatum (Leckman et al., 1997). Inhibitory striato–pallidal and pallido–thalamic projections are represented with blue arrows. Excitatory thalamo–cortical projections are not shown.

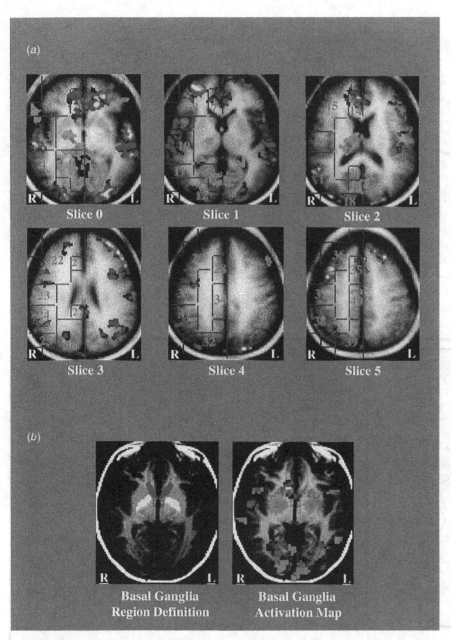

Fig. 14.3. Tic suppression. (*a*) Group-averaged activations in Talairach space: red indicating increased activity during tic suppression and blue decreased activity. Intersubject averaging is an imperfect visual representation of regional significance testing because of the variability between subjects in the location of anatomic regions such as the basal ganglia, and variability in the spatial location of activation within subcortical and stereotactically defined cortical regions. This is especially evident in the left basal ganglia, where the group-average map fails to indicate activation (Peterson et al., 1998). The Talairach stereotactic definitions of cortical regions of interest are shown in green outline. Anterior cingulate: 1, 7, 14, 21, 28, 35; posterior cingulate: 20, 27, 34, 40; frontal cortex: 2, 8, 15, 22, 29, 36; superior temporal gyrus: 3, 10, 17; middle temporal gyrus: 4, 11, 25; precentral gyrus: 9; sensorimotor cortex: 16, 23, 30, 37; inferior parietal cortex: 24, 31, 38; occipital cortex: 5, 12, 18, 26, 32; hippocampus/parahippocampus: 6; cuneus: 13, 19; and precuneus: 33, 39. (*b*) Basal ganglia definition and activation in a single subject. Region definitions are shown for the inferior-most slice, where basal ganglia activation was seen. In the basal ganglia definitions on the left, yellow indicates putamen, blue indicates globus pallidus, and red indicates caudate. In the activation map on the right, decreased activity of the putamen and globus pallidus is seen bilaterally (blue); activity during tic suppression in the caudate nucleus is increased on the right (red).

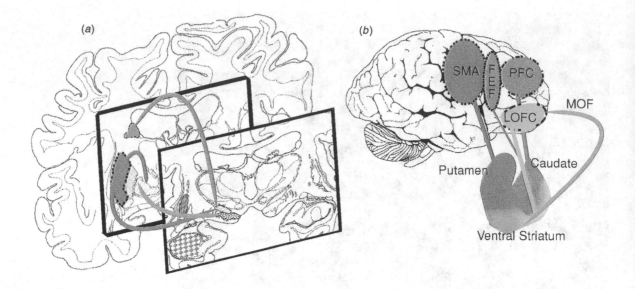

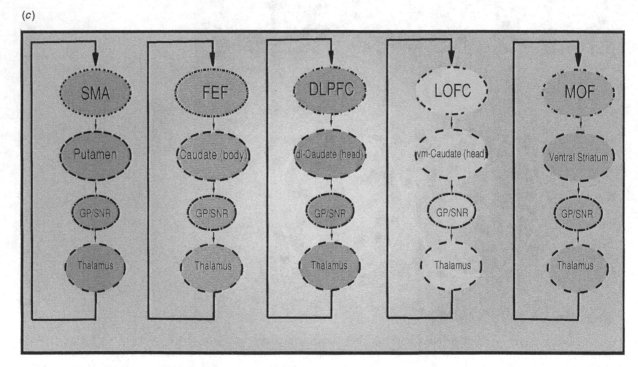

Fig. 16.1. Basal ganglia loops. (*a*) General representation of the motor cortico–striatal loop encompassing the putamen and the prefrontal caudate loop (background slice) in relation to the subthalamic nucleus and substantia nigra (foreground slice). (*b*) Cortical projections to rostral frontal section of the basal ganglia (dashed line style corresponds to loops in (*c*). (*c*) The five major cortico–striatal loops: the motor circuit serving sensorimotor area (SMA) integration; the oculomotor composed of the frontal eye fields (FEF) projecting to the head and body of the caudate in the attentional control of eye movements; the prefrontal cognitive/association pathway composed of the dorsolateral prefrontal cortex (DLPFC), dorsolateral (dl) head of the caudate; the orbitofrontal pathway composed of the lateral orbitofrontal cortex (LOFC), which projects to the ventromedial (vm) head of the caudate; and the ventral striatal pathway composed of the anterior cingulate (not shown), medial orbitofrontal (MOF) cortex and ventromedial caudate and nucleus accumbens. GP/SNR, global pallidus/substantia nigra pars reticulata, PFC, prefrontal cortex. (Based on Fig. 3 in Alexander et al., 1986.)

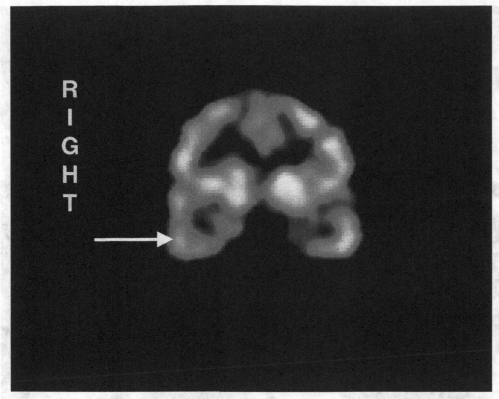

Fig. 17.1. SPECT image: coronal section of the brain showing unilateral temporal lobe hypoperfusion in patient with early-onset anorexia nervosa.

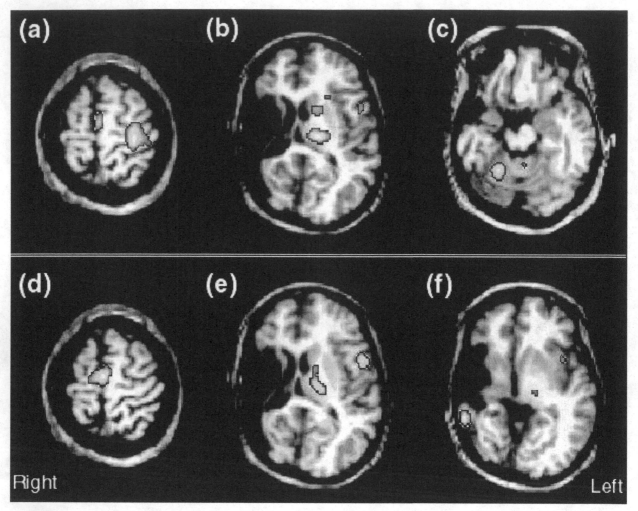

Fig. 20.2. Regional cerebral blood flow (rCBF) increases >20% ($p < 0.001$; uncorrected) for unilateral finger movement in a 20-year-old patient with history of intrauterine or perinatal middle cerebral artery infarction in the right hemisphere (from Müller et al., 1998e). The activations from the $H_2^{15}O$ PET subtraction images are superimposed onto the patient's structural MRI. (*a–c*) A normal pattern of activations for finger movement of the unaffected right hand is seen in primary motor cortex and the supplementary motor area (*a*), as well as in the thalamus, basal ganglia, and premotor cortex of the left hemisphere (*b*), and in the right anterior cerebellum (*c*). (*d–f*) Activations for movement of the hemiparetic left hand. Activations in the supplementary motor area (*d*) are enhanced and are more bilateral compared with movement of the unaffected hand, but there is no activation in primary motor cortex. (*e*) Atypical activations are also seen in the hemisphere *ipsilateral* to the side of movement in premotor cortex and in the thalamus. (*f*) An unexpected activation is found in residual temporal cortex of the lesioned hemisphere. The activations for movement of the hemiparetic hand suggest that multiple regions are involved in reorganization, with the exception of the primary motor cortex.

differences in sex composition of the patient and control groups, studies must be carefully designed to avoid sex differences in the composition of the groups and to avoid confounding the findings of the study.

Comorbid illnesses

Patients with TS are often plagued by recurrent, intrusive thoughts, mental images, and urges to action of classically defined obsessive-compulsive disorder (OCD). Family studies have shown that at least one form of OCD is a manifestation of the putative genes that confer vulnerability to and transmission of TS (Pauls et al., 1986). Similarly, attention-deficit hyperactivity disorder (ADHD) is diagnosed in approximately 50% of all clinically identified patients with TS. Evidence from a recent family genetic study suggests that at least some of the ADHD in TS families may be caused by the TS genes (Pauls et al., 1993).

A spectrum of semi-involuntary behaviors

Superficially, the behavioral phenotypes of TS, OCD, and ADHD differ dramatically: one consists of motor and vocal tics, another consists of obsessions and compulsions, and yet another consists of inattention, hyperactivity, and impulsivity. It is astounding that a single genetic vulnerability can produce these vastly different phenotypes. The genetic relatedness of certain subtypes of these disorders raises the question of whether their phenotypes might be more intimately related than their surface appearance would suggest. The resemblance between OCD symptoms and complex tics suggests, for example, that the symptoms of TS and OCD lie on a spectrum of "compulsory" behaviors. Those symptoms that have a prominent ideational component belong to OCD on the one end and those with little or no ideational component belong to the simple tics of TS on the other; complex tics belong somewhere between these two extremes. Similarly, the symptoms of ADHD share some of the features of tics. Tics, for example, can be thought of as "hyperkinesia", and motoric hyperactivity is a prominent feature of ADHD. Patients with TS can inhibit their tics for only brief periods of time, and the impaired inhibition of impulses is a hallmark of ADHD. In this way, both children with ADHD and those with TS have excessive motor activity and difficulty inhibiting specific behaviors.

It may be that a given genetic vulnerability to TS can produce not three behaviorally unrelated disorders but instead an entire spectrum of related semi-involuntary behaviors. Genes, however, do not code for a behavior or even a spectrum of behaviors. They code for proteins, and

those proteins are expressed in specific cells in a regionally specific fashion. The brain regions whose function the proteins affect then produce the predisposition to the specified behaviors. This suggests that the region or regions of the CNS in which disordered functioning produces the symptoms of TS, OCD, and ADHD could be related because of the expression of the TS gene product in those regions. Therefore, the phenomenologic similarities and the genetic relatedness of these conditions may provide important clues in the search for their shared neurobiologic substrate. The substrates of TS, OCD, and ADHD cannot be identical, however, because the disorders are still phenomenologically distinct, and those distinctions ultimately must be brain based.

Frequent confounds in studies of Tourette's syndrome

The phenomenology of TS introduces numerous potential confounds that can seriously impair our ability to interpret adequately the findings from functional imaging studies. These confounds include the effects of chronic illness when studying adolescents and adults, differences in age between patient and control groups, underlying structural differences between groups, and selection of inappropriate methods of regional normalization.

Effects of chronic illness

Perhaps the most serious limitation of radiotracer studies is the ethical concern of exposing younger children to radioactivity. Because the modal onset of tic symptoms is 6 years of age, imaging investigations of adolescents and adults will necessarily be studying in large part the effects of chronic illness. The brain is a tremendously plastic organ and its primary function can be viewed as one of adaptation to maintain homeostasis. Tics and comorbid illnesses are a tremendous burden for children to carry, and adaptation to them will probably alter broadly distributed neural systems throughout the brain. We will see, for instance, that the voluntary suppression of tics, an activity that for many children with TS occupies an inordinate amount of time in their waking life, activates broad expanses of cerebral cortex and basal ganglia. Repeated and chronic activation of these brain regions is likely to induce plastic changes in the underlying neuronal structural and functional architecture. If we are to understand TS pathophysiology better, it is, therefore, imperative that we find ways to study its neural substrate in the absence of chronic compensatory change. This involves somehow pushing our imaging techniques to progressively younger age groups. It could also involve studying unaffected but genetically vulnerable family members to identify trait or risk factors rather than state markers of the CNS functioning that are specific to TS.

Age-related changes

As yet, it has not been possible to control adequately for the effects of simple age-related changes in measures followed by imaging studies. It is likely, for instance, that metabolism, blood flow, and dopaminergic transmission in the basal ganglia all demonstrate their own specific developmental profiles (Shaywitz et al., 1980; Riddle et al., 1986; Seeman et al., 1987). Inadequately controlling for these age-related changes will produce variable and conflicting findings. Although individual matching of patient and subject groups helps to address this problem, this is still not a satisfactory substitute for knowing the developmental characteristics of the experimental measure. The same is true for sex-specific effects, which assumes greater importance in TS because of the much higher prevalence of TS in males than in females. The exclusive study of adults with these disorders also introduces important ascertainment biases that may skew findings and severely limit how the results generalize to the larger population of patients who have TS. Follow-up studies of TS, for instance, suggest that approximately one third of children with TS will be symptom-free as adults, and another one third will have only mild symptoms that do not require clinical attention (Erenberg et al., 1987; Bruun, 1988; Leckman et al., 1998). Therefore, adults who have symptoms severe enough to be ascertained clinically are unusual representatives of all subjects who have a lifetime diagnosis of TS. Either they have a relatively unusual neurobiologic substrate that determines tic persistence (dopaminergic hyperinnervation of their striatum, for instance), or they may have a second disease process (an early dementing illness, for example) that releases the tic symptoms from the inhibitory influences that typically come into play in late adolescence and early childhood. These adult subjects, moreover, are very likely to have received psychotropic medications in their lifetime, either for the treatment of tics or for comorbid OCD, ADHD, depression, or anxiety (Goetz et al., 1992; Park et al., 1993), which are likely to affect brain structure and function and confound study results. Therefore, although studies of adults with TS are important for hypothesis generation and for studies of more severe outcome, they are nevertheless fraught with methodologic limitations that severely limit our ability to interpret and generalize the

findings. Longitudinal imaging studies of children who either have TS or who are at risk for developing TS are, therefore, imperative to improve understanding of this disorder.

Comorbid illnesses

Another confound in functional imaging studies of TS is the high rate of comorbid illness associated with this disorder: OCD affects as many as 60% and ADHD affects approximately 50% of TS clinical populations, while affective illness and anxiety disorders affect even more patients. Despite these extraordinarily high rates of comorbid illness, TS functional imaging studies have rarely assessed the potential presence of these disorders in the patients studied, let alone examined their findings to determine whether these comorbidities were responsible for the findings.

Structure–function relationships

Another potential confound that no functional imaging study in TS has yet addressed is the possibility that group differences in functional measures are largely driven by underlying differences between groups in brain structure. The obvious example in TS is basal ganglia hypometabolism. It is possible, for instance, that the frequently reported reduction in metabolism and blood flow to the basal ganglia is simply a consequence of the previously reported volume reductions in those same areas. Similarly, the normal relationship between morphologic characteristics of the basal ganglia and their neurotransmitter and neuroreceptor profiles is unknown. It is possible that volume reductions in the basal ganglia may account for the greater density and, therefore, elevated levels of presynaptic transporter, postsynaptic dopamine D_2 receptor, and DOPA decarboxylase enzyme that have been reported in TS. Aristotle posited that structure determines function (Kirwan, 1971). Although the direction of causality may not be this clear in the brain, it seems likely that measures of structure and function are at the very least correlated. Future studies should assess these relationships in normal subjects to improve our ability to interpret deviations from those relationships in disease states. Longitudinal studies will also be able to assess how changes in structure and function are related and thereby will allow us to understand better those relationships in temporal cross-section. At the very least, structural indices should be used as covariates in the testing of statistical significance of functional indices. This argues strongly for multimodal imaging studies in TS.

Normalization of metabolism and blood flow

One last potential confound for many imaging studies of TS is the need for normalization of regional metabolic rates. Most metabolism and blood flow studies so far have used measures of blood flow or metabolism in either the visual or the cerebellar cortex as the basis for normalization. The investigators argue that these regions are unlikely to be involved in TS pathophysiology and should, therefore, serve as an adequate reference by which to quantify measures in regions of interest (ROIs) of more central interest to the study. However, activations seen during tic suppression are also likely to be present in metabolism and blood flow studies of TS and this would call into question the use of visual cortex for normalization purposes. We attribute the activations in visual association cortex during tic suppression to the strategy that many subjects use to help to suppress their tics during the scanning session, that of reallocating attentional resources to visual stimuli. This attentional reallocation is thought to "tune" neurons in the visual cortices to visual stimuli as a general mechanism for enhancing task performance. Tuning of the neurons in visual cortex increases their activity and blood flow (Moran and Desimone, 1985; Spitzer, 1988; Petersen et al., 1990; Heinze et al., 1994; Gratton, 1997; Shulman et al., 1997a). Normalizing regional metabolism and blood flow by the values in a region that is itself hypermetabolic relative to normal controls will produce false reports of reduced metabolism and blood flow in other ROIs in the TS patient group. The cerebellum also seems to be a dubious choice by which to normalize, since it is increasingly identified as active in attentional tasks. It also has well-known connections with other motor systems that may be abnormal in TS. These anatomic connections and functional characteristics of the cerebellum may produce differences in its metabolism and blood flow in TS subjects compared with normal controls.

Candidate neural systems in the etiology of tics

Contemporary models of parallel distributed information processing recognize a general modularity in CNS organization. Rather than requiring a temporally serial processing of stimuli, these models suggest that processing in the different modules occurs simultaneously in an iterative, reverberating manner. Effective information processing requires the integrity and interaction of all regional modules, without a strict one-to-one correspondence between regional location, neural computation, and overt behavior. The neural substrate of behavior, therefore, is neither holistic nor phrenologic. Despite the general recognition that brain function is fundamentally based on parallel distributed processing, investigators still tend to localize pathologic brain functioning to relatively small, discrete brain regions. So, although mental functioning is, in part, regionally specified within the modules of the CNS, in our investigations of the neural substrate of tic symptoms we must remember that regional functioning also depends on brain function at spatially distributed sites. In fact, it seems probable at face value that the product of the putative TS vulnerability genes, rather than producing a discrete, localized lesion in the brain is more likely to be expressed and, therefore, more likely to produce disordered functioning within a distributed neural circuit.

The leading candidate system in the search for the neural substrate of TS (along with the substrates of OCD and ADHD comorbidity) is the circuit that loops between cortical and subcortical brain regions (Leckman et al., 1991). Named by the successive structural components within the loops, it is referred to as the cortico–striato–thalamo–cortical (CSTC) circuitry. The hypothesized function of this circuitry is consistent with the frequent co-occurrence of TS, OCD, and ADHD. Involvement of motor portions of the circuit may subserve tics and hyperkinesia. Dysfunction in portions of the circuitry that subserve higher cognitive and ideational processes may produce the premonitory urges of TS and the obsessions of OCD. The involvement of inhibitory portions of the circuit may produce the difficulties with inhibiting inappropriate, impulsive behaviors that is seen in ADHD. In short, the CSTC circuit comprises motor, associational, and inhibitory neural systems that are likely to subserve the symptoms of TS-related illnesses.

CSTC pathways

Multiple, partially overlapping, but largely parallel circuits compose the CSTC circuitry. By directing information from the cerebral cortex to the subcortex, and then back again to specific cortical regions, these circuits form multiple cortical–subcortical loops (Fig. 14.1, p. 242). The loops are considered parallel by virtue of their microscopic segregation from other circuits that course through the same macroscopic structures, the basal ganglia and thalamus. Multiple anatomically and functionally connected cortical regions provide input to particular subcortical portions of the circuit; these subcortical portions then project back to a limited subset of the cortical regions initially contributing to the circuit's input.

The number of anatomically discrete subdivisions of these circuits is controversial. Nevertheless, CSTC circuitry

Table 14.1. The components of the cortico–striatal–thalamo–cortical circuit (CSTC)

CSTC component	Sensorimotor pathways	Orbitofrontal pathways	Association pathways	Limbic system pathway
Cortical afferents	Somatosensory Primary motor Supplementary motor	Orbitofrontal Superior temporal gyrus Inferior temporal gyrus Anterior cingulate	Dorsolateral prefrontal Posterior parietal Arcuate premotor	Anterior cingulate Hippocampal cortex Entorhinal cortex Superior temporal gyrus Inferior temporal gyrus

Striatum	Dorsolateral putamen
	Dorsolateral caudate
	  (dorsolateral subthalamic
	  nucleus)
		Ventral caudate
		Ventral putamen
			Dorsolateral caudate	Ventral caudate
				Ventral Putamen
				Nucleus accumbens
				Olfactory tubercle

Pallidum substantia nigra pars reticulata (SNr)	Ventrolateral globus pallidus internal segment (GPi) Caudolateral SNr	Dorsomedial GPi Rostromedial SNr	Dorsomedial GPi Rostrolateral SNr	Rostrolateral GPi Ventral pallidum Rostrodorsal SNr

Thalamus	Ventrolateral nucleus
	Centromedian intralaminar
	  nucleus
		Medial dorsal nucleus
		  (parvocellular portion)
			Ventral anterior nucleus
			  (parvocellular portion)
				Medial dorsal nucleus
				  (posteromedial portion)

Cortical projections	Supplementary motor	Orbitofrontal	Dorsolateral prefrontal	Anterior cingulate

Sources: Alexander et al., 1990; Parent and Hazrati, 1995a,b.

seems to include four major subcomponents: those loops originating from and projecting back to the sensorimotor, orbitofrontal, association, or temporolimbic cortices (Table 14.1) (Alexander et al., 1990; Parent and Hazrati, 1995a,b). Each of these expanses of cortex projects either to the caudate or putamen, which together comprise the striatum. The projections to the striatum are organized in parasagittally elongated, somatotopic domains. The information leaves these basal ganglia regions primarily through the internal segment of the globus pallidus and its brainstem counterpart, the substantia nigra pars reticulata. The loops then ascend to the thalamus and finally back again to the cortex. This organization is referred to as the direct pathway, which stands in contrast to the indirect pathway. In this latter circuit, the striatum projects first to the external segment of the globus pallidus and then to the reticular portion of the thalamus, as well as to the subthalamic nucleus and the internal segment of the globus pallidus (see Fig. 14.3a, below). This indirect pathway is considered an intrinsic modulator of activity in the direct pathway, since the reticular thalamic nucleus exerts powerful gamma-aminobutyric acid (GABA)-mediated inhibitory influences on circuit elements of the direct pathway in other nuclei of the thalamus (Parent and Hazrati, 1995a). The projection from the external to the internal segment of the globus pallidus, moreover, may similarly modulate direct pathway activity in the internal segment of the globus pallidus.

Subcortical nuclei

Single-cell recordings of the functioning of normal basal ganglia neurons provide circumstantial evidence that these structures may be involved in TS pathophysiology. The recordings indicate that activity in individual neurons in the putamen is correlated with specific aspects of limb movement, including velocity and direction. Motor portions of the CSTC circuitry, therefore, appear to be implicated in controlling the direction of movement as well as scaling its force and speed. Tics show features of normal behavioral repertoires but are executed more frequently, rapidly, and forcefully than their normal behavioral counterparts. It is possible, therefore, that locally disinhibited functioning of CSTC circuits within the basal ganglia could produce tic-like phenomena. Further evidence for this hypothesis comes from chemical or electrical stimulation of the basal ganglia, which produce tic-like stereotypies in animal and human subjects (McLean and Delgado, 1953; Baldwin et al., 1954; Alexander and Delong, 1985; Kelley et al., 1988). Conversely, the clinical efficacy of neuroleptic medications is thought to derive from blocking dopaminergic influences on the basal ganglia from nigrostriatal neurons projecting from the brainstem. Similarly, dopamine-depleting agents, such as α-methyl-p-tyrosine and tetrabenazine, have been reported to suppress tic symptoms in some patients (Sweet et al., 1976; Jankovic et al., 1984), while L-DOPA and stimulant medications, which are dopaminergic agonists, can with varying reliability exacerbate tic symptoms (Golden, 1974; Lowe et al., 1982; Gadow et al., 1995). Finally, human studies and autopsy structural imaging studies suggest the importance of basal ganglia in TS pathophysiology. These studies have been reasonably consistent in demonstrating reduced volumes and abnormal asymmetries in the putamen and globus pallidus nuclei of children and adults with TS (Balthazar, 1956; Richardson, 1982; Peterson et al., 1993; Singer et al., 1993; Castellanos et al., 1994).

Thalamic portions of the CSTC circuit have been implicated in TS largely in the context of tic symptom changes resulting from either space-occupying or neurosurgical lesions (Leckman et al., 1993; Rauch et al., 1995; Peterson et al., 1996). While irritative space-occupying lesions in ventral thalamic nuclei may increase tic symptoms (Peterson 1996), surgical lesions to ventral, medial, and intralaminar thalamic nuceli may attenuate symptoms in some patients (Cooper, 1969; Hassler and Dieckmann, 1970; de Divitiis et al., 1977; Korzen et al., 1991; Rauch et al., 1995). Further evidence for thalamic involvement comes from intraoperative microelectrode stimulation of the ventral intermediate and ventral oralis posterior thalamic nuclei, which produces sensations similar to the premonitory urges that occur in patients with TS prior to the performance of their tics (Tasker and Dostrovsky, 1993).

Sensorimotor pathways

The sensorimotor pathways originate in part from and project back to the supplementary motor area (Table 14.1). Electrical stimulation of the supplementary motor area produces, in some patients, complex movements, vocalizations, and speech arrest, in addition to sensations that in some patients are described as an "urge" to move the somatotopically stimulated contralateral body region (Fried et al., 1991; Lim et al., 1994). These urges to move are reminiscent of the premonitory "urges" that adolescents and adults with TS describe prior to the performance of their tics (Leckman et al., 1993). Electroencephalographic (EEG) recordings have demonstrated potential changes preceding normal voluntary movements that are localized to supplementary motor areas bilaterally. The first EEG study of this kind in six patients with TS was unable to detect premotor movement potentials associated with tics, although they were detected when patients mimicked their own tics (Obeso et al., 1981). Similar results were seen in a second study of five TS patients using a similar experimental design, although premotor movement potentials were discerned before the tics in two of the subjects (Karp

et al., 1996). These results suggest that the neural circuits that produce tics may involve the supplementary motor areas in some patients.

Orbitofrontal pathways

The orbitofrontal cortex is interconnected with the anterior cingulate and other limbic structures. The orbitofrontal cortex may contribute to the capacity for such tasks as successive discrimination, go-no-go and response reversal tasks (Rosvold and Mishkin, 1961; Drewe, 1975; Diamond and Goldman-Rakic, 1989). Lesions of this region appear to interfere with the ability to generate the internal cues that are needed to guide goal-directed behaviors (Goldman-Rakic, 1987). Lesions of the orbitofrontal cortex interfere with an animal's capacity to make appropriate changes in its behavioral set (Divac et al., 1967; Iverson and Mishkin, 1970; Mishkin and Manning, 1978); they typically disrupt the regulation of affect, and they can produce impulsive, socially inappropriate behaviors (Luria, 1980).

Temporolimbic pathways

The limbic system consists of the amygdala and hippocampus in the temporal lobe, the cingulum, the caudate nucleus and other basal ganglia structures in the subcortex, the hypothalamus and periaqueductal gray matter in the brainstem, and connections with the associated frontal cortex. Despite the hypothesized involvement of the temporal lobe in TS pathophysiology, neurobiologic investigations of these regions are remarkably few (Jadresic, 1992; Peterson et al., 1992). The sexual and aggressive content of many complex motor and vocal tics, and of many obsessions and compulsions, also suggest the involvement of the amygdala and related circuitry. Moreover, steroid hormone receptors densely populate the human amygdala and related portions of the limbic circuitry and may mediate sex-specific differences in the prevalence of tic symptoms in the general population, as well as the sexual and aggressive content of tics in some individuals. A neuroimaging study of T_2 relaxation times found evidence of abnormal tissue characteristics in the left and right amygdalae of adults with TS compared with those in normal controls (Peterson et al., 1994).

Cingulate cortex

The cingulate cortex is a heterogeneous structure that probably is a component in most of the major CSTC pathways: the supplementary motor area, orbitofrontal cortex and temporolimbic circuits. The cingulate receives input from the thalamus, amygdala, and motor cortex to its anterior region. It sends projections primarily to motor cortex, striatum, periaqueductal gray, and brainstem motor nuclei (Vogt et al., 1992; Bates and Goldman-Rakic, 1993). The anterior cingulate cortex is thought to subserve, among other things, attentional and executive functioning (Pardo et al., 1990; Peterson et al., 1999), and impairment of these functions probably account for some of the inattention, impulsivity, and motoric dyscontrol that commonly characterizes the TS phenotype. Electrical stimulation of the anterior cingulate in humans can produce semi-voluntary movements resembling complex motor tics (Talairach et al., 1973), and there are reports of anterior cingulotomies alleviating tic symptoms in some patients, although these were uncontrolled studies (Kurlan et al., 1990; Robertson et al., 1990).

Brainstem neuromodulators and motor nuclei

Finally, the brainstem has been implicated as one possible component of the neural substrate of TS. The various brainstem centers that generate catecholamine and indoleamine neurotransmitters are thought to play important neuromodulatory roles in the disorder. These centers project to the basal ganglia and may thereby influence tic symptoms. One suspected modulator of tic symptoms, for instance, includes the dopaminergic afferent systems ascending to the basal ganglia from the midbrain substantia nigra. In addition, noradrenergic projections from the locus ceruleus modulate midbrain dopamine and frontal inhibitory centers; these effects indirectly influence basal ganglia function and may thereby help to suppress tic-related behaviors. Noradrenergic systems may also mediate the exquisite stress responsivity seen in the disorder (Chappell et al., 1994). Aside from these neurotransmitter systems, limbic regions presumably have a modulating effect via direct afferent projections to the ventral striatum, and indirectly through projections to midbrain dopaminergic neurons. The limbic regions are hypothesized to be important in modulating the sexual and aggressive content of tic symptoms (Jadresic, 1992; Peterson et al., 1992).

Descending projections from the motor cortex and basal ganglia nuclei regulate the motor discharge of brainstem interneurons and motor nuclei. Abnormalities associated with this regulation could produce motor and vocal tics having the somatotopy characteristics of TS. A study supporting this hypothesis found an increased amplitude of one component of the blink reflex in patients with TS compared with normal controls, suggesting the presence of

increased excitability of TS brainstem regulatory interneurons (Smith and Lees, 1989). Abnormalities in these regulatory interneurons could affect functioning of brainstem motor nuclei, which innervate the musculature most commonly affected by tics. These nuclei innervate the muscles of the face (motor nucleus of cranial nerve VII in the midpons), neck and shoulders (spinal accessory cranial nerve XI in the medulla), larynx and pharynx (nucleus ambiguus, a portion of the vagus cranial nerve X in the medulla), tongue (hypoglossal nucleus of cranial nerve XII in the medulla), and diaphragm (descending brainstem control of high cervical spinal cord). All of these brainstem nuclei are situated closely to one another and could easily be involved in a relatively discrete pathologic process in the brainstem. Consistent with this hypothesis, the neural basis for conscious control of musculature in the extremities resides largely in the motor cortex, and the extremities are much less commonly affected by tics than are the facial, vocal, and diaphragmatic musculature.

The basal ganglia and descending dopaminergic systems from the midbrain are also known to influence the activity of brainstem sensory pathways, another possible contributor to tic symptoms. For instance, disturbing the relay of proprioceptive information from the face to the mesencephalic nucleus of cranial nerve V in the pons could produce the clonus-like activity of muscle groups affected by tics (Lawrence and Redmond, 1985; Larumbe et al., 1993).

Functional neuroimaging studies

The neural systems described above have been identified as candidates for the substrate of tic-related behaviors primarily through consideration of a vast preclinical literature on the normal structural and functional organization of the CNS, TS-related phenomenology, and human lesion studies. One goal of our review will be to assess which of these candidate systems are most strongly implicated in TS pathophysiology.

Resting metabolism and blood flow studies

In vivo positron emission tomography (PET) and single photon emission computed tomography (SPECT) studies generally report a hypometabolism in cortical and subcortical brain regions of patients who have TS. These studies, however, typically do not adequately relate the implications of these results to the current knowledge of the neural circuitry and neurophysiology of TS. More importantly, in failing to make explicit the demands of their scanning protocol, these studies usually overlook the effects that either spontaneous tics or the suppression of tics may have on brain metabolism (Tables 14.2 and 14.3). We will review functional imaging studies of TS in chronological order of their publication.

The first preliminary fluorodeoxyglucose (FDG) PET study of 12 adults with TS (10 males, two females; mean age 33 ± 2 years) and an equal number of normal control subjects (eight males, four females; mean age 31 ± 2 years) reported a 15% average reduction of absolute glucose utilization rates in the frontal, cingulate, and insular cortices and in the inferior corpus striatum ($p<0.01$) (Chase et al., 1986). An inverse correlation ($p<0.01$) was seen between the severity of tics (both vocal and motor) and glucose rates in these same areas. The authors did not specify whether instructions were given to the patients to suppress their tics during scanner uptake. Additionally, the normal controls and subjects with TS were unevenly sex-matched, which may have affected group comparisons.

Significant differences between patients and controls were found only at horizontal levels 8.4–8.8 cm caudal to the brain vertex. This orientation bears an approximate correspondence to the level of the anterior commissure–posterior commissure (AC–PC) line in Talairach coordinates. The absence of a standard anatomic reference scheme, however, renders impossible any accurate alignment with Talairach coordinates and hence also any accurate anatomic comparison with other studies. The investigators did not specify whether the medication-free status of the 12 untreated patients was for lifetime or only recent status, and subject handedness was not reported. Finally and most importantly, the methods employed for statistical analysis were not described.

In a report published only in abstract form, brain perfusion deficits were also found in a hexamethyl-propyle-neamine oxime (HMPAO) SPECT study of 25 patients with TS (19 males, six females; 7–48 years old) compared with 10 normal subjects whose scans were selected from a pre-existing library of normal scans (Hall et al., 1990). Hypoperfusion of the basal ganglia and thalamus was seen in the patients with TS relative to the controls. Perfusion deficits were also seen in the frontal and temporal cortices. The poorly matched controls, whose scans were selected only by convenience, and the absence of methodologic details makes critical appraisal of the study impossible.

Another HMPAO SPECT study of 20 patients with TS (17 males, three females; mean age 34.7 ± 12 years; 18/20 right-handed; 10 with comorbid OCD) and five normal controls (five males, three females; mean age 34.7 ± 12.5 years; five right-handed) failed to detect group differences in basal ganglia blood flow (George et al., 1992). Instead,

the investigators noted an increased right frontal activity compared with control subjects when this region was normalized to regional cerebral blood flow (rCBF) in the visual cortex. Yet the small number of controls and limitations in scanner resolution (7–9mm full width half maximum (FWHM) limit the generalizability of these negative findings. Moreover, as our discussion of subsequent studies will make clear, the choice of the visual cortex for normalization may have been misguided in that blood flow to the region may have been affected by the demands of the scanning protocol. Tic behaviors during tracer uptake were not described. Other investigators conducted an HMPAO SPECT study of nine patients with TS (six males, three females; mean age 29.6 ± 7 years) and nine individually sex- and age-matched controls (Riddle et al., 1992). HMPAO uptake was reduced by 4% in the left putamen and globus pallidus of the patients with TS compared with control values, although the p-value for this group comparison was not provided. In addition, a paired t-test was used to perform between-group comparisons when an unpaired test may have been more appropriate, since matching on age and sex does not control sufficiently for the biological determinants of HMPAO-assessed blood flow. The unpaired analysis probably would have eliminated the statistical significance of the 4% reduction in the rCBF to the basal ganglia.

Several case reports of HMPAO SPECT blood flow abnormalities have been reported in TS. One, published as an abstract, is that of an 11-year-old girl who had TS and who demonstrated hypoperfusion only in the region of her left basal ganglia (Sieg et al., 1992). Despite its obvious limitations, this study is consistent with others demonstrating regional hypoperfusion in patients with TS. A second case report documents the metabolic effects of a limbic leucotomy in a 45-year-old patient with TS and OCD (Sawle et al., 1993). This patient underwent a PET scan 15 months before and 21 months after his leucotomy. His data were compared with data from six age-matched, male normal controls. Preoperatively, the caudate appeared to be the most hypermetabolic, as was the thalamus. Postoperatively, the greatest reductions in metabolic rate occurred in the caudate and anterior cingulate. Reduction in cingulate metabolism would be expected as a consequence of the surgical lesion, which is typically placed in the anterior- and inferior-most portion of the anterior cingulate gyrus beneath the genu of the corpus callosum (Rauch et al., 1995). This lesion also typically interrupts projections from orbitofrontal cortex to caudate and thalamic nuclei, which probably accounts for the reduction in caudate metabolism.

The largest and methodologically finest FDG PET imaging study compared normalized metabolic rates

Table 14.2. Design features of metabolic studies and blood flow-related studies in Tourette's syndrome

Investigator	Modality and resolution	Sample size		Age (years)		Sex		Comorbidity	Handedness	
		TS	NC	TS	NC	TS	NC		TS	NC
Chase et al. (1986)	FDG PET; 5 mm FWHM	12	12	33±2	31±2	10M, 2F	8M, 4F	N/A	N/A	N/A
Hall et al. (1990)	HMPAO SPECT	25	10 (from library)	7–48	–	19M, 6F	–	N/A	N/A	N/A
George et al. (1992)	HMPAO SPECT	20	8	23.8±12	34.7±13	17M, 3F	5M, 3F	10 OCD	18R, 2L	5R, 0L
Riddle et al. (1992)	HMPAO SPECT; 8 mm in-plane, 16 mm through-plane	9	9	29.6+6.9	Matched within 2 years	6M, 3F	6M, 3F	N/A	N/A	N/A
Sieg et al. (1992)	HMPAO SPECT	1	–	9		1F		N/A	N/A	N/A
Sawle et al. (1993)	^{15}O PET	1	6	45	Age matched	1M	6M	TS+OCD	N/A	N/A
Stoetter et al. (1992) and Braun et al. (1993)	FDG PET; 6–7 mm in-plane, 11–12 mm through-plane	18	16	33±7 (23–49)	34±10 (20–50)	16M, 2F	11M, 5F	N/A	N/A	N/A
Moriarty et al. (1995)	HMPAO SPECT (2 scanners)	50	20	24 (7–65)	23	38M, 12F	9M, 12F	27/50 OCB	N/A	N/A
Moriarty et al. (1997)	HMPAO SPECT	Families of 5 TS children (8 had TS)			8–57	N/A		4 OCB	N/A	N/A
Klieger et al. (1997)	HMPAO SPECT	6	9	36 (26–54)	70 (56–81)	3M, 3F	4M, 5F	N/A	N/A	N/A
Eidelberg et al. (1997)	FDG PET	10	10	4.5±12.7	42.5±11.5	9M, 1F	5M, 5F	N/A	10R, 0L	10R, 0L
Peterson et al. (1998)	fMRI; 7 mm through-plane, 3.1 mm × 3.1 mm in-plane	22	–	35.7±10.9 (18–55)	–	11M, 11F	–	10 OCD	14R, 8L	–

Notes: NC, normal controls; TS, Tourette's syndrome; OCD, obsessive-compulsive disorder; L, left-handedness; R, right-handedness; N/A, not available. FDG-PET, [18F]-fluorodeoxyglucose PET; FWHM, full width half maximum; HMPAO SPECT, hexamethyl-propyleneamine oxime SPECT.

Table 14.3. Reported results of metabolic studies and blood flow-related studies of Tourette's syndrome

Study	Sensorimotor pathways	Orbitofrontal pathways	Association pathways	Temporolimbic pathways	Subcortical portions
Chase et al. (1986)[a]			− Bilateral mid frontal[a]	− Anterior cingulate[b] − Insular cortex[c]	− Inferior striatum
Hall et al. (1990)					− Basal ganglia
George et al. (1992)			+ Right midfrontal[d]		
Riddle et al. (1992)					− Left putamen − Globus pallidus
Stoetter et al. (1992) and Braun et al. (1993)[e]	Supplementary motor area + Lateral premotor + Sensorimotor	− Orbitofrontal	+ Superior parietal lobule	− Inferior insular[c] − Parahippocampal region	− Ventral striatum
Moriarty et al. (1995)			− Left dorsolateral prefrontal cortex	− Anterior cingulate	− Left basal ganglia
Kleiger et al. (1997)					+ Asymmetry of basal ganglia
Eidelberg et al. (1997)	+ Factor 1 in TS group[f]			Factor 2[f], correlates with symptom severity	Factor 2[f], correlates with symptom severity
Peterson et al. (1998)	− Left sensorimotor	+ Left sensorimotor	+ Right midfrontal cortex + Right middle temporal gyrus + Superior temporal gyrus bilaterally + Both inferior occipital regions[g] − Cuneus bilaterally[f] − Left inferior parietal	+ Right anterior cingulate − Right posterior cingulate − Parahippocampus − Left hippocampus	+ Ventral head of right caudate − Ventral globus pallidus − Ventral putamen − Midbody of each hemithalamus

Notes:

Regional activations are grouped according to the different pathways within cortico–striatal–thalamo–cortical (CSTC) circuit. Increased metabolism, blood flow, or signal intensity indicated by "+" and decreases by "−". The case reports of Sieg et al. (1992) and Sawle et al. (1993) and the preliminary family study of Moriarty et al. (1997) are not included here because the small number of subjects might bias interpretations of the table and the circuits most commonly implicated in TS. These omitted studies, despite their limitations, are also suggestive of basal ganglia hypometabolism.

[a] Cortical region of interest assignments are only approximate as imaging planes were not acquired in Talairach coordinates, making impossible a precise comparison with other studies.

[b] The hypometabolism of the anterior cingulate is cited as located 8.4–8.8 cm caudal to the brain vertex. Approximating this location within the Talairach coordinate system would suggest that it was located near the anterior–posterior commissure line.

[c] Because of limitations in scanner resolution, it is unclear whether this area of decreased metabolism is located in the insular cortex, as the authors contend, or whether it is instead in the lateral putamen and claustrum.

[d] The authors' description (given only as "frontal") does not permit accurate localization. Based on the figure provided in the paper, we tentatively identify this as "midfrontal".

[e] The Stoetter et al. (1992) and Braun et al. (1993) studies differ by only two subjects. We, therefore, cite them as a single study here.

[f] Factors 1 and 2 are the products of a principle components analysis that load primarily on motor regions and right-sided temporal cortices, respectively.

[g] The inferior occipital and cuneate regions belong to visual association systems and are here assigned to belonging as association pathways.

between 16 patients with TS (14 males, two females; mean age 33 ± 7 years) and 16 normal controls who were matched well for age but not for sex (11 males, five females; mean age 34 ± 10 years) (Braun et al., 1993). Global cerebral metabolism showed no differences between groups. Increased relative metabolic rates were seen in superior sensorimotor cortices of the subjects with TS. Reduced metabolism was seen in the inferior limbic-associated areas, especially in paralimbic, ventral prefrontal, striatal, and brainstem regions. The largest reductions were located generally in the left hemisphere (Fig. 14.2). The basal ganglia subregions in which metabolic activity was most reduced appeared to be the limbic-associated regions of the ventral striatum. Although typically the ventral striatum is considered to comprise the nucleus accumbens and caudate, the large size of the ROI, as well as the limited scanner resolution, make it likely that activity in this ROI derived from all basal ganglia nuclei, including the putamen and globus pallidus.

Despite the many strengths of this study, it has several important limitations. Four of the patients with TS in this study were on neuroleptics and three were on other medications within 8 weeks of their scans. The remaining nine patients had a history of medication of some type. It is possible, therefore, that prior medication exposure may have contributed to the findings. In addition, it is possible that the patterns of metabolic differences in those with TS relative to controls may be explained by the implicit and explicit need to remain still or to suppress tic symptoms during radiotracer uptake. The patients, in fact, were noted to tic rarely during the period of FDG uptake, which is not uncommon for TS patients during novel and attention-demanding experiences. Finally, the image analytic methods used in this study can be questioned. Eight slices were analyzed for significance. The investigators used two methodologies to identify the ROIs. One employed 164 pie-shaped ROIs in the entire axial cross-sections, while the other used 112 circular ROIs placed only in the cortex. Of all statistical tests that were performed using either method of region definition, 22 regions were significant using both methods. Another 32 ROIs were significant in one or the other analysis but not in both. The authors note that the significance of regions in both analyses support claims for the reliability of their image analytic methods. Although this is true, the reliability of the findings (in terms of their independent test–retest reproducibility) would be more rigorously demonstrated if the same regional group differences were identified using the two analytic methods on different data sets – either between two different subject groups or the between scans obtained on a single subject group at two different times. Moreover, the authors did not correct their p values for multiple comparisons; consequently the risk of type I error (false-positive group differences) is considerable.

Additional analyses were performed on this same data set after adding two subjects to the group of patients with TS, bringing it to a total of 18 (16 males, two females; mean age 33 ± 7 years) (Stoetter et al., 1992). The new analysis examined the correlations between all combinations of significantly activated regions. Significantly different interregional correlations were seen in the patients compared with controls. In the correlations involving the frontal lobe, group differences were seen most frequently in those with the orbitofrontal cortex. In those involving the limbic regions, group differences were seen most frequently in regions around the insula. The most frequent group differences, however, involved the ventral striatum (seen in 35% of all possible correlations). Of all the correlation analyses, those that the authors singled out for discussion were those between the ventral striatum and sensorimotor cortices. These regions were inversely correlated in the controls but positively correlated in the TS group, suggesting a disturbed functional relationship between the ventral striatum and sensorimotor cortices in the TS group. Although these altered functional relationships may represent inherent disturbances in the connectivity of the brain in TS subjects, it is also possible that the altered relationships may be caused by implicitly different group behavioral demands, such as requiring subjects to remain still or to suppress tics during the scan. These demands will be greater in the TS group and may specifically alter relationships between ventral striatum and sensorimotor cortices.

The largest HMPAO SPECT study to date compared 50 patients with TS (38 males, 12 females; mean age 24 years; age range 7–65 years; 27 had significant OCD symptoms) with 20 normal controls (nine males, 11 females; mean age 23 years) (Moriarty et al., 1995). Subjects were scanned for 30 min, although patients with TS who could not suppress their disruptive tics were scanned for a shorter period of time. Consistent with previous TS neuroimaging studies, the results indicated hypoperfusion in the left caudate and anterior cingulate, as well as hypoperfusion in the left dorsolateral prefrontal cortex. Because the resolution of the scans did not allow the investigators to differentiate reliably between perfusion of the caudate and lenticular nuclei, the blood flow reductions that are reported as located in the left caudate should instead be more accurately described as being located in the left basal ganglia. Additional limitations of the study include the failure to take into consideration the effects of age on regional blood flow values. The age range of the patients with TS

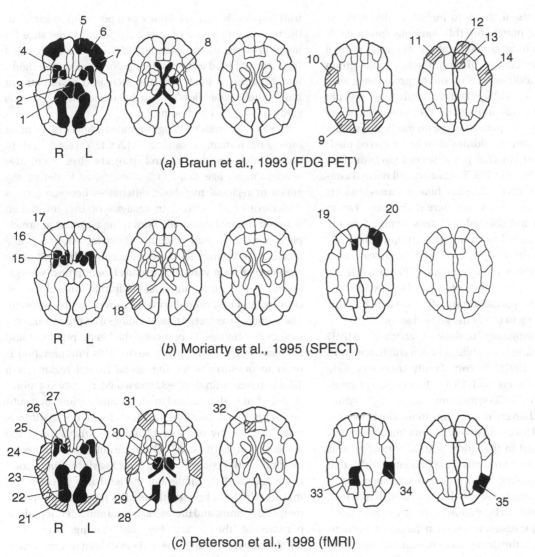

Fig. 14.2. Comparison of the largest functional imaging studies in Tourette's syndrome using PET, SPECT, and fMRI. The results are presented using five representative slices. Regions of interest (ROI) hatched represent increased activity while those colored black represent regional decreases in activity. (a, b) In the PET and SPECT study, these are increases and decreases in the patient groups relative to normal control values. (c) In the fMRI study, the changes are relative to baseline signal intensities. The key for numbered ROIs (below) identifies ROIs in any of the three studies that have significantly increased or decreased activity. Note that these representations are not strictly comparable, as decisions had to be made in the assignment of certain ROIs. In ROI 4 of study (a), for instance, we have assigned to the putamen the decreased activity that was originally reported in the right insula, since the regions cannot be distinguished with the limited scanner resolution. Similar considerations of scanner resolution prompted us to assign to the basal ganglia in general the reduced metabolism originally reported in the caudate and inferior insula regions in study (b). We were unsure where in the anterior/posterior extent of the cingulate to place ROI 19, as it was labeled in study (b) only as "cingulum". 1, hippocampus/parahippo-campus; 2, midbrain; 3, ventral striatum; 4, inferior insula; 5, medial orbital cortex; 6, lateral orbital cortex; 7, opercular orbital cortex; 8, putamen; 9, superior lateral occipital cortex; 10, inferior sensorimotor ("Rolandic") cortex; 11, inferior lateral premotor cortex; 12, inferior lateral premotor cortex; 13, anterior supplementary motor cortex; 14, superior sensorimotor ("Rolandic") cortex; 15, globus pallidus; 16, inferior insula/putamen; 17, caudate; 18, anterior inferior temporal cortex; 19, superior anterior cingulate; 20, superior lateral prefrontal cortex; 21, occipital cortex; 22, hippocampus/parahippocampus; 23, middle temporal gyrus; 24, superior temporal gyrus; 25, putamen; 26, globus pallidus; 27, caudate; 28, cuneus; 29, superior temporal gyrus; 30, thalamus; 31, frontal cortex; 32, anterior cingulate; 33, posterior cingulate; 34, sensorimotor cortex; 35, inferior parietal cortex. L, left; R, right.

(7–65 years) and the inability to include children in the control group to match on this variable (presumably because of the ethical concerns about exposing normal children to radioactivity) likely influenced the group comparisons. In addition, the TS and control groups were not matched by sex, and apparently handedness was not assessed, further confounding the interpretation of the findings. Sixteen of the patients were on medication at the time of the scan, and an additional 10 had received medications in the past. Another possible confound concerns the use of two different SPECT scanners. All normal controls were scanned on a single machine, whereas subjects with TS were imaged on two different scanners. Group membership was not blinded for scans acquired on the machine that scanned both subject groups, effectively unblinding the entire study. Even though the investigators did not find evidence for systematic differences in the results from the two scanners, they could not exclude the possibility of greater partial volume effects in data from the patient group owing to use of the second scanner.

The same investigators undertook another HMPAO SPECT study on parents or siblings of five children with TS (Moriarty et al., 1997). Twenty family members were scanned: eight subjects had TS (eight males: age range 8–57 years); four had OCD symptoms; one had OCD symptoms and tics, and seven had no symptoms. The ROIs were visually inspected for qualitative abnormalities. No control group was included in the study, and "abnormality" was not defined. In the seven scans from patients with TS that had acceptable quality, hypoperfusion was seen in the caudate in five subjects (although again, this should read "basal ganglia" owing to limitations in scanner resolution). In addition, hypoperfusion was seen in the parietal or temporal lobe in five, in the thalamus in two and in the frontal lobe and brainstem in one. Abnormalities were not seen in any of the family members who were symptom free. Despite the limitations of small subject numbers and the reliance on qualitative data, these results again suggest the presence of reduced blood flow to the basal ganglia in TS.

Yet another HMPAO SPECT study of six adults with TS (three males; three females; mean age 36 years) and nine normal elderly control subjects (four males, five females; mean age 70 years) reported an increased asymmetry of basal ganglia blood flow in the TS group (reported as a right/left ratio, $p < 0.001$) (Klieger et al., 1997). The abnormally large asymmetry of basal ganglia blood flow seemed to be driven by a relatively large (12.6%) decrease in flow to the right-sided structures, a decrease that in itself was not statistically significant (normalized to cerebellar blood flow; $p = 0.11$). The limitations of this study include a small number of subjects, poor matching of patients and con-

trols (especially on age), failure to report comorbidities in the patient group, use of only a single transaxial slice for image analysis, and nonstandard ROI definition (left-sided ROIs were defined as mirror images of those on the right). Finally, it seems likely that the increased asymmetry of basal ganglia blood flow seen in the patients with TS in this study was a post-hoc finding.

An FDG PET study of 10 right-handed adults with TS (nine men, one woman; mean age 41.5 ± 12.7 years) and 10 normal right-handed control subjects (five men, five women; mean age 42.5 ± 11.5 years) failed to detect any global or regional metabolic differences between groups (Eidelberg et al., 1997). An analysis of the covariation between regional metabolic rates using a variant of principle components analysis identified two factors, or regional metabolic groupings, that together accounted for 29% of the subject-by-region variance. Regions loading most strongly on the first factor included lateral frontal, medial frontal, cuneate, and paracentral cortices, as well as the midbrain. The authors interpreted these loadings as representing cortical motor circuits, in particular the lateral premotor and supplementary motor area systems. This interpretation is open to question, since the lateral frontal regions at a Talairach z-coordinate of $+32$ mm would indicate not motor systems but prefrontal and medial frontal regions that subserve attentional functions. Factor scores for the TS subjects were significantly elevated compared with those of the normal controls ($p < 0.01$), which the authors attributed to motor activity. Regions loading most heavily on the second factor included the midbrain; the lenticular nucleus and thalamus in the subcortex; the medial, lateral, and superior temporal regions; and the lateral frontal and inferior parietal portions of the cortex. Regional loadings were predominantly right-sided. The authors did not interpret what circuits the loadings on this factor may represent, and the TS subjects did not differ significantly from controls on their loadings for this factor. The scores for the subjects with TS did, however, correlate positively and significantly with one measure of symptom severity from the (now nonstandard) Tourette Syndrome Global Scale ($r = 0.85$; $p < 0.005$). Although these findings are interesting, they must be regarded as preliminary and in need of rigorous replication, since they are undoubtedly post hoc and exploratory. Interpretation of the findings is also potentially confounded by the failure to assess cormorbid illness in the TS group, the unequal sex compositions of the two groups, and the greater degree of motion artifact in the TS group. Finally, the abnormal correlation patterns seen in the TS group could have been a consequence of the need to suppress tics during tracer uptake, an implicit behavioral demand not required of the normal controls.

A functional MRI study of voluntary tic suppression

Our recent functional MRI (fMRI) study investigated the effects of voluntary tic suppression on fMRI signal changes (Peterson et al., 1998). These signal changes are produced by a change in regional deoxyhemoglobin content, which is itself induced by a local change in neuronal activity and metabolic demand (see Chapter 3). In the study, 22 patients with TS (11 males and 11 females; mean age 35.7 ± 10.9 years; 10 comorbid OCD; 14/22 right-handed) were asked to alternate 40 s epochs of allowing themselves to tic freely with 40 s epochs of suppressing their tics voluntarily, for a total of eight tic/suppression cycles. Signal intensity decreased significantly during tic suppression epochs in the ventral globus pallidus, ventral putamen, midbody of each hemithalamus, right posterior cingulate, left hippocampus and parahippocampus, the cuneus bilaterally, left sensorimotor cortex, and left inferior parietal region. Increased signal intensity during tic suppression occurred in the ventral portion of the right caudate nucleus, right midfrontal cortex, right middle temporal gyrus, superior temporal gyrus bilaterally, right anterior cingulate cortex, and bilateral inferior occipital regions (Fig. 14.3, p. 242).

The severity of tic symptoms outside of the scanner correlated with the change in signal intensity associated with tic suppression inside of the scanner much more frequently in subcortical (8/8 regions) than in cortical regions (2/15 regions). Moreover, the direction of correlation between symptom severity and signal change in the subcortex suggested that as symptom severity increases, the absolute value of the magnitude of signal change in the subcortex decreases. This suggests that the subcortical signal changes – increases in the right caudate and decreases in the rest of the subcortex – participate in the suppression of these unwanted behaviors. When these braking mechanisms begin to fail and subcortical signal change is reduced, tics are progressively more likely to escape inhibition. Motion artifact, assessed in several different ways, did not seem to account for the observed correlations. These findings suggest that the pathogenesis of TS involves dysfunction of subcortical portions of CSTC circuitry. An additional interpretation is that the most important determinant of clinical phenotype and symptom severity may not be the genetic vulnerability to tic disorders. Rather, the stronger determinant of symptom severity may be the degree to which the control system either suppresses or unmasks the inherent diathesis to tic. The functional integrity of this control system itself may be under genetic control, or it may be a manifestation of other nongenetic pathophysiologic determinants.

Radioligand studies

Other preliminary functional studies have focused on quantifying various functional indices of the dopaminergic neurotransmitter system in the striatum in subjects with TS (Table 14.4). An [^{18}F]-fluorodopa study of three patients with TS, six with OCD, and 30 normal control adults found no difference between patient and control groups for the influx constants of fluorodopa (Brooks et al., 1992). A [^{11}C]-raclopride PET investigation from the same laboratory studied three patients with TS and eight normal adults and found no group differences in [^{11}C]-raclopride binding (Singer et al., 1992). These PET studies were then expanded to include 10 patients with TS and 34 controls in the fluorodopa study, and five patients with TS and nine controls in the [^{11}C]-raclopride study (Turjanski et al., 1994). Again, no group differences were found. The negative fluorodopa findings indicate normal fluorodopa uptake and decarboxylation, while the negative [^{11}C]-raclopride findings indicate normal numbers of available dopamine D_2 and D_3 postsynaptic receptor-binding sites in these patients with TS. The patient and control groups in these studies, however, were inadequately matched (Table 14.4); 7 of the 10 TS subjects in the fluorodopa study were on neuroleptic medication at the time of scanning, and the patient numbers in each study were still relatively small. In addition, fluorodopa has limited signal-to-noise properties ($<2:1$) mainly because the peripheral radiolabeled fluorodopa metabolite (3-O-methyl-6-F-DOPA) is present in the striatum (Garnett et al., 1983). All of these considerations may have limited the statistical power to detect potential group differences (Table 14.4).

Although these initial studies suggested normal synaptic dopamine transmission in TS, a subsequent pilot study of striatal [^{123}I]-β-CIT (2β-carboxymethoxy-3β-[4-iodophenyl]tropane) uptake suggested the presence of elevated presynaptic dopamine transporter levels in TS (Malison et al., 1995). Transporter levels were 37% higher in five patients with TS (mean age 27 ± 8 years) than in five normal controls who were individually matched by age (28 ± 8 years) and sex: 10.4 ± 2.3 versus 7.7 ± 1.4 (mean $\pm$ SD) ratio of striatal to occipital uptake, respectively. The limitations of the study included small subject numbers, the use of paired t-tests (age- and sex-matching do not account for all confounding biological variability), and the inclusion of TS subjects who had prior neuroleptic exposure. Despite these limitations, the findings are intriguing, and they are consistent with one autopsy study of three adults with TS and six normal controls that reported increased numbers of presynaptic dopamine-uptake sites in the caudate nucleus and putamen of the former (Singer

Table 14.4. Design features and results of radioligand studies in Tourette's syndrome

Investigator	Modality and resolution	Sample size TS	Sample size NC	Age (years) TS	Age (years) NC	Sex TS	Sex NC	Finding	Interpretation
Brooks et al. (1992)	[18F]-Fluorodopa PET; 7 mm × 8.5 mm × 8.5 mm FWHM	3	30	24–46	N/A	3M	N/A	No differences	Normal striatal DOPA metabolism
Brooks et al. (1992)	[11C]-Raclopride PET; 7 mm × 8.5 mm × 8.5 mm FWHM	3	8	18–46	N/A	3M	N/A	No differences	Normal D$_2$-like site density
Turjanski et al. (1994)	[18F]-Fluorodopa PET; 7 mm × 8.5 mm × 8.5 mm	10	34	30 (18–48)	58 (20–77)	8M, 2F	N/A	No differences	Normal striatal DOPA metabolism
Turjanski et al. (1994)	[11C]-Raclopride PET; 7 mm × 8.5 mm × 8.5 mm FWHM	5	9	33 (18–46)	50 (24–74)	5M	N/A	No differences	Normal D$_2$-like site density
Malison et al. (1995)	β-CIT SPECT; 8–12 mm FWHM	5	5	27 ± 8	28 ± 8	2M, 3F	2M, 3F	37% elevation in striatal β-CIT binding	Increased presynaptic dopamine transporter levels
Wolf et al. (1996)	IBZM SPECT; 11.5 mm FWHM	Five pairs of monozygotic twins		29 ± 4 (18–42)	–	4M, 1F	–	17% increase in caudate binding in more severely affected co-twin	Increased D$_2$ receptor levels in caudate produce dopaminergic supersensitivity to explain phenotypic variation
Wong et al. (1997)[a]	NMSP PET; 8 mm in-plane, 12–14 mm axial	9	44	27	19–73	N/A	22M, 22F	No differences	Normal D$_2$-like receptor densities
		20	24	36.2 ± 8.9	18–83	16M, 4F	N/A	No differences	Normal D$_2$-like receptor densities
Ernst et al. (1999)	[18F]-Fluorodopa PET; 5.2 mm in-plane, 11.8 mm axial	11	10	15.2 ± 1.9	14.8 ± 1.7	8M, 3F	7M, 3F	Higher fluorodopa accumulation in left caudate nucleus (25%) and right midbrain (53%)	Regionally specific increase in DOPA decarboxylase enzyme activity

Note:

[a] Two protocols, see text for details.

Source: Abbreviations as in Table 14.2 and β-CIT, 2β-carboxymethoxy-3β-[4-iodophenyl]tropane; IBZM, [123I]-iodobenzamide; NMSP, [11C]-3-*N*-methylspiperone.

et al., 1991). In this same study, levels of dopamine and its metabolites in the subjects with TS were not significantly different from control levels. Whereas the autopsy study found higher transporter levels in the putamen, the SPECT study suggested that transporter levels were particularly elevated in the caudate nucleus.

A subsequent [^{123}I]-iodobenzamide (IBZM, a D$_2$-like receptor ligand) SPECT study of five monozygotic twin pairs (four male and one female twin pairs; mean age 29 ± 4 years; all currently medication free) reported an increase of IBZM binding in the caudate of all five of the more severely affected co-twins (Wolf et al., 1996). No differences in IBZM binding were seen in the putamen. The group differences did not appear to be a result of differences in blood flow between groups, since blood flow values from HMPAO SPECT scans in the same twin pairs did not reveal any group differences. Intrapair differences in IBZM binding correlated highly with the corresponding differences in overall symptom severity between co-twins ($r = 0.99$; $p < 0.001$). The investigators suggested that a variation in D$_2$ receptor availability in the caudate nucleus might have accounted for the differing severity of symptom expression between siblings who have the same genetic vulnerability. Although these initial findings are exciting, it is important to remember that they are based on a sample of five twin pairs, rendering the statistical tests highly unstable. In addition, the possible discordance of comorbid illnesses is not considered as a possible confound. Neither is the possibility considered that the greater D$_2$ receptor availability in the more severely affected twin could represent either a compensatory response to the presence of more severe tics or an epiphenomenon owing to greater neuroleptic exposure in the more severely affected twin.

The D$_2$-like receptors were again studied with [^{11}C]-3-N-methylspiperone ([^{11}C]-NMSP) in two different PET protocols (Wong et al., 1997). All patients were medication free for at least 6 months. The first protocol measured only caudate-to-cerebellar ratio of radioligand binding at 45 min postinjection in nine patients with TS (mean age 27 years; five with prior neuroleptic use) and 44 neurologically normal control subjects (22 males, 22 females; age 19–73 years). The second, applied in 20 TS subjects (16 males, 4 females; mean age 36.2 ± 8.9 years) and 24 normal adults (mean age not provided; range 18–83 years) was designed to provide an absolute measure of available receptor density (B'_{max}), which they hypothesized would suggest the presence of elevated D$_2$-like dopamine receptors in TS. After their first scan, this second group of subjects received a dose of unlabeled haloperidol, which in part displaced [^{11}C]-NMSP from its D$_2$-like receptors. They then underwent a second scan to determine the degree of

radioligand displacement. In the first protocol, the caudate-to-cerebellar ratio of radioligand binding did not differ significantly between the TS and control groups. In the second protocol, B_{max} binding potential values also did not differ between groups. These results are consistent with prior studies that show the postsynaptic D$_2$-like receptors in TS to be similar to those of normal control subjects. If the findings of the previously described IBZM monozygotic twin study are correct, then these NMSP findings would have two primary implications. First, D$_2$-like receptor levels must determine a relatively small portion of between-subject variance in clinical symptom severity in singletons with TS, even though the levels may account for much of the variability in symptom severity between monozygotic co-twins. Second, nongenetic factors must account for a small portion of the normal individual variability in D$_2$ receptor levels.

Finally, a relatively recent fluorodopa PET study of 11 adolescents with TS (mean age 15.2 ± 1.9 years) and 10 sex-matched normal controls (mean age 14.8 ± 1.7 years) found higher fluorodopa accumulation in the left caudate nucleus (25%) and the right midbrain (53%) of the former (Ernst et al., 1999). Subjects watched a videotape during the first 80 min of tracer uptake and were not specifically told to suppress tics. It should be noted that activities that engage attention, even relatively simple ones such as watching videotapes, often alter tic frequency (typically reducing it). The investigators, however, recorded motor activity of the patients during tracer uptake and scanning, but they found no correlation with fluorodopa levels. While intriguing and consistent with the growing number of studies implicating the right caudate nucleus in TS pathophysiology (Table 14.3), these results must nevertheless be interpreted with caution. Had the p values been correlated for multiple comparisons, the analyses for fluorodopa accumulation would not have retained their statistical significance. In addition, if the findings are correct, it is still unclear whether the regionally specific increase in DOPA decarboxylase enzyme activity is a consequence of a larger number of dopaminergic synapses or enzyme upregulation in those regions. Altered levels of dopamine (from medication blockade, increased presynaptic uptake, or altered release and catabolism) can produce enzyme upregulation. The prior preliminary findings of increased presynaptic transporter in singletons with TS and increased postsynaptic D$_2$ receptor availability in more severely affected monozygotic co-twins could both be consistent with reduced levels of extracellular dopamine leading to upregulation of DOPA decarboxylase. Reduced extracellular dopamine, in turn, can reflect downregulation of dopamine release from either increased GABAergic or reduced glutamatergic input to the striatum (Fig. 14.4). Thus, the explanations consistent with the known circuitry or the basal ganglia are many, complex, and varied.

Implications of imaging studies

Which brain systems are most implicated in pathophysiology?

A careful review of the findings of each of the metabolism and blood flow-related studies (Table 14.3) shows the consistency with which the basal ganglia are implicated in the pathophysiology of TS. Only the HMPAO SPECT study of George and colleagues (1992) failed to show abnormalitites in this region. Nearly all other PET and SPECT studies demonstrated reduced metabolism or blood flow to the basal ganglia in TS subjects relative to controls, most frequently in the ventral striatum and most often in the left hemisphere. Two studies failed to show regional group differences in basal ganglia blood flow or metabolism but did detect other evidence for abnormal asymmetry in basal ganglia blood flow (Klieger et al., 1997) or correlations between measures of activity in basal ganglia circuitry and symptom severity (Eidelberg et al., 1997). Most studies lacked the spatial resolution needed to differentiate individual nuclei within the basal ganglia, and two of the studies that reported hypometabolism in the inferior insular cortex (Chase et al., 1986; Braun et al., 1993) may actually have inadvertently measured instead the activity in the lateral aspect of the putamen, which is in close proximity to the insular cortex.

The radioligand studies also generally implicate the basal ganglia in TS pathophysiology, though perhaps less consistently than do the metabolism and blood flow studies. This is likely because of the specificity of the information that these radioligand studies provide regarding particular neurochemical characteristics of the basal ganglia and because of the complexity of the physiologic regulation of dopamine metabolism and dopamine receptor system. Radioligand studies that have examined synaptic dopamine activity and D_2-like receptor levels in TS have been variously hampered by the inclusion of medicated subjects, small numbers of participants, and age and sex mismatches between groups. Nevertheless, the positive findings thus far indicate abnormalities of dopaminergic innervation to the caudate nucleus. Increased D_2 receptor levels in the caudate nucleus appear to account for some of the nongenetic determinants of variance in symptom severity. DOPA decarboxylase levels and presynaptic dopamine transport levels may be elevated in this region.

These preliminary results may indicate a hyperinnervation of the striatum by dopaminergic neurons. This striatal hyperinnervation could result in increased thalamocortical activity by stimulating the direct and further inhibiting the indirect pathway through CSTC circuits, as follows (Leckman et al., 1997). Evidence from both rodents (Girault et al., 1986) and primates (Filion and Tremblay, 1991; Filion et al., 1991) indicates that stimulation of D_1 and D_2 receptors produces opposing behavioral effects, with D_1 stimulation increasing and D_2 stimulation decreasing behavioral activity. In addition, stimulation of D_1 receptors facilitates the release of GABA whereas stimulation of D_2 receptors inhibits it. Figure 14.4b may help to understand the model supporting these opposite behavioral effects based on the anatomic connectivity within CSTC circuits. In the *direct pathway*, dopaminergic hyperinnervation activates D_1 receptors (located postsynaptically, particularly on GABA postsynaptic neurons). GABA neurons, which project from the internal segment of the globus pallidus/substantia nigra pars reticulata to the thalamus will in turn block inhibitory interneurons, resulting in enhanced the glutamatergic (GLU) tone of thalamic glutamatergic neurons projecting to the cortex. This enhanced thalamocortical GLU tone will result in an excessive motor output. The role of the *indirect pathway* and D_2 receptors in motor dyscontrol with respect to dopaminergic hyperinnervation is unclear. Presumably, the inhibitory effect of GABAergic projection neurons from the external segment of the globus pallidus to the reticular nucleus, internal segment of the globus pallidus/substantia nigra, and subthalamic nucleus would be reinforced. This increased GABAergic tone of the projections to these other three basal ganglia nuclei would have a threefold effect (Fig. 14.4b), all of which would tend to produce a net increase in thalamic cortical excitation and an increased propensity for movement. First, it would suppress activity in the GABAergic projections from the thalamic reticular nucleus to other thalamic nuclei, thereby disinhibiting thalamocortical excitation. Second, it would suppress activity in the GABAergic inhibitory projections from the internal segment of the globus pallidus/substantia nigra to thalamic nuclei, further disinhibiting thalamocortical excitation. Third, it would suppress excitatory activity in glutamatergic projections from subthalamic nuclei to the internal segment of the globus pallidus/substantia nigra, which again would ultimately produce thalamocortical disinhibition. It can be appreciated that, in this scheme, striatal hyperinnervation by dopaminergic neurons would overdetermine, through multiple effects on the direct and indirect pathways, a functional and neurochemical syndrome of *disinhibition* in TS. This could account for much

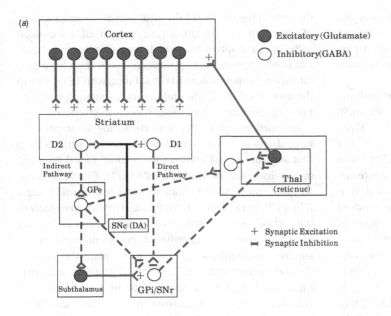

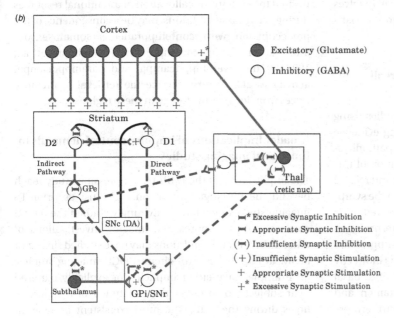

Fig. 14.4. Effects of postulated dopaminergic hyperinnervation of the striatum. Although some studies have reported normal integrity of striatal dopamine metabolism and D_2 receptor site density in patients with Tourette's syndrome (Brooks et al., 1992; Turjanski et al., 1994), others have reported increased transporter level abnormalities in the striatum (Malison et al., 1995) and higher fluorodopa accumulation in portions of the caudate nucleus and midbrain (Ernst et al., 1999). Autopsy data have also suggested higher levels of presynaptic dopamine uptake sites in the caudate nucleus and putamen. These preliminary results suggest a hyperinnervation of the striatum by dopaminergic neurons. (a) Normal cortico–striato–thalamo–cortical circuits. (b) Hypothesized hyperinnervation of the striatum in TS by dopaminergic neurons. Dopaminergic hyperinnervation could produce multiple effects in the direct and indirect pathways through the basal ganglia (see text), all of which may predispose to disinhibition of thalamocortical excitatory projections and the concomitant disinhibition of behavior seen in TS-related conditions. Excitatory (glutamatergic) projections are indicated by solid lines and inhibitory (GABAergic) projections by dotted lines. SNc (DA), dopaminergic projections from the substantia nigra pars compacta; GPi/SNr, internal segment of the globus pallidus or the substantia nigra pars reticulata; GPe, external segment of the globus pallidus; Thal, thalamus; retic nuc, reticular nuclei of the thalamus.

of the phenomenology of TS-related conditions – not just tics, but also recurrent obsessional thoughts, compulsions, and impulsive behaviors – depending upon which portions of the striatal, pallidal, or thalamic nuclei were disinhibited.

The blood flow and metabolism studies, along with the radioligand findings, therefore, quite strongly implicate in TS pathophysiology the basal ganglia portions of CSTC circuitry, in particular the caudate nucleus portions of the ventral striatum. As we have seen, however, the basal ganglia are conduits for information-processing streams that serve multiple and diverse functions. The ventral striatum, and particularly the ventral caudate nucleus, tends to subserve temporolimbic and orbitofrontal portions of CSTC circuitry (Alexander et al., 1990). Of these systems, regions belonging to the temporolimbic system – the anterior cingulate, parahippocampal, and possibly insular cortices in particular – appear to differ most consistently between groups in studies of metabolism and blood flow (Table 14.3). The other CSTC system in which regions differ frequently in TS from normals is the one that involves numerous association cortices, particularly frontal, parietal, and superior temporal regions.

What were the functional imaging studies really imaging?

This overlap in findings between different studies using various imaging modalities provide converging evidence that CSTC circuits are probably involved in TS pathophysiology. The usual and most obvious interpretation of this overlap is that dysfunction in the basal ganglia and related cortical portions of the CSTC circuit gives rise to the symptoms of TS. Our study of the brain regions involved in tic suppression, however, offers an alternative interpretation of the overlap between imaging studies. Tic suppression produces a decrease in signal intensity (which is indirectly related to changes in neuronal activity) in ventral basal ganglia regions, particularly the ventral putamen and globus pallidus. PET and SPECT studies furthermore suggest that "resting" metabolism and blood flow are reduced in subjects with TS relative to normal controls in the "ventral striatum", and this tends to be used by the respective investigators as synonymous with "ventral caudate nucleus". These imaging modalities, however, rarely if ever have provided sufficient spatial resolution to discriminate ventral caudate from the lenticular nucleus, or to discriminate "inferior insular cortex" from "inferior lateral putamen". Furthermore, subjects in most PET and SPECT studies may have either intentionally or unintentionally suppressed their tics during tracer uptake. This is a

time when the novelty of the situation or the engagement of attention in the procedure may itself have been sufficient to suppress tics, which is a well-recognized clinical phenomenon. Tic suppression would then have produced a hypometabolism in the subjects with TS relative to the control subjects, who did not have the burden of suppressing these unwanted behaviors during the scan.

The cortical regions that activate during tic suppression have also been reported to differ in subjects with TS from that seen in normal controls in "resting" blood flow and metabolism studies. These PET and SPECT findings in the cortex are more variable than are those in the basal ganglia (Fig. 14.2). In our fMRI study, we have interpreted many of the cortical regions involved in tic suppression as deriving from the intensive attentional requirements that tic suppression requires. This may also explain the variable cortical findings in the PET and SPECT studies, particularly those involving frontal, superior temporal, and anterior cingulate cortices. The decrease in metabolism and blood flow to hippocampal and parahippocampal cortices, posited to result from reallocation of attentional resources during active task conditions, may be a consequence of the preoccupation with contemporaneous somatosensory information during tic suppression (Shulman et al., 1997b). The lower hippocampal and parahippocampal activity would, in turn, reduce the retrieval of memory traces from long-term storage in these regions.

Broader implications of impulse control demands in functional imaging studies

The implications of the fMRI tic suppression study reach beyond the investigations of only TS. Just as prior TS imaging studies may have unwittingly studied the neural correlates of tic suppression, imaging investigations of other disorders and conditions may have studied similar or identical impulse control circuits. OCD imaging studies, for example, have either implicitly or explicitly required their subjects to suppress the enactment of compulsive urges during the scan. The most consistent findings in OCD imaging studies thus far have been hypermetabolism and increased blood flow to the inferior frontal cortex, right caudate nucleus (Baxter et al., 1987, 1988; Rauch et al., 1994; Breiter et al., 1996), and anterior cingulate cortex (Swedo et al., 1989; Rauch et al., 1994; Breiter et al., 1996): regional changes; these were also induced by tic suppression. If these findings in OCD were, in fact, a result of the suppression of obsessions and compulsions during the scan, then it is of little surprise that these differences normalized after successful antiobsessional therapy (Benkelfat et al., 1990; Baxter et al., 1992; Swedo et al., 1992;

Rubin et al., 1995; Schwartz et al., 1996), when the need to suppress less-severe compulsions would have attenuated.

It seems likely that other functional neuroimaging protocols may also have implicitly studied the suppression of unwanted impulses. The subjective experience of pain, for instance, has of late become an area of great interest and intensive investigation. Painful stimuli typically produce widespread areas of cerebral activation in the perigenual portion of the anterior cingulate cortex, related mesial frontal cortex, midprefrontal and inferior parietal areas, and somatosensory cortex (Talbot et al., 1991; Derbyshire et al., 1997, 1998). Decreases may be seen in the amygdala, hippocampus, or thalamus (Hsieh et al., 1995; Derbyshire et al., 1997). We believe that these diverse areas of activation represent not only the subjective experience of pain but also the suppression during the scan of the powerful impulse to withdraw from the painful stimulus. The possibility that these diverse imaging protocols implicitly studied the suppression of unwanted impulses is bolstered by a PET study that purported to investigate the sensation of itch and the urge to scratch in response to the subcutaneous injection of histamine. We postulate that the study did not only image the urge to scratch, it also imaged the concomitant cerebral activation that is the neural correlate of the suppression of the scratch (Hsieh et al., 1994). This postulate is supported by the similiarities of many of the activations – which include anterior cingulate cortex, supplementary motor and premotor areas, and inferior parietal cortex – with the areas that activate during the suppression of tics, compulsions, and the withdrawal to painful stimuli.

The possibility that diverse functional imaging paradigms may have unwittingly studied the suppression of unwanted impulses underscores a profound and fundamental difficulty with functional imaging studies in general. The CNS is a dynamic entity whose raison d'être is to sense and react. These two domains of experience – sensing both internal and external stimuli and reacting appropriately (or not) to them – are not so easily separated as we would want and suppose them to be for our imaging protocols. The subtraction paradigms that are now so popular in PET and fMRI may not be able to subtract out completely sensation from response to the sensation. And the between-group comparisons of resting brain blood flow and metabolism in disease processes all assume that the disease process in question is an entity isolated from the rest of experience and CNS functioning. Studies of schizophrenia are a prime example. The subjective responses to the presence of positive symptoms, such as hallucinations, delusions, and thought disorganization, must involve a wide range of compensatory mechanisms

that may confound the interpretation of functional imaging data. The patients but not their controls are likely during the scanning procedure to attempt to make sense of the fragmentation of their sensory experience, to test the reality of hallucinations and delusions, and to cope with the intense anxieties during the procedure that normal subjects usually do not have. Imaging studies of subjects with TS may have similar confounds. The patients usually have to suppress their tics during the scan, which normal subjects do not have to do. Even if not suppressing their tics, the TS subjects at least have the experience of them during the scan, whereas normal subjects do not. And of course they will have the premonitory urges associated with their tics. Finally, subjects with TS are likely to have more thoughts during the scan about whether they have complied or not with instructions to hold their head and neck still during the procedure, even if they are allowed to tic.

Chronic adaptive responses are likely to have diverse effects on structural and neurochemical features of the brain that affect the findings from our functional imaging studies. Learning and experience also have long-term plastic effects on brain structure and function (Merzenich et al., 1983; Black et al., 1990; Elbert et al., 1995). It is possible, then, that the radioligand findings in TS may not represent a process central to the pathophysiology of TS in the sense of causing symptoms. They could instead represent a compensatory response to the presence of tics.

We have already suggested several ways to help to determine what is cause and what is compensatory effect in functional imaging data in TS. Imaging protocols must include young children, and perhaps even genetically vulnerable children prior to disease onset. If adults are studied exclusively, the patient groups should be representative of the general population of subjects who have lifetime histories of TS, not just those who continue to be symptomatic. Imaging protocols should increasingly be longitudinal in design; they should include studies of age-related changes in normal children and adults, and they should collect in the same individuals data from other imaging modalities. Studies of trait vulnerabilities in family members will also be valuable in sorting out what is cause (i.e., a trait) and what is compensatory (i.e., a state) effect. Thorough characterization of comorbid neuropsychiatric diagnoses and the accounting for their effects in the imaging data is now mandatory. Finally, it is necessary in study design to assess both the implicit and explicit demands of the scanning protocols. This will require isolating to the degree possible those features of the imaging data that are a result of tic behaviors and those (such as inhibitory control mechanisms in tic suppression) that compensate for them. Distinguishing what in our data is causal to tics and what is an epiphenomenon or compensatory for them will perhaps be our greatest future methodologic and scientific challenge.

References

Alexander, G. and Delong, M. (1985). Microstimulation of the primate neostriatum. II. Somatotopic organization of striatal microexcitable zones and their relation to neuronal response properties. *J. Neurophysiol.*, **53**, 1417–30.

Alexander, G., Crutcher, M. and DeLong, M. (1990). Basal ganglia-thalamocortical circuits: parallel substrates for motor, oculomotor, 'prefrontal', and 'limbic' functions. *Prog. Brain Res.*, **85**, 119–46.

Apter, A., Pauls, D. L., Bleich, A. et al. (1993). An epidemiologic study of Gilles de la Tourette's syndrome in Israel. *Archiv. Gen. Psychiatry*, **50**, 734–8.

Baldwin, M., Frost, L. L. and Wood, C. D. (1954). Investigation of the primate amygdala. Movements of the face and jaws. *Neurology*, **4**, 596–8.

Balthazar, K. (1956). Uber das anatomishe substrat der generalisierten tic-krankeit (maladie des tics, Gilles de la Tourette): Entwicklungshemmung des corpus striatum. *Arch. Psychiatr. Nervenkr.*, **195**, 531–9.

Bates, J. F. and Goldman-Rakic, P. S. (1993). Prefrontal connnections of medial motor areas in the rhesus monkey. *J. Comp. Neurol.*, **336**, 211–28.

Baxter, L., Schwartz, J., Mazziotta, J. et al. (1988). Cerebral glucose metabolic rates in nondepressed patients with obsessive-compulsive disorder. *Am. J. Psychiatry*, **145**, 1560–3.

Baxter, L., Jr, Schwartz, J. M. Bergman, K. S. et al. (1992). Caudate glucose metabolic rate changes with both drug and behavior therapy for obsessive-compulsive disorder. *Arch. Gen. Psychiatry*, **49**, 681–9.

Baxter, L. R. Jr, Phelps, J. M., Mazziotta, J. C., Guze, B. H. and Schwartz, J. M. (1987). Local cerebral glucose metabolic rates in obsessive-compulsive disorder: a comparison with rates in unipolar depression and normal controls. *Arch. Gen. Psychiatry*, **44**, 211–18.

Benkelfat, C., Nordahl, T. E., Semple, W. E., King, A. C., Murphy, D. L. and Cohen, R. M. (1990). Local cerebral glucose metabolic rates in obsessive-compulsive disorder. Patients treated with clomipramine. *Arch. Gen. Psychiatry*, **47**, 840–8.

Black, J. F., Isaacs, K. R., Anderson, B. J., Alcantara, A. A. and Greenough, W. T. (1990). Learning causes synaptogenesis, whereas motor activity causes angiogenesis, in cerebellar cortex of adult rats. *Proc. Natl. Acad. Sci. USA*, **87**, 5568–72.

Braun, A. R., Stoetter, B., Randolph, C. et al. (1993). The functional neuroanatomy of Tourette's syndrome: an FDG-PET study. I. Regional changes in cerebral glucose metabolism differentiating patients and controls. *Neuropsychopharmacology*, **9**, 277–91.

Breiter, H. C., Rauch, S. L., Kwong, K. K. et al. (1996). Functional magnetic resonance imaging of symptom provocation in obsessive-compulsive disorder. *Arch. Gen. Psychiatry*, **53**, 595–606.

Brooks, D. J., Turjanski, N., Sawle, G. V., Playford, E. D. and Lees, A. J. (1992). PET studies on the integrity of the pre and postsynaptic dopaminergic system in Tourette syndrome. *Adv. Neurol.*, **58**, 227–31.

Bruun, R. D. (1988). The natural history of Tourette's syndrome. In *Tourette's Syndrome and Tic Disorders: Clinical Understanding and Treatment*, eds. D. J. Cohen, R. D. Bruun and J. F. Leckman, pp. 21–39. New York: Wiley.

Burd, L., Kerbeshian, J., Wikenheiser, M. and Fisher, W. (1986). A prevalence study of Gilles de la Tourette syndrome in North Dakota school-age children. *J. Am. Acad. Child Psychiatry*, **25**, 552–3.

Castellanos, F. X., Giedd, J. N., Eckburg, P. et al. (1994). Quantitative morphology of the caudate nucleus in attention deficit hyperactivity disorder. *Am. J. Psychiatry*, **151**, 1791–6.

Chappell, P., Riddle, M., Anderson, G. et al. (1994). Enhanced stress responsivity of Tourette syndrome patients undergoing lumbar puncture. *Biol. Psychiatry*, **36**, 35–43.

Chase, T. N., Geoffrey, V., Gillespie, M. and Burrows, G. H. (1986). Structural and functional studies of Gilles de la Tourette syndrome. *Rev. Neurol.*, **142**, 851–5.

Comings, D. E., Himes, J. A. and Comings, B. G. (1990). An epidemiologic study of Tourette's syndrome in a single school district. *J. Clin. Psychiatry*, **51**, 463–9.

Cooper, I. S. (1969). *Involuntary Movement Disorders.* New York: Harper and Row.

Craig, A. D., Reiman, E. M., Evans, A. and Bushnell, M. C. (1996). Functional imaging of an illusion of pain. *Nature*, **384**, 258–60.

de Divitiis, E., D'Errico, A. and Cerillo, A. (1977). Stereotactic surgery in Gilles de la Tourette syndrome. *Acta Neurochirurg.*, **24**, 73.

Derbyshire, S. W. G., Jones, A. K. P., Gyulai, F., Clark, S., Townsend, D. and Firestone, L. L. (1997). Pain processing during three levels of noxious stimulation produces differential patterns of central activity. *Pain*, **73**, 431–45.

Derbyshire, S. W. G., Vogt, G. A. and Jones, A. K. P. (1998). Pain and Stroop interference tasks separate processing modules in anterior cingulate cortex. *Exp. Brain Res.*, **118**, 52–60.

Diamond, A. and Goldman-Rakic, P. S. (1989). Comparison of human infants and rhesus monkeys on Piaget's AB task: evidence for dependence on dorsolateral prefrontal cortex. *Exp. Brain Res.*, **74**, 24–40.

Divac, I., Rosvold, H. and Szwarcbart, M. (1967). Behavioral effects of selective ablation of the caudate nucleus. *J. Comp. Physiol. Psychol.*, **63**, 184–90.

Drewe, E. (1975). Go-no-go learning after frontal lobe lesions in humans. *Cortex*, **11**, 8–16.

Eidelberg, D., Moeller, J. R., Antonini, A. et al. (1997). The metabolic anatomy of Tourette's syndrome. *Neurology*, **48**, 927–34.

Elbert, T., Pantev, C., Wienbruch, C., Rockstroh, B. and Taub, E. (1995). Increased cortical representation of the fingers of the left hand in string players. *Science*, **270**, 305–7.

Erenberg, G., Cruse, R. P. and Rothner, A. D. (1987). The natural history of Tourette syndrome: a follow-up study. *Ann. Neurol.*, **22**, 383–5.

Ernst, M., Zametkin, A. J., Jons, P. H., Matochik, J. A., Pascualvaca, D. and Cohen, R. M. (1999). High presynaptic dopaminergic activity in children with Tourette's disorder. *J. Am. Acad. Child Adolesc. Psychiatry*, **38**, 86–94.

Filion, M. and Tremblay, L. (1991). Abnormal spontaneous activity of the globus pallidus neurons in monkeys with MPTP-induced parkinsonism. *Brain Res.*, **547**, 147–51.

Filion, M., Tremblay, L. and Bedard, P. J. (1991). Effects of dopamine agonists on the spontaneous activity of the globus pallidus neurons in monkeys with MPTP-induced parkinsonism. *Brain Res.*, **547**, 152–61.

Fried, I., Katz, A., McCarthy, G., Sass, K., Spencer, S. and Spencer, D. (1991). Functional organization of human supplementary motor cortex studies by electrical stimulation. *J. Neurosci.*, **11**, 3656–66.

Gadow, K. D., Sverd, J., Sprafkin, J., Nolan, E. E. and Ezor, S. N. (1995). Efficacy of methylphenidate for attention-deficit hyperactivity disorder in children with tic disorder. *Arch. Gen. Psychiatry*, **52**, 444–55.

Garnett, E., Firnau, G., Nahmias, C. and Chirakal, R. (1983). Striatal dopamine metabolism in living monkeys examined in positron emission tomography. *Brain Res.*, **280**, 169–71.

George, M. S., Trimble, M. R., Costa, D. C., Robertson, M. M., Ring, H. A. and Ell, P. J., (1992). Elevated frontal cerebral blood flow in Gilles de la Tourette syndrome: a 99Tcm-HMPAO SPECT study. *Psychiatr. Res.*, **45**, 143–51.

Girault, J. A., Spampinato, U., Glowinski, J. and Besson, M. J. (1986). In vivo release of [³H]-gamma-aminobutyric acid in the rat neostratum. II. Opposing effects of D_1 and D_2 dopamine receptor stimulation in the dorsal caudate putamen. *Neuroscience*, **19**, 1109–17.

Goetz, C. G., Tanner, C. M., Stebbins, G. T., Leipzig, G. and Carr, W. C. (1992). Adult tics in Gilles de la Tourette's syndrome: description and risk factors. *Neurology*, **42**, 784–8.

Golden, G. S. (1974). Gilles de la Tourette's syndrome following methylphenidate administration. *Dev. Med. Child Neurol.*, **16**, 76–8.

Goldman-Rakic, P. (1987). Circuitry of primate prefrontal cortex and regulation of behavior by representational memory. In *Handbook of Physiology, The Nervous System*, eds. V. Mountcastle, F. Plum and S. Geiger, pp. 373–414. Bethesda, MD: American Physiological Society.

Gratton, G. (1997). Attention and probability effects in the human occipital cortex: an optical imaging study. *Neuroreport*, **8**, 1749–53.

Hall, M., Costa, D. C., Shields, J., Heavens, J., Robertson, M. and Ell, P. J. (1990). Brain perfusion patterns with Tc-99m-HMPAO/SPET in patients with Gilles de la Tourette syndrome. *Eur. J. Nucl. Med.*, **16**, WP18.

Hassler, R. and Dieckmann, G. (1970). Stereotaxic treatment of tics and inarticulate cries or coprolalia considered as motor obsessional phenomena in Gilles de la Tourette's disease. *Rev. Neurol.* **123**, 89–100.

Heinze, H. J., Mangun, G. R., Burchert, W. et al. (1994). Combined spatial and temporal imaging of brain activity during visual selective attention in humans. *Nature*, **372**, 543–6.

Hsieh, J. C., Hagermak, O., Stahle-Backdahl, M. et al. (1994). Urge to scratch represented in the human cerebral cortex during itch. *J. Neurophysiol.*, **72**, 3004–8.

Hsieh, J.-C., Belfrage, M., Stone-Elander, S., Hansson, P. and Ingvar, M. (1995). Central representation of chronic ongoing neuropathic pain studied by positron emission tomography. *Pain*, **63**, 225–36.

Iverson, S. and Mishkin, M. (1970). Perseverative interference in monkeys following selective lesions of the inferior prefrontal cortex. *Exp. Brain Res.*, **11**, 376–86.

Jadresic, D. (1992). The role of the amygdaloid complex in Gilles de la Tourette's syndrome. *Br. J. Psychiatry*, **161**, 532–4.

Jankovic, J., Glaze, D. G. and Frost, J., Jr (1984). Effect of tetrabenazine on tics and sleep of Gilles de la Tourette's syndrome. *Neurology*, **34**, 688–92.

Karp, B. I., Porter, S., Toro, C. and Hallett, M. (1996). Simple motor tics may be preceded by a premotor potential. *J. Neurol. Neurosurg. Psychiatry*, **61**, 103–6.

Kelley, A. E., Lang, C. G. and Gauthier, A. M. (1988). Induction of oral stereotypy following amphetamine microinjection into a discrete subregion of the striatum. *Psychopharmacology*, **95**, 556–9.

Kirwan, C. (ed.) (1971). *Aristotle's Metaphysics*. Oxford: Clarendon Press.

Klieger, P. S., Fett, K. A., Dimitsopulos, T. and Kurlan, R. (1997). Asymmetry of basal ganglia perfusion in Tourette's syndrome shown by Technetium-99m-HMPAO SPECT. *J. Nucl. Med.*, **38**, 188–91.

Korzen, A. V., Pushkov, V. V., Kharitonov, R. A. and Shustin, V. A. (1991). Stereotaxic thalamotomy in the combined treatment of Gilles de la Tourette's disease. *Zh. Nevrotpatol. Psykhiatri*, **91**, 100–1.

Kurlan, R., Kersun, J., Ballantine, H., Jr and Caine, E. D. (1990). Neurosurgical treatment of severe obsessive-compulsive disorder associated with Tourette's syndrome. *Movement Disord.*, **5**, 152–5.

Larumbe, R., Vaamonde, J., Artieda, J., Zubieta, J. L. and Obeso, J. A. (1993). Reflex blepharospasm associated with bilateral basal ganglia lesion. *Movement Disord.*, **8**, 198–200.

Lawrence, M. and Redmond, D. (1985). MPTP lesions and dopaminergic drugs alter eye blink rate in African green monkeys. *Pharmacol. Biochem. Behav.*, **38**, 869–74.

Leckman, J. F., Knorr, A. M., Rasmusson, A. M. and Cohen, D. J. (1991). Basal ganglia research and Tourette's syndromes. [Letter] *Trends Neurosci.*, **14**, 94.

Leckman, J. F., Walker, D. E. and Cohen, D. J. (1993). Premonitory urges in Tourette's syndrome. *Am. J. Psychiatry*, **150**, 98–102.

Leckman, J. F., Peterson, B. S., Anderson, G. M., Arnsten, A. F. T., Pauls, D. L. and Cohen, D. J. (1997). Pathogenesis of Tourette's syndrome. *J. Child Psychol. Psychiatry*, **38**, 119–42.

Leckman, J. F., Zhang, H., Vitale, A. et al. (1998). Course of tic severity in Tourette's syndrome: the first two decades. *Pediatrics*, **102**, 14–19.

Lim, S. H., Dinner, D. S., Pillay, P. K. et al., (1994). Functional anatomy of the human supplementary sensorimotor area: results of extraoperative electrical stimulation. *Electroencephalogr. Clin. Neurophysiol.*, 91, 179–93.

Lowe, T. L., Cohen, D. J., Detlor, J., Kremenitzer, M. W. and Shaywitz, B. A. (1982). Stimulant medications precipitate Tourette's syndrome. *J. Am. Med. Assoc.*, 247, 1168–9.

Luria, A. R. (1980). *Higher Cortical Functions in Man*. New York: Basic Books.

Malison, R. T., McDougle, C. J., van Dyck, C. H. et al. (1995). ^{123}IBeta-CIT SPECT imaging demonstrates increased striatal dopamine transporter binding in Tourette's syndrome. *Am. J. Psychiatry*, 152, 1359–61.

McLean, P. and Delgado, J. (1953). Electrical and chemical stimulation of frontotemporal portion of limbic system in the waking animal. *Electroencephalogr. Clin. Neurophysiol.*, 5, 91–100.

Merzenich, M. M., Kaas, J. H., Wall, J. T., Sur, M., Nelson, R. J. and Felleman, D. J. (1983). Progression of change following median nerve section in the cortical representation of the hand in areas 3b and 1 in adult owl and squirrel monkeys. *Neuroscience*, 10, 639–65.

Mishkin, M. and Manning, F. (1978). Nonspatial memory after selective prefrontal lesions in monkeys. *Brain Res.*, 143, 313–23.

Moran, J. and Desimone, R. (1985). Selective attention gates visual processing in the extrastriate cortex. *Science*, 229, 782–4.

Moriarty, J., Campos Costa, D., Schmitz, B., Trimble, M. R., Ell, P. J. and Robertson, M. M. (1995). Brain perfusion abnormalities in Gilles de la Tourette's syndrome. *Br. J. Psychiatry*, 167, 249–54.

Moriarty, J., Eapen, V., Costa, D. C. et al. (1997). HMPAO SPET does not distinguish obsessive-compulsive and tic syndromes in families multiply affected with Gilles de la Tourette's syndrome. *Psychol. Med.*, 27, 737–40.

Nomoto, F. and Machiyama, Y. (1990). An epidemiological study of tics. *Jap. J. Psychiatr. Neurol.*, 44, 649–55.

Obeso, J. A., Rothwell, J. C. and Marsden, C. D. (1981). Simple tics in Gilles de la Tourette's syndrome are not prefaced by a normal premovement EEG potential. *J. Neurol. Neurosurg. Psychiatry*, 44, 735–8.

Pardo, J. V., Pardo, P. J., Janer, K. W. and Raichle, M. E. (1990). The anterior cingulate cortex mediates processing selection in the Stroop attentional conflict paradigm. *Proc. Natl. Acad. Sci. USA*, 87, 256–9.

Parent, A. and Hazrati, L. (1995a). Functional anatomy of the basal ganglia. I. The cortico-basal ganglia-thalamo-cortical loop. *Brain Res. Rev.*, 20, 91–127.

Parent, A. and Hazrati, L.-N. (1995b). Functional anatomy of the basal ganglia: II. The place of subthalamic nucleus and external pallidum in basal ganglia circuitry. *Brain Res. Rev.*, 20, 128–54.

Park, S., Como, P. G., Cui, L. and Kurlan, R. (1993). The early course of the Tourette's syndrome clinical spectrum. *Neurology*, 43, 1712–15.

Pauls, D. L., Towbin, K. E., Leckman, J. F., Zahner, G. E. and Cohen, D. J. (1986). Gilles de la Tourette's syndrome and obsessive-com- pulsive disorder. Evidence supporting a genetic relationship. *Arch. Gen. Psychiatry*, 43, 1180–2.

Pauls, D. L., Raymond, C. L., Stevenson, J. M. and Leckman, J. F. (1991). A family study of Gilles de la Tourette syndrome. *Am. J. Hum. Genet.*, 48, 154–63.

Pauls, D. L., Leckman, J. F. and Cohen, D. J. (1993). Familial relation- ship between Gilles de la Tourette's syndrome, attention deficit disorder, learning disabilities, speech disorders, and stuttering. *J. Am. Acad. Child Adolesc. Psychiatry*, 32, 1044–50.

Petersen, S. E., Fox, P. T., Snyder, A. Z. and Raichle, M. E. (1990). Activation of extrastriate and frontal cortical areas by visual words and word-like stimuli. *Science*, 249, 1041–4.

Peterson, B. S., Leckman, J. F., Scahill, L. et al. (1992). Steroid hor- mones and CNS sexual dimorphisms modulate symptom expression in Tourette's syndrome. *Psychoneuroendocrinology*, 17, 553–63.

Peterson, B., Riddle, M. A., Cohen, D. J. et al. (1993). Reduced basal ganglia volumes in Tourette's syndrome using three-dimen- sional reconstruction techniques from magnetic resonance images. *Neurology*, 43, 941–9.

Peterson, B. S., Gore, J. C., Riddle, M. A., Cohen, D. J. and Leckman, J. F. (1994). Abnormal magnetic resonance imaging T_2 relaxation time asymmetries in Tourette's syndrome. *Psychiatr. Res. Neuroimaging*, 55, 205–21.

Peterson, B. S., Bronen, R. A. and Duncan, C. C. (1996). Three cases of Gilles de la Tourette's syndrome and obsessive-compulsive disorder symptom change associated with paediatric cerebral malignancies. *J. Neurol. Neurosurg. Psychiatry*, 61, 497–505.

Peterson, B. S., Skudlarski, P., Anderson, A. W. et al. (1998). A func- tional magnetic resonance imaging study of tic suppression in Tourette syndrome. *Arch. Gen. Psychiatry*, 55, 326–33.

Peterson, B. S., Skudlarski, P., Zhang, H., Gatenby, J. C., Anderson, A. W. and Gore, J. C. (1999). An fMRI study of Stroop word-color interference: evidence for cingulate subregions subserving multiple distributed attentional systems. [Priority Communi- cation] *Biol. Psychiatry*, 45, 1237–58.

Price, R. A., Kidd, K. K., Cohen, D. J., Pauls, D. L. and Leckman, J. F. (1985). A twin study of Tourette syndrome. *Arch. Gen. Psychiatry*, 42, 815–20.

Rauch, S. L., Jenike, M. A., Alpert, N. M. et al. (1994). Regional cere- bral blood flow measured during symptom provocation in obsessive-compulsive disorder using oxygen 15-labeled carbon dioxide and positron emission tomography. *Arch. Gen. Psychiatry*, 51, 62–70.

Rauch, S. L., Baer, L., Cosgrove, G. R. and Jenike, M. A. (1995). Neurosurgical treatment of Tourette's syndrome: a critical review. *Compr. Psychiatry*, 36, 141–56.

Richardson, E. P. (1982). Neuropathological studies of Tourette syn- drome. In *Gilles de la Tourette Syndrome*, eds. A. J. Friedhoff and T. N. Chase, pp. 83–7. New York: Raven.

Riddle, M. A., Anderson, G. M., McIntosh, S., Harcherik, D. F., Shaywitz, B. A. and Cohen, D. J. (1986). Cerebrospinal fluid monoamine precursor and metabolite levels in children treated for leukemia: age and sex effects and individual variability. *Biol. Psychiatry*, 21, 69–83.

Riddle, M. A., Rasmusson, A. M., Woods, S. W. and Hoffer, P. B. (1992). SPECT imaging of cerebral blood flow in Tourette syndrome. *Adv. Neurol.*, **58**, 207–11.

Robertson, M., Doran, M., Trimble, M. and Lees, A. J. (1990). The treatment of Gilles de la Tourette syndrome by limbic leucotomy. *J. Neurol. Neurosurg. Psychiatry*, **53**, 691–4.

Rosvold, H. and Mishkin, M. (1961). Nonsensory effects of frontal lesions on discrimination learning and performance. In *Brain Mechanisms and Learning*, ed. J. Delafresnaye. Oxford: Blackwell.

Rubin, R. T., Ananth, J., Villanueva-Meyer, J., Trajmar, P. G. and Mena, I. (1995). Regional [133]Xenon cerebral blood flow and cerebral ^{99m}Tc-HMPAO uptake in patients with obsessive-compulsive disorder before and during treatment. *Biol. Psychiatry*, **38**, 429–37.

Sawle, G. V., Lees, A. J., Hymas, N. F., Brooks, D. J. and Frackowiak, R. S. (1993). The metabolic effects of limbic leucotomy in Gilles de la Tourette syndrome. *J. Neurol. Neurosurg. Psychiatry*, **56**, 1016–19.

Schwartz, J. M., Stoessel, P. W., Baxter, L. R., Martin, K. M. and Phelps, M. E. (1996). Systematic changes in cerebral glucose metabolic rate after successful behavior modification treatment of obsessive-compulsive disorder. *Arch. Gen. Psychiatry*, **53**, 109–13.

Seeman, P., Bzowej, N. H., Guan, H. C. et al. (1987). Human brain dopamine receptors in children and aging adults. *Synapse*, **1**, 399–404.

Shaywitz, B. A., Cohen, D. J., Leckman, J. F., Young, J. G. and Bowers, M., Jr (1980). Ontogeny of dopamine and serotonin metabolites in the cerebrospinal fluid of children with neurological disorders. *Dev. Med. Child Neurol.*, **22**, 748–54.

Shulman, G. L., Corbetta, M., Buckner, R. L. et al. (1997a). Top-down modulation of early sensory cortex. *Cereb. Cortex*, **7**, 193–206.

Shulman, G. L., Fiez, J. A., Corbetta, M. et al. (1997b). Common blood flow changes across visual tasks: II. Decreases in cerebral cortex. *J. Cogn. Neurosci.*, **9**, 648–63.

Sieg, K. G., Buckingham, D., Gaffney, G. R., Preston, D. F. and Sieg, K. G. (1992). Tc-99m HMPAO SPECT brain imaging of Gilles de la Tourette's syndrome. *Clin. Nucl. Med.*, **18**, 255.

Singer, H. S., Hahn, I. H. and Moran, T. H. (1991). Abnormal dopamine uptake sites in postmortem striatum from patients with Tourette's syndrome. *Ann. Neurol.*, **30**, 558–62.

Singer, H. S., Wong, D. F., Brown, J. E. et al. (1992). Positron emission tomography evaluation of dopamine D-2 receptors in adults with Tourette syndrome. *Adv. Neurol.*, **58**, 233–9.

Singer H. S., Reiss, A. L., Brown, J. E. et al. (1993). Volumetric MRI changes in basal ganglia of children with Tourette's syndrome. *Neurology*, **43**, 950–6.

Smith, S. J. M. and Lees, A. J. (1989). Abnormalities of the blink reflex in Gilles de la Tourette syndrome. *J. Neurol. Neurosurg. Psychiatry*, **52**, 895–8.

Spitzer, H., Desimone, R. and Moran, J. (1988). Increased attention enhances both behavioral and neuronal performance. *Science*, **240**, 338–40.

Stoetter, B., Braun, A. R., Randolph, C. et al. (1992). Functional neuroanatomy of Tourette syndrome. Limbic-motor interactions studied with FDG PET. *Adv. Neurol.*, **58**, 213–26.

Swedo, S. E., Schapiro, M. B., Grady, C. L. et al. (1989). Cerebral glucose metabolism in childhood-onset obsessive-compulsive disorder. *Arch. Gen. Psychiatry*, **46**, 518–23.

Swedo, S. E., Pietrini, P., Leonard, H. L. et al. (1992). Cerebral glucose metabolism in childhood-onset obsessive-compulsive disorder. Revisualization during pharmacotherapy. *Arch. Gen. Psychiatry*, **49**, 690–4.

Sweet, R. D., Bruun, R., Shapiro, E. and Shapiro, A. K. (1976). Presynaptic catecholamine antagonists as treatment for Tourette syndrome: effects of alpha-methyl-para-tyrosine and tetrabenazine. *Arch. Gen. Psychiatry*, **31**, 857–61.

Talairach, J., Bancaud, J., Geier, S. et al. (1973). The cingulate gyrus and human behavior. *Electroenceph. Clin. Neurophys.*, **34**, 45–52.

Talbot, J. D., Marrett, S., Evans, A. C., Meyer, E., Bushnell, M. C. and Duncan, G. H. (1991). Multiple representations of pain in human cerebral cortex. *Science*, **251**, 1355–8.

Tasker, R. R. and Dostrovsky, J. O. (1993). What goes on in the motor thalamus? *Stereotact. Funct. Neurosurg.*, **60**, 121–6.

Turjanski, N., Sawle, G. V., Playford, E. D. et al. (1994). PET studies of the presynaptic and postsynaptic dopaminergic system in Tourette's syndrome. *J. Neurol. Neurosurg. Psychiatry*, **57**, 688–92.

Vogt, B. A., Finch, D. M. and Olson, C. R. (1992). Functional heterogeneity in cingulate cortex: the anterior executive and posterior evaluative regions. *Cereb. Cortex*, **2**, 435–43.

Wolf, S. S., Jones, D. W., Knable, M. B. et al. (1996). Tourette syndrome: prediction of phenotypic variation in monozygotic twins by caudate nucleus D_2 receptor binding. *Science*, **273**, 1225–7.

Wong, D. F., Singer, H. S., Brandt, J. et al. (1997). D_2-like dopamine receptor density in Tourette syndrome measured by PET. *J. Nucl. Med.*, **38**, 1243–7.

15

Dyslexia: conceptual issues and psychiatric comorbidity

Frank B. Wood and D. Lynn Flowers

Introduction

Until the advent of technology for direct imaging of localized anatomically specific brain function became available in the 1970s, the clinico-pathologic correlation method of Charcot and his contemporaries, whereby CNS lesions on autopsy were correlated with behavioral deficits in life, formed the gold standard of clinical neurology. To this day, if a neurologist claims that a patient's behavioral deficit arises from a focal lesion, and if there is dispute over that claim, only an autopsy can settle the issue with satisfactory certainty. Structural imaging by computed tomography (CT) and especially by magnetic resonance imaging (MRI), of course, has become a widely acceptable substitute for the autopsy. It is nonetheless also widely accepted (and vigorously asserted whenever a lesion that is proposed to explain a patient's deficit is not visualized on MRI) that some "true" lesions can be invisible by MRI and hence will only "show up" on autopsy. Against this, technological advances mean that demonstration of a structural lesion by imaging or at autopsy may no longer be essential, as it is possible to show dysfunction of a brain region(s). A lesion might certainly still be implied, but the range of possible lesions could be much broader, to include subtler derangements of functional anatomy on levels of scale as small as the synapse itself, where the abnormality would only express itself when large aggregates of these synapses, or their associated neurons, functioned deviantly (thus making themselves visible to functional imaging). Similarly, abnormalities of neurotransmitter function would fall within this enlarged class of "lesion" since they do represent ultrastructural variations at the cellular and synaptic level. These and similar abnormalities might never be visible on autopsy, not simply because of the microscopic scale but because the abnormality itself might only be observable in living tissue.

Psychiatric disorders – a substantial subset of which have defied consensual clinicopathologic correlational analysis on autopsy – would be expected to yield their functional neuroanatomic secrets to investigation by the new technology. The basic changes in the brain might now be objectively demonstrated. To do this, clinico pathologic correlates between disordered behavior and altered functional imaging landscapes would need to be drawn, a process involving a number of difficulties: individual differences in cellular or synaptic physiology are incompletely understood, the relationships of such physiological events to overt behavior are not fully known, and the necessary mathematical descriptions are complex at best.

Models of cognitive deficits

The range of neurobehavioral disorders that have been investigated by this technology has reflected two rather different theoretical perspectives, seldom reconciled. The difference between these two perspectives can be highlighted by asking: what could happen to the brain that would create the appearance of selective cognitive deficit, as in selective reading disability? There are two distinctly different possibilities described by a modular cognitive model and an anatomic model.

The modular cognitive model

The modular cognitive model postulates that a circumscribed, relatively specific cognitive process is disrupted in relative isolation from other processes. To use Pennington's (1997) analogy, a Swiss Army knife breaks one of its blades. While there are plausible neurobehavioral examples (e.g., weakness in the left leg arising from a high cortical motor strip lesion), this notion is ordinarily considered crude and oversimplified when applied to more complex cognitive and behavioral processes. The modestly more elaborate version of this concept, however, is more acceptable; it stresses the disruption of some particular process or system that is involved in several behaviors of a general cognitive class, all of which are to some extent affected. It seems fair to say that the present state in dyslexia research tends to adopt this view. It expects that one or a few relatively circumscribed cognitive impairments selectively impede the learning and execution of a range of reading and reading-related skills and that the "disorder" in dyslexia is limited to those impairments. Whether phonological, visual, or other processes are presumed to underlie dyslexia, the theories put forward all share this common modular cognitive assumption – that dyslexia reflects the selective disruption of a cognitively identifiable, appropriately delimited system. (Note that this does not necessarily imply explicit subtyping, only different mechanisms any one or several of which would affect a given dyslexic individual.) The major current multiple mechanism theory, Wolf's (Wolf and Obregon, 1992) two-factor model, does stress separate phonological and rapid naming (fluency) components, which may operate jointly or separately in particular individuals. Such multiple mechanism models do allow for more heterogeneity of deficits among dyslexics, but in the larger scheme of things they still imply, at most, a relatively few circumscribed underlying deficits that are cognitively defined.

Genetic investigations of dyslexia have followed a similar pattern toward differentiation of underlying mechanism. Initially, the linkages to a putative gene that conferred risk for reading disability were pursued with relatively global reading phenotypes that used a combination of tests to define generalized impairment in reading. This approach was fruitful in establishing linkages involving general reading ability on chromosome 15 (Smith et al., 1983) and chromosome 6 (Cardon et al., 1994). Heterogeneity, however, was strongest in our report (Grigorenko et al., 1997) in which the linkage on chromosome 6 was most strong if the phenotype was phonemic awareness (defined by tests such as isolating a single phoneme within a word), less strong but still significant if the phenotype was phonologic decoding (defined as nonword reading), and only barely significant if the phenotype was defined as single word reading. Conversely, the linkage on chromosome 15 involved a phenotype that could only be defined by single word reading skill, not involving phonemic awareness or phonologic decoding at all. Subsequently, we have demonstrated yet another strong linkage on chromosome 1 involving a putative gene best characterized by a phenotype of phonologic decod-ing, operationally defined as nonword reading (E. L. Grigorenko et al., unpublished data). Such findings naturally suggest heterogeneity of underlying mechanisms, but the data also suggest overlaps or interactions among these mechanisms.

In general, whether the underlying mechanisms are one or many, and regardless of whether they are molecular (genetic) or molar (anatomic), the modular cognitive model views them as behaviorally specific. The predictions from this model are, therefore, inherently specific: cognitive competencies will have a one-to-one mapping to biological mechanisms.

The anatomic model

The anatomic model postulates that a definable anatomic territory in the brain suffers damage, disease, or other compromise of its structure or function, either mild or severe, and all behavioral processes depending on tissue in that territory are to some extent affected. A simple example of this concept is a stroke. Vascular territories do not follow functional maps, so a stroke – especially a large one – impairs a diverse collection of processes that are unified only by their separate dependence on the affected tissue. In milder lesions, it is often the case that one of the symptoms is more obvious, and that is what brings the patient to clinical attention. A mild left frontal stroke, for example, may induce halting, dysfluent speech as the main symptom, but an observant clinician would readily detect the mild but definite right upper extremity weakness as well and might also detect the depression that often arises in the aftermath of such lesions (Robinson and Price, 1982). The underlying mechanism of dysfluent speech might be sought and carefully characterized as to behavioral subtypes and critical loci of lesion, and this would be instructive for cognitive neuroscience. Nonetheless, no explanation of the mechanism of the speech disorder, however sophisticated, could explain the hemiparesis or even the depression, which is independent of the severity or even the presence of associated motor, language, or cognitive deficit. At another level of analysis, the underlying mechanism is the stroke itself, and science also does well to search for such mechanisms. If applied to the case of dyslexia, this model would stress that the lesion causing dyslexia is likely also to be causing other comorbid deficits.

As in the cognitive modular model above, there are also more complex and subtle versions of the anatomic model. One familiar version of this model in dyslexia research is the Galaburda et al. (1985) tradition stressing the diffuse changes in neuronal connectivity that can arise from circumscribed cortical ectopias of prenatal origin in humans: inherent in this view has always been the proviso that the resultant cognitive deficits would be diverse, unpredictable, and likely to extend well beyond any particular cognitive process. Another version of a subtle anatomic model would be a lesion in a specific neurotransmitter projection system that has diffuse consequences throughout the brain for a wide range of its functional capabilities. The degree to which an anatomic disruption is local, regional, or diffuse is seldom predictable a priori: location of lesion, therefore, becomes the fundamental empirical question that is a prerequisite to understanding the disease mechanism itself, as well as its behavioral consequences. Here, too, the symptom that comes to clinical attention may not be the only one that is present or important to the patient's life. Indeed, such additional unnoticed symptoms may be of particular importance precisely because they have impact on the patient's life without the patient's awareness. If there are comorbid deficits, perhaps in the psychiatric domain, that accompany dyslexia, then the anatomic model assumes that it may not necessarily be possible to understand comorbidity to be arising from a common underlying "processing" disorder. Instead, it may well be the case – as in the above example of poststroke depression – that the reading deficit and the psychiatric comorbidity are independent expressions of the same general anatomic locus of dysfunction.

In contrast to the modular cognitive model then, the anatomic model predicts that the mappings from biology to behavior are always one to many, i.e., a given biological "lesion" always results in several different types and levels of behavioral profiles.

Psychiatric comorbidity

Central to a consideration of reading disability is the prospect of a different perspective on the issue of comorbidity. Comorbidity is often considered in psychiatric nosology as a problem that threatens the accuracy and specificity of diagnosis. However, the anatomic model reviewed above suggests at least that the goal of specificity needs to be balanced with a goal of comprehensiveness. From our own work, we can formulate the following general suggestions for achieving that balance both in clinical and research situations. We will use two specific subtypes of dyslexia to illustrate that differential brain dysfunctions in specific subtypes of dyslexia have differential primary psychiatric consequences as well.

The subtypes or phenotypes in this illustration are (i) a primary phonemic awareness deficit involving the inabil-

ity to segment spoken words orally into their constituent parts and (ii) a decoding deficit involving the inability to pronounce written nonwords, despite intact phonemic awareness. (Grigorenko et al. (1997) gives a full description of the tests operationalizing these two phenotypes.) For the purposes of this analysis, the overlap between these two subtypes must be resolved since a phonemic awareness deficit is itself one cause of decoding deficit. Here anyone with a phonemic awareness deficit is classified as affected with the first phenotype, regardless of whether they have a decoding deficit. The second phenotype is reserved for those with a decoding deficit without a phonemic awareness deficit. Figures 15.1 and 15.2 show our present knowledge of the loci of anatomic hypometabolism in the two phenotypes.

The anatomic hypometabolism profiles could not differ more: the phoneme awareness deficit phenotype is associated with left posterior hypometabolism while the phonologic decoding deficit phenotype is associated with right frontal hypometabolism. The heterogeneity is unambiguous, without overlap.

We next must ask whether other differential, anatomically plausible behavioral deficits are also found. We find that the phonemic awareness deficit phenotype is often accompanied by symptoms of attention-deficit hyperactivity disorder (ADHD), especially symptoms of the inattentive subtype, whereas the phonological decoding deficit phenotype is accompanied only by some self-reported social withdrawal and shyness. We also find the patients with phonemic awareness tend to have a variety of other perceptual inefficiencies, including visual ones, whereas those with decoding problems may be somewhat more motorically clumsy. Further testing is obviously required to confirm the reliability and validity of these behavioral–anatomic associations, including their generalizability to other activating tasks or conditions of rest. (Note that if both types of dyslexic subject are combined into a single group, and this group is compared with normal control subjects, then the picture is simply a composite of the two regional syndromes and the simple contrast is statistically weakened because of the heterogeneity within dyslexia.)

The illustration permits the following broader suggestions:

1 When children have deficits involving the perception or isolation of phonemes (the children who cannot, for example, say what remains of a word after removing the initial consonant sound), it is as though they lack the elementary building blocks of reading. They are also likely to be unaware of other types of detail in the environment and may simulate or actually have a comorbid deficit of ADHD, inattentive subtype. More broadly still, the inat-

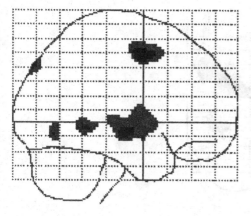

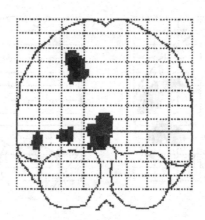

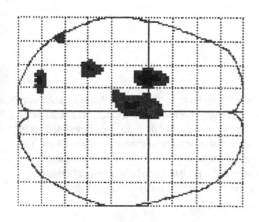

Fig. 15.1. Statistical parametric maps for the phonemic awareness subgroup showing regions of reduced glucose utilization during letter identification, as measured with PET, in adults with a history of dyslexia and current deficits in phonemic awareness ($n = 16$) relative to unaffected controls ($n = 30$). The regions shown reflect foci of at least 27 spatially contiguous voxels having a $p < 0.001$ pixelwise group difference in metabolic rate following normalization for whole brain metabolism.

tentive subtype should be considered as a major risk whenever a learning disability involves inadequate perception.

2 When children have a particular and relatively isolated deficit in decoding without a phonemic awareness deficit (the children who can decode the individual sounds but have difficulty blending them), it is as though they have a gestalt formation problem. They may be particularly prone to show this same problem in social relationships, seeming shy or clumsy. More generally, when children cannot integrate the components of written language, they may be at risk for a broad variety of coping deficits. These are sometimes termed executive function deficits, but that term may be too broad. In the present case at least, it looks more particularly like a gestalt formation problem or at least an organizational weakness. Still, such a deficit alone can carry a major adaptive burden of inadequate coping, the symptoms of which would extend far beyond reading.

In the light of this example, we will now review current results and the prospects for future progress. This essay argues caution: although there has been important progress already, and some results could even be considered definitive, nevertheless there are still serious hazards to progress.

Progress and problems

The evidence for a genetic, and presumed neuroanatomic, basis for dyslexia is strong. There is abundant evidence to support a familial form of dyslexia (e.g., Hallgren, 1950; DeFries and Decker, 1982; DeFries et al., 1987; Wolff and Melngailis, 1994), and there is ongoing investigation into the differential transmission of underlying reading acquisition skills (e.g., Olson et al., 1989; DeFries et al., 1991; Hohnen and Stevenson, 1995). Genetic linkage has further been demonstrated for global dyslexia phenotypes using markers on chromosome 15 (Smith et al., 1983; Fulker et al., 1991) and chromosome 6 (Cardon et al., 1994). Recent work shows that the linkages may involve more specific reading-related cognitive

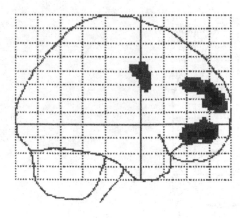

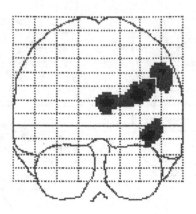

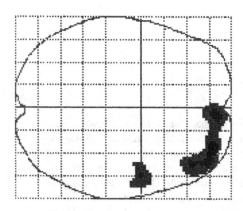

Fig. 15.2. Statistical parametric map for the phonological decoding subgroup showing regions of reduced glucose utilization during letter identification, as measured with PET, in adults with a history of dyslexia and current deficits in phonological decoding (but normal phonemic awareness) ($n = 8$) relative to unaffected controls ($n = 30$). The regions shown reflect foci of at least 27 spatially contiguous voxels having a $p < 0.001$ pixelwise group difference in metabolic rate following normalization for whole brain metabolism.

phenotypes: phonemic awareness describes the chromosome 6 linkage especially well, single word reading the chromosome 15 linkage (Grigorenko et al., 1997), and phonologic decoding the chromosome 1 linkage (E. L. Grigorenko et al., unpublished data).

The apparent genetic heterogeneity of dyslexia raises the strong possibility that there are heterogeneous neurofunctional bases for dyslexia as well. By the term "neurofunctional" we mean "pertaining to mechanisms whereby specific brain processes yield specific behavioral results". Given heterogeneity, then serious methodologic problems follow as a direct consequence. There are three distinct possibilities, which can be described as three paradigms.

1 The strong heterogeneity paradigm. This simplest case assumes that different genetic subtypes inflict different lesions, however subtle, each having different neurofunctional consequences and each capable in its own right of inducing reading impairment. Any two-group normal versus dyslexic subject imaging study could fail, therefore, because the dyslexic group is not appropriately subtyped and the underlying mechanisms are obscured in the group comparison. This paradigm

assumes that reading can be poor for any of several distinct reasons, any one of which is a sufficient condition. Further investigation of this paradigm requires genetically relevant subgrouping, and it predicts the neurofunctional correlates to be distinctive to that subgrouping.

2 The converging pathway paradigm. This next case assumes that there are different genetic mechanisms, but that they are nevertheless expressed in the same final common pathway toward the same neuroanatomic lesion. In this case, a common localized functional deficit is found across different genetic subtypes. All subtypes impair the same process, which by definition and inexorable logic must then be a process required for adequate reading. This paradigm claims to have disclosed a common neuroanatomic mechanism or pathway from brain to reading disorder, but its further pursuit requires genetic subtyping for elucidation of the multiple pathways from genes to a common neuroanatomic mechanism. In this model, therefore, different genes could impair the same anatomic locus in the brain, with identical behavioral results.

3 The tautology paradigm. This last case assumes underlying genetic and neuroanatomic heterogeneity, just as in the strong heterogeneity paradigm. In spite of that granted assumption, however, a common neurofunctional deficit may nonetheless be shown, regardless of genetic subtype. The deficit is by definition unrelated to the underlying genetic or neuroanatomic mechanism and, therefore, must be related only to the defining attribute (reading disability) of the dyslexic versus normal comparison. If a localized functional deficit is shown during reading task activation, then the case is a pure tautology: "people who read poorly activate their brain reading mechanisms during tasks in an abnormal fashion, compared with those who read well". (How could it be otherwise, if the brain is the pathway to behavior?) To be sure, if several regions (i.e., a network) activate during normal reading and dyslexic subjects activate some portions of this network normally and others not at all, then, at least the search for important sites is narrowed. For example, Rumsey et al. (1997b) report that dyslexic subjects activate many portions of the neural networks that subserve reading as much as do normal subjects (e.g., some visual cortex and left inferior frontal cortex) and activate other regions (e.g., insula) even more than normal subjects. The abnormally activated areas are, in such a case, more interesting than the normally activated areas, although it remains unclear whether the abnormality is cause or consequence.

Problems with the paradigms

As it stands, the tautology paradigm cannot disclose the mechanism of dyslexia. As an example, let us assume that a phonological analysis task such as rhyming judgment, when competently performed, activates the left posterior superior perisylvian region. By definition, this means that in normal subjects the phonologic task causes more activation than a control task such as musical similarity judgments or than a resting baseline condition. Let us assume also that dyslexic subjects are known to be deficient on this task, consistent with the general notion that most dyslexic subjects have some kind of phonologic processing problems. If dyslexic subjects show less than normal activity of Wernicke's area during rhyming task performance, then their brain activation profile resembles that of controls who are performing either a nonphonologic task or are in a resting baseline condition. That might be simply because the dyslexic subjects were voluntarily not doing the phonologic task at all (refutable only if the experimenter monitors task performance) or were doing it carelessly with little

motivation or "set" for the task (refutable only if motivation, strategy, and accuracy of performance were not only monitored but demonstrably fully equal between normals and dyslexics). For all we know in such a case, the observed brain activation deficit in dyslexia could have been environmentally induced by years of poor reading experience. In any case, the brain activation finding in itself means no more than the fact that the dyslexic subjects did not select Wernicke's area for activation. It specifically does not prove that they could not do so, still less that they were somehow prevented from doing so by a lesion in Wernicke's area.

When the tautology paradigm is pursued further, the issue of task specificity looms. If no neurofunctional deficit is shown except on specific reading activation tasks, then the tautology is severe: it means simply that poor readers do not activate to reading tasks. If a neurofunctional deficit is also shown on other tasks or states (e.g., music activation), and if this deficit is nonetheless still independent of genetic subtypes, then some interesting content can be added to the tautology, which then becomes: "poor readers, whatever their etiology, are also deficient in other areas, so they not only fail to activate certain brain mechanisms during reading but also during other tasks (e.g. music activation)". The more such tasks are shown to differentiate the groups, the less confidence there is in the specificity of the group classification. In turn, adding to the list of deficits leads to an unenlightening statement to the effect that reading disabled individuals are simply less able in many ways. While this expands the content of the tautology, it certainly does not escape it. Historians of psychology will recognize the formal similarity of the tautology paradigm to the faculty psychology paradigm of the eighteenth century ("a person is logical or musical according to the relative strength of his or her logical or musical faculties") or the phrenology paradigm of the nineteenth century ("a person is logical or musical according to the relative size of his or her logical or musical brain area").

Both the converging pathway and tautology paradigms present an additional severe difficulty: although they are conceptually distinct, the two paradigms are indistinguishable without additional supporting evidence. In the example just discussed, the finding of a specific neurofunctional difference between normal and dyslexic subjects, on a reading-related task, was in itself no more than a tautology whereby poor readers activate their brains differently when engaged in a reading-related task. The neuroanatomic reason, if any, for that difference in activation remains completely obscure, and other approaches are required to elucidate it. There is no escape (i.e., no evidence with which to invoke a converging pathway paradigm and reject the tautology paradigm) unless evidence about specific pathways from different genes to a common neuroanatomic deficit can be adduced. One example of such evidence might be the demonstration that genetically defined subgroups of poor readers not only share common neurofunctional deficits but also have separate additional traits specific to their genetic subtype. Consequently, in the literature review that follows, not only are the above explanatory paradigms generally at issue, but they are particularly so where an otherwise interesting finding may be no more than a neurobehavioral tautology.

Studies of normal language and reading

Logically, interest first focuses on studies involving normal language processing. These show numerous examples of nonreading disabled subjects with left temporal activation during the execution of language tasks: word meaning tasks (Vanderberghe et al., 1996), phoneme monitoring (Sergent et al., 1992; Demonet et al., 1994a), rhyme judgments (Shaywitz, et al., 1995), word repetition (Herholz et al., 1994; Karbe et al., 1995), and reading aloud (Small et al., 1996). Left inferior parietal regions are also implicated in normal phonetic processing (Petersen et al., 1989; Demonet et al., 1994a; Zatorre et al., 1996), word retrieval (Warburton et al., 1996), viewing words (Menard et al., 1996), and oral reading (Bookheimer et al., 1995). A century of neurobehavioral theory and evidence leads to this expectation, and the expectation is confirmed. Even in normal subjects, however, the broader relationships of tasks to regions are far from simple. On the one hand, some of the same regions show deactivation to relevant verbal tasks (e.g., oral pronunciation or lexical decision, Rumsey et al., 1997a). On the other hand, a wide variety of other regions is also activated by language stimuli. Numerous left hemisphere regions, other than temporal, respond to language processing: viewing words (Menard et al., 1996), reading pseudowords (Frith et al., 1995), speech from memory (Tamas et al., 1993), rhyme judgment (Paulesu et al., 1993; Shaywitz et al., 1995; Zatorre et al., 1996), and phoneme monitoring (Demonet et al., 1992, 1994b) all activate Broca's and related frontal areas, which is not surprising. Somewhat more surprising is a consistent but less commonly advertised finding: left or bilateral lingual and neighboring extrastriate cortex is also activated by a variety of language-related tasks: by reading, pronouncing, naming, or making phonologic or orthographic judgments about words, nonwords, idiosyncratically spelled words, or objects (Price, 1977; Bookheimer et al., 1995; Frith et al., 1995; Kiyosawa et al. 1996; Rumsey et al., 1997a). It is espe-

cially interesting that the nonvisual task of monitoring of speech and nonspeech sounds for the occurrence of target phonemes (Demonet et al., 1994b) also activates the lingual gyri. Other nonlexical visual–verbal tasks such as face identification and categorizing visual objects (Sergent et al., 1992) also activate this region.

Language tasks also activate right hemisphere regions, confirming that the left hemisphere is not alone in the processing of language-related stimuli. There is right hemisphere or bilateral participation in tasks requiring word repetition (Herholz et al., 1994; Karbe et al., 1995), phoneme monitoring (Demonet et al., 1994a), exemplar generation (Shaywitz et al., 1995), speech from memory (Tamas et al., 1993), listening to distorted spoken words (Howard et al., 1992), and executive functions involving naming or reading, such as the Stroop test (Bench et al., 1993). Speaking or reading aloud also activates sensorimotor cortices and supplementary motor areas of both hemispheres (e.g., Herholz et al., 1994; Price et al., 1994; Warburton et al., 1996). Furthermore, tasks requiring nonlexical processing also activate some of the same left hemisphere regions as are activated by language tasks in normal subjects: attending to shape is found to activate the left inferior parietal lobule (Corbetta et al., 1991) and processing pictures for meaning activates the left posterior inferior temporal sulcus (Vanderberghe et al., 1996). Silent naming of pictures also activates basal temporal cortex and the parietal operculum (Bookheimer et al., 1995).

Generally then, different types of language tasks may activate the same left hemisphere regions – whether classic language areas or not – and a language task may activate bilateral or isolated right hemisphere regions as well. Nonlanguage tasks may also activate left hemisphere regions, overlapping with those seen in language activation tasks. To be sure, some of the variance is certainly accounted for by stimulus parameters (Ingvar et al., 1993), some by registration technique (Watson et al., 1993; Grabowski et al., 1995), and some by the nearly universal use of subtraction techniques (Poeppel, 1996; but see Demonet et al., 1993).

Additionally, as has been suggested (Poeppel, 1996), some of the variance in findings could be explained by the fact that it may be impossible to avoid engaging the whole of the language apparatus when presenting subjects with lexical materials. See Petersen and Fiez (1993) for a comprehensive review of their important series on processes involved in single word reading in normal subjects, illustrating many of these and other complexities and Demonet et al. (1993) for a review of broader language processing studies in normal subjects using positron emission tomography (PET).

Dyslexia studies

To date, the published functional neuroimaging studies of dyslexia have studied adult subjects virtually exclusively. Functional imaging work on dyslexia begins conceptually with an early PET study (Lubs et al., 1988) that followed logically from the genetic studies of the early 1980s implicating a linkage on chromosome 15 involving familial dyslexia (Smith et al., 1983). Lubs et al. (1988) compared the brain glucose profiles of six familial dyslexic subjects as they read aloud with the profiles of unaffected subjects who either read aloud or viewed pictures. The dyslexic subjects had lower left perisylvian and higher occipital glucose metabolism when compared with the oral reading control group, dyslexic subjects having a profile more similar to that of control subjects who viewed pictures, suggesting that familial dyslexic subjects process less of the lexical or phonetic characteristics and more of the visual or pictorial characteristics of words. The same group (Gross-Glenn et al., 1991), also using PET assessment of glucose, found greater right than left prefrontal activity in both familial dyslexic subjects and controls, less prefrontal asymmetry in the dyslexic group, and greater bilateral activity in the lingual gyri of the occipital lobe in the dyslexic subjects, especially pronounced on the left. This was interpreted as inefficient, hence metabolically more demanding, visual word form processing within the primary visual to temporal lobe pathway and suggested a visual system impairment in dyslexia. Visual pathway abnormalities in dyslexia have also been reported by Eden et al. (1996). The regions of excess or deficient activity in the left hemisphere in dyslexia in all these studies have extended beyond the left perisylvian region to include more posterior regions of cortex usually implicated in visual rather than auditory processing. (See Kinsbourne et al. (1991) for the analogous behavioral finding of considerable breadth of dyslexic deficit, not at all limited to phonologic or even to verbal processes.) Nonetheless, perisylvian and related regions have certainly also been implicated. In another relatively early study from our own group (Flowers et al., 1991), subjects performed an auditory-orthographic task during the measurement of blood flow using xenon inhalation, and the dyslexic subjects showed abnormal task-related activity in the left hemisphere. In that study, however, lower than normal left posterior superior temporal activation was accompanied by greater than normal activation in the left angular gyrus regions. Interestingly, there were also right hemisphere group distinctions in anterior and posterior perisylvian regions that were unrelated to task performance measures, with the posterior one being related to a measure of anxiety in the dyslexia sample. In a subsequent PET study using a phoneme discrimination task, we found another abnormality of excess: in the bilateral medial posterior temporal lobes of dyslexic subjects (Hagman et al., 1992). Measures of regional cerebral blood flow (rCBF) using xenon in the same phoneme discrimination task in a larger number of subjects showed that, while there were no group mean differences in task performance or blood flow values, left superior temporal lobe activation was positively correlated with task accuracy in dyslexic subjects but negatively correlated with task accuracy in controls: as though dyslexic subjects actually depended more on the left temporal language cortex than normal readers (Wood et al., 1991). (See Wood (1990) for a review of this and related interpretive issues including abnormalities of excess.)

Ingvar et al. (1995) also reported lower than normal activation in the middle temporal gyrus of dyslexic subjects during a different task, that of reading either aloud or silently. Paulesu et al. (1996) reported that compensated dyslexic subjects did not show normal activation of the left insular area during either a rhyming task or a visual letter memory task; they also showed abnormal hypoactivation of the right hemisphere during a phonologic memory task. However, they did find Broca's area activation during a rhyming task and temporoparietal activation during a letter memory task in dyslexic subjects. While nonreading disabled control subjects activated the anterior and posterior perisylvian areas simultaneously, the compensated dyslexic group did not. That fact and the lack of insular activity suggested to them that dyslexia is a "disconnection syndrome", or at least a disorder in which activation is fragmented and not as unified as in normals. More recently, Shaywitz (1998) has reported a somewhat similar dissociation in dyslexia of anterior and posterior excess and deficit, respectively, involving phonologic activation using fMRI subtraction.

In all the above studies, however, there is little hard evidence with which to refute a tautology paradigm or compel adoption of a converging pathway paradigm; the absence of explicit heterogeneity of brain activation profiles within dyslexia eliminates the strong heterogeneity paradigm. Although abnormalities of excess represent a degree of additional complexity in the interpretation of the underlying deficits, they still are vulnerable to the circular interpretation that dyslexic individuals fail to activate left hemisphere regions because they are dyslexic (or dysphonologic, hypoverbal, etc.).

Rumsey and colleagues have made the major sustained, contribution to date in a series of studies in the investigation of dyslexia brain profiles. Their series of PET rCBF studies has demonstrated a specific temporoparietal deficit in severely reading-disabled men in spite of partial compensation. In comparing nonaffected controls with dyslexic men on a rhyme detection task, they found the dyslexic men to have lower activation in the left superior posterior perisylvian region and supramarginal/angular gyrus regions as well as in a posterior frontal region (near Broca's area); however, the two groups did not differ in those regions during rest or tone detection conditions (Rumsey et al., 1992). The finding partly replicates Flowers et al. (1991) in showing posterior superior temporal hypometabolism in dyslexia. In its general implication of abnormal activation of left hemisphere language regions, this finding standing alone is tautologic as discussed above. However, several other features of the work preserve the larger Rumsey series from at least the narrowest forms of tautology.

In the first place, in this work, normal versus dyslexic differences also extend to right hemisphere regions and to rest conditions. Normal left hemisphere, but lower right temporal and posterior frontal activation in dyslexic subjects during a tonal memory task (Rumsey et al., 1994a) suggest that inefficiency of nonverbal functions may also be involved in developmental dyslexia (Rumsey et al., 1994b), possibly related to rapid serial processing. Resting state conditions showed group differences as well, as when Rumsey et al. (1992) reported that during an eyes closed rest condition the dyslexic subjects had lower blood flow in the right perisylvian area and concomitant higher blood flow in the medial frontal region. Notably, in a finding strongly suggestive of heterogeneity, many but not all of the same subjects who were hypoactive at rest were also hypoactive in right anterior areas during the tonal memory task. While this finding by itself might seem to implicate a generalized deficit notion for dyslexia, already criticized above as unenlightening, it also escapes from that pitfall, as shown by the following finding.

Rumsey et al. (1994b) showed that dyslexic men do not differ from controls in activation of the left temporal and posterior frontal areas during performance of a sentence comprehension task (a finding interpretable as consistent with the typical case of intact comprehension in the compensated dyslexic individual who remains phonologically impaired). In fact, on this task the dyslexic subjects showed normal levels of activation of the same left perisylvian region that was abnormally hypoactive during the rhyme detection task, described above. A generalized deficit explanation is thereby contradicted, nor is it possible to dismiss this finding as tautologic, since the task that had elicited the deficient activation was narrow (rhyme detection) and a cognitively "higher" use of language (for sentence comprehension) evoked normal activation in this region. Finally, Rumsey et al. (1997b) showed a range of abnormalities that included a replication of the earlier Gross-Glenn et al. (1991) finding of lingual gyrus excess in dyslexic adults on a pseudoword reading task. This tends to secure a major locus sufficiently different from the traditional language activation areas and implies the prospect of true heterogeneity within dyslexics. Though the Rumsey series has never explicitly investigated the heterogeneity issue, the very multiplicity and scope of their findings across studies, sometimes replicating earlier work, plausibly suggests the possibility of heterogeneity.

A number of studies, therefore, implicate a considerable variety of brain regions, not only the left posterior perisylvian cortex but also the extrastriate visual pathway including lingual gyri and the frontal lobes, and they imply the possibility of relevant individual differences within dyslexia. It is their very imprecision that preserves the current findings from tautology. Their demonstration of a variety of brain regional abnormalities, sometimes involving abnormalities of excess as well as of deficit, in some studies but not others suggests something considerably more complex is at work than "simple" language failure.

Summary and future directions

If the complexity of the data described above suggests that a strong heterogeneity paradigm or at least a converging pathway paradigm would be viable, then they are conversely antithetical to any simple notion of a single underlying information-processing malfunction that characterizes all dyslexia. As this review indicates, and as others have argued (Poeppel, 1996), the prospect of isolating specific phonologic or other cognitive mechanisms is beset with numerous complexities, confounds, and conflicting findings. While the effort to isolate cognitive mechanisms is nonetheless defensible and well worth pursuing (Demonet et al., 1996), it is clear that its pursuit – like any other in science – is a cost–benefit question that must take the larger research goals into account. In the case of dyslexia, there is abundant evidence in the above review that brain metabolism or blood flow in dyslexia can be abnormal in a wide variety of task or control conditions, even at rest. The evidence also strongly suggests that there may be heterogeneity across dyslexic subjects in the functional neuroanatomy of these abnormalities. On the assumption that the tautology paradigm can be excluded and that some degree of neuroanatomic specificity can plausibly be sought using the strong heterogeneity paradigm or at least a converging pathway paradigm, we may then suggest the following directions for functional neuroimaging research in dyslexia.

To account for valid genetic or behavioral subtypes

Genetic heterogeneity is at least so probable (if not certain) that it no longer suffices to define dyslexic groups simply by their reading disability. Designs that consider all dyslexics as a single group expected to share a single deficit run the serious risk of the tautology paradigm (by considering only those neurofunctional characteristics that are similar across genetic variance). Furthermore, by ignoring the genetically related variance the true underlying mechanisms will not even be investigated, much less clarified. Subtyping need not be explicitly genetic (though that is desirable when possible): subtyping can be based upon behavioral phenotypes, so long as they have plausible genetic validity. (See Grigorenko et al. (1997) for operational definitions of four such candidate phenotypes.)

To test the anatomic model

The assumption that dyslexia is "nothing but" a circumscribed cognitive deficit is at least questionable. If a given brain region, no matter how subtle or diffusely represented, is implicated in dyslexia, then it is naive to think that dyslexia would be the only consequence. Others, including those within the psychiatric domain, should at least be sought.

To avoid exclusive reliance on subtraction methods

Subtraction methodology compares a given cognitive activation task with a control condition in an effort to isolate a particular cognitive mechanism that is impaired. Usually this means that a given comparison of two tasks is found to generate metabolic activation in a given region in normal controls but not in dyslexic subjects. Beyond the obvious problem of the overriding of subtypes, this procedure inherently risks tautology if the task difference is plausibly related to reading or language and if it activates brain regions generally accepted to be substantially involved in language. If an anatomic region is shown to be hypoactive during a language- or reading-related task, but not during a control task, then at the very least certain further clarifications should be sought. Task accuracy, effort, anxiety, and related confounds should be explicitly equalized between the two conditions (since the essence of the subtraction method depends on the isolation of a particular cognitive task difference). Other subtractions or single task conditions, which on a priori grounds are likely to reflect dysfunction in the relevant anatomic area, should also be attempted in the effort to test whether the brain region in question is dysfunctional on tasks other than dyslexia-related ones. (The noninvasive and relatively inexpensive nature of fMRI can be exploited to permit multiple studies using a variety of tasks, thus capitalizing on what is otherwise a limitation, i.e., fMRI's virtual dependence on subtraction methods.) Finally, with some technologies, chiefly PET studies of glucose metabolism, and in selected situations where task activation differences have already been demonstrated, the strongest test of chronic dysfunction in a localized region can be attempted: comparisons between two groups during rest. Rest conditions offer a particularly stringent test, since the only demand that is made on the brain is that it should comply with the rest instruction. Failure to demonstrate group differences at rest is, therefore, not particularly compelling; however, successful demonstration of differences at rest offers particularly strong evidence of a group difference that is anatomically based.

To consider longitudinal studies in children

Longitudinal studies are possible with fMRI and may allow data to be acquired early enough in childhood to capture the genetic heterogeneity at a time when it is less subtle and more readily demonstrable. Variance in reading-related mechanisms often occurs surprisingly early in the school career, changing rapidly thereafter. (See Meyer et al. (1998) for an illustration involving rapid automatized naming ability, an important underlying ability in reading.)

Summary

Present data acquired by functional neuroimaging in dyslexia suggests a diverse range of neurofunctional deficits, not well described by current models stressing an isolated cognitive deficit in dyslexia. Since it is likely that part of the variance across this range is genetically based, the next generation of studies in dyslexia will need to take this variance into account in experimental design and also will need to test the convergence of varied functional activation deficits on given brain regions or processes. As always, the expectation of a single *experimentum crucis* is unrealistic: only a systematic, programmed effort in these directions is likely to be productive.

References

Bench, C. J., Frith, C. D., Grasby, P. M. et al. (1993). Investigations of the functional anatomy of attention using the Stroop test. *Neuropsychologia*, 31, 907–22.

Bookheimer, S. Y., Zeffiro, T. A., Blaxton, T., Gaillard, W. and

Theodore, W. (1995). Regional cerebral blood flow during object naming and word reading. *Hum. Brain Map.*, **3**, 93–106.

Cardon, L. R., Smith, S. D., Fulker, D. W., Kimberling, W. J., Pennington, B. F. and DeFries, J. C. (1994). Quantitative trait locus for reading disability on chromosome 6. *Science*, **26**, 276–9.

Corbetta, M., Miezin, F. M., Dobmeyer, S., Shulman, G. L. and Petersen, S. E. (1991). Selective and divided attention during visual discriminations of shape, color, and speed: functional anatomy by positron emission tomography. *J. Neurosci.*, **11**, 2382–402.

DeFries, J. C. and Decker, S. N. (1982). Genetic aspects of reading disability: a family study. In *Reading Disorders: Varieties and Treatments*, ed. R. N. Malatesha and P. G. Aaron, pp. 255–79. New York: Academic Press.

DeFries, J. C., Fulker, D. W. and LaBuda, M. C. (1987). Evidence for a genetic aetiology in reading disability in twins. *Nature*, **329**, 537–9.

DeFries, J. C., Olson, R. K., Pennington, B. F. and Smith, S. D. (1991). Colorado Reading Project: an update. In *The Reading Brain: The Biological Basis of Dyslexia*, ed. D. D. Duane and D. B. Gray, pp. 53–88. Parkton, MD: York Press.

Demonet, J. F., Chollett, F., Ramsay, S. et al. (1992). The anatomy of phonological and semantic processing in normal subjects. *Brain*, **115**, 1753–68.

Demonet, J. F., Wise, R. and Frackowiak, R. S. J. (1993). Language functions explored in normal subjects by positron emission tomography: a critical review. *Hum. Brain Map.*, **1**, 39–47.

Demonet, J. F., Price, C., Wise, R. and Frackowiak, R. S. J. (1994a). A PET study of cognitive strategies in normal subjects during language tasks. Influence of phonetic ambiguity and sequence processing on phoneme monitoring. *Brain*, **117**, 671–82.

Demonet, J. F., Price, C., Wise, R. and Frackowiak, R. S. J. (1994b). Differential activation of right and left posterior sylvian regions by semantic and phonological tasks: a positron-emission tomography study in normal human subjects. *Neurosci. Lett.*, **182**, 25–8.

Demonet, J. F., Fiez, J., Paulesu, E., Petersen, S. and Zatorre, R. (1996). PET studies of phonological processing: a critical reply to Poeppel. *Brain Lang.*, **55**, 352–79.

Eden, G. F., van Meter, J. W., Rumsey, J. M., Maisog, J. Ma., Woods, R. P. and Zeffiro, T. A. (1996). Abnormal processing of visual motion in dyslexia revealed by functional brain imaging. *Nature*, **382**, 66–9.

Flowers, D. L., Wood, F. B. and Naylor, C. E. (1991). Regional cerebral blood flow correlates of language processes in reading disability. *Arch. Neurol.*, **48**, 637–43.

Frith, C. D., Kapur, N., Friston, K. J., Liddle, P. F. and Frackowiak, R. S. J. (1995). Regional cerebral activity associated with the incidental processing of pseudo-words. *Hum. Brain Map.*, **3**, 153–60.

Fulker, D. W., Cardon, L. R., DeFries, J. C., Kimberling, W. J., Pennington, B. F. and Smith, S. D. (1991). Multiple regression analysis of sib-pair data on reading to detect quantitative trait loci. *Reading Writing Interdisc. J.*, **3**, 299–313.

Galaburda, A. M., Sherman, G. F., Rosen, G. D., Aboitiz, F. and Geschwind, N. (1985). Developmental dyslexia: four consecutive patients with cortical anomalies. *Ann. Neurol.*, **18**, 222–33.

Grabowski, T. J., Damasio, H., Frank, R. J. et al. (1995). Neuroanatomical analysis of functional brain images: validation with retinotopic mapping. *Hum. Brain Map.*, **2**, 134–48.

Grigorenko, E. L., Wood, F. B., Meyer, M. S. et al. (1997). Susceptibility loci for distinct components of developmental dyslexia on chromosomes 6 and 15. *Am. J. Hum. Genet.*, **60**, 27–39.

Gross-Glenn, K., Duara, R., Barker, W. W. et al. (1991). Positron emission tomographic studies during serial word-reading by normal and dyslexic adults. *J. Clin. Exp. Neuropsychol.*, **13**, 531–44.

Hagman, J. O., Wood, F., Buchsbaum, M. S., Tallal, P., Flowers, L. and Katz, W. (1992). Cerebral brain metabolism in adult dyslexic subjects assessed with positron emission tomography during performance of an auditory task. *Arch. Neurol.*, **49**, 734–9.

Hallgren, B. (1950). Specific dyslexia ("congenital word blindness"): a clinical and genetic study. *Act. Psychiat. Neurolog. Scand.*, **65**, 1–287.

Herholz, K., Pietrzyk, U., Karbe, H., Wurker, M., Wienhard, K. and Heiss, W. D. (1994). Individual metabolic anatomy of repeating words demonstrated by MRI-guided positron emission tomography. *Neurosci. Lett.*, **182**, 47–50.

Hohnen, B. and Stevenson, J. (1995). Genetic effects in orthographic ability: a second look. *Behav. Genet.*, **25**, 271.

Howard, D., Patterson, K., Wise, R. et al. (1992). The cortical localization of the lexicons. *Brain*, **115**, 1769–82.

Ingvar, M., Greitz, T., Eriksson, L., Stone-Elander, S., Trampe, P. and Euler, C. (1995). Developmental dyslexia studied with PET. *Hum. Brain Map.*, Suppl. 1, 378.

Karbe, H., Wurker, M., Herholz, K., Ghaemi, M., Pietrzyk, U., Kessler, J. and Heiss, W. D. (1995). Planum temporale and Brodmann's area 22. *Arch. Neurol.*, **52**, 869–74.

Kinsbourne, M., Rufo, D. T., Gamzu, E., Palmer, R. L. and Berliner, A. K. (1991). Neuropsychological deficits in adults with dyslexia. *Devel. Med. Child Neurol.*, **33**, 763–75.

Kiyosawa, M., Inoue, C., Kawasaki, T. et al. (1996). Functional neuroanatomy of visual object naming: a PET study. *Graef. Arch. Clin. Emp. Ophthalmol.*, **234**, 110–15.

Lubs, H. A., Smith, S., Kimberling, W., Pennington, B., Gross-Glenn, K. and Duara, R. (1988). Dyslexia subtypes: genetics, behavior, and brain imaging. In *Language, Communication, and the Brain*, ed. F. Plum, pp. 139–47. New York: Raven Press.

Menard, M. T., Kosslyn, S. M., Thompson, W. L., Alpert, N. M. and Rauch, S. L. (1996). Encoding words and pictures: a positron emission tomography study. *Neuropsychologia*, **34**, 185–94.

Meyer, M. S., Wood, F. B., Hart, L. and Felton, R. H. (1998). Selective predictive value of rapid automatized naming within poor readers. *J. Learn. Disabil.*, **31**, 106–17.

Olson, R., Wise, B., Conners, F., Rack, J. and Fulker, D. (1989). Specific deficits in component reading and language skills: genetic and environmental influences. *J. Learn. Disabil.*, **22**, 339–48.

Paulesu, E., Frith, C. D. and Frackowiak, R. S. J. (1993). The neural correlates of the verbal component of working memory. *Nature*, 362, 342–4.

Paulesu, E., Frith, U., Snowling, M. et al. (1996). Is developmental dyslexia a disconnection syndrome? Evidence from PET scanning. *Brain*, 119, 143–57.

Pennington, B. F. (1997). Using genetics to dissect cognition. [Editorial comment] *Am. J. Hum. Genet.*, 60, 13–16.

Petersen, S. E. and Fiez, J. A. (1993). The processing of single words studied with positron emission tomography. *Annu. Rev. Neurosci.*, 16, 509–30.

Petersen, S. E., Fox, P., Posner, M., Mintun, M. and Raichle, M. (1989). Positron emission tomographic studies of the processing of single words. *J. Cogn. Neurosci.*, 1, 153–70.

Poeppel, D. (1996). A critical review of PET studies of phonological processing. *Brain Lang.*, 55, 317–51.

Price, C. J. (1977). Functional anatomy of reading. In *Human Brain Function*, ed. R. S. J. Frackowiak, K. J. Friston, C. D. Frith, R. J. Dolan and J. C. Mazziotta, pp. 301–27. London: Academic Press.

Price, C. J., Wise, R. J. S., Watson, J. D. G., Patterson, K., Howard, D. and Frackowiak, R. S. J. (1994). Brain activity during reading. The effects of exposure duration and task. *Brain*, 117, 1255–69.

Robinson, R. G. and Price, T. R. (1982). Post-stroke depressive disorders: a follow-up study of 103 outpatients. *Stroke*, 13, 635–41.

Rumsey, J. M., Andreason, P., Zametkin, A. J. et al. (1992). Failure to activate the left temporoparietal cortex in dyslexia. An oxygen 15 positron emission tomographic study. *Arch. Neurol.*, 49, 527–34.

Rumsey, J. M., Andreason, P., Zametkin, A. J. et al. (1994a). Right frontotemporal activation by tonal memory in dyslexia, an O^{15} PET study. *Biol. Psychiatry*, 36, 171–80.

Rumsey, J. M., Zametkin, A. J., Andreason, P. et al. (1994b). Normal activation of frontotemporal language cortex in dyslexia, as measured with oxygen 15 positron emission tomography. *Arch. Neurol.*, 51, 27–38.

Rumsey, J. M., Horwitz, B., Donohue, B. C., Nace, A. K., Maisog, J. M. and Andreason, P. (1997a). Phonological and orthographic components of word recognition: a PET – rCBF study. *Brain*, 120, 739–59.

Rumsey, J. M., Nace, K., Donohue, B., Wise, D., Maisog, J. M. and Andreason, P. (1997b). A positron emission tomographic study of impaired word recognition and phonological processing in dyslexic men. *Arch. Neurol.*, 54, 562–73.

Sergent, J., Ohta, S. and MacDonald, B. (1992). Functional neuro-anatomy of face and object processing. *Brain*, 115, 16–36.

Shaywitz, S. E. et al. (1998). Functional disruption in the organization of the brain for reading in dyslexia. *Proc. Natl. Acad. Sci USA*, 95, 2636–41.

Shaywitz, B. A., Pugh, K. R., Constable, R. T. et al. (1995). Localization of semantic processing using functional magnetic resonance imaging. *Hum. Brain Map.*, 2, 149–58.

Small, S. L., Noll, D. C., Perfetti, C. A., Hlustik, P., Wellington, R. and Schneider, W. (1996). Localizing the lexicon for reading aloud: replication of a PET study using fMRI. *Neuroreport*, 7, 961–5.

Smith, S. D., Kimberling, W. J., Pennington, B. F. and Lubs, H. A. (1983). Specific reading disability: identification of an inherited form through linkage analysis. *Science*, 219, 1345–7.

Tamas, L. B., Shibasaki, T., Horikoshi, S. and Ohye, C. (1993). General activation of cerebral metabolism with speech: a PET study. *Int. J. Psychophysiol.*, 14, 199–208.

Vandenberghe, R., Price, C., Wise, R., Josephs, O. and Frackowiak, R. S. J. (1996). Functional anatomy of a common semantic system for words and pictures. *Nature*, 383, 254–5.

Warburton, E., Wise, R. J. S., Price, C. J. et al. (1996). Noun and verb retrieval by normal subjects. Studies with PET. *Brain*, 119, 159–79.

Watson, J. D. G., Myers, R., Frackowiak, R. S. J. and Haynal, J. V. (1993). Area V5 of the human brain: evidence from a combined study using positron emission tomography and magnetic resonance imaging. *Cerebr. Cortex*, 3, 79–94.

Wolff, M. and Obregon, M. (1992). Early naming deficits, developmental dyslexia and a specific deficit hypothesis. *Brain Lang.*, 42, 217–47.

Wolf, P. H. and Melngailis, I. (1994). Family patterns of developmental dyslexia. *Am. J. Med. Genet. (Neuropsychiatr. Genet.)*, 54, 122–31.

Wood, F. (1990). Functional neuroimaging in neurobehavioral research. In *Neuromethods*, Vol. 17: *Neuropsychology*, ed. A. A. Boulton, G. B. Baker and M. Hiscock, pp. 107–25. Clifton NJ: Humana Press.

Wood, F., Flowers, L., Buchsbaum, M. and Tallal, P. (1991). Investigation of abnormal left temporal functioning in dyslexia through rCBF, auditory evoked potentials, and positron emission tomography. *Reading Writing Interdisc. J.*, 3, 379–93.

Zatorre, R. J., Meyer, E., Gjedde, A. and Evans, A. C. (1996). PET studies of phonetic processing of speech: review, replication, and reanalysis. *Cereb. Cortex*, 6, 21–30.

16

Attention-deficit hyperactivity disorder: neuroimaging and behavioral/cognitive probes

Julie B. Schweitzer, Carl Anderson and
Monique Ernst

Clinical phenomenology and epidemiology

Attention-deficit hyperactivity disorder (ADHD) is characterized by persistent inattention and/or situationally excessive motor activity, and impulsive behavior (Barkley, 1990). According to the current *Diagnostic and Statistical Manual of Mental Disorder* (4th edition (DSM-IV); American Psychiatric Association, 1994), individuals must exhibit symptoms for at least 6 months and must express the symptoms by 7 years of age. The symptoms must be developmentally inappropriate and exhibited in at least two settings. DSM-IV specifies three subtypes: predominantly inattentive (ADHD-I), predominantly hyperactive–impulsive (ADHD-HI), and combined type (ADHD-C). The number and nature of items endorsed within lists of inattentive and hyperactive/impulsive symptoms determines the specific diagnostic subtype.

ADHD is the most prevalent childhood psychiatric disorder and is estimated to affect 3–11% of the school-age population, depending on the source of the sample (American Psychiatric Association, 1994; Wolraich et al., 1996). There is a much higher incidence rate in boys, who are 2.5–9 times more likely than girls to be diagnosed with ADHD (Szatmari et al., 1989; Barkley, 1990; Wolraich et al., 1996). The disorder often has a chronic course, with 30–50% of affected children exhibiting ADHD symptoms into adulthood (Barkley et al., 1990; Weiss and Hechtman, 1993). Numerous problems are associated with childhood and adulthood ADHD, including poor academic performance, learning disabilities, conduct disorders, antisocial personality disorder, lower occupational success, poor social relationships, frequent car accidents, and a higher incidence of anxiety and depression (Barkley et al., 1990, 1996; Biederman et al., 1993; Weiss and Hechtman, 1993; Murphy and Barkley, 1996; Mannuzza et al., 1998).

Theoretical perspectives

Diagnostic labels

The diagnostic label for ADHD has changed several times during the twentieth century, reflecting the continuously evolving conceptualization of the disorder. The metamorphosis in the labels, from "minimal brain dysfunction", to "hyperkinetic impulse disorder", to "attention-deficit disorder", mirrors the changing emphasis on brain, motor, and attentional dysfunction. Recent theoretical models of ADHD, however, are less likely to focus on "attention deficits" and more likely to highlight neurobehavioral dysfunction affecting response inhibition, working memory, and the implementation of organizational strategies subsumed under the term of "executive functions" (Denckla, 1996; Barkley, 1997a,b). In these models, problems with sustained attention, distractibility, and reduced motor control are secondary to disrupted response inhibition and interference control. The deficient response inhibition ultimately results in behavior that is less internally guided (i.e., less able to follow verbal rules and less goal-directed). (See Barkley (1997a) and Denckla (1996) for a more in-depth discussion of these models.) These ADHD models implicate the dysfunction of discrete neural circuits the functional integrity of which can be examined in neuroimaging studies.

To examine these circuits in ADHD, it is critical to study clinically homogeneous samples, such as the ADHD-I, ADHD-HI, or ADHD-C subtypes specified in DSM-IV. Subjects who are free of comorbid disorders can be studied as relatively homogeneous behavioral subgroups with objectively quantified motor and/or attentional dysfunction. For example, as hyperactivity is primarily thought to stem from an inability to inhibit motor acts, the use of imaging paradigms that require subjects to inhibit responses (e.g., performance of go-no-go tasks) may be exploited to reveal functional neuroanatomic differences between healthy controls and subtypes of ADHD.

Functional neuroanatomy

Recently, studies indicating a role for the basal ganglia in a variety of neuropsychiatric conditions involving motor and attentional dysfunctions (Mega and Cummings, 1994; Rauch and Savage, 1997; Peterson et al., 1998) have suggested the differential involvement in ADHD of five functionally interconnected subcortical structures: the caudate nucleus, putamen, globus pallidus, subthalamic nucleus, and ventral mesencephalon. In addition, five parallel basal ganglia–thalamocortical circuits have been proposed (Alexander et al., 1986, 1990) to convey the output of these subregions through specific thalamic zones to different parts of the frontal cortex. These functionally segregated striato–thalamo–cortico–striatal loops contribute respectively to motor, somatosensory, oculomotor, executive, emotion, and motivation functions: (i) a motor circuit involving the arcuate premotor area, supplementary motor area, somatosensory cortex, superior parietal lobe, and motor cortex, all of which project to the posterior putamen, subserving sensorimotor integration; (ii) an oculomotor pathway involving the frontal eye fields, as well as the supplementary eye fields, both of which project to the head and body of the caudate and subserve the attentional control of eye movements; (iii) the prefrontal cognitive/association pathway, composed of the dorsolateral prefrontal cortex (DLPFC), the dorsolateral head of the caudate, and the anterior putamen, regions involved in working memory and the planning of voluntary movements; (iv) the orbitofrontal pathway, which is composed of the lateral orbitofrontal cortex and its projections to both the head and body of the caudate, and which is less involved in working memory and spatial processing than the prefrontal pathway and more involved with response inhibition and emotion; and (5) the ventral striatal pathway, composed of the anterior cingulate, medial orbitofrontal cortex, ventromedial caudate, and the nucleus accumbens, which subserves motivational processes and influences the other pathways via extensive projections back to the ventral mesencephalic dopamine system; this, in turn, modulates all of the dorsal striatum (Heimer et al., 1997). The motor and prefrontal basal ganglia–thalamocortical circuits are depicted in Fig. 16.1a (p. 242) and the regional cortico–striatal pathways are illustrated in Fig. 16.1b (p. 242).

Since the late 1980s, a large number of functional imaging studies (see Tables 16.1–16.3) have implicated various components of these pathways in the pathophysiology of ADHD. Functional imaging studies of ADHD tend to follow a dimensional rather than a categorical approach and focus on a combination of behavioral- and circuit-specific paradigms to elucidate neural abnormalities specific to behavioral subtypes.

How do these functionally segregated circuits exchange information to enable the smooth flow of motor and attentional functions? One view is that regions of the striatum such as the putamen contain a combinatorial map of body regions allowing extensive overlap and interdigitation between body-part elements (Brown et al., 1998). The functional connectivity of this cortico-striatal gridwork appears to be regulated by dopamine levels. The putamen projects somatotopically to both the external and internal segments of the globus pallidus and to the substantia nigra pars reticulata (SNR). In general, striatal projections to the external segment are inhibitory on movement and considered part of the "indirect pathway," whereas projections to the internal segment facilitate movement and are part of the "direct pathway" to the SNR (Smith et al., 1998). The SNR, in turn, regulates the dopaminergic inputs from the substantia nigra pars compacta back to the putamen and other striatal regions. In addition, both the SNR and the internal segment of the globus pallidus project directly to the thalamus, which somatotopically innervates the frontal motor cortical areas (supplementary motor area and motor cortex). Normal dopaminergic tone in the putamen facilitates independent firing patterns of globus pallidus neurons (Bergman et al., 1998).

The hallmark of the loss of dopaminergic tone in the basal ganglia is Parkinson's disease, which is characterized by difficulty initiating and executing movements and by a breakdown of independent firing within the globus pallidus. In Parkinson's disease, contiguous neurons in the internal segment of the globus pallidus fire in highly synchronized oscillations in phase with behavioral tremor (Bergman et al., 1998), and inhibitory output from the external segment predominates. Therefore, dopamine appears to modulate the cross-linkage between different pathways in the gridwork of cortico–striatal projections regulating the balance between indirect and direct striato-pallidal outflow to thalamic and frontal cortical networks.

To summarize, the striatum (caudate nucleus, putamen, and ventral striatum or nucleus accumbens) is divided into functional domains based on cortical projections (Heimer et al., 1997). Prefrontal cortical and associative areas including primary and secondary visual and auditory cortical regions project to the dorsolateral head of the caudate and the anterior putamen. The sensorimotor cortex projects to

Table 16.1. Frontal neurocircuits implicated by neuroimaging research in attention-deficit hyperactivity disorder (ADHD)

Study	Modality	Condition[a]	Subjects	Findings
Zametkin et al. (1990)	FDG PET	Normalized	Adults	Reduced normalized regional metabolic activity in left premotor and somatosensory areas in subjects with ADHD
Matochik et al. (1993)	FDG PET	Normalized	Adults	Increases and decreases (in different regions) in metabolic activity in left and right frontal areas with dextroamphetamine and methylphenidate
Teicher et al. (1996)[b]	fMRI steady-state technique	Rest	Children	Hyperactivity associated with lower perfusion in the left dorsolateral prefrontal cortex; methylphenidate increases perfusion in the dorsolateral prefrontal cortex in objectively hyperactive only and decreases perfusion in the left dorsolateral prefrontal cortex in nonhyperactive children
Casey et al. (1997a)	Structural MRI/task correlation	N/A	Children	Response inhibition accuracy correlated with right prefrontal cortex volume for normal but not subjects with ADHD
Schweitzer et al. (2000)	$H_2^{15}O$ PET	Stress	Adults	Absence of right dorsolateral prefrontal cortex activation in subjects with ADHD during working memory task
Schweitzer et al. (1998)[b]	$H_2^{15}O$ PET	Stress	Adults	Absence of right dorsolateral prefrontal cortex activation in subjects with ADHD during working memory task
Flowers et al. (1997)[b]	FDG PET	Normalized	Adults	Decreased right superior frontal and increased normalized metabolic activity in left inferior frontal regions in subjects with ADHD
Vaidya et al. (1998)	fMRI	Stress	Children	Greater frontal activation in subjects with ADHD in response-controlled condition; equivalent frontal activation in the stimulus-controlled condition
Ernst et al. (1998)	[18F]-Fluorodopa PET	N/A	Adults	Lower fluorodopa ratios in subjects with ADHD in the medial and left prefrontal areas
Ernst et al. (1999)	[18F]-Fluorodopa PET	N/A	Children	Lower fluorodopa ratios in subjects with ADHD in the anterior medial frontal cortex

Notes:

N/A, not applicable; FDG, [18F]-fluorodeoxyglucose.

[a] Condition refers to the behavioral state during the scanning with rest indicating no behavioral task, normalized indicating a task used to control for extraneous stimulation and internal mental activity, and stress indicating a task used to activate putative neural circuits related to ADHD.

[b] Abstract only available.

large regions of the putamen (Graybiel et al., 1994). The ventral striatum or nucleus accumbens receives extensive projections from the anterior cingulate and medial orbito-frontal cortex. How do the findings of recent functional imaging studies of ADHD fit with this current model of basal ganglia function?

Neuroimaging studies linked to functional neuroanatomy

As a general caveat to the interpretation of the following studies, the reader must keep in mind that most pediatric studies are conducted in children who have a history (past or current) of exposure to stimulant treatment, whereas adult studies usually involve individuals who did not have the opportunity to be treated for ADHD as children and have no prior history of exposure to stimulant treatment. Generally, stimulant treatment is suspended between 48 h to 2 weeks prior to an imaging study, depending on the study protocol and the requirements of Institutional Review Boards. The contribution of past or current exposure of stimulants to deviance in brain function is not clear. Information about stimulant treatment is not always available and not systematically indicated in this review of the literature.

Table 16.2. Anterior cingulate findings in neuroimaging research in attention-deficit hyperactivity disorder (ADHD)

Study	Modality	Condition[a]	Subjects	Findings
Schweitzer et al. (2000)	H$_2$^{15}O PET	Stress	Adults	Absence of anterior cingulate activation in subjects with ADHD with increased practice on working memory task
Bush et al. (1999)	fMRI	Stress	Adults	Absence of anterior cingulate activation in subjects with ADHD during cognitive interference task
Rubia et al. (1999)	fMRI	Stress	Adolescents	Absence of right anterior cingulate activation during motor timing task in subjects with ADHD
Steinberg et al. (1998)[b]	^{133}Xe SPECT	Stress	Children	Absence of left anterior cingulate during target detection task in subjects with ADHD
Vaidya et al. (1998)	fMRI	Stress	Children	Greater anterior cingulate activation in subjects with ADHD during response-controlled condition; equivalent activation during stimulus-controlled condition; methylphenidate increased activation for ADHD group only during response-controlled condition; both groups increased cingulate activation during stimulus-controlled condition

Notes:
[a] Stress condition refers to the behavioral state during the scanning with a task used to activate putative neural circuits related to ADHD.
[b] Abstract only available.

The same studies may be mentioned several times throughout the text, according to the structure being discussed, but the description of their methodology will not be repeated.

Prefrontal cortex

The starting point of functional basal ganglia loops are motor commands initiated by frontal regions. The frontal lobe is divided into posterior motor regions and anterior prefrontal regions, particularly the DLPFC. Evidence for dysfunction in the DLPFC circuit comes from the growing number of studies showing abnormalities in the prefrontal cortex of subjects with ADHD. Cognitive and higher level processes are thought to be dependent on the functional connections between frontal regions and basal ganglia, particularly the caudate nucleus (Alexander et al., 1990). The frontal lobes receive input relayed by the thalamus from the subcortical nuclei of the basal ganglia, including the caudate and globus pallidus. The largest morphometric MRI study (subjects with ADHD: $n = 57$; mean age 11.7 years, range 5.8–17.8; controls: $n = 55$; mean age 12.0 years, range 5.5–17.8) (Castellanos et al., 1996) reported that boys with ADHD had a significantly smaller right, but not left, prefrontal volumes than control boys.

Following work by Lou et al. (1984, 1989) reporting regional cerebral blood flow (rCBF) abnormalities in the striatum of children with ADHD (small and heterogeneous samples including children with history of neonatal neuro-logic insults), Zametkin et al. (1990) demonstrated functional abnormalities in the brain of adults with ADHD. This study used positron emission tomography (PET) and [^{10}F]-flurodeoxyglucose (FDG), and was remarkable for its thorough assessment of the subjects with ADHD, and its clean (no comorbidity) and relatively large sample sizes (25 adults with ADHD, 50 controls). Zametkin and colleagues (1990) reported lower absolute metabolic rate of glucose (CMRGlu) in many brain regions, including the prefrontal cortex, in adults with ADHD compared with controls. PET measures were collected while subjects performed a continuous performance test (CPT) that was used to standardize the mental and motoric state of the subjects.

Given this strong finding, Zametkin initiated studies in adolescents after refining the PET methodology to minimize radiation exposure (Chapter 6) (Zametkin et al., 1993; Ernst et al., 1994a). In contrast to the extensive reduction of CMRGlu in adults with ADHD compared with controls, adolescents (ADHD: $n = 20$; mean age 14.7 ± 1.7 years; healthy controls: $n = 19$; mean age 14.4 ± 1.4 years) showed regionally limited differences between boys with ADHD (15) and control boys (13). In contrast, girls with ADHD (5) showed a statistically significant 15% reduction of global CMRGlu compared with that in control girls (6) (Ernst et al., 1994a). When regional CMRGlu (rCMRGlu) was normalized (divided by whole-brain CMRGlu), the left frontal cortex was the region most affected in adults (Zametkin et al., 1990) and adolescents with ADHD (left anterior middle prefrontal gyrus) (Ernst et al., 1994a).

Table 16.3. Basal ganglia neurocircuits implicated by neuroimaging research in attention-deficit hyperactivity disorders (ADHD)

Study	Modality	Condition[a]	Subjects	Findings
Lou et al. (1989)	^{133}Xe SPECT	Rest	Children	Right striatal regions hypoperfused in ADHD subjects; methylphenidate increased flow in left striatum
Lou et al. (1990)	^{133}Xe SPECT	Rest	Children	Striatum hypoperfused in ADHD subjects
Zametkin et al. (1990)	FDG PET	Normalized	Adults	Reduced global metabolism in right caudate of ADHD subjects
Matochik et al. (1993)	FDG PET	Normalized	Adults	Increased metabolism in right caudate with dextroamphetamine
Casey et al. (1997a)	Structural MRI/task correlation	N/A	Children	Response inhibition performance in subjects correlated with right caudate volume, caudate symmetry, and left globus pallidus volume
Flowers et al. (1997)[b]	FDG PET	Normalized	Adults	Right caudate significantly more activated in ADHD subjects
Teicher et al. (1996)[b]	fMRI (steady-state technique)	Rest	Children	Motor activity negatively correlated with right caudate perfusion in ADHD subjects; high doses of methylphenidate increased perfusion in right caudate
Teicher et al. (2000)	fMRI (steady-state technique)	Rest	Children	Hyperactivity associated with lower bilateral perfusion in the putamen, primarily left; methylphenidate increased bilateral perfusion of the putamen in the objectively hyperactive only; methylphenidate decreased bilateral perfusion in nonhyperactive
Schweitzer et al. (1998)[b]	H$_2$^{15}O PET	Stress	Adults	Increased activation of left globus pallidus during working memory task in ADHD subjects; activations decreased with methylphenidate
Vaidya et al. (1998)	fMRI	Stress	Children	Caudate and putamen activations lower in ADHD subjects during stimulus-controlled condition; caudate and putamen activations marginally higher ($p = 0.08$) in ADHD during response-controlled condition; methylphenidate increased caudate and putamen activations in ADHD subjects and decreased activations in control subjects in stimulus-controlled condition; no methylphenidate effects during response-controlled condition in ADHD or in control subjects

Notes:

N/A, not applicable; FDG, [^{18}F]-Fluorodeoxyglucose.

[a] Condition refers to the behavioral state during the scanning with rest indicating no behavioral task, normalized indicating a task used to control for extraneous stimulation and internal mental activity, and stress indicating a task used to activate putative neural circuits related to ADHD.

[b] Abstract only available.

Because of the encouraging results in the girl sample, and the difficulty in generalizing them owing to small sample size, a larger independent sample of girls with (10) and without (11) ADHD was studied (Ernst et al., 1997a). This study did not replicate the abnormally low CMRGlu in girls with ADHD. However, although of similar age, the girls of the initial study (Ernst et al., 1994a) were more sexually mature than those of the second study (Ernst et al., 1997a). Because the data showed a negative association between sexual maturation and CMRGlu (more mature, lower CMRGlu), the absence of differences between ADHD and control girls may have been masked in sexually immature girls. The role of sexual maturation on CMRGlu, as well as potential CMRGlu deviance in girls with ADHD compared with controls, remains to be determined. The difficulty in conducting such studies makes it difficult to examine these questions in a timely fashion.

The findings of decreased CMRGlu in adults with ADHD were partially replicated in a more recent study using FDG PET (Flowers et al., 1997). This study also used a CPT performance to standardize the mental and motoric state of the subjects (11 subjects with attention-deficit disorder (ADD) with and without hyperactivity based on DSM-III; 10 nonADD with reading disability; no data on gender available). Similar to findings reported by Zametkin et al. (1990), Flowers et al. (1997) reported lower absolute rCMRGlu in the frontal lobes in adults with ADD compared with a control group of adults without ADD but with a reading disability. In contrast to the report of abnormally low frontal rCMRGlu (Zametkin et al., 1990), Flowers et al. (1997) found higher normalized rCMRGlu in the left inferior frontal cortex relative to controls with dyslexia. The differences between Zametkin's study and Flower's study in the control samples (healthy versus reading disabled) and in the subtypes of ADHD included in the patient sample may have accounted for the discrepant findings.

Further evidence for the presence of functional differences between ADHD and control subjects in frontal lobe comes from activation studies of PET and $H_2{}^{15}O$ using a cognitive challenge in the form of an auditory working memory task in adult males. In two independent studies (Schweitzer et al., 1998, 2000) control subjects (nine in the 1998 study, six in that of 2000), showed activation of the right dorsolateral prefrontal cortex (Brodmann areas 46 and 9), which has been reported to be active during retrieval in memory (Tulving et al., 1994; Andreasen et al., 1995). In contrast, adults with ADHD-C type and no comorbidity (12 in the 1988 study, and six in that of 1999) showed no activation of these regions, suggesting a disruption in the use of retrieval function. While the ADHD groups evidenced diminished activation in frontal regions, they displayed increased activation in other brain regions (e.g., occipital and cerebellar), suggesting that these non-frontal regions may be activated to compensate for the underfunctioning frontal regions. Such hypothesis could be tested using connectivity analysis with larger samples.

Studies using PET and FDG have detected only limited effects of stimulants on the frontal lobes in ADHD. Stimulant administration (acute oral, chronic oral, and intravenous) did not raise prefrontal rCMRGlu as was expected given the abnormally low CMRGlu of untreated adults with ADHD (Matochik et al., 1993, 1994; Ernst et al., 1994b, 1997b). Such negative finding suggests that CMRGlu may not be the appropriate variable to examine.

In contrast, blood flow studies using fMRI have been more sensitive to the effects of stimulant medications. Using steady-state fMRI relaxometry, Teicher et al. (1996) found that low oral doses (0.5 mg/kg) methylphenidate in children with ADHD (13 males, two females; mean age 9.93 ± 0.45 years; all subtypes) increased perfusion in the left dorsolateral prefrontal cortex and the right caudate and putamen

during a resting state condition. Using fMRI with a response inhibition task (go-no-go task), Vaidya et al. (1998) studied the acute effects of methylphenidate on frontal lobe cerebral blood flow (CBF) in 10 boys with ADHD (aged 10.5 ± 1.4 years; eight combined type, two inattentive type) and six control boys (aged 9.3 ± 1.5 years). The authors state, however, that ratings of three (not including the two diagnosed as ADHDI) of the ten did not reach significance on the hyperactivity index on an ADHD rating scale. In patients, methylphenidate was administered at the regular prescribed dose (7.5–30 mg) and was discontinued for 36 h prior to scanning for the off-drug session; controls were scanned off-drug and 2.0–2.5 h after the administration of a 10 mg dose. Methylphenidate improved task performance and increased perfusion in frontal regions in children with ADHD, as well as in normal controls (Vaidya et al., 1998). However, the effects of methylphenidate differed in the striatum as a function of group (increase in ADHD, decrease in controls). The authors concluded that the stimulant modulates frontal activation in a similar way in ADHD and controls and suggested that dysfunction in ADHD more likely involves the striatum and striato–frontal connections.

Caudate nuclei

The strongest evidence of disruption of the DLPFC loop in ADHD comes from a growing body of structural MRI findings. Decreased volume and altered asymmetries of the caudate nucleus in children with ADHD have been reported in several studies (Hynd et al., 1993; Castellanos et al., 1996; Filipek et al., 1997). However, less consistent are the directions of lateralization observed in the caudate nucleus of children with and without ADHD. In the first study to examine the caudate volumes in ADHD, Hynd and colleagues (1993) studied 11 children with ADHD (eight males and three females; ages not reported) and 11 normal controls (six males and five females; ages not reported) and found a decrease in the size of the head of the left caudate nucleus. The control children evidenced a left-larger-than-right pattern of asymmetry, whereas the children with ADHD evidenced a right-greater-than-left asymmetry. Filipek and colleagues (1997) compared the volume of total caudates and caudate heads in 15 boys with ADHD (aged 12.4 ± 3.4 years) without comorbid diagnosis with 15 healthy control subjects (aged 14.4 ± 3.4 years). The subjects with ADHD had smaller left total caudate and caudate head volumes, with a loss of the normal left-predominant asymmetry seen in controls. An exploratory analysis suggested that the stimulant responders in the ADHD group evidenced the smallest bilateral caudate volumes. In the currently largest structural MRI study of ADHD,

Castellanos and colleagues (1996) compared the caudate volumes of 57 boys with ADHD (mean age 11.7 years; range 5.8–17.8 years) with 55 healthy control subjects (mean age 12.0 years; range 5.5–17.8 years). They found a reduced right caudate volume for the subjects with ADHD, with a loss of the right-predominant asymmetry seen in their normal control subjects. Differences in methodology, subject selection, measurement techniques and equipment, as well as the subtlety of these asymmetries and the limited knowledge of normal age-related anatomic variability in this structure, may all contribute to the contradictory findings.

Morphometric and functional findings implicating the caudate nucleus in the pathophysiology of ADHD have also been correlated with symptomatic behaviors in ADHD. Response inhibition in tasks conducted outside of a scanner was reported to be correlated with caudate volume and symmetry in 26 boys with ADHD (aged 9.69 ± 1.99 years) with faster reaction times and higher accuracy associated with larger caudate volumes in ADHD and caudate symmetry (right greater than left) (Casey et al., 1997a). Greater motor hyperactivity assessed out of the scanner has also been found to be correlated with lower perfusion, assessed with resting state fMRI, in the right caudate (Teicher et al., 1996) in children with ADHD (13 male, two female; mean age 9.93 ± 0.45 years).

Further evidence for caudate dysfunction in ADHD comes from studies of integrated neural activity (CBF or CMRGlu). The earliest studies evaluated resting CBF using ^{133}Xe inhalation and computed tomography (CT) in children with ADHD. Three studies with overlapping samples of children with ADHD and other neurologic problems reported hypoperfusion in the striatum (i.e., caudate and putamen) (Lou et al., 1984, 1989, 1990), and two of these studies reported that oral administration of methylphenidate increased striatal CBF (Lou et al., 1984, 1989). Limitations in the interpretation of these findings included the substantial overlap in the samples studied, the lack of use of standard structured diagnostic instruments, the inclusion of subjects with significant neurologic and developmental delays, the inclusion of siblings of those with ADHD as control subjects, and poor matching of the groups for age and gender. Resolution of the images in these studies was 17 mm and only a single axial slice through the striata and thalamus was examined.

The two studies in adults using FDG and PET during the performance of a CPT found significant differences in caudate activity between adults with ADHD and controls. In the first study (Zametkin et al., 1990), reduced absolute rCMRGlu was found in subjects with ADHD in the right caudate, while in the second study (Flowers et al., 1997),

increased normalized rCMRGlu was found in the right caudate in the ADHD group. As mentioned earlier, comparison of these studies is limited by the use of different diagnostic criteria for the ADHD groups, differences in the control groups, and the use of absolute CMRGlu values in one study and normalized ones in the other study.

A recent fMRI study (Vaidya et al., 1998) that compared the brain activity of children with ADHD and a group of normal controls during the performance of two go-no-go tasks found that differences in caudate activity between groups of children with ADHD and normal controls varied depending on the task requirements. In a condition that controlled for the rate of stimulus presentation, subjects with ADHD showed reduced caudate activation relative to controls. In a condition that controlled for the rate of responses, subjects with ADHD showed a trend ($p = 0.08$) toward increased caudate activation compared with controls. This study suggests that caudate activation may vary with the type and degree of cognitive demands placed on the subjects.

Effects of psychostimulants on caudate activity have been documented in several studies (Matochik et al., 1993; Teicher et al., 1996; Vaidya et al., 1998). An acute oral dose of dexamfetamine (dextroamphetamine, dexamphetamine) administered to adults with ADHD significantly altered rCMRGLu in seven brain regions, including the right caudate nucleus, which showed elevated rCMRGlu (Matochik et al., 1993) (nine males, four females). Chronic methylphenidate treatment increased perfusion in the right caudate of children with ADHD as assessed by steady-state fMRI relaxometry (Teicher et al., 1996), and in a fMRI study using a stimulus-controlled activation (go-no-go task: rate of presentation similar in the go and the no-go task blocks) (Vaidya et al., 1998). In this latter study, when a response-controlled condition (number of key presses similar in the go and the no-go task blocks) was used, methylphenidate did not significantly activate the caudate nucleus. In normal controls, caudate perfusion decreased during the stimulus-controlled condition and was unchanged during the response-controlled condition (Vaidya et al., 1998). The results suggested that methylphenidate may affect the caudate nucleus in a different way in children with ADHD than in controls, although the influence of chronic (1–3 years in patients) versus acute (controls) exposure to stimulants could not be controlled.

Putamen

As behavioral hyperactivity is a fundamental characteristic of ADHD, this section will emphasize findings associated primarily with the putamen and sensorimotor activity. The putamen is somatotopically organized into an array of overlapping regions for integrating leg, arm, and orofacial movements with sensorimotor information about target location, limb kinematics, and muscle patterns (Alexander et al., 1990; Brown et al., 1998).

Teicher et al. (1996, 2000) proposed that the putamen was among the primary structures involved in ADHD. This hypothesis is based on their fMRI findings, where rCBF was not only lower selectively in the putamen of boys with ADHD (11; mean age 9.3 ± 1.6 years) compared with controls (six; mean age 10.02 ± 1.5 years) (no group differences in thalamus or caudate), it was also associated with measures of attention and activity (Teicher et al., 2000). This effect was more pronounced on the right than on the left side. In addition, methylphenidate seemed to alter rCBF in putamen differentially as a function of unmedicated activity level (to which putamen rCBF was correlated) (Teicher et al., 2000). It is not clear whether this influence of basal activity on stimulant effects could be confounded by differences in treatment of children with worse pathology (e.g., longer treatment at higher doses for more severe pathology). Given gender-related differences in basal levels of activity (girls generally less motorically active than boys), the study of girls would be particularly informative. In fact, Ernst et al. (1994a) in their PET and FDG study of girls reported that rCMRGlu of the right anterior putamen was higher in girls with ADHD (10; mean age 14.10 ± 1.91 years) than in control girls (11; mean age 14.3 ± 1.70 years), and mean rCMRGlu of the left anterior putamen tended to be lower. The larger the asymmetry in rCMRGlu of the anterior putamen (left < right), the more hyperactive were the girls with ADHD. Comparable differences were not found in PET studies involving adolescent boys (Ernst et al., 1994a; Zametkin et al., 1993). Although these findings are difficult to reconcile with those of Teicher et al. (1996, 2000), it is clear that girls need to be involved in future studies of ADHD.

Globus pallidus

The direct and indirect pathways of the globus pallidus (Smith et al., 1998) allow convergence between "motor" cortico–striatal loops and thalamo–tegmental–brainstem outflow and have been implicated by a number of imaging studies of ADHD (Aylward et al., 1996; Castellanos et al., 1996; Schweitzer et al., 1998). Alterations in globus pallidus structure and function have been observed in boys with ADHD compared with normal control boys (Aylward et al., 1996; Castellanos et al., 1996), boys with ADHD and comorbid Tourette's syndrome (TS) (Aylward et al., 1996), and between adult men with ADHD and normal control men

(Schweitzer et al., 1998). Aylward et al. (1996) found decreases in the total and left globus pallidus volumes (smaller than the right) in boys with ADHD (10; mean age 11.26 ± 1.62 years) compared with normal control boys (11; mean age 10.71 ± 1.98 years), with no significant differences seen between boys with ADHD and boys with ADHD and TS (16; mean age 11.32 ± 1.46 years), although the globus pallidus volumes in the subjects with ADHD and TS were intermediate in size between those in the normal controls and those in boys with ADHD. Castellanos et al. (1996) found a significant reduction in the volume of the right globus pallidus in boys with ADHD compared with control boys.

Functional imaging with PET found significant activation in adults with ADHD in the globus pallidus (left greater than right) during a working memory task compared with controls, who showed no significant activation in the globus pallidus. Methylphenidate administration removed the globus pallidus activation from the subjects with ADHD, thus normalizing activation in the globus pallidus (Schweitzer et al., 1998).

Anterior cingulate

Whereas abundant evidence suggests dysfunction in the DLPFC loop, there is also increasing evidence implicating dysfunction in the anterior cingulate loop, also recognized as the limbic loop, a circuit associated with attention, emotion, and motivation. The anterior cingulate circuit originates in the anterior cingulate gyrus and orbitofrontal gyri with projections to the ventral striatum, including the ventromedial caudate, ventral putamen, nucleus accumbens, and olfactory tubercle (Mega and Cummings, 1994). The ventral striatum also receives projections from temporal lobe structures such as the amygdala and hippocampus (Heimer et al., 1997). The ventral striatum projects to the globus pallidus and the medial dorsal thalamus. The globus pallidus projects to parts of the magnocellular mediodorsal thalamus. The magnocellular mediodorsal thalamus projects back to the anterior cingulate and orbitofrontal gyri. A number of recent studies (Steinberg et al., 1998; Bush et al., 1999; Rubia et al., 1999; Schweitzer et al., 2000) implicated dysfunction in the anterior cingulate in subjects with ADHD.

Reduced task-related activation in the anterior cingulate has been consistently noted in subjects with ADHD compared with controls in functional neuroimaging studies (Bush et al., 1999; Rubia et al., 1999; Schweitzer et al., 2000). This consistency is worthy of further exploration of the function of the anterior cingulate using tasks mediated by this structure, such as tasks of preparatory states (Murtha et al., 1996), inhibition (Casey et al., 1997a), and motivation.

The globus pallidus, which is part of the anterior cingulate loop, may also be relevant to this circuit. As temporal and spatial resolution improve in neuroimaging, it might become possible to specify the areas of abnormality within the globus pallidus further and the corresponding striato–cortical circuits (DLPFC versus the anterior cingulate loops). Tasks that target selective circuits may also be used in activation studies to separate abnormalities in the DLPFC and anterior cingulate loops.

Cerebellum

The cerebellum is a critical but often neglected component of the motor system, with wide-ranging feedforward and feedbackward connections to the DLPFC and anterior cingulate circuits (Schmahmann and Pandya, 1997). This structure is increasingly recognized as contributing to cognitive and emotional functioning (Daum and Ackerman, 1995; Schmahmann, 1998) and possibly to the developmental psychopathology associated with ADHD (Berquin et al., 1998). Middleton and Strick (1994) demonstrated a link between the globus pallidus, cerebellum, and Brodmann area 46 in primates. This linkage suggests that the abnormalities found in the cerebellum, basal ganglia, and prefrontal cortex in ADHD may reflect a circuit-wide dysfunction in prefrontal–basal ganglia loops. Along these lines, Berquin et al. (1998) proposed, based on recent anatomic findings in children with ADHD, that cerebello–thalamo–prefrontal dysfunction may underlie the motor, inhibition, and executive function deficits that characterize ADHD.

Recent theories of cerebellar function point to a critical role in monitoring and adjusting the acquisition of multimodal sensory data in cognitive processes (Bower, 1997). Schmahmann's concept of cognitive "dysmetria" (Schmahmann and Pandya, 1997; Schmahmann, 1998; Schmahmann and Sherman, 1998), which proposes that the refinement of coordination imparted by the cerebellum to the motor system can also be applied to the regulation of ". . . [the] speed, capacity, consistency, and appropriateness of mental or cognitive processes", embraces many of the deficits characteristic of ADHD. This proposal is in agreement with the observation of Levinson (1990) of cerebellar-vestibular (CV) dysfunction in most learning disabled students (82.9%), who also exhibited ADD-like symptoms. Children and adults with ADHD have often been characterized as "clumsy" and "lacking social graces", features that may result from deficits in sensorimotor integration, reminiscent of symptoms produced by cerebellar lesions (Ratey and Johnson, 1997).

Two studies (Castellanos et al., 1996; Mostofsky et al., 1998) reported smaller cerebellar volumes in subjects with ADHD ($n = 57$; mean age 11.7 years; range 5.8–17.8 years; and $n = 12$; mean age 11.3 years, range 8.2–14.6 years) compared with controls ($n = 55$; mean age 12.0 years, range, 5.5–17.8 years; and $n = 23$; mean age 11.3 years, range 6.6–24.6 years). In addition, diminished overall vermal volume and posterior inferior lobe volume were observed in boys with ADHD (46; mean age 11.7 years) compared with normal controls (47; mean age 11.8 years) (Berquin et al., 1998).

Although the cerebellar findings reported by Berquin et al. (1998) primarily involved the posterior inferior lobules (VIII–X) of the vermis, recent functional imaging studies using $H_2^{15}O$ PET have indicated rCBF differences in the anterior vermial lobes of the cerebellum (I–V) in adults (Schweitzer et al., 1998). In this study, the main activation during a working memory task was in frontal and temporal regions in normal adults, and in the anterior vermis of the cerebellum in adults with ADHD. The cerebellar activation decreased after methylphenidate administration. The on-medication group was given methylphenidate for a minimum of 3 weeks at a dosage that resulted in significant clinical improvement, and this also improved performance on the working memory task.

In addition, preliminary findings using steady-state fMRI by one of the authors (C. Anderson, personal communication) indicate methylphenidate dose-dependent decreases in anterior vermis blood flow in two boys with ADHD with aggressive traits. The anterior vermis, termed the "limbic vermis" in light of its neuroanatomic and neurochemical connections with limbic structures (Snider and Maiti, 1976; Nieoullon et al., 1978; Dempsey and Richardson, 1987; Haines et al., 1997), has a long history of association with psychopathology states of aggression (Heath, 1992; Berman, 1997), autism (Kates et al., 1998), anxiety (Reiman, 1997), depression (Drevets, 1998), and schizophrenia (Andreasen et al., 1998). The recent interest (e.g., Middleton and Strick, 1994; Allen et al., 1997; Houk, 1997; Schmahmann and Pandya, 1997) in the roles of the cerebellum and basal ganglia in higher cognitive function should stimulate further basic work of relevance to the neurobiology of ADHD.

Hemispheric asymmetries and the corpus callosum

A number of hemispheric asymmetries that characterize normal brain anatomy, as well as deviations in the morphology of the corpus callosum (which contributes to brain lateralization), appear to be altered in ADHD. In healthy adults (19; aged 18–49 years), Peterson et al. (1993)

volumetrically reconstructed the basal ganglia and found that right-handed men and women had larger left total basal ganglia than did left-handed subjects, who demonstrated no asymmetry. Asymmetries favoring the right frontal lobe in normal subjects have also been reported (Weinberger et al., 1982). In children with ADHD, as discussed earlier, studies have noted abnormalities in caudate asymmetry (Hynd et al., 1993; Castellanos et al., 1996; Filipek et al., 1997).

Measurements of the cross-sectional area of the anterior corpus callosum are roughly proportional to the size of homotopic regions of the premotor and orbital prefrontal cortex and have been found to be significantly smaller in boys with ADHD than in controls (Giedd et al., 1994). The early work of Hynd et al. (1990, 1991) in single-slice axial measurements of the width of anterior cortical regions revealed a lack of normal asymmetry and a smaller anterior corpus callosum in boys with ADHD. Taken together, these studies suggest that the right cortico–striato–thalamic loop in children with ADHD may be dysfunctional and that hemispheric integration between right and left prefrontal dorsolateral and orbitofrontal cortical areas could be more limited.

Conclusion

This review of structural and functional anatomy related to ADHD suggests the involvement of cortico–striato–thalamo–cortical loops in ADHD. There is some indication of lateralization of dysfunction, although no clear consensus is evidenced. A much needed approach is the application of methods designed to examine functional interactions between various brain regions (Horwitz, 1998) to delineate more closely the neural circuits underlying the psychopathology. Another approach, briefly addressed above, is the use of therapeutic intervention in an attempt to reverse brain abnormalities as symptoms abate.

The dopaminergic hypothesis

Our understanding of ADHD can be furthered by testing theories of dopaminergic dysfunction in the disorder with neuroimaging techniques. In addition to the above imaging findings implicating the involvement of the basal ganglia in ADHD, the following observations support a dopaminergic hypothesis in ADHD: (i) ADHD symptomatology involves the motor and attentional systems that are known to be regulated by dopamine; (ii) stimulant medications, the treatment of choice of ADHD, enhance intrasynaptic dopamine concentrations; (iii) abnormal dopamine

metabolites in body fluids have been reported in individuals with ADHD, albeit inconsistently; (iv) animal models of ADHD based on dopaminergic dysfunction have been developed; (v) genetic linkage has been found between ADHD and dopaminergic genes, particularly the sevenfold repeat allele of the dopamine D_4 receptor gene (Solanto, 1984; Zametkin and Rapoport, 1987; Levy, 1991; for review see Ernst, 1998).

Although considerable evidence points to a role of the dopaminergic system in ADHD, the underlying mechanism remains unclear. PET methodology permits the direct examination of the dopaminergic function in vivo. Initial PET studies have used the tracer [18F]-fluorodopa (FDOPA).

Studies conducted by the same investigators using identical methodologies in adolescents with ADHD (Ernst et al., 1999) and adults with ADHD (Ernst et al., 1998) indicate dopaminergic abnormalities that are age dependent. In adolescents, the right midbrain FDOPA activity was significantly higher (48%) in ADHD (10, eight males, 2 females; mean age 13.8 ± 1.9 years) than in control subjects (10; seven males, three females; mean age 14.8 ± 1.7 years) (Ernst et al., 1999), suggesting abnormal dopamine synthesis or storage in the dopaminergic nuclei of children with ADHD. No other regions differed significantly between groups. Of note, the anterior medial frontal cortex FDOPA activity was 17% lower in the ADHD than the control adolescents. In adults, medial and lateral prefrontal FDOPA activity were, respectively, 52% and 51% lower in subjects with ADHD (significant difference; eight males, nine females; mean age 39.3 ± 6.2 years) than in healthy controls (13 males, 10 females; mean age 33.7 ± 10.5 years) (Ernst 1998). No other regions differed between groups. Taken together, these findings suggest a shift of dopaminergic dysfunction from the midbrain during adolescence to the anterior frontal cortex during adulthood, a finding in need of further investigation using a longitudinal design.

The authors hypothesized that ADHD is a progressive neurodevelopmental disorder in which the initial deficit is at the site of dopaminergic cell bodies (midbrain). This initial deficit progresses into a deficit in the prefrontal dopaminergic terminal field. Such a change with development is likely to result from interactions between (i) adaptive changes of ADHD symptoms (environmentally engendered, e.g., behaviorally or pharmacologically), (ii) normal brain physiologic changes (maturation, aging), (iii) hormonal influences, and (iv) genetic programs. The task of further identifying the molecular mechanisms underlying dopamine dysfunction represents an important next challenge.

Neurobehavioral probes

Another step in investigating ADHD using neuroimaging involves the use of cognitive/behavioral activation tasks that place demands on the neurobiochemical systems that are putatively dysfunctional in ADHD. Because this strategy offers great promise, we felt that a discussion of the cognitive/behavioral probes that are most appropriate in ADHD research may help the readers to understand better the factors critical to the choice of such activation tasks and may assist investigators in their choice of tasks for use in future imaging studies.

Task development

The tools (e.g., tasks) and models of brain functioning that can be applied to testing specific models of ADHD can be found in the psychologic (clinical, experimental, developmental, and neuropsychologic), neurologic, and psychiatric literature. Research based on normal and aberrant functioning in animal (e.g., Goldman-Rakic, 1987, 1995; Sagvolden et al., 1992; Ungerleider et al., 1998) and human models (Fiez et al., 1996; Braver et al., 1997; Cohen et al., 1997; O'Craven et al., 1997; Badgaiyan and Posner, 1998; Buchel et al., 1998) has produced behavioral and neuroanatomic predictions useful in the study of ADHD. The rapidly expanding field of cognitive neurosciences is responsible for the development of many tests of models that are applicable to ADHD.

A number of tasks may prove to be useful neurobehavioral probes to study ADHD in functional imaging paradigms. Many of these tasks have already been used in imaging studies or have potential for being easily altered for presentation in imaging studies (see Chapters 9, 21, and 22). The tasks described here have been selected because they have been shown to be reliably sensitive to behavioral deficits in ADHD or because they can be used to help to test specific behavioral and/or neuroanatomic models of ADHD (Table 16.4). Tasks and data from both the pediatric and adult literature will be presented. Many of them can be used in both adults and children (by adjusting difficulty level) and, thus, may also provide clues about the developmental changes in the expression of ADHD and compensatory skills.

Continuous Performance Tasks

Several CPTs have been used in functional neuroimaging studies of attention and frontal lobe function in normal subjects (Cohen et al., 1996), ADHD (Zametkin et al., 1990), and schizophrenia (O'Leary et al., 1996). CPTs are used frequently in research to assess deficits in sustained attention in individuals with ADHD. Generally, these vigilance tasks require the detection of target stimuli. A series of letters, numbers, or shapes are presented to subjects who are instructed to respond only to a predetermined target (e.g., the single letter "X") or to a sequence of targets (e.g., "AX", not "GX" or "FT"). Missed targets constitute omission errors and are interpreted as signs of inattention. Responses to nontargets constitute commission errors and measure impulsivity. In recent years, signal detection analyses have been applied to the CPT, yielding more elaborate performance measures (e.g., Conners, 1995). On an individual level, these tasks are not diagnostic of ADHD. However, numerous studies suggest that children with ADHD make significantly more errors of omission and commission than normal children (Corkum and Siegel, 1993; Losier et al., 1996). Errors are significantly reduced in children with ADHD when they are treated with methylphenidate (Losier et al., 1996).

A number of variables can influence the performance and level of difficulty of the CPTs. Research in normal control subjects suggests that auditory presentations are more difficult than visual presentations (Baker et al., 1995). CPTs that use shorter stimulus durations, relatively short interstimulus intervals, and a higher percentage of targets are better at discriminating between children with ADHD and normal control subjects (Corkum and Siegel, 1993). The presence of an experimenter in the room (as opposed to his/her absence) during CPT performance decreases the ability of CPTs to discriminate between control and subjects with ADHD (Draeger et al., 1986; van der Meere et al., 1995). The wide availability, extensive use, ease in application to imaging situations, and theoretical links between deficits in vigilance and ADHD made the CPTs an early favorite for functional imaging studies. However, changing conceptualizations of the deficits associated with ADHD suggest a need for additional neurobehavioral probes.

Working memory/short-term memory

As noted above, ADHD has been recently conceptualized as a disorder of behavioral inhibition that can produce deficits in short-term and working memory (Barkley, 1997a). The interest of cognitive neuroscientists in short-term memory has produced a proliferation of tasks that may prove useful in functional neuroimaging studies. Tasks of working memory require individuals to keep information on-line while manipulating new information (Baddeley, 1992; D'Esposito and Grossman, 1996). Many of the regions implicated in working memory studies are those hypothesized to be linked to ADHD, including prefrontal regions

Table 16.4. Neuroimaging probes for attention-deficit hyperactivity disorder

Task	Function	Normative Data Yes/No	Child (C)/Adult (A)	Adjustable levels of difficulty
Forward Digit Span (Wechsler Intelligence scale for children (WISC) and Wechsler Adult Intelligence scale (WAIS))	Auditory recall, working memory with longer strings	Yes	C and A	Not with norms, can increase or decrease string length
Backward digit span (WISC and WAIS)	Auditory working memory	Yes	C and A	Not with norms, can increase or decrease string length
Letter-Number Sequencing (WAIS)	Auditory working memory, sequencing	Yes	A	Not with norms, can increase or decrease string length
PASAT (Paced Auditory Serial Addition Task)	Auditory working memory, inhibition, observable active manipulation of stimuli	Yes	A	Yes
CHIPASAT (children's PASAT)	Auditory working memory, inhibition, observable active manipulation of stimuli	Yes, smaller sample	C	Yes
N-back	Short-term recall, working memory with longer delays and sequences, verbal and spatial tasks available	No, several studies available for comparison, however	C and A	Yes
CVLT (California Verbal Learning Test)	Verbal short-term recall	Yes	A	Not with norms
CVLT-C (children's version of CVLT)	Verbal short-term recall	Yes	C	Not with norms
Concentration Endurance Test (d2 test)	Selective attention, response inhibition	Yes	C and A	No
Continuous performance tests (CPTs)	Vigilance, sustained attention	Yes	C and A	Yes
Choice paradigms contrasting reward size and delays	Impulsivity, ability to evaluate reward size versus delay, integration of responding over time	No	C and A; easier in younger children	Yes by varying delays and reward size
Stop-signal task	Response inhibition	No	C and A	Yes
Go-no-go	Response inhibition	No	C and A	Yes
Counting Stroop task	Cognitive interference	No	A, could be used with older children	No
Tower of London	Planning	Yes	C and A (norms available for adults)	Yes

(e.g., D'Esposito et al., 1995; Braver et al., 1997) and cerebellum (Desmond et al., 1997). Theories regarding right hemisphere deficits (Heilman et al., 1991) in ADHD might be best tested using visuospatial working memory tasks, which activate preferentially right-hemisphere regions (Smith et al., 1995, 1996). Indeed, the ability to keep information on-line is more likely to activate the right prefrontal cortex than the left (Kapur et al., 1995).

The perceptual demands of the working memory task will also influence which regions and reciprocal connections are activated. Therefore, the selection of the sensory/cognitive modality of the memorized objects (cues) may also influence how well the task can test a specific neural model of ADHD. For example, color and object cues will more likely activate ventral prefrontal regions; spatial cues will more likely activate dorsal prefrontal regions (Martin et al., 1995; Ungerleider, 1995), and verbal cues will more likely activate left hemisphere regions (e.g., Broca's area; Smith et al., 1996). The specificity of the neural circuits underlying memory processes of different types of object is more complex and will not be further discussed here.

A number of working memory tests can be used in imaging paradigms. These tasks have excellent normative data and are sensitive to the behavioral impairment of ADHD. Examples include the backward repetition of digits on the Wechsler Intelligence Scale for Children-Third Edition (WISC-III; Wechsler, 1991) and the Wechsler Adult Intelligence Scale-Third Edition (WAIS-III; Tulsky et al., 1997), mental arithmetic problems, and the Paced Auditory Serial Addition Task (PASAT; Ackerman et al., 1986; Tannock et al., 1995; Barkley et al., 1996; Mariani and Barkley, 1997).

Performance by children with ADHD on the child version of the PASAT, the childrens' PASAT (CHIPASAT) has been found to be impaired and to improve after methylphenidate relative to placebo administration (Tannock et al., 1995). Adults diagnosed with current ADHD and childhood ADHD by self- and parent-report evidenced impairment on the PASAT (Schweitzer et al., 1998, 2000), in contrast with control subjects. Methylphenidate was found to ameliorate performance deficits in the subjects with ADHD (Schweitzer et al., 1998), resulting in equivalent performance to normal controls.

The PASAT (Gronwall, 1977; Stuss et al., 1987) is a particularly useful working memory task because of its ease of administration and the availability of both adult and child norms (Dyche and Johnson, 1991; Spreen and Strauss, 1991). It consists of a series of 50 single digit numbers (1 to 9) presented auditorily in different random sequences. Subjects are instructed to add each number to the preceding number and to verbalize each answer. The speed at which the numbers are delivered is consistent within each series with interstimulus intervals usually set at 2.8, 2.4, 2.0, 1.6, or 1.2 s. The level of difficulty has been found to increase for adults with ADHD at the 1.6 s interval (J. Schweitzer and C. D. Kilts, personal communication). The task can be readily readministered, permitting an evaluation of practice effects on rCBF.

The new WAIS-III (Tulsky et al., 1997) includes another working memory subtest that may prove to be useful in neuroimaging paradigms. The Letter-Number Sequencing subtest presents a random series of letters and numbers to the subject and requires the subject to sequentially reorganize the series by number first, into ascending order, and then by letters into alphabetical order. Presumably, this task could be used with children of elementary school age by presenting shorter series. However, norms are only currently available for individuals 16 years and older.

Short-term recall tests are memory tests that require less active manipulation of information than the PASAT or Letter-Number Sequencing, while still yielding relevant data. The working memory aspect is more inferred in these tests because the manipulation of the stimuli cannot be directly observed by the experimenter. These memory tasks have a temporal gap and/or distractor between the stimulus and response, and covert strategies are used by the subjects to maintain the memory of the stimulus before the response is required. These paradigms are often referred to as "n-back" or "item recognition tasks" (Sternberg, 1966). The subject typically has to recall a stimulus presented one to three trials back ("2-back" or "3-back" memory task) (Casey et al., 1995; Chapter 9). The length of the delay and the presentation of interfering stimuli during the delay are thought to increase the effort and need for subsidiary neural systems to help to remember the initial stimulus.

Spatial n-back tasks have been studied extensively in both primates (Wilson et al., 1993) and humans (e.g., Jonides et al., 1993; Courtney et al., 1998), providing a solid basis with which to interpret results. Spatial memory tasks may be particularly well-suited for testing theories that link ADHD to right-hemisphere dysfunction. PET investigations that have compared working memory tasks using spatial stimuli with those using object and verbal stimuli have found activations for the spatial memory tasks primarily in the right hemisphere and activations for object and verbal memory tasks primarily in the left hemisphere (Smith et al., 1995, 1996). Descriptions of spatial tasks can be found in the work of Goldman-Rakic and her colleagues (e.g., Goldman-Rakic, 1987; Funahashi et al., 1989) and Smith and his colleagues (Smith et al., 1995, 1996).

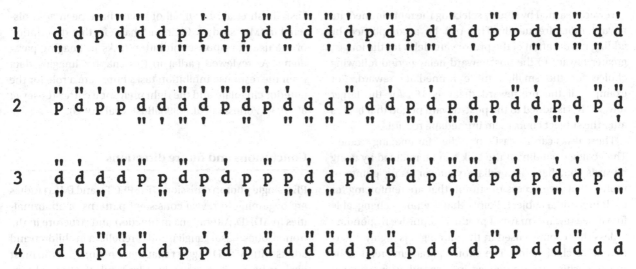

Fig. 16.2. Sample of stimuli presented in the Concentration Endurance Test (d2 Test of Attention; Brickenkamp, 1981). Subjects are instructed to identify the letter "d" with two marks above, below, or separated by the letter with one mark below and mark above the letter.

Other short-term memory tests with excellent normative data are available for use in imaging studies. Children with ADHD have been shown to have significant difficulty performing short-term memory tests involving the repetition of numbers (forward digit span) (WISC-III, (Wechsler, 1991)) and the identification of spatial locations (Milich and Loney, 1979; Anastopoulos et al., 1994). The children's version of the California Verbal Learning Test (CVLT-C; Delis et al., 1994), a word list learning task, has normative data for children and may also be sensitive to deficits in ADHD. Adults with ADHD perform poorly on the Digit Span subtest of the WAIS-III (Tulsky et al., 1997) and on verbal list learning and sequencing in tests such as the California Verbal Learning Test (CVLT; Delis et al., 1994; Downey et al., 1997; Holdnack et al., 1995).

Cancellation tests of attention

The Concentration Endurance Test (d2 Test; Brickenkamp, 1981) may be useful in testing prefrontal models of ADHD (Fig. 16.2). The cancellation task assesses the capacity for maintaining attention, accurate visual scanning, and activation and inhibition of rapid responses. It could easily be modified for PET or fMRI imaging paradigms. Low scores on cancellation tasks may reflect difficulty filtering out irrelevant stimuli, general response slowing, poor shifting of responses, or unilateral spatial neglect. In this task, 14 lines of randomly sequenced letters "p" and "d" are presented. The target is the letter "d" with two marks above, below, or one mark below and one mark above the letter.

Distractors include the letter "d" with one, three, or four marks or the letter "p" with one to four marks in any arrangement. The subject is instructed to identify targets as quickly as possible with a limit of 20 s per line. This commercially available test provides normative data from large samples, ages 9–60 years ($n = 3132$), including norms for practice effects (Brickenkamp, 1981; Spreen and Strauss, 1991).

Impulsivity

Problems in impulsivity appear to be one of the core deficits of ADHD (Barkley, 1990). Choice paradigms have been used successfully to detect significant differences in impulsivity between children with and without ADHD (Rapport et al., 1986; Sonuga-Barke et al., 1992; Schweitzer and Sulzer-Azaroff, 1996). Preferences for smaller, more immediate rewards over larger, delayed rewards are defined as "impulsive" responses (i.e., the converse of self-control; Ainslie, 1974). Variations of these paradigms have assessed the subject's ability to choose the most advantageous (i.e., the greatest payoff) response within a trial or over several trials within a session using money, points, or small toys as the rewards. Schweitzer and Sulzer-Azaroff (1996) were able to demonstrate differences in responding between 5- and 6-year-old boys with and without ADHD using delays of 16 s for the larger reward (three nickels) versus 0 s for the smaller reward (one nickel). The session length and number of trials need to be held constant in these tasks so that subjects cannot maximize the amount of rewards earned by simply selecting the more immediate reward more frequently. This can be accomplished by adding the duration of the pre-reward delay for the longer, greater reward to the post-reward delay period following choice for the smaller, more immediate reward. For example, if the pre-reward delay is 16s for the larger reward, 16s is added to the post-reward period that occurs after the subject chooses an immediate reward.

These tasks can be easily modified for imaging studies. The ecologic validity of the task can be retained by using rewards that have immediate value or using points or money that give access to stimuli that are reinforcing for each individual subject. Points that are not exchangeable for valued rewards may not produce impulsive responding unless the response used in the paradigm is highly entertaining or challenging. The choice paradigms tend to be most sensitive to differences in responding in younger children, and it may be difficult to elicit impulsive responding in these paradigms in adolescents and adults with ADHD, depending on the type of reward used.

Impulsive responding in delay-choice tasks may reflect difficulty in integrating and evaluating behavioral responses over time (Fuster, 1997). Fuster (1997) proposed a theory of prefrontal lobe function that suggests that attainment of long-term goals is dependent on the ability to integrate behavioral responses over time. According to Fuster, reward tasks with a delay can assess how successful an organism will be at inhibiting impulsive behavior by linking single behavioral units into chains of behavioral units directed toward fulfilling long-term goals. Lesions in the dorsolateral prefrontal cortex are associated with impaired performance on delayed response tasks that could reflect an inability to integrate behavioral sequences over time (Fuster, 1997). Therefore, it can be hypothesized that choice for the smaller, more immediate rewards seen in children with ADHD are associated with functional impairment in the dorsolateral prefrontal cortex.

Tasks of response inhibition

Whereas reward/delay tasks assess one aspect of impulsivity, tasks of response inhibition measure another aspect of self-control deficits in ADHD. Poor response inhibition in children with ADHD has been consistently noted in behavioral descriptions of the disorder (Still, 1902; Quay, 1988; Iaboni et al., 1995; Denckla, 1996; Barkley, 1997a,b). In general, response inhibition tasks instruct subjects to inhibit responding to particular stimuli. Variations of these tasks include the go-no-go paradigm (Casey et al., 1997a), the stop–signal paradigm (i.e., Schachar et al., 1995; Pliszka et al., 1997; Ponesse et al., 1998), and the Counting Stroop

Task (Bush et al., 1999), all of which have been administered in fMRI studies. Chapter 9 has a further description of the use of response inhibition tasks in imaging paradigms. As reviewed earlier in this chapter, imaging data from the response inhibition tasks implicate a role for the anterior cingulate and the right prefrontal cortex (Casey et al., 1995; Ponesse et al., 1998; Bush et al., 1999).

Conclusions and future directions

PET, single photon emission CT (SPECT), and fMRI studies are beginning to reveal consistent patterns of abnormalities in ADHD. Alterations in function and structure in the frontal lobes, basal ganglia, and cerebellum in children and adults with ADHD suggest that these regions are the most likely to be involved in the disorder. While the general consistency between studies is promising, there remains substantial variability from study to study regarding the involvement and role of specific brain regions, and further replication is crucial. Issues related to circuitry and the examination of functional interactions among brain regions using neuroimaging (e.g., Horwitz, 1998) will undoubtedly enhance our understanding of ADHD.

The heterogeneous nature of the existing studies with respect to clinical symptoms, imaging techniques and conditions, age of the subjects, and perhaps medication history are likely to account for some of the variability in findings. One of the major limitations to the generalization of the current findings is the variability in the clinical and diagnostic characterization of ADHD and the nature of the control groups both within and across studies. In the future, researchers will need to use more rigorous methods to diagnose subjects with ADHD (e.g., inter-rater reliability between diagnosticians) and to characterize their control groups. Researchers will need to be more explicit in their descriptions of the severity and type of symptom present and to rely on objective measures of behavioral traits. Research reports also need to be consistent in detailing the presence or absence of comorbid psychiatric disorders in subjects with ADHD. Subtyping of ADHD is also essential, with studies examining differences and similarities in brain functional activity between subjects with the inattentive, hyperactive/impulsive, or combined types of ADHD. Relationships between ADHD and learning disabilities, such as dyslexia, should also be examined using functional neuroimaging because of the significant clinical overlap of these disorders (Barkley, 1990). In conclusion, we anticipate significant progress in understanding ADHD through the use of improved methodologic rigor and the application of novel imaging techniques.

Acknowledgements

Julie Schweitzer was supported in part by the National Institutes of Mental Health (NIMH) K08MH-01053, and Carl Anderson by NIMH R01MH-53636-01 (Principal Investigator: M. Teicher).

References

Ackerman, P. T., Anhalt, J. M. and Dykman, R. A. (1986). Arithmetic automatization failure in children with attention and reading disorders: associations and sequela. *J. Learn. Disabil.*, **19**, 222–32.

Ainslie, G. W. (1974). Impulse control in pigeons. *J. Exp. Anal. Behav.*, **21**, 485–9.

Alexander, G. E., de Long, M. R. and Strick, P. L. (1986). Parallel organization of functionally segregated circuits linking basal ganglia and cortex. *Annu. Rev. Neurosci.*, **9**, 357–81.

Alexander, G., Crutcher, M. and DeLong, M. (1990). Basal ganglia-thalamocortical circuits: parallel substrates for motor, oculomotor, 'prefrontal' and 'limbic' functions. *Prog. Brain Res.*, **85**, 119–46.

Allen, G., Buxton, R. B., Wong, E. C. and Courchesne, E. (1997). Attentional activation of the cerebellum independent of motor involvement. *Science*, **275**, 1940–3.

American Psychiatric Association (1994). *Diagnostic and Statistical Manual of Mental Disorders*, 4th edn. Washington, DC: American Psychiatric Association.

Anastopoulos, A., Spisto, M. and Maher, M. (1994). The WISC-III freedom from distractibility factor: its utility in identifying children with attention deficit hyperactivity disorder. *Psychol. Assess.*, **2**, 368–71.

Andreasen, N. C., O'Leary, D. S., Arndt, S. et al. (1995). Short-term and long-term verbal memory: a positron emission tomography study. *Proc. Natl. Acad. Sci. USA*, **92**, 5111–15.

Andreasen, N. C., Paradiso, S. and O'Leary, D. S. (1998). 'Cognitive dysmetria' as an integrative theory of schizophrenia: a dysfunction in cortical-subcortical-cerebellar circuitry? *Schizophr. Bull.*, **24**, 203–18.

Aylward, E., Reiss, A., Reader, M., Singer, H., Brown, J. and Denckla, M. (1996). Basal ganglia volumes in children with attention-deficit hyperactivity disorder. *J. Child Neurol.*, **11**, 112–15.

Baddeley, A. (1992). Working memory. *Science*, **255**, 556–9.

Badgaiyan, R. D. and Posner, M. I. (1998). Mapping the cingulate cortex in response selection and monitoring. *Neuroimage*, **7**, 255–60.

Baker, D. B., Taylor, C. J. and Leyva, C. (1995). Continuous performance tests: a comparison of modalities. *J. Clin. Psychol.*, **51**, 548–51.

Barkley, R. A. (1990). *Attention Deficit Hyperactivity Disorder*. New York: Guildford Press.

Barkley, R. A. (1997a). Behavioral inhibition, sustained attention, and executive functions: constructing a unifying theory of ADHD. *Psychol. Bull.*, **121**, 65–94.

Barkley, R. A. (1997b). Attention-deficit/hyperactivity disorder, self-regulation, and time: toward a more comprehensive theory. *J. Dev. Behav. Pediatr.*, **18**, 271–9.

Barkley, R. A., Fischer, M., Edelbrock, C. S. and Smallish, L. (1990). The adolescent outcome of hyperactive children diagnosed by research criteria. I: an 8-year prospective follow-up study. *J. Am. Acad. Child Adolesc. Psychiatry*, **29**, 546–57.

Barkley, R. A., Murphy, K. R. and Kwasnik, D. (1996). Psychological adjustment and adaptive impairments in young adults with ADHD. *J. Attent. Disord.*, **1**, 41–54.

Bergman, H., Feingold, A., Nini, A. (1998). Physiological aspects of information processing in the basal ganglia of normal and parkinsonian primates. *Trends Neurosci.*, **21**, 32–8.

Berman, A. J. (1997). Amelioration of aggression: response to selective cerebellar lesions in the rhesus monkey. *Int. Rev. Neurobiol.*, **41**, 111–19.

Berquin, P. C., Giedd, J. N., Jacobsen, L. K. et al. (1998). Cerebellum in attention-deficit hyperactivity disorder: a morphometric MRI study. *Neurology*, **50**, 1087–93.

Biederman, J., Faraone, S. V., Spencer, T. et al. (1993). Patterns of psychiatric comorbidity, cognition, and psychosocial functioning in adults with attention deficit hyperactivity disorder. *Am. J. Psychiatry*, **150**, 1792–8.

Bower, J. M. (1997). Control of sensory data acquisition. *Int. Rev. Neurobiol.*, **41**, 489–513.

Braver, T. S., Cohen, J. D., Nystrom, L. E., Jonides, J., Smith, E. E. and Noll, D. C. (1997). A parametric study of prefrontal cortex involvement in human working memory. *Neuroimage*, **5**, 49–62.

Brickenkamp, R. (1981). Test d2: Aufmerksamkeits-Belastungs-Test [Test d2: Concentration-Endurance Test: Manual], 5 edn. Götteningen: Verlag für Psychologie.

Brown, L. L., Smith, D. M. and Goldbloom, L. M. (1998). Organizing principles of cortical integration in the rat neostriatum: corticostriate map of the body surface is an ordered lattice of curved laminae and radial points. *J. Comp. Neurol.*, **392**, 468–88.

Buchel, C., Josephs, O., Rees, G., Turner, R., Frith, C. D. and Friston, K. J. (1998). The functional anatomy of attention to visual motion. A functional MRI study. *Brain*, **121**, 1281–94.

Bush, G., Frazier, J. A., Rauch, S. L. et al. (1999). Anterior cingulate cortex dysfunction in attention deficit/hyperactivity disorder revealed by fMRI and the counting Stroop. *Biol. Psychiatry*, **45**, 1542–52.

Casey, B. J., Cohen, J. D., Jezzard, P. et al. (1995). Activation of prefrontal cortex in children during a nonspatial working memory task with functional MRI. *Neuroimage*, **2**, 221–9.

Casey, B. J., Castellanos, F., Giedd, J. et al. (1997a). Implication of right frontostriatal circuitry in response inhibition and attention-deficit/hyperactivity disorder. *J. Am. Acad. Child Adolesc. Psychiatry*, **36**, 374–83.

Casey, B. J., Trainor, R., Giedd, et al. (1997b). The role of the anterior cingulate in automatic and controlled processes: a developmental neuroanatomical study. *Dev. Psychobiol.*, **30**, 61–9.

Castellanos, F., Giedd, J., Marsh, W. et al. (1996). Quantitative brain magnetic resonance imaging in attention-deficit hyperactivity disorder. *Arch. Gen. Psychiatry*, 53, 607–16.

Cohen, J. D., Perlstein, W. M., Braver, T. S. et al. (1997). Temporal dynamics of brain activation during a working memory task. *Nature*, 386, 604–8.

Cohen, M., Kosslyn, S., Breiter, H. et al. (1996). Changes in cortical activity during mental rotation. A mapping study using functional MRI. *Brain*, 119, 89–100.

Conners, C. K. (1995). *Connors' Continuous Performance Test: User's Manual*. Toronto: Multi-Health Systems.

Corkum, P. V. and Siegel, L. S. (1993). Is the continuous performance task a valuable research tool for use with children with attention-deficit-hyperactivity disorder? *J. Child Psychol. Psychiatry*, 34, 1217–39.

Courtney, S. M., Petit, L., Maisog, J. M., Ungerleider, L. G. and Haxby, J. V. (1998). An area specialized for spatial working memory in human frontal cortex. *Science*, 279, 1347–51.

Daum, I. and Ackerman, H. (1995). Cerebellar contributions to cognition. *Behav. Brain Res.*, 67, 201–10.

Delis, D. C. Kramer, J. H., Kaplan, E. and Ober, B. A. (1994). *The California Verbal Learning Test – Children's Version*. San Antonio, TX: The Psychological Corporation, Harcourt Brace.

Dempsey, C. W. and Richardson, D. E. (1987). Paleocerebellar stimulation induces in vivo release of endogenously synthesized [³H]dopamine and [³H]norepinephrine from rat caudal dorsomedial nucleus accumbens. *Neuroscience*, 21, 565–71.

Denckla, M. B. (1996). Biological correlates of learning and attention: what is relevant to learning disability and attention-deficit hyperactivity disorder? *J. Dev. Behav. Pediatr.*, 17, 114–19.

Desmond, J. E., Gabrieli, J. D., Wagner, A. D., Ginier, B. L. and Glover, G. H. (1997). Lobular patterns of cerebellar activation in verbal working-memory and finger-tapping tasks as revealed by functional MRI. *J. Neurosci.*, 17, 9675–85.

D'Esposito, M. and Grossman, M. (1996). The physiological basis of executive function and working memory. *Neuroscientist*, 2, 345–52.

D'Esposito, M., Detre, J. A., Alsop, D. C., Shin, R. K., Atlas, S. and Grossman, M. (1995). The neural basis of the central executive system of working memory. *Nature*, 378, 279–81.

Downey, K. K., Stelson, F. W., Pomerleau, O. F. and Giordoni, B. (1997). Adult attention deficit hyperactivity disorder: psychological test profiles in a clinical population. *J. Nerv. Mental Dis.*, 185, 32–8.

Draeger, S., Prior, M. and Sanson, A. (1986). Visual and auditory attention performance in hyperactive children: competence or compliance. *J. Abnorm. Child Psychol.*, 14, 411–24.

Drevets, W. C. (1998). Functional neuroimaging studies of depression: the anatomy of melancholia. *Annu. Rev. Med.*, 49, 341–61.

Dyche, G. M. and Johnson, D. A. (1991). Development and evaluation of CHIPASAT, an attention test for children. II. Test–retest reliability and practice effect for a normal sample. *Percept. Mot. Skills*, 72, 563–72.

Ernst, M. (1998). Dopaminergic function in ADHD. In *Proceedings of the IBC International Symposium on Dopaminergic Disorders*, pp. 235–60.

Ernst, M., Liebenauer, L., Fitzgerald, G., Cohen, R. and Zametkin, A. J. (1994a). Reduced brain metabolism in hyperactive girls. *J. Am. Acad. Child Adolesc. Psychiatry*, 33, 858–68.

Ernst, M., Zametkin, A. J., Matochik, J. A., Liebenauer, L., Fitzgerald, G. A. and Cohen, R. M. (1994b). Effects of intravenous dextroamphetamine on brain metabolism in adults with attention-deficit hyperactivity disorder (ADHD). Preliminary findings. *Psychopharmacol. Bull.*, 30, 219–25.

Ernst, M., Cohen, R. M., Liebenauer, L. L., Jons, P. H. and Zametkin, A. J. (1997a). Cerebral glucose metabolism in adolescent girls with attention-deficit/hyperactivity disorder. *J. Am. Acad. Child Adolesc. Psychiatry*, 36, 1399–406.

Ernst, M., Zametkin, A. J. Matochik, J. A., Jons, P. H. and Cohen, R. M. (1998). DOPA decarboxylase activity in attention deficit hyperactivity disorder adults. A [fluorine-18]fluorodopa positron emission tomographic study. *J. Neurosci.* 18, 5901–7.

Ernst, M., Zametkin, A. J., Matochik, J. et al. (1997b). Intravenous dextroamphetamine and brain glucose metabolism. *Neuropsychopharmacology*, 17, 391–401.

Ernst, M., Zametkin, A. J., Matochik, J. A., Pascualvaca, D., Jons, P. H. and Cohen, R. M. (1999). High midbrain [¹⁸F]DOPA accumulation in children with attention deficit hyperactivity disorder. *Am. J. Psychiatry*, 156, 1209–15.

Fiez, J. A., Raife, E. A., Balota, D. A., Schwarz, J. P., Raichle, M. E. and Petersen, S. E. (1996). A positron emission tomography study of the short-term maintenance of verbal information. *J. Neurosci.*, 16, 808–22.

Filipek, P., Semrud-Clikeman, M., Steingard, R., Renshaw, P. and Kennedy, D. (1997). Volumetric MRI analysis comparing subjects having attention-deficit hyperactivity disorder with normal controls. *Neurology*, 48, 589–601.

Flowers, D. L., Wood, F. B., Price, N. J. and Absher, J. R. (1997). Regional cerebral blood flow and brain metabolism in adults with childhood diagnosed with attention deficit disorder. *Soc. Neurosci. Abst.*, 23, 1837.

Funahashi, S., Bruce, C. J., Goldman-Rakic, P. S. (1989). Mnemonic coding of visual space in the monkey's dorsolateral prefrontal cortex. *J. Neurophysiol.*, 61, 331–49.

Fuster, J. M. (1997). *The Prefrontal Cortex: Anatomy, Physiology, and Neuropsychology of the Frontal Lobe*, 3rd edn. New York: Lippencott-Raven.

Giedd, J. N., Castellanos, F. X., Casey, B. J. et al. (1994). Quantitative morphology of the corpus callosum in attention deficit hyperactivity disorder. *Am. J. Psychiatry*, 151, 665–9.

Goldman-Rakic, P. S. (1987). Circuitry of primate prefrontal cortex and regulation of behavior by representational memory. In *Handbook of Physiology*, ed. F. Blum, pp. 373–417. Bethesda, MD: American Physiological Society.

Goldman-Rakic, P. S. (1995). Architecture of the prefrontal cortex and the central executive. *Ann. N. Y. Acad. Sci.*, 769, 71–83.

Graybiel, A. M., Aosaki, T., Flaherty, A. W. and Kimura, M. (1994). The basal ganglia and adaptive motor control. *Science*, 265, 1826–31.

Gronwall, D. (1977). Paced auditory serial addition task: a measure of recovery from concussion. *Percep. Mot. Skills*, 44, 367–73.

Haines, D. E., Dietrichs, E., Mihailoff, G. A. and McDonald, E. F.

(1997). The cerebellar–hypothalamic axis: basic circuits and clinical observations. *Int. Rev. Neurobiol.*, **41**, 83–107.

Heath, R. G. (1992). Correlation of brain activity with emotion: a basis for developing treatment of violent-aggressive behavior. *J. Am. Acad. Psychoanal.*, **20**, 335–46.

Heilman, K., Voeller, K. and Nadeau, S. (1991). A possible pathophysiological substrate of attention deficit hyperactivity disorder. *J. Child Neurol.*, **6**, 74–9.

Heimer, L., Alheid, G. F., de Olmos, J. S. et al. (1997). The accumbens: beyond the core-shell dichotomy. *J. Neuropsychiatry Clin. Neurosci.*, **9**, 354–81.

Holdnack, J., Moberg, P., Arnold, S. and Gur, R. (1995). Speed of processing and verbal learning deficits in adults diagnosed with attention deficit disorder. *Neuropsychiatry, Neuropsychol. Behav. Neurol.*, **8**, 282–92.

Horwitz, B. (1998). Using functional imaging to understand human cognition. *Complexity*, **3**, 39–52.

Houk, J. C. (1997). On the role of the cerebellum and basal ganglia in cognitive signal processing. *Prog. Brain Res.*, **114**, 543–52.

Hynd, G. W., Semrud-Clikeman, M., Lorys, A. R., Novey, E. S. and Eliopulos, D. (1990). Brain morphology in developmental dyslexia and attention deficit disorder/hyperactivity. *Arch. Neurol.*, **47**, 919–26.

Hynd, G. W., Semrud-Clikeman, M., Lorys, A. R., Novey, E. S., Eliopulos, D. and Lyytinen, H. (1991). Corpus callosum morphology in attention deficit-hyperactivity disorder: morphometric analysis of MRI. *J. Learn. Disabl.*, **24**, 141–6.

Hynd, G. W., Hern, K., Novey, et al. (1993). Attention deficit hyperactivity disorder and asymmetry of the caudate nucleus. *J. Child Neurol.*, **8**, 339–47.

Iaboni, F., Douglas, V. I. and Baker, A. G. (1995). Effects of reward and response costs on inhibition in ADHD children. *J. Abnorm. Psychol.*, **104**, 232–40.

Jonides, J., Smith, E. E., Koeppe, R. A., Awh, E., Minoshima, S. and Mintun, M. A. (1993). Spatial working memory in humans as revealed by PET. *Nature*, **363**, 623–5.

Kapur, S., Craik, F., Jones, C., Brown, G., Houle, S. and Tulving, E. (1995). Functional role of the prefrontal cortex in retrieval of memories: a PET study. *Neuroreport*, **6**, 1880–4.

Kates, W. R., Mostofsky, S. H., Zimmerman, A. W. et al. (1998). Neuroanatomical and neurocognitive differences in a pair of monozygous twins discordant for strictly defined autism. *Ann. Neurol.*, **43**, 782–91.

Levinson, H. N. (1990). The diagnostic value of cerebellar-vestibular tests in detecting learning disabilities, dyslexia, and attention deficit disorder. *Percept. Mot. Skills*, **71**, 67–82.

Levy, F. (1991). The dopamine theory of attention deficit hyperactivity disorder (ADHD). *Aust. N. Z. J. Psychiatry*, **25**, 277–383.

Losier, B. J., McGrath, P. J. and Klein, R. M. (1996). Error patterns on the continuous performance test in non-medicated and medicated samples of children with and without ADHD: a meta-analytic review. *J. Child Psychol. Psychiatry*, **37**, 971–87.

Lou, H., Henriksen, L. and Bruhn, P. (1984). Focal cerebral hypoperfusion in children with dysphasia and/or attention deficit disorder. *Arch. Neurol.*, **41**, 825–9.

Lou, H., Henriksen, L., Bruhn, P., Borner, H. and Nielsen, J. (1989). Striatal dysfunction in attention deficit and hyperkinetic disorder. *Arch. Neurol.*, **46**, 48–52.

Lou, H., Henriksen, L. and Bruhn, P. (1990). Focal cerebral dysfunction in developmental learning disabilities. *Lancet*, **335**, 8–11.

Mannuzza, S., Klein, R. G., Bessler, A., Malloy, P. and La Padula, M. (1998). Adult psychiatric status of hyperactive boys grown up. *Am. J. Psychiatry*, **155**, 493–8.

Mariani, M. and Barkley, R. (1997). Neuropsychological and academic functioning in preschool boys with attention deficit hyperactivity disorder. *Dev. Neuropsychol.*, **13**, 111–29.

Martin, A., Haxby, J. V., Lalonde, F. M., Wiggs, C. L. and Ungerleider, L. G. (1995). Discrete cortical regions associated with knowledge of color and knowledge of action. *Science*, **270**, 102–5.

Matochik, J. A., Nordahl, T. E., Gross, M. et al. (1993). Effects of acute stimulant medication on cerebral metabolism in adults with hyperactivity. *Neuropsychopharmacology*, **8**, 377–86.

Matochik, J., Liebenauer, L., King, C., Szymanski, H., Cohen, R. and Zametkin, A. (1994). Cerebral glucose metabolism in adults with attention deficit hyperactivity disorder after chronic stimulant treatment. *Am. J. Psychiatry*, **151**, 658–64.

Mega, M. S. and Cummings, J. L. (1994). Frontal-subcortical circuits and neuropsychiatric disorders. *J. Neuropsychiatry Clin. Neurosci.*, **6**, 358–70.

Middleton, F. A. and Strick, P. L. (1994). Anatomical evidence for cerebellar and basal ganglia involvement in higher cognitive function. *Science*, **266**, 458–61.

Milich, R. and Loney, J. (1979). The factor composition of the WISC for hyperkinetic/MBD males. *J. Learn. Disab.*, **12**, 67–70.

Mostofsky, S. H., Reiss, A. L., Lockhart, P. and Denckla, M. B. (1998). Evaluation of cerebellar size in attention-deficit hyperactivity disorder. *J. Child Neurol.*, **13**, 434–9.

Murphy, K. R. and Barkley, R. A. (1996). ADHD adults: comorbidities and adaptive impairments. *Compr. Psychiatry*, **37**, 393–401.

Murtha, S., Chertkow, H., Beauregard, M., Dixon, R. and Evans, A. (1996). Anticipation causes increased blood flow to the anterior cingulate cortex. *Hum. Brain Map.*, **4**, 103–12.

Nieoullon, A., Cheramy, A. Glowinski, J. (1978). Release of dopamine in both caudate nuclei and both substantia nigra in response to unilateral stimulation of cerebellar nuclei in the cat. *Brain Res.*, **148**, 143–52.

O'Craven, K. M., Rosen, B. R., Kwong, K. K., Treisman, A. and Savoy, R. L. (1997). Voluntary attention modulates fMRI activity in human MT-MST. *Neuron*, **18**, 591–8.

O'Leary, D. S., Andreasen, N. C., Hurtig, R. R. et al. (1996). Auditory attentional deficits in patients with schizophrenia. A positron emission tomography study. *Arch. Gen. Psychiatry*, **53**, 633–41.

Peterson, B. S., Riddle, M. A., Cohen, D. J., Katz, L. D., Smith, J. C. and Leckman, J. F. (1993). Human basal ganglia volume asymmetries on magnetic resonance images. *Magn. Reson. Imaging*, **1**, 493–8.

Peterson, B. S., Skudlarski, P., Anderson, A. W. et al. (1998). A functional magnetic resonance imaging study of tic suppression in Tourette syndrome. *Arch. Gen. Psychiatry*, **55**, 326–33.

Pliszka, S. R., Borcherding, S. H., Spratley, K., Leon, S. and Irick, S. (1997). Measuring inhibitory control in children. *J. Dev. Behav. Pediatr.*, **18**, 254–9.

Ponesse, J. S., Logan, W. J., Schachar, R. S., Tannock, R., Crawley, A. P. and Mikulus, D. J. (1998). Functional neuroimaging of the inhibition of a motor response. In *Proceedings of an International Conference on Functional Mapping of the Human Brain*, Montreal, Canada.

Quay, H. C. (1988). The behavioral reward and inhibition systems in childhood behavior disorder. In *Attention Deficit Disorder*: III. *New Research in Treatment, Psychopharmacology, and Attention*, ed. L. M. Bloomingdale, pp. 176–86. New York: Pergammon Press.

Rapport, M. D., Tucker, S. B., DuPaul, G. J., Merlo, M. and Stoner, G. (1986). Hyperactivity and frustration: the influence of control over and size of rewards in delaying gratification. *J. Abnorm. Child Psychol.*, **14**, 191–204.

Ratey, J. and Johnson, C. (1997). *Shadow Syndromes: The Mild Forms of Major Mental Disorders That Sabotage Us.* New York: Bantam.

Rauch, S. L. and Savage, C. R. (1997). Neuroimaging and neuropsychology of the striatum. Bridging basic science and clinical practice. *Psychiatr. Clin. North Am.*, **20**, 741–68.

Reiman, E. M. (1997). The application of positron emission tomography to the study of normal and pathologic emotions. *J. Clin. Psychiatry*, **58**, 4–12.

Rubia, K., Overmeyer, S., Taylor, E. et al. (1999). Hypofrontality in attention deficit hyperactivity disorder during higher-order motor control: a study with functional MRI. *Am. J. Psychiatry*, **156**, 891–6.

Sagvolden, T., Metzger, M. A., Schiorbeck, H. K., Rugland, A. L., Spinnangr, I. and Sagvolden, G. (1992). The spontaneously hypertensive rat (SHR) as an animal model of childhood hyperactivity (ADHD): changed reactivity to reinforcers and to psychomotor stimulants. *Behav. Neural. Biol.*, **58**, 103–12.

Schachar, R., Tannock, R., Marriott, M. and Logan, G. (1995). Deficient inhibitory control in attention deficit hyperactivity disorder. *J. Abnorm. Child Psychol.*, **23**, 411–37.

Schmahmann, J. D. (1998). Dysmetria of thought: clinical consequences of cerebellar dysfunction on cognition and affect. *Trends Cogn. Sci.*, **2**, 362–71.

Schmahmann, J. D. and Pandya, D. N. (1997). The cerebrocerebellar system. *Int. Rev. Neurobiol.*, **41**, 31–60.

Schmahmann, J. D. and Sherman, J. C. (1998). The cerebellar cognitive affective syndrome. *Brain*, **121**, 561–79.

Schweitzer, J. B. and Sulzer-Azaroff, B. (1996). Self-control in boys with attention deficit hyperactivity disorder: effects of distractors and time. *J. Child Psychol. Psychiatr. Allied Disciplines*, **36**, 671–86.

Schweitzer, J. B., Lee, D. O., Ely, T. D. et al. (1998). The effects of methylphenidate on the functional neuroanatomy of working memory in ADHD. *Soc. Neurosci. Abst.*, **24**, 958.

Schweitzer, J. B., Faber, T. L., Grafton, S. T., Tune, L. E., Hoffman, J. M., Kilts, C. D. (2000). Alterations in the functional anatomy of working memory in adult-attention deficit/hyperactivity disorder. *Am. J. Psychiatry*, **157**, 278–80.

Smith, E. E., Jonides, J., Koeppe, R. A. et al. (1995). Spatial versus object working memory: PET investigations. *J. Cogn. Neurosci.*, **7**, 337–56.

Smith, E. E., Jonides, J. and Koeppe, R. A. (1996). Dissociating verbal and spatial working memory using PET. *Cereb. Cortex*, **6**, 11–20.

Smith, Y., Bevan, M. D., Shink, E. and Bolam, J. P. (1998). Microcircuitry of the direct and indirect pathways of the basal ganglia. *Neuroscience*, **86**, 353–87.

Snider, R. S. and Maiti, A. (1976). Cerebellar contributions to the Papez circuit. *J. Neurosci. Res.*, **2**, 133–46.

Solanto, M. V. (1984). Neuropharmacological basis of stimulant drug action in attention deficit disorder with hyperactivity: a review and synthesis. *Psychol. Bull.*, **95**, 387–409.

Sonuga-Barke, E. J., Taylor, E., Sembi, S. and Smith, J. (1992). Hyperactivity and delay aversion – I. The effect of delay on choice. *J. Child Psychol. Psychiatry*, **33**, 387–98.

Spreen, O. and Strauss, E. (1991). *A Compendium of Neuropsychological Tests: Administration, Norms, and Commentary.* New York: Oxford University Press.

Steinberg, B., McLaughlin, T., Lou, H. C., Andresen, J. and Friberg, L. (1998). Anterior cingulate and supramodal attention in ADHD children. In *Proceedings of an International Conference on Functional Mapping of the Human Brain*, Montreal, Canada.

Sternberg, S. (1966). High-speed scanning in human memory. *Science*, **153**, 652–4.

Still, G. F. (1902). Some abnormal psychical conditions in children. *Lancet*, i:1008–12, 1077–82, 1163–80.

Stuss, D. T., Stetham, L. L. and Poirier, C. A. (1987). Three tests of attention and rapid information processing: an extension. *Clin. Neuropsychol.*, **2**, 246–50.

Szatmari, P., Offord, D. R. and Boyle, M. H. (1989). Ontario Child Health Study: prevalence of attention deficit disorder with hyperactivity. *J. Child Psychol. Psychiatry*, **30**, 219–30.

Tannock, R., Ickowicz, A. and Schachar, R. (1995). Differential effects of methylphenidate of working memory in ADHD children with and without comorbid anxiety. *J. Am. Acad. Child Adolesc. Psychiatry*, **34**, 886–96.

Teicher, M. H., Polcari, A., Anderson, C. H. et al. (1996). Dose dependent effects of methylphenidate on activity, attention, and magnetic resonance measures in children with ADHD. *Soc. Neurosci. Abst.*, **22**, 1191.

Teicher, M. H., Anderson, C. M., Polcari, A. et al. (2000). Functional deficits in basal ganglia of children with attention-deficit/hyperactivity disorder revealed using fMRI relaxometry. *Nat. Med.*, in press.

Tulsky, D., Zhu, J. and Ledbetter, M. (1997). *WAIS-III and WMS-III Technical Manual.* San Antonio, TX: The Psychological Corporation, Harcourt Brace.

Tulving, E., Kapur, S., Craik, F. I. M., Moscovitch, M. and Houle, S. (1994). Hemispheric encoding/retrieval asymmetry in episodic memory: positron emission tomography findings. *Proc. Natl. Acad. Sci. USA*, **91**, 2016–20.

Ungerleider, L. G. (1995). Functional brain imaging studies of cortical mechanisms for memory. *Science*, **270**, 769–75.

Ungerleider, L. G., Courtney, S. M. and Haxby, J. V. (1998). A neural system for human visual working memory. *Proc. Natl. Acad. Sci. USA*, **95**, 883–90.

Vaidya, C. J., Austin, G., Kirkorian, G. et al. (1998). Selective effects of methylphenidate in attention deficit hyperactivity disorder: a functional magnetic resonance study. *Proc. Natl. Acad. Sci. USA*, **95**, 14494–9.

van der Meere, J., Shalev, R., Borger, N. and Gross-Tsur, V. (1995). Sustained attention, activation and MPH in ADHD: a research note. *J. Child Psychol. Psychiatry*, **36**, 697–703.

Wechsler, D. (1991). *Wechsler Intelligence Scale for Children*, 3rd edn. San Antonio, TX: The Psychological Corporation, Harcourt Brace.

Weinberger, D. R., Luchins, D. J., Morihisa, J. and Wyatt, R. J. (1982). Asymmetrical volumes of the right and left frontal and occipital regions of the human brain. *Ann. Neurol.*, **11**, 97–100.

Weiss, G. and Hechtman, L. (1993). *Hyperactive Children Grown Up*. Guilford New York: Guilford Press.

Wilson, F. A., Scalaidhe, S. P. and Goldman-Rakic, P. S. (1993). Dissociation of object and spatial processing domains in primate prefrontal cortex. *Science*, **260**, 1955–58.

Wolraich, M., Hannah, J., Pinnock, T., Baumgaertel, A. and Brown, J. (1996). Comparison of diagnostic criteria for attention-deficit hyperactivity disorder in a county-wide sample. *J. Am. Acad. Child Adolesc. Psychiatry*, **35**, 319–24.

Zametkin, A. J. and Rapoport, J. L. (1987). Neurobiology of attention deficit disorder with hyperactivity: where have we come in 50 years? *J. Am. Acad. Child Adolesc. Psychiatry*, **26**, 676–86.

Zametkin, A. J., Nordahl, T., Gross, M. et al. (1990). Cerebral glucose metabolism in adults with hyperactivity of childhood onset. *N. Engl. J. Med.*, **323**, 1361–6.

Zametkin, A. J., Liebenauer, L., Fitzgerald, G. et al. (1993). Brain metabolism in teenagers with attention-deficit hyperactivity disorder. *Arch. Gen. Psychiatry*, **50**, 333–40.

17

Eating disorders

Uttom Chowdhury, Isky Gordon and Bryan Lask

Introduction

Eating disorders are defined as those disorders in which there is excessive concern with the control of body weight and shape, accompanied by grossly inadequate, irregular, or chaotic food intake. It is widely accepted that eating disorders occur in young adults and adolescents, but their occurrence in younger children has received little attention. Recently, a number of reports have described series of young patients, ages 8 years and above, with eating disorders (Fosson et al., 1987; Higgs et al., 1989; Gowers et al., 1991; Bryant-Waugh and Lask, 1995). The range of these disorders in children include selective eating, food avoidance emotional disorder, functional dysphagia, and pervasive refusal syndrome (discussed later in this chapter), as well as the more common conditions of anorexia nervosa and bulimia nervosa. In the medical literature, there have been an increasing number of studies published involving functional brain imaging in adults with eating disorders, and some of these studies have also included older adolescent subjects. There have been relatively few reports of functional imaging studies in children with eating disorders.

In this chapter, we will first provide background information, including theories of etiology concerning early-onset anorexia nervosa and bulimia nervosa. We will then review some of the structural and functional neuroimaging studies of eating disorders in the adult population. Finally, we will describe in detail the recent neuroimaging studies in children with anorexia nervosa.

Anorexia nervosa

Diagnostic considerations

DSM-IV criteria for anorexia (American Psychiatric Association, 1994) include (i) refusal to maintain body weight at or above a minimally normal weight for age and height (e.g., weight loss leading to the maintenance of body weight less than 85% of expected or failure to make weight gain during a growth period); (ii) an intense fear of gaining weight or becoming fat, even though underweight; (iii) a disturbance in the way in which body weight and shape is experienced, undue influence of body weight or shape on self-evaluation, or denial of the seriousness of current low body weight; and (iv) the absence of at least three consecutive menstrual cycles. Subtypes include a "restricting type" without regular binge eating or purging behavior, and a "binge-eating/purging type".

These criteria, intended primarily for use with older patients, fail to address the identification of anorexia nervosa in children adequately. For example, criterion (iv) specifying the absence of menstrual cycles applies only to postmenarcheal females and is clearly inapplicable to children, most of whom are premenarcheal. Equally unhelpful is the statement that weight should be maintained at less than 85% of that expected, for expected weight can only be calculated on the basis of height and age; yet growth may also be impaired because of poor nutrition.

For these reasons, the Eating Disorders Team at Great Ormond Street Hospital for Sick Children in London, UK developed more practical diagnostic criteria for early-onset anorexia nervosa (Lask and Bryant-Waugh, 1986). The Great Ormond Street diagnostic criteria for early-onset anorexia nervosa (Lask and Bryant-Waugh, 1999) include (i) determined weight loss (e.g., food avoidance, self-induced vomiting, excessive exercising, abuse of laxatives), (ii) abnormal cognition regarding weight and/or shape, and (iii) morbid preoccupation with weight and/or shape.

Since children should be growing, static weight may be regarded as equivalent to weight loss in adults. Weight loss is a real cause for concern in children, since they have lower total body fat deposits and, therefore, less fat to lose. One measurement for weight loss uses the Tanner–Whitehouse Standards (Tanner et al., 1966) where 100% represents the desired weight for a child's sex, age, and height, and 80% or less is classified as wasting.

As with later-onset anorexia, in early-onset anorexia, weight is controlled through food avoidance, self-induced vomiting, and excessive exercise; less commonly it can occur through laxative abuse. Children most often attribute food avoidance to a fear of becoming obese. Other reasons for food refusal are feelings of nausea or fullness, abdominal pain, appetite loss and difficulty swallowing (Fosson et al., 1987). In their study of early-onset anorexia nervosa, Fosson et al. (1987) reported that at least 40% of the 48 children included were known to be vomiting at presentation. Excessive exercising is not uncommon in children. Daily workouts may be a feature, with exercise sometimes carried out in secret in the privacy of a bedroom or bathroom. Perhaps because children have little access to laxatives, their abuse is not common in early-onset anorexia.

Cognition regarding weight and/or shape focuses around a distortion of body image, although it must be acknowledged that body image is difficult to assess reliably. Many children with anorexia nervosa will report that they consider themselves fat even when severely underweight, not unlike the image suggested by clinical observations in adult patients with the same condition. Closely related to their fear of fatness, children with anorexia nervosa tend to be preoccupied with their own body weight and are often experts at calorie counting.

Physical aspects

The majority of physical changes in anorexia nervosa are predominantly related to the effects of starvation and dehydration. These include slow pulse rate, low blood pressure, and poor circulation leading to cold hands and feet. Often there is excess fine hair, known as lanugo, especially on the back. Teeth may be pitted, eroded, and decayed from their exposure to gastric acid during vomiting.

Although there is little information specifically relating to children, a wide range of biochemical and endocrine changes have been described in anorexia nervosa. These include low hemoglobin and white cell count, low levels of potassium and chloride, raised liver enzymes such as alanine transaminase and alkaline phosphatase, and low levels of plasma zinc and serum iron. Endocrine changes, which are likely secondary to starvation, include increased cortisol, growth hormone, and cholecystokinin, and decreased luteinizing hormone, follicle-stimulating hormone, estrogen, triiodothyronine, and thyroid-stimulating hormone.

Comorbidity

Herzog et al. (1992) reported that major depressive disorder was the most prevalent comorbid disorder, occurring in 37% of patients with anorexia nervosa. Obsessional behaviors in anorexia nervosa are also common and are usually focused around food, eating, and exercise. Kaye et al. (1992) showed that patients with anorexia nervosa had elevated scores on the Yale–Brown Obsessive–Compulsive Scale even after compulsive eating behaviors and obsessive concerns about weight were excluded. This clinical characteristic is important to consider in the interpretation of brain imaging data.

Bulimia nervosa

Diagnostic considerations

DSM-IV criteria (American Psychiatric Association, 1994) include (i) recurrent episodes of binge eating (e.g., eating large amounts of food in 2 h and a sense of lack of control during the episodes), (ii) regular use of methods of weight control (e.g., vomiting, laxatives, diuretics, fasting/strict diet, vigorous exercise), (iii) a minimum of two binges per week for 3 months, (iv) self-evaluation being unduly influenced by body shape and weight, and (v) these disturbances are not limited to episodes of anorexia nervosa. Subtypes include a "purging type", with regular self-induced vomiting or misuse of laxatives, diuretics, or enemas and a "nonpurging type" with other inappropriate compensatory behaviors (e.g., fasting or excess exercise) but without use of the methods used by the purging type.

Until recently, very few cases of bulimia nervosa with onset below the age of 14 years were reported (Schmidt et al., 1992). During the 1990s, there has been a gradual increase in referrals of such children to the eating disorders clinic at the Great Ormond Street Hospital, but reported cases of bulimia remain relatively rare in children under 12 years. The clinical features do not seem to differ from those found in adult patients with bulimia nervosa. The physical manifestations of bulimia nervosa are initially less dramatic than those of anorexia nervosa because weight is usually maintained within normal range. However, self-induced vomiting can lead to complications such as fluid and electrolyte disturbance and gastrointestinal bleeding. Other physical complications include dental erosions, enlargement of the salivary glands, and muscle weakness.

Comorbidity

Studies in adult patients with bulimia nervosa have shown that depressive and anxiety symptoms are prevalent (Laessle et al., 1987). Drug and alcohol abuse are also common, as are disorders of impulse control such as self-mutilation (Treasure, 1997). This comorbidity holds implications for the subtyping of patients in order to achieve homogeneous study samples.

Other eating disorders in children

A number of other eating disorders have been identified in children (additional information on these can be obtained from Lask and Bryant-Waugh (1999)).

Food avoidance emotional disorder

First introduced by Higgs et al. (1989), food avoidance emotional disorder describes a group of underweight children who present with inadequate food intake and emotional disturbance and who do not meet the criteria for anorexia nervosa. An operational definition used by us has evolved from Higgs and colleagues' original description together with our own clinical experience. Included are (i) food avoidance not accounted for by a primary affective disorder, (ii) weight loss, (iii) mood disturbance not meeting criteria for primary affective disorder, (iv) lack of abnormal cognition regarding weight or shape, (v) lack of morbid preoccupation regarding weight or shape, (vi) no morbid preoccupation regarding weight or shape, and (vii) no organic, brain disease or psychosis.

Selective eating

Selective eaters are a group of children who present with very restricted eating habits in terms of the range of foods they will accept. Their characteristics include (i) having eaten a narrow range of foods for at least 2 years, (ii) an unwillingness to try new foods, (iii) a lack of abnormal cognition regarding weight or shape, (iv) a lack of fear of choking or vomiting, and (v) weight loss that may be low, normal, or high.

Pervasive refusal syndrome

The term pervasive refusal syndrome was first used by Lask et al. (1991) to describe children with (i) a profound refusal to eat, drink, walk, talk or engage in self-care; and (ii) a determined resistance to the efforts of others to help.

Initially these children present with features fairly typical of anorexia nervosa, but their food avoidance is gradually followed by a more generalized avoidance with marked fear responses.

Functional dysphagia

Children with functional dysphagia generally present with complaints of difficulty or pain on swallowing. Features include (i) food avoidance; (ii) a fear of swallowing, choking, or vomiting; (iii) no abnormal cognition regarding weight or shape; (iv) no morbid preoccupation regarding weight or shape; and (v) no organic brain disease or psychosis.

For additional information on the above eating disorders in children, the reader is referred to Lask and Bryant-Waugh (1999).

Epidemiology of eating disorders

For a number of reasons, the incidence and prevalence of childhood-onset anorexia are unknown. There have been no epidemiologic studies that have focused specifically on this age group, and the use of strict diagnostic criteria in epidemiologic studies may lead to a substantial underestimate of the true incidence of these disorders (Bryant-Waugh and Lask, 1995). However, studies in adolescent populations estimate the prevalence to be in the order of 0.1–0.2% (Bentovim and Morton, 1990; Whitaker et al., 1990), and it is likely to be even lower in children. Although debatable, an increase in the referral rate of child cases of anorexia nervosa has been reported (Bryant-Waugh and Lask, 1995). With regard to gender distribution, only 5–10% of cases of anorexia nervosa in adolescents and young adults occur in males (Barry and Lippmann, 1990). However, studies have reported that between 19 and 30% of children with anorexia nervosa have been boys (Hawley, 1985; Jacobs and Isaacs, 1986; Fosson et al., 1987; Higgs et al., 1989). At present, there is little epidemiologic information on the other disorders in children.

Etiology of eating disorders

Although the etiology of anorexia nervosa is unknown, a number of interacting factors, including biological, psychologic, familial, and sociocultural factors, appear to contribute to its development. Contributing biological factors include genetics, neurotransmitter levels, and endocrine dysfunction, as well as mechanisms of appetite regulation and malnutrition. Biological variables that influence eating behavior include various CNS structures, central and peripheral neurotransmitters, neuropeptides, and neurohormones.

Brain structures implicated in the regulation of eating

A number of CNS structures have been implicated in the regulation of eating behavior. Discoveries in the early 1950s supported for a time a "dual-center theory" of the control of eating (Anand and Brobeck, 1951). According to this theory, the hypothalamus contained the primary control centers for hunger and satiety. Experiments showed that bilateral lesions of the ventromedial hypothalamus caused rats to become obese. This area was, therefore, called the satiety center. It had also been shown that bilateral destruction of the lateral hypothalamus caused rats to stop eating; consequently this area was called the feeding center. It was proposed that the ventromedial hypothalamus normally acted as a brake on feeding by inhibiting the lateral hypothalamus. Informations from the rest of the brain and from other factors (e.g., hormones) that influence eating were presumed to act through these hypothalamic control centers.

Several subsequent observations challenged this dual center hypothesis. Studies showed that following bilateral damage to the ventromedial hypothalamus, rats began to increase food consumption. After a few weeks, body weight stabilized at an obese level and food intake was not much above normal. Similarly, with bilateral destruction of the lateral hypothalamus, the resulting aphagia was not permanent, and a few rats began to eat spontaneously after about a week (Teitelbaum and Stellar, 1954). The ability of animals with these lesions to regulate their weights around higher or lower than normal points casts doubt on the simple dual center theory.

Clinical evidence in humans has shown that hypothalamic lesions, both neoplastic (Lewin et al., 1972; Heron and Johnston, 1976; Goldrey, 1978) and degenerative (White and Hain, 1959), have been associated with undereating and emaciation. De Vile et al. (1995) described two boys who initially presented with features of anorexia nervosa but were found to have tumors affecting the hypothalamus. Other clinical examples of organic brain disease in humans have highlighted other parts of the brain that may have a role in feeding. Overeating has been described in patients with lesions of the amygdala (Terzian and Ore, 1955) and of the orbitofrontal cortex (Erb et al., 1989).

Neuroendocrine aspects

Russell (1985) postulated the existence of a primary hypothalamic disorder manifested by endocrine disturbances involving the hypothalamus and pituitary gland as a basis for eating disorders. This hypothesis was based on the endocrine changes seen in anorexia nervosa (see above). However, the endocrine changes are similar to those found in starvation from other causes and tend to normalize after the patient's weight returns to normal (Casper, 1984). So far, therefore, the hope of finding an endocrinologic cause for anorexia nervosa has not materialized.

Neurotransmitter system

The mechanisms whereby the above brain structures regulate food intake involve neurotransmitters of both central and peripheral origin that stimulate and inhibit eating behavior. At least three neurotransmitters have been implicated in eating disorders: serotonin, noradrenaline (norepinephrine), and dopamine. Serotonergic agents cause a reduction in food intake in animals and humans. Injection of serotonergic agents directly into the medial hypothalamus in animals is followed by the suppression of food intake. In contrast, injection of noradrenaline into the medial hypothalamus causes an increase in food intake. Dopamine appears to act via the lateral hypothalamus to produce a decrease in feeding. Dopamine blockers such as chlorpromazine and haloperidol have the opposite effect (Hsu, 1990). Dopamine has also been implicated in reward and reinforcement processes (Wise and Rompre, 1989) that could constitute a core symptom in eating disorders.

It has also been suggested that anorexia nervosa could be viewed as a state of dependence on starvation, similar to alcohol dependence (Szmukler and Tam, 1984), and that during starvation there would be increased central opioid activity. In fact, elevated opioid activity has been found in the cerebrospinal fluid of patients with anorexia nervosa (Kaye et al., 1982; Jonas and Gold, 1986), but as yet the hypothesis remains untested.

Genetics

It is important to consider genetic contributions when discussing the biological factors related to the possible pathogenesis of eating disorders. Strober et al. (1990) have shown that the frequency of anorexia nervosa in female relatives of patients with anorexia nervosa is about eight times higher than that in the general population. Holland et al. (1988), in a study of 45 twin pairs, showed a concordance rate for anorexia nervosa in dizygotic twins of 5%

compared with 56% for monozygotes. In identical twin pairs discordant for anorexia nervosa, the affected twin had higher levels of stress related to significant life events prior to onset.

Molecular genetic studies have attempted to identify genes contributing to eating disorders. Although unreplicated (Hinney et al., 1997; Campbell et al., 1998), an association between a polymorphism of the serotonin 5-HT$_{2A}$ receptor gene and anorexia nervosa has recently been reported (Collier et al., 1997; Sorbi et al., 1998). A lack of association between polymorphisms and anorexia has been found for serotonin transporter (Hinney et al., 1997) and the dopamine D$_3$ receptor gene (Bruins-Slot et al., 1998).

Neuropsychology

A number of studies in adults and adolescents with anorexia nervosa provide evidence of cognitive impairment in anorexia nervosa. Although an early study by Dally (1969) showed that patients with anorexia nervosa had above average IQs, recent studies have reported mean IQ scores to be within an average range (Szmukler et al., 1992; Gillberg et al., 1996; Kingston et al., 1996). None of these studies looked at a younger prepubertal population. However, Christie et al. (1998) recently reported a pilot study looking at IQ, memory, and attainments in a group of 12 girls with anorexia nervosa (age range, 10.6–16.5 years). They found that three cognitive factors that contribute to IQ score (verbal comprehension, perceptual organization, and freedom from distractibility) were within the average range. In contrast, the girls showed a relative increase in a fourth factor: processing speed. The implication of this finding is not yet known and further research is needed.

There have been conflicting reports of attentional dysfunction in adult and adolescent patients with anorexia nervosa. Szmukler et al. (1992) found that patients at low weight were impaired on tests of attention, perceptual-motor functions, visuospatial construction, and problem-solving. Weight gain resulted in significant improvements in performance. Pendleton-Jones et al. (1991) found deficits in underweight anorexic women on tests assessing the focusing and execution aspects of attention (in verbal, memory, and visuospatial domains). Witt et al. (1985), however, found that patients with anorexia nervosa performed as well as normal healthy controls on measures of attention but not on an associative learning task. Visuospatial processing has also been found to be impaired (Szmukler et al., 1992; Maxwell et al., 1984; Kingston et al., 1996). A follow-up study by Kingston et al. (1996) found that attention, but not visuospatial ability, improved significantly with weight gain, suggesting that

attention deficits are state related while visuospatial deficits are trait-related findings in anorexia nervosa.

Overall, neuropsychologic profiles are still poorly characterized in the adult and adolescent populations. There is also inadequate documentation of the impact of low body weight associated with the psychopathology of anorexia nervosa on the development of intellectual functioning, school performance, and cognitive processing in children whose brains are still developing.

The theories and hypotheses regarding the neurobiology of eating disorders are still at a relatively early stage. This may account for the few hypothesis-driven functional imaging studies in this field. The next section reviews first structural studies and then moves on to functional imaging studies.

Structural neuroimaging studies

A number of computed tomography (CT) and magnetic resonance imaging (MRI) studies in female adult and adolescent patients with anorexia nervosa have shown structural abnormalities in the brain. Although some studies have shown changes in subcortical areas of the brain, such as a reduction in size of the thalamus and midbrain (Husain et al., 1992) and a decreased size in the pituitary (Doriaswamy et al., 1991), the most consistent finding has been sulcal widening and/or ventricular enlargement (Artmann et al., 1985; Krieg et al., 1988). These changes were to a large extent reversible after weight gain and, therefore, appeared to be secondary to the effects of starvation. However, in the majority of studies, the brain did not entirely return to complete normality following weight gain (Krieg et al., 1988). Furthermore, cross-sectional CT studies of normal-weight bulimic patients have revealed morphologic brain changes similar to those in anorexia nervosa (i.e., ventricular dilatation and sulcal widening; Krieg et al., 1987).

A recent MRI study involving 12 female patients with anorexia nervosa (age range 11.7–37.6 years; mean age 18.9 years) showed that there were significant reductions in both total gray matter and total white matter volumes compared with controls (Lambe et al., 1997). A longitudinal study by the same team showed that the gray matter volume changes persisted in patients who recovered their weight, suggesting that anorexia nervosa had a reversible and an irreversible component in relation to structural brain changes with weight recovery (Katzman et al., 1997).

Some researchers have examined the relationship between brain alterations and cognitive impairment in a series of patients with anorexia nervosa (Laessle et al.,

1989; Palazidou et al., 1990; Kingston et al., 1996). Palazidou et al. (1990) reported a negative correlation between sulcal width and scores on a symbol-digit coding task. A study by Kingston et al. (1996) reported cognitive deficits in a large group of patients with anorexia nervosa (mean age 22.1 years) both before and after treatment. Deficits on memory tasks and on cognitive flexibility and response inhibition tasks persisted despite substantial weight recovery, but relationships between morphologic brain changes and cognitive impairments were weak.

In summary, the majority of findings using structural imaging techniques appear to be secondary to the effects of starvation and contribute little to the understanding of the pathogenesis of eating disorders.

Functional neuroimaging studies

Caveats and methodologic limitations

Several methodologic problems present special challenges for functional neuroimaging studies of patients with eating disorders. The timing of the scan needs to be considered in the experimental designs, as changes in brain function may vary around mealtimes. Abnormally high plasma levels of ketone bodies have been observed in patients with anorexia nervosa (Pirke et al., 1985). Such high ketone bodies levels may influence cerebral glucose metabolic rates (CMRGlu) measured by positron emission tomography (PET) and [18F]-fluorodeoxyglucose (FDG) (Krieg et al., 1991). Hawkins and Biebuyck (1979) have reported that uptake of ketone bodies is higher in the cerebral cortex than in the basal ganglia. Therefore, if there were a global change in brain metabolism in anorexia nervosa, such as an increased, preferential utilization of ketone compounds in the cerebral cortex, this could actually lead to the appearance of an increased CMRGlu in the basal ganglia (Herholz et al., 1987). Consequently, at the time of FDG-PET studies, patients should ideally be in a stable metabolic state, assessed by the absence of ketone bodies in urine and by normal plasma glucose levels. However, the chronic effect of ketoacidosis on the brain following chronic starvation cannot be totally excluded. Herholz (1996) has suggested that malnutrition may affect the uptake of tracers in the brain through changes in tissue amino acids, leading to an artifactual difference in brain function between controls and starved patients.

Other problems with functional imaging studies in patients with eating disorders include the selection of a suitable control group. Some adult studies have used healthy volunteers as a control group, though this is clearly

difficult in child studies. Other informative comparison groups could include patients with low weight for reasons other than anorexia nervosa; however, it is likely that the numbers would be small, especially in childhood studies. In addition, such low-weight comparison groups might introduce confounding effects of the other etiologies for low weight.

Few functional imaging studies in adults with eating disorders have been published to date and only a single study of children. Not only are the number of studies relatively few, but the patient sample sizes involved in the studies are small. Other limitations include the use of mixed age groups, suboptimal control groups, inadequate details concerning patient characteristics (e.g., chronicity of illness, nutritional state, therapy involved prior to or at the time of the study, handedness). Study designs vary; there is little or no consistency in the states in which patients are at the time of study (e.g., resting condition, eyes closed, eyes open, during task performance). Finally, there is a shortage of longitudinal studies. Well-controlled studies with larger sample sizes are needed to provide a better understanding of eating disorders.

Some of the main findings in this patient group are now described (Table 17.1).

PET studies of anorexia nervosa in adults and adolescents

The PET studies described below have measured regional CMRGlu (rCMRGlu). The first published study using PET in anorexia nervosa was carried out in Germany by Herholz et al. (1987). In this study, five females with anorexia nervosa (aged 17–21 years) were scanned when their weight ranged from 66% to 74% of their ideal body weight and then rescanned after a period of behavior therapy and an average weight gain of 16% of their ideal body weight. Because of legal constraints in Germany on the exposure of young women of reproductive age to PET procedures, the researchers were unable to use a healthy female control group. Young healthy males (n = 15; mean age 23–35 years) were, therefore, used for comparison. The results showed that the patients with active anorexia nervosa had significant higher absolute CMRGlu in the caudate and temporal cortex prior to weight gain compared with post-weight gain. The hypermetabolism in the caudate nucleus was also significantly higher in patients with active anorexia compared with the control group. Global CMRGlu tended to be higher in patients prior to weight gain, relative to postweight gain, and also higher compared with healthy males. The authors suggested that global hypermetabolism, with accentuation in the caudate nucleus,

Table 17.1. Functional imaging studies in patients with anorexia nervosa

Study	Sample Size		Gender		Mean age (years)		Technique	Results
	AN	C	AN	C	AN	C		
Herholz et al. (1987)	5	15	F	M	19.0	29	FDG PET	Bilateral caudate and temporal hypermetabolism before weight gain
Krieg et al. (1989)	12	12 (Clinical contrast group)	5F; 7M	5F; 7M	21.3	31	^{133}Xe SPECT	No change in rCBF after eating or compared with control group
Nozoe et al. (1993)	7	5	F	F	19.0	–	^{99m}Tc-HMPAO SPECT	Increase in rCBF in response to food intake in left inferior cortex
Nozoe et al. (1995)	8	9	F	F	24.1	20.3	^{99m}Tc-HMPAO SPECT	Decrease in rCBF in left parietal region before eating compared with control group
Delvenne et al. (1995)	20	10	F	F	20.5	24	FDG PET	Global and regional hypometabolism of glucose especially in frontal and parietal cortices
Delvenne et al. (1996)	10	10	F	F	20.0	23.8	FDG PET	Hypometabolism in parietal and superior frontal cortices; relative hypermetabolism in caudate and inferior frontal cortex
Delvenne et al. (1997a)	10 (underweight depressed)	10 (normal-weight depressed)	F	F	24.5	29.3	FDG PET	Caudate hypermetabolism in patients with AN compared with that in low- and normal-weight depressed group; absolute hypometabolism of glucose found in AN and low-weight depressed group
Gordon et al. (1997)	15	–	14F; 1M	–	13.0	–	^{99m}Tc HMPAO and ^{99m}Tc-ECD SPECT	Unilateral temporal lobe hypoperfusion in 13 patients

Notes: AN, anorexia nervosa; C, healthy control group; PET, positron emission tomography; SPECT, single photon emission computed tomography; FDG, [^{18}F]-fluoro-2-deoxyglucose; ^{99m}Tc-HMPAO, [^{99m}Tc]-labeled hexamethylpropyleneamine oxime; ECD, ethyl cysteineate dimer; rCBF, regional cerebral blood flow.

may contribute to the increased vigilance seen in patients with anorexia nervosa, since stimulation of the caudate influences alertness and responses to external stimuli. The head of the caudate may also be important in anorexia nervosa because it receives afferents from not only the frontal cortex but also the limbic system. However, the small patient sample size involved and the use of a male control group make it difficult to interpret the findings. Indeed, most PET studies (Baxter et al., 1987; Yoshii et al., 1988; Andreason et al., 1994; Ernst et al., 1998) but not all (Miura et al.,1990; Gur et al., 1995), report higher global CMRGlu in women than in men.

Delvenne et al. (1995) observed global and regional absolute cerebral glucose hypometabolism in 20 underweight female patients with anorexia nervosa (14–33 years; mean age 20.5 years; <85% normal body weight) compared with 10 healthy female volunteers (18–30 years; mean age 24 years). All patients were under 85% of normal weight. The abnormally low CMRGlu was particularly significant in the frontal and parietal cortices bilaterally. The effect of age was not addressed. In addition, there was no correlation between rCMRGlu and depression or anxiety levels.

To assess the reversibility of this hypometabolism, Delvenne et al. (1996) measured rCMRGlu in 10 female patients with anorexia nervosa (aged 14–29 years; mean age 20.0 years) five of whom had participated in the 1995 study and rescanned them after weight gain. All patients with anorexia nervosa were under 85% normal weight at the time of the first scan and had an average weight gain of 20% at the time of the second scan. Compared with 10 female controls (same controls as in the 1995 study), the patients with anorexia nervosa had global and regional absolute glucose hypometabolism (i.e., not normalized to global metabolism) significant in the superior frontal and parietal cortices. This finding was associated with relative hypermetabolism (after normalization to global metabolism) in the caudate nuclei and inferior frontal cortex. After weight gain, the absolute hypometabolism returned to normal in all regions, whereas relative rCMRGlu remained low in the parietal cortex and high in the inferior frontal cortex (orbitofrontal gyri). The authors suggested that parietal cortex hypometabolism might reflect a primary cerebral dysfunction or a particular regional sensitivity to the consequences of starvation. Cognitive studies in anorexia nervosa have also shown low performances in arithmetic (Fox, 1981; Hamsher et al., 1981), consistent with parietal dysfunction. Abnormalities in orbitofrontal cortex and caudate nucleus were reminiscent of CMRGlu patterns found in obsessive-compulsive patients, suggesting their possible involvement with obsessive thoughts about food,

weight, and body shape, which remained in weight-restored anorexic patients.

In a further study, Delvenne et al. (1997a) compared PET brain images from 10 female patients with anorexia nervosa (mean age 24.5 years; from the previous 1985 study group) and 20 female depressed patients, 10 of whom were underweight as a direct consequence of depression (normal-weight group mean age 29.3 years; underweight group mean age 23.4 years). The mean body mass index (BMI: weight over squared height ratio, used as a measure of body size) of the patients with anorexia nervosa was 14.29, while that of the depressed group who were underweight was 16.52. Ten healthy female volunteers were also scanned as controls. It is unclear whether the sample of patients and controls were the same as in the previous study. Nevertheless, the results showed that absolute hypometabolism of glucose appeared to be a consequence of low weight, as it was found in both low-weight patients with anorexia nervosa and low-weight patients with depression. In relative values, patients with anorexia nervosa showed significant hypometabolism in the parietal lobe and significant hypometabolism in the caudate nuclei. It was also noted that the influence of depressive symptoms did not influence absolute metabolism, as depressed patients without low weight did not differ from controls.

Although one has to apply a degree of caution when interpreting the above results, it is notable that two different research centers have reported caudate hypermetabolism in patients with anorexia nervosa. Whether other research groups replicate the finding of parietal hypometabolism seen in the work by Delvenne et al. (1995, 1996) remains to be seen.

PET studies of bulimia nervosa in adults

Patients with bulimia nervosa tend to maintain a relatively normal body weight, thus avoiding the confounds introduced by weight loss. Wu et al. (1990) compared PET images of CMRGlu of eight female adults with bulimia nervosa (mean age 28.6 years; six right-handed, two left-handed) with those of eight female healthy controls (all right-handed; mean age 28.9 years). All were evaluated with the Hamilton Rating Scale for Depression, and all performed a visual continuous performance task, a measure of sustained attention. The use of an attention task was designed to control the state in which subjects were scanned. The healthy control group showed relatively higher rCMRGlu in the right hemisphere, whereas patients with bulimia nervosa lacked this asymmetry. Also, the right parietal/temporal region and the cingulate and ventral putamen appeared to show a reversal of the normal "right greater than left" pattern in the patients with bulimia nervosa.

In contrast to an earlier study of anorexia nervosa (Herholz et al., 1987), Wu et al. (1990) did not find abnormally high rCMRGlu in the caudate or temporal lobes in patients with bulimia nervosa. The authors suggested that bulimia nervosa and anorexia nervosa were likely to be mediated by different neural pathways and that the loss of right-predominant temporal lobe asymmetry in patients with bulimia raised questions about the possible role of aberrant hemispheric lateralization in the etiology of bulimia nervosa. In support of this hypothesis, the authors cited a PET study by Mayberg et al. (1988) that found that lateralized changes in brain function caused by stroke damage had differential effects on mood and serotonin receptor density. Wu et al. (1990) proposed that this may have some implications for bulimia nervosa since the serotonin system has been shown to be involved in this disorder.

Andreason et al. (1992) studied 11 adult female inpatients with bulimia nervosa (mean age 25.5 years) and 18 healthy matched volunteers (mean age 25.3 years). Obsessive-compulsive symptoms were assessed using the Maudsley Obsessive Compulsive Inventory. The Hamilton Rating Scale was used to measure depression. All subjects were scanned 2–3 h after a light meal and performed a continuous auditory discrimination task for 30 min to control state during scanning. The results showed no difference between the global metabolic rates of patients with bulimia nervosa and normal control subjects. There was a left-predominant hemispheric asymmetry in the temporal lobes of patients with bulimia nervosa that was not observed in comparison subjects and a relative bilateral inferior temporal lobe hypermetabolism.

Orbitofrontal regions were analyzed to compare the results with the studies of Nordahl et al. (1989) and Baxter et al. (1987), which found that patients with obsessive-compulsive disorder had increased orbitofrontal metabolic rates. There was no difference in mean rCMRGlu nor was there a positive correlation between rCMRGlu and obsessive-compulsive symptoms in the orbitofrontal regions.

Metabolism in the left anterior and posterior lateral prefrontal cortical areas correlated negatively with Hamilton Depression Scale scores. When patients with scores of 15 or greater were considered separately, mean rCMRGlu values in the left anterior and posterior lateral prefrontal cortex were found to be significantly lower than those of comparison subjects. Andreason et al. (1992) concluded that left anterior lateral prefrontal cortex hypometabolism varied with the depressive symptoms observed in bulimia

nervosa. In contrast, the lack of correlation between temporal CMRGlu and depressive symptoms in the patient group suggested that temporal lobe hypermetabolism and asymmetries were independent of the mood state.

Delvenne et al. (1997b) investigated CMRGlu in patients with bulimia nervosa at rest. Eleven female patients with bulimia nervosa (mean age 26.2 years) and 11 healthy matched controls underwent brain PET imaging. Compared with the control group, the patients with bulimia showed hypometabolism in most of the cerebral regions and relative hypometabolism in the parietal cortex. Since previous studies (Delvenne et al., 1995, 1996) demonstrated similar findings in patients with anorexia nervosa, the authors suggested that the observations might support a possible primary cerebral dysfunction or a particular regional sensitivity to the consequences of nutritional deficiencies. They cited previous works by Bowden et al. (1989) and Horne et al. (1991) showing that patients with anorexia and bulimia nervosa present with disturbed body image perception. Therefore, the findings of parietal involvement in bulimia would be consistent with the proposed involvement of the parietal cortex in the perception of body image.

SPECT studies of adults and older adolescents with eating disorders

In an early study using inhaled ^{133}Xe to measure regional cerebral blood flow (rCBF), Krieg et al. (1989) compared SPECT (single photon emission CT) images of 12 female inpatients with anorexia nervosa (aged 16–27 years) with a control group of five female and seven male patients (aged 19–17 years) whose rCBF had been measured to exclude cerebrovascular disease. The authors do not give the diagnosis of the control group but state that these patients showed no signs of a neuropsychiatric disorder after clinical examination. Eleven of the patients with anorexia nervosa were rescanned after discharge, an average of 102 days after admission. At this time, the mean weight gain after behavioral therapy was 11% of ideal body weight. The results showed that the mean global rCBF rate assessed at the first examination did not differ significantly from the second examination or from those of the control group.

Using technetium-99m-labeled hexamethylpropyleneamine oxime (^{99m}TC-HMPAO) to measure rCBF, Nozoe et al. (1993) measured rCBF in a single session before eating and again during eating and at an average interval of 71 days before therapy and again after therapy. The authors hypothesized that when patients with anorexia nervosa ate, the rCBF in "certain cortical areas would increase" because of the abnormal sensitivity of patients to food stimuli. Seven female adults with anorexia nervosa (mean age 19.0 years) were scanned prior to eating their breakfast. The procedure involved injecting a dose of ^{99m}TC-HMPAO and scanning the subjects at rest and with eyes closed. After the first scan, the subjects were asked to eat a piece of cake with their left hand with their eyes remaining closed. During this time, another dose of isotope was injected and 5 min later the patients were rescanned. The same procedure was applied to five healthy female volunteers.

Only five symmetrical pairs of cortical regions were analyzed (superior frontal, inferior frontal, temporal, parietal, and occipital). All regional values were normalized to the cerebellum by using the ratio of the region of interest to the cerebellar activity. Unfortunately, whether the cerebellar metabolism is affected by the disorder is unknown and, therefore, normalization using this region as a reference structure may have introduced some artifacts. The authors repeated the procedure in the patients following therapy but did not identify the type of therapy. The results showed that the patients' eating increased rCBF in the left inferior frontal cortex compared with that in the resting condition (8.9% increase).

Other methodologic issues include the potential influence of the motor and sensory variables involved in eating on brain activity. The involvement of the left inferior frontal lobe in the eating process may be related to the role of the dorsolateral prefrontal cortex in complex learned feeding behavior elicited in monkeys (Ono et al., 1984) or the influence of emotional state and arousal on this brain region (Nauta, 1971).

Nozoe et al. (1995) conducted a second SPECT brain imaging study of five female patients with bulimia nervosa (mean age 21.0 years), eight females with anorexia nervosa (mean age 24.1 years) (although it is not clear whether there was any overlap between this sample and that of the previous study), and nine healthy female volunteers (mean age 20.3 years). Using the same procedure as in their previous study (Nozoe et al., 1993), they measured values for rCBF in 10 cerebral cortical regions before and after eating. Patients with bulimia nervosa showed higher rCBF values before eating in inferior frontal and left temporal regions compared with the other groups. The patients with anorexia nervosa showed significantly lower rCBF values in the left parietal region compared with the control group. There were no significant differences among the three groups following food intake. The authors suggested that differences in cerebral function of patients with bulimia nervosa and anorexia nervosa could be characterized through SPECT imaging. Given the small numbers involved, as well as the design and methodologic issues mentioned above, interpretation of these studies is problematic.

Kuruoglu et al. (1998) reported on two female teenagers (aged 16 and 18 years) with anorexia nervosa who underwent SPECT brain imaging using ^{99m}TC-HMPAO. Both presented with a history of intentional weight loss, for 14 and 16 months, respectively, and both were diagnosed with anorexia nervosa of the binge eating and purging type. Neither was depressed according to the Hamilton Depression Rating Scale. They were both scanned 4–6 weeks following diagnosis. Scanning was repeated after 1.5 years of treatment when the patients had remained free of symptoms for at least 3 months. No control subjects were included in the study.

The pretreatment SPECT scan showed diffuse bilateral hypoperfusion in frontal, parietal, and frontotemporal areas. It is unclear how "abnormality" was defined. These abnormalities were judged to be more prominent in the left hemisphere. Post-treatment SPECT studies showed normal brain perfusion in both patients.

Overall, SPECT studies in adults and adolescents with eating disorder have failed to yield consistent and conclusive results. In the following section, we will discuss the only SPECT study published to date in children with anorexia nervosa.

SPECT in early-onset anorexia nervosa

Using SPECT, Gordon et al. (1997) measured rCBF in 15 children and adolescents (14 girls, one boy; age range 8–16 years) with a DSM-IV diagnosis of anorexia nervosa. Three of the patients had a follow-up scan after returning to normal weight. Initially, ^{99m}TC-HMPAO was the radiotracer of choice used by the hospital, but it was later replaced by ^{99m}TC-ECD (ethyl cysteinate dimer). Since the study was carried out during this period of change, only the first few patients received an injection of ^{99m}TC-HMPAO; the remainder received ECD. The comparison group included five children who underwent rCBF as part of an investigation for cerebrovascular disease because of hypertension. Their SPECT rCBF scans and cerebral angiograms were considered normal. These control SPECT scans showed either no asymmetry of rCBF or an asymmetry below 5% (Gordon, 1996).

The scans of the patients with early-onset anorexia nervosa were evaluated clinically by nuclear medicine physicians, who judged them to be abnormal if there was an asymmetry above 10% between the two sides of the brain on more than one contiguous slice. By this criterion, 13 of 15 patients showed an abnormal degree of temporal lobe asymmetry (Fig. 17.1, p. 242). Temporal lobe rCBF was decreased on the left in eight patients and on the right side in five patients. In the follow-up study of the three children who had regained weight, all continued to show asymmetries of rCBF in the temporal lobe that fell in the same direction as that seen on their initial scans. The magnitude of the asymmetry in the repeat scans was not indicated by the authors. Since publication of the above study, an additional 9 of 14 children studied by this group have asymmetry in the temporal lobes on SPECT images (I. Gordon, personal communication).

Further support for the above finding comes from a similar SPECT study carried out by the Childrens' Hospital in Sydney, Australia, which has shown unilateral reduced temporal lobe rCBF in three of four children with anorexia nervosa (Howman-Giles, personal communication). Some of the patients in the study by Gordon et al. (1997) had rCBF measured with ^{99m}TC-HMPAO, while others had rCBF measured with ^{99m}TC-ECD. This change in tracers makes comparison between subjects difficult, because the tracers will have varying properties, such as the rate of uptake. Nonetheless, the frequency of the finding of temporal lobe asymmetry is striking.

This, together with the persistence of an abnormality in those patients re-scanned by Gordon et al. (1997) after weight restoration, suggests that the data cannot be explained as being secondary to starvation. Changes in rCBF that are purely secondary to starvation would be likely to produce global and symmetrical changes. Therefore, such asymmetry may reflect an underlying primary cerebral abnormality that is contributing to the development of anorexia nervosa in these young patients. The abnormality in the temporal lobe (although it is not clear which part of the temporal lobe is involved) might be associated with functional imbalance in the limbic system. Such imbalance in the limbic system may lead to a disturbance in the hypothalamic–pituitary axis, which is thought to be responsible for the clinical changes seen in anorexia nervosa.

Summary and future directions

Structural neuroimaging studies in patients with anorexia nervosa have revealed abnormalities such as sulcal widening and ventricular enlargement that appear to be related to the consequences of anorexia nervosa, rather than to the cause. Results of PET studies in adults and older adolescents with anorexia nervosa have not yielded consistent findings; however some of these, too, have been linked to consequences of anorexia nervosa rather than to its causes (Delvenne et al., 1997a).

The majority of functional imaging studies in adults were discordant with rCBF studies in children. Studies in adults with anorexia nervosa found abnormalities in the caudate (Herholz et al., 1987; Delvenne et al., 1996) and parietal lobe (Delvenne et al. 1997a,b). Technical variations may account for the discrepancy in the findings, but the effects of a maturing and developing brain may be the critical factors. In addition, there may be a dissociation between rCBF and glucose metabolism in anorexia nervosa. Gordon et al. (1997) has pointed out a number of other possible explanations for the discrepancy in findings: childhood-onset anorexia nervosa may represent a biologically distinct group or a subgroup of patients with more severe involvement than is typically seen in patients with later onsets or childhood-onset anorexia nervosa may be a separate illness with a different etiology from that in adult populations. This seems unlikely as the clinical syndrome is similar no matter what the age of onset. And finally, it is possible that rCBF abnormalities result from a lesion that is influenced by age or chronicity.

The findings of asymmetrical temporal lobe hypoperfusion in a large percentage of the children (13/15) studied by Gordon et al. (1997) and by the team at the Childrens' Hospital in Sydney, Australia, who found it in three of four children studied, suggest that the temporal lobe may be involved in anorexia nervosa. This hypothesis is further strengthened by the observation that following full weight restoration in the Gordon et al. (1997) study, the focal rCBF abnormality persisted in all three children who were re-scanned. The continuation of this longitudinal study presently shows three of five children with unilateral temporal lobe hypoperfusion. One child continues to show rCBF assymetry in the temporal lobe almost 4 years after her first SPECT scan despite weight gain (I. Gordon, unpublished data). These findings may reflect an underlying biological factor contributing to the development and/or maintenance of anorexia nervosa.

Current understanding of the physical symptoms of anorexia nervosa suggests a hypothalamic–pituitary abnormality, but whether this abnormality is a primary or secondary event remains unclear. The limbic system has clear connections between the frontal and temporal lobes and the hypothalamic–pituitary axis. The work of MacLean (1955) and Papez (1937) suggest a close interdependent role of portions of the temporal lobe, including the amygdala, and hippocampus, in maintaining equilibrium of the limbic system and so allowing normal hypothalamic function. Dysfunction in the limbic system provides a possible mechanism that links disturbances in cortical functioning, emotional processes, and appetite control. Such an underlying cerebral vulnerability may be of genetic origin and may help to explain the heritability of anorexia nervosa (Holland et al., 1988). An important question arising from the studies of early-onset anorexia nervosa is whether asymmetry in the temporal lobe reflects a primary abnormality or a vulnerability, i.e., an underlying limbic system imbalance that, if exposed to emotional stress, could lead to the development of anorexia nervosa.

As noted above, the SPECT study of Gordon et al. (1997) is the first published functional imaging study involving children with anorexia nervosa. Additional controlled imaging studies using larger samples and examining relationships of functional imaging findings to clinical and neuropsychologic profiles are needed. Longitudinal studies will be important for monitoring the effects of treatment, as well as CNS maturational effects on the clinical expression of these disorders. Cognitive activation studies using fMRI or PET may further our understanding of the interaction of cognitive and emotional processing in relationship to eating disorders, e.g., the role of fear or disgust in anorexia nervosa. The investigation of neurotransmitter systems using PET may elucidate the role of serotonin, dopamine, noradrenaline, and the opioids in these disorders.

Acknowledgements

We would like to thank the Eating Disorders Team at Great Ormond Street Hospital who have helped with the SPECT study, especially Rachel Bryant-Waugh, Deborah Christie, Dasha Nicholls, and Kate Wigley. We would also like to thank the Gordon Carlton Memorial Fund for financial support.

References

American Psychiatric Association (1994). *Diagnostic and Statistical Manual of Mental Disorders*, 4th edn. Washington, DC: American Psychiatric Association.

Anand, B. K. and Brobeck, J. R. (1951). Localisation of a "feeding centre" in hypothalamus of the rat. *Proc. Soc. Exp. Biol. Med.*, **77**, 323–4.

Andreason, P. J., Altemus, M., Zametkin, A. J., King, A. C., Lucinio, J. and Cohen, R. M. (1992). Regional cerebral glucose metabolism in bulimia nervosa. *Am. J. Psychiatry*, **149**, 1506–13.

Andreason, P. J., Zametkin, A. J., Guo, A. C., Baldwin, P. and Cohen, R. M. (1994). Gender-related differences in regional cerebral glucose metabolism in normal volunteers. *Psychiatr. Res.*, **51**, 175–83.

Artmann, H., Grau, H., Adelmann, M. and Schleiffer, R. (1985). Reversible and non-reversible enlargement of cerebrospinal fluid space in anorexia nervosa. *Biol. Psychiatry*, **23**, 377–87.

Barry, A. and Lippman, B. (1990). Anorexia in males. *Postgrad. Med.*, **87**, 161–5.

Baxter, L. R., Phelps, M. E., Mazziotta, J. C., Guze, B. H., Schwartz, J. M. and Selin, C. E. (1987). Local cerebral glucose metabolism rates in obsessive compulsive disorder. *Arch. Gen. Psychiatry*, **44**, 211–18.

Bentovim, D. and Morton, J. (1990). Anorexia in males. *Postgrad. Med.*, **87**, 161–5.

Bowden, P. K., Touyz, S. W., Rodriguez, P. J., Hensely, R. and Beumont, P. J. V. (1989). Distorting patient or distorting instrument? *Br. J. Psychiatry*, **155**, 196–201.

Bruins-Slot, L., Gorwood, P., Bouvard, M. et al. (1998). Lack of association between anorexia nervosa and D3 dopamine receptor gene. *Biol. Psychiatry*, **43**, 76–8.

Bryant-Waugh, R. and Lask, B. (1995). Annotation: Eating disorders in children. *J. Child Psychol. Psychiatry*, **36**, 191–202.

Campbell, D. A., Sundaramurthy, D., Markham, A. F. and Pieri, L. F. (1998). Lack of assoication between 5-HT$_{2A}$ gene promoter polymorphism and susceptibility to anorexia nervosa. (Letter) *Lancet*, **351**, 499.

Casper, R. C. (1984). Hypothalamic dysfunction and symptoms of anorexia nervosa. *Psychiatr. Clin. North Am.*, **7**, 201–13.

Christie, D., Lambert, S., Wigley, K. et al. (1998). IQ, memory and attainments in childhood onset anorexia nervosa. In *Proceedings of the 8th International Conference on Eating Disorders*, New York.

Collier, D. A., Arranz, M. J., Li, T., Mupita, D., Brown, N. and Treasure, J. (1997). Association between 5-HT$_{2A}$ gene promoter polymorphism and anorexia nervosa. (Letter) *Lancet*, **350**, 412.

Dally, P. (1969). *Anorexia Nervosa*. London: Heinemann Medical.

De Vile, C. J., Sofrraz, R., Lask, B. D. and Stanhope, R. (1995). Occult intracranial tumours masquerading as early onset anorexia nervosa. *BMJ*, **311**, 1359–60.

Doraiswamy, P. M., Krishnan, K. R., Bogko, O. B. et al. (1991). Pituitary abnormalies in eating disorders: further evidence from MRI studies. *Prog. Neuropsychopharmacol. Biol. Psychiatry*, **15**, 351–6.

Delvenne, V., Lotstra, F., Goldman, S. et al. (1995). Brain hypometabolism of glucose in anorexia nervosa: a PET-scan study. *Biol. Psychiatry*, **37**, 161–9.

Delvenne, V., Goldman, S., de Maertelaer, V., Simon, Y., Luxen, A. and Lotstra, F. (1996). Brain hypometabolism in anorexia nervosa; normalization after weight gain. *Biol. Psychiatry*, **40**, 761–8.

Delvenne, V., Goldmann, S., de Maertelaer, V., Wikler, D., Damhaut, P. and Lostra, F. (1997a). Brain glucose metabolism in anorexia nervosa and affective disorders: influence of weight loss or depressive symptomatology. *Psychiatr. Res.*, **74**, 83–92.

Delvenne, V., Goldman, S., Simon, Y., de Maertelaer, V. and Lostra, F. (1997b). Brain hypometabolism of glucose in bulimia nervosa. *Int. J. Eating Disord.*, **21**, 313–20.

Erb, J. L., Gwirtsman, H. E., Fuster, J. M. and Richeimer, S. H. (1989). Bulimia associated with frontal lobe lesions. *Int. J. Eating Disord.*, **8**, 117–21.

Ernst, M., Zametkin, A. J. Phillips, R. L. and Cohen, R. M. (1998). Age-related changes in brain glucose metabolism in adults with attention-deficit/hyperactivity disorder and control subjects. *J. Neuropsychiatry Clin. Neurosci.*, **10**, 168–77.

Fosson, A., Knibbs, J., Bryant-Waugh, R. and Lask, B. (1987). Early onset anorexia nervosa. *Arch. Dis. Childhood*, **621**, 114–18.

Fox, C. F. (1981). Neuropsychological correlates of anorexia nervosa. *Int. J. Psychiatr. Med.*, **11**, 285–90.

Garfinkel, P. E. (1974). The perception of hunger and satiety in anorexia nervosa. *Psychol. Med.*, **4**, 309–15.

Gillberg, C. (1995). *Clinical Child Neuropsychiatry*. Cambridge, UK: Cambridge University Press.

Gillberg, I. C., Gillberg, C., Rastam, M. and Johansson, M. (1996). The cognitive profile of anorexia nervosa: a comparative study including a community-based sample. *Compr. Psychiatry*, **37**, 23–30.

Goldrey, R. D. (1978). Craniopharyngioma simulating anorexia nervosa. *J. Nerv. Mental Dis.*, **166**, 533–6.

Gordon, I. (1996). Cerebral blood flow imaging in paediatrics: a review. *Nuc. Med. Commun.*, **17**, 1021–9.

Gordon, I., Lask, B., Bryant-Waugh, R., Christie, D. and Timimi, S. (1997). Childhood-onset anorexia nervosa: towards identifying a biological substrate. *Int. J. Eating Disord.*, **22**, 159–65.

Gowers, S., Crisp, A., Joughin, N. and Bhat, A. (1991). Premenarcheal anorexia nervosa. *J. Child Psychol. and Psychiatry*, **32**, 515–24.

Gur, R. C., Mozley, L. H., Mozley, P. D. et al. (1995). Sex differences in regional cerebral glucose metabolism during a resting state. *Science*, **267**, 528–31.

Hamsher, K. S., Halmi, K. A. and Benton, A. L. (1981). Prediction of outcome of anorexia nervosa from neuropsychological status. *Psychiatr. Res.*, **4**, 79–88.

Hawkins, R. A. and Biebuyck, J. F. (1979). Ketone bodies are selectively used by individual brain regions. *Science*, **205**, 325–7.

Hawley, R. (1985). The outcome of anorexia nervosa in younger subjects. *Brit. J. Psychiatry*, **146**, 657–60.

Herholz, K. (1996). Neuroimaging in anorexia nervosa. *Psychiatr. Res.*, **62**, 105–10.

Herholz, K., Krieg, J. C., Emrich, H. M. et al. (1987). Regional cerebral glucose metabolism in anorexia nervosa measured by positron emission tomography. *Biol. Psychiatry*, **22**, 43–51.

Heron, G. B. and Johnston, D. A. (1976). Hypothalamic tumour presenting as anorexia nervosa. *Am. J. Psychiatry*, **133**, 580–2.

Herzog, D., Keller, M. B., Sacks, N. R., Yeh, C. J. and Lavori, P. W. (1992). Psychiatric comorbidity in treatment-seeking anorexics and bulimics. *J. Am. Acad. Child Adolesc. Psychiatry*, **31**, 810–18.

Higgs, J., Goodyer, I. and Birch, J. (1989). Anorexia nervosa and food avoidance emotional disorder. *Arch. Dis. Childhood*, **64**, 346–51.

Hinney, A., Barth, N., Ziegler, A. et al. (1997). Serotonin transporter gene-linked polymorphic region: allele distributions in relationship to body weight and in anorexia nervosa. *Life Sci*, **61**, 295–303.

Holland, A., Sicotte, N. and Treasure, J. (1988). Anorexia nervosa: evidence for a genetic basis. *J. Psychosomat. Res.*, **32**, 549–54.

Horne, R. L., van Vactor, J. C. and Emerson, S. (1991). Disturbed body image in patients with eating disorders. *Am J. Psychiatry*, **148**, 211–15.

Hsu, L. K. G. (1990). *Eating Disorders*. New York: Guilford Press.

Husain, M. M., Black, K. J., Doraiswamy, P. M. et al. (1992). Subcortical brain anatomy in anorexia and bulimia. *Biol. Psychiatry*, **31**, 735–8.

Jacobs, B. and Isaacs, S. (1986). Pre-pubertal anorexia nervosa. A retrospective controlled study. *J. Child Psychol. Psychiatry*, **27**, 237–50.

Johnson, R. D. (1995). Opioid involvement in feeding behavior and the pathogenesis of certain eating disorders. *Med. Hypoth.*, **45**, 491–7.

Jonas, J. M. and Gold, M. S. (1986). Naltrexone reverses bulimic symptoms. *Lancet*, **1**, 807.

Katzmann, D. K., Zipursky, R. B., Lambe, E. K. and Mikulis, D. J. (1997). A longitudinal magnetic resonance imaging study of brain changes in adolescents with anorexia nervosa. *Arch. Paediatr. Adolesc. Med.*, **151**, 793–7.

Kaye, W. H., Pickar, D., Nabar, D. and Ebert, M. H. (1982). Cerebrospinal fluid opioid activity in anorexia nervosa. *Am. J. Psychiatry*, **139**, 643–5.

Kaye, W., Weltzin, T. E., Hsu, L. K. G., Bulik, C., McConaha, C. and Sobkiewicz, T. (1992). Patients with anorexia nervosa have elevated scores on Yale–Brown Obsessive Compulsive Scale. *Int J. Eating Disord.*, **12**, 57–62.

Kingston, K., Szmukler, G., Andrewes, D., Tress, B. and Desmond, P. (1996). Neuropsychological and structural brain changes in anorexia nervosa before and after refeeding. *Psychol. Med.*, **26**, 15–28.

Krieg, J. C., Backmund, H., Pirke, K. M. (1987). Cranial computed tomography findings in bulimia. *Acta Psychiatr. Scand.*, **75**, 144–9.

Krieg, J. C., Pirke, K. M., Lauer, C. and Backmund, H. (1988). Endocrine, metabolic, and cranial computed tomographic findings in anorexia nervosa. *Biol. Psychiatry*, **23**, 377–87.

Krieg, J. C., Lauer, C., Leinsinger, G. et al. (1989). Brain morphology and regional cerebral blood flow in anorexia nervosa. *Biol. Psychiatry*, **25**, 1041–8.

Krieg, J. C., Holtoff, V., Schreiber, W., Pirke, K. M. and Herholz, K. (1991). Glucose metabolism in the caudate nuclei of patients with eating disorders, measured by PET. *Eur. Arch. Psychiatry Clin. Neurosci.*, **240**, 331–3.

Kuruoglu, A. C., Kapucu, O., Atasever, T., Arikan, Z., Isik, E. and Unlu, M. (1998). Technetium-99m-HMPAO brain SPECT in anorexia nervosa. *J. Nucl. Med.*, **39**, 304–6.

Laessle, R. G., Zoettl, H. and Pirke, K. (1987). Meta-analysis of treatment studies for bulimia. *Int. J. Eating Disord.*, **11**, 97–110.

Laessle, R. G., Krieg, J. C., Fichter, M. M., Pirke, K. M. (1989). Cerebral atrophy and vigilance performance in patients with anorexia nervosa and bulimia nervosa. *Neuropsychobiology*, **21**, 187–91.

Lambe, E. K., Katzman, D. K., Mikulis, D. J., Kennedy, S. H. and Zipursky, R. B. (1997). Cerebral grey matter volume deficits after weight recovery from anorexia nervosa. *Arch. Gen. Psychiatry*, **54**, 537–42.

Lask, B. and Bryant-Waugh, R. (1986). Childhood onset anorexia nervosa. In *Recent Advances in Paediatrics*, No. 8, ed. R. Meadow, pp. 21–31. London: Churchill Livingstone.

Lask, B. and Bryant-Waugh, R. (eds.) (1999). *Anorexia Nervosa and Related Eating Disorders in Childhood and Adolescence*, 2nd edn. Hove, UK: Psychology Press.

Lask, B., Britten, C., Kroll, L., Magagna, J. and Tranter, M. (1991). Pervasive refusal in children. *Arch. Dis. Childhood*, 66, 866–9.

Lewin, K., Mattingley, D. and Millin, R. R. (1972). Anorexia nervosa associated with hypothalamic tumour. *BMJ*, 2, 629–30.

Mayberg, H. S., Robinson, R. G. and Wong, D. F. (1988). PET imaging of cortical S$_2$ serotonin receptors after stroke: lateralized changes and relationship to depression. *Am. J. Psychiatry*, 145, 937–43.

Maxwell, J. K., Tucker, D. M. and Towes, B. D. (1984). Asymmetric cognitive function in anorexia nervosa. *Int. J. Neurosci.*, 24, 37–44.

MacLean, P. (1955). The limbic system and emotional behaviour. *Arch. Neurol. Psychiatry*, 73, 130–4.

Miura, S. A., Schapiro, M. B., Grady, C. L. et al. (1990). Effect of gender on glucose utilization rates in healthy humans: a positron emission tomography study. *J. Neurosci. Res.*, 27, 500–4.

Nauta, W. J. H. (1971). The problem of the frontal lobe: a reinterpretation. *J. Psychiatry*, 147, 838–49.

Nordahl, T. E., Benkelfat, C., Semple, W. E., Gross, M., King, A. C. and Cohen, R. M. (1989). Cerebral glucose metabolic rates in obsessive compulsive disorder. *Neuropsychopharmacology*, 2, 23–8.

Nozoe, S., Naruo, T., Nakabeppu, Y., Soejima, Y., Nakajo, M. and Tanaka, H. (1993). Changes in regional cerebral blood flow in patients with anorexia nervosa detected through single photon emission tomography imaging. *Biol. Psychiatry*, 34, 578–80.

Nozoe, S., Naruo, T., Yonekura, R. et al. (1995). Comparison of regional cerebral blood flow in patients with eating disorders. *Brain Res. Bull.*, 36, 251–5.

Ono, T., Nishino, H., Fukunda, M., Sasaki, K. and Nishijo, H. (1984). Single neuron activity in dorsolateral prefrontal cortex of monkey during operant behaviour sustained by food reward. *Brain Res.*, 311, 332.

Palazidou, E., Robinson, P. and Lishman, W. (1990). Neuroradiological and neuropsychological assessment in anorexia nervosa. *Psychol. Med.*, 20, 521–7.

Papez, J. (1937). A proposed mechanism of emotion. *Arch. Neurol. Psychiatry*, 38, 725–43.

Pendleton-Jones, B., Duncan, C., Browers, P. and Mirsky, A. F. (1991). Cognition in eating disorders. *J. Clin. Exp. Neuropsychol.*, 13, 711–28.

Phillipp, E., Pirke, K. M., Keller, M. and Krieg, J. (1991). Disturbed cholecystokinin secretion in patients with eating disorders. *Life Sci.*, 48, 2443–50.

Pirke, K. M., Pahl, J., Schweiger, U. and Warnoff, M. (1985). Metabolic and endocrine indices of starvation in bulimia: a comparison with anorexia nervosa. *Psychiatr. Res.*, 15, 33–9.

Russell, G. (1985). Anorexia and bulimia nervosa. In *Child and Adolescent Psychiatry*, 2nd edn, eds. M. Rutter and Hersov, pp. 625–37. Oxford: Blackwell Scientific.

Schmidt, U., Hodes, M. and Treasure, J. (1992). Early onset bulimia nervosa-who is at risk? *Psychol. Med.*, 22, 623–8.

Sorbi, S., Nacmias, B., Tedde, A., Ricca, V., Mezzani, B. and Rotella, C. M. (1998). 5-HT$_{2A}$ promoter polymorphism in anorexia nervosa. (Letter) *Lancet*, 351, 1785.

Silver, A. J. and Morley, J. E. (1991). The role of CCK regulation of food intake. *Prog. Neurobiol.*, 36, 23–34.

Strober, M., Lampert, C., Morrell, W., Burroughs, J. and Jacobs, C. (1990). A controlled family study of anorexia nervosa. *Int. J. Eating Disord.*, 9, 239–54.

Szmukler, G. I. and Tam, D. (1984). Anorexia nervosa: starvation dependence. *Br. J. Med. Psychol.*, 57, 303–10.

Szmukler, G. I., Andrewes, D., Kingston, K., Chen, L., Stargatt, R. and Stanley, R. (1992). Neuropsychological impairment in anorexia nervosa before and after refeeding. *J. Clin. Exp. Neuropsychol.*, 14, 347–52.

Tanner, J., Whitehouse, R. and Takaishi, M. (1966). Standards from birth to maturity for height, weight, height velocity and weight velocity: British children, 1965, Parts 1 and 2. *Arch. Dis. Childhood*, 41, 454–71, 613–35.

Teitelbaum, P. and Stellar, E. (1954). Recovery from failure to eat produced by hypothalamic lesions. *Science*, 120, 894–5.

Terzian, H. and Ore, G. (1955). Syndrome of Kluver and Bucy reproduced in man by bilateral removal of the temporal lobes. *Neurology*, 15, 373 80.

Treasure, J. (1997). Eating disorders. In *Essentials of Postgraduate Psychiatry*, 3rd edn, eds. R. Murray, P. Hill and P. McGuffin, pp. 192–221. Cambridge, UK: Cambridge University Press.

Treasure, J. and Campbell, I. (1994). The case for biology in the aetiology of anorexia nervosa. *Psychol. Med.*, 24, 3–8.

Whitaker, A., Johnson, J., Shaffer, D., Rapoport, J. and Kalikow, K. (1990). Uncommon troubles in young people: prevalence estimates of selected psychiatric disorders in a non-psychiatric population. *Arch. Gen. Psychiatry*, 47, 487–96.

White, L. E. and Hain, R. F. (1959). Anorexia in association with a destructive lesion of the hypothalamus. *Arch. Pathol.*, 68, 275–81.

Wise, R. A. and Rompre, P. P. (1989). Brain dopamine and reward. *Annu. Rev. Psychol.*, 40, 191–255.

Witt, E. D., Ryan, C. and Hsu, E. (1985). Learning deficits in adolescents with anorexia nervosa. *J. Nerv. Mental Dis.*, 173, 182–4.

Wu, J. C., Hagman, J., Buchsbaum, M. S. et al. (1990). Greater left cerebral hemispheric metabolism in bulimia assessed by positron emission tomography. *Am. J. Psychiatry*, 147, 309–12.

Yoshii, F., Barker, W. W., Chang, J. Y. et al. (1988). Sensitivity of cerebral glucose metabolism to age, gender, brain volume, brain atrophy, and cerebrovascular risk factors. *J. Cereb. Blood Flow Metab.*, 8, 654–61.

Part 5

Future directions

Genetics, development of tasks and paradigms for neuroimaging, and conceptual/interpretative issues are leitmotifs in the review of neuroimaging applications in child psychiatry. Clearly, future research will draw on the rapid developments in genetics and seek to integrate genetic and neuroimaging methods. The readers will find in this section two chapters on genetics. In Chapter 18, Vandenbergh describes the techniques and methods of molecular genetics. These techniques may enable researchers to identify genes underlying neuroimaging phenotypes and playing a role in brain function. In Chapter 19, Pauls discusses specific issues in the genetic study of complex neurobehavioral conditions and stresses the need for a developmental focus in this work.

A conceptual framework for viewing neuroimaging studies of childhood disorders is provided by Müller and Courchesne (Chapter 20), who bring development to the forefront in their discussion of plasticity and its potentially detrimental, as well as beneficial, effects. Models of the range of developmental paths from neuropathology to behavioral outcomes, and implications for the design and interpretation of imaging studies, are highlighted.

Finally, the need for well-validated neuropsychologic tools for use with functional neuroimaging is addressed with two chapters on the Cambridge Neuropsychological Testing Automated Battery (CANTAB), which may serve as a model for task and paradigm development. In Chapter 21, Lee and his colleagues describe the development of this instrument and its utility in functional neuroimaging. The decomposition of complex cognitive functions, hypotheses concerning their neural substrates informed by animal research, and validation of behavioral tests as probes for examining the integrity of brain circuits in human adults with focal or circumscribed neuropathology provide a basis for using the battery in conjunction with neuroimaging to extend our knowledge of the neural substrates of psychiatric disorders.

Extending this work to children, Luciana and Nelson discuss the use and validation of the CANTAB as a tool for measuring frontal lobe and other functions in neurodevelopmental studies (Chapter 22). Emerging applications in children whose development has been impaired by a variety of conditions, many of which are less focal in nature than are adult-acquired lesions, are described. The availability of neuropsychologic measures that span a wide age range, from childhood into adulthood, offers promise for probing phenotypic variability (e.g., milder variants) in family genetic studies.

In Chapter 23, the editors address topics not covered in this book, such as promising new techniques, the combined uses of different imaging modalities, and advances in research design and image analysis that allow for improved exploitation of exist- ing imaging modalities. They highlight the need for integration with other aspects of clinical neuroscience and emphasize the focus within child psychiatry on executive and attentional dys- functions, on emotion, and their interrelationships and neuro- chemistry. Emerging contributions of neuroimaging studies to child psychiatry are highlighted, and directions for future research proposed.

18

Techniques of molecular genetics

David J. Vandenbergh

Introduction

The fields of functional brain imaging and molecular genetics are at the forefront of biomedical research because these techniques are rapidly identifying new questions to be addressed and increasing the depth to which old questions can be addressed. The purpose of this chapter is to describe the techniques that will facilitate new understanding of neuroimaging results by adding a molecular genetic approach to examining neuroimaging phenotypes. It is hoped that these genetic techniques will enable researchers to identify the genes that play a role in the processes that underlie brain function.

What is meant by a neuroimaging phenotype, or trait? Examples include receptor density measured by ligands in positron emission tomography (PET) or the location and size of a brain region activated in response to a cognitive task measured by cerebral blood flow techniques. A phenotype could also be a psychiatric diagnosis that has some relationship to neuroimaging measurements. Defined broadly, a phenotype, or trait, is any observable characteristic that has a heritable component. In fact, it is the quantitative nature of neuroimaging that may provide an essential element for making significant progress in finding the genes that underlie the biochemical and molecular pathways of brain function. The choice of the definition of the phenotype in a genetic study is of paramount importance for the success of the research enterprise, as is discussed in Chapter 19. The search for the genes responsible for a given phenotype needs to be guided by hypotheses, given that more than half of the 50–100000 human genes are expressed in the brain (Lewin, 1997).

A brief example of Mendelian genetics is provided initially to highlight the point that variation in a single gene can affect many of the phenotypes measured in neuroimaging. This is followed by a description of complex genet-

ics – the most likely to be encountered in neuroimaging studies – in which several genes contribute to the phenotype of interest. The types of study design that are needed for complex genetics are then described, followed by the methods necessary to collect the genomic DNA, which is required for a genetic analysis of neuroimaging results. A glossary is provided at the end of the chapter for quick reference to the genetic terms encountered either within this chapter or within the material referred to during the chapter. Some readers may benefit by referring to a general textbook of human genetics (e.g., Gelerter et al., 1998; Strachan and Read, 1996) to help to understand the following material.

Mendelian genetics: single gene mutations alter brain function

First, an important point of clarification: the terms altered genes or gene variants are used to avoid the common misnomer of a "disease gene". The term disease gene suggests that an individual with the disease has a gene that nondiseased individuals do not. Rather, it is intended to refer to a mutated variant of the same gene that is inherited in a "normal" form by nondiseased individuals. This mutated variant is responsible for the inherited disease.

As of March 1998, about 46800 genes have been described in the human genome database (www.gdb.org), and 1325 genetic diseases have been mapped to chromosomal sites. Many human genes have been cloned and sequenced, including those that, when mutated, give rise to diseases relevant to neuroimaging, such as Huntington's disease (chromosome 4), Alzheimer's disease (chromosomes 1, 14, 21), neurofibromatosis (chromosomes 17, 22), fragile X syndrome (chromosome X), and Lesch–Nyhan disease (chromosome X).

Lesch–Nyhan disease is a well-known example of a Mendelian disorder in which a mutated form of a single gene can cause a neuropsychiatric syndrome of motor and compulsive self-injurious symptoms (McKusick, 1990). At its simplest, a Mendelian disorder is one in which an individual can be defined as either having, or not having, the disorder. The inheritance pattern is thus categorical – one either inherits a mutated form (allele) of the gene or a non-mutated form. In the case of Lesch–Nyhan disease, the causative mutation is an inactive allele of the hypoxanthine-guanine phosphoribosyl transferase (HPRT) gene, where, most frequently, one base pair of the gene is deleted (a point mutation). This single alteration causes the gene to encode a nonfunctional protein. The mutation is recessive, i.e., for the disease to be expressed, both inherited genes (one from each parent) need to be mutated; as a corollary, an individual that inherits one active allele from one parent and one inactive allele from the other parent is unaffected. In Lesch–Nyhan disease, the gene is located on the X chromosome. Therefore, females who carry only one affected gene (carrier) do not express the disease but will pass the gene, and thus the disease, to 50% of their male offspring. The mutation can also occur de novo during the gametogenesis. HPRT is a key enzyme in the nucleotide salvage pathway, and in the absence of active HPRT, uric acid accumulates to toxic levels. A result of this build up of uric acid is the development of multiple symptoms, including choreathetosis and self-destructive behavior. The relationship of the HPRT gene and brain function is not clear; however, it has been shown by neuroimaging that individuals with Lesch–Nyhan disease have reduced levels of the DOPA decarboxylase enzyme activity (Ernst et al., 1996) and the dopamine transporter (Wong et al., 1996).

The relationship of an inactive HPRT gene with decreased levels of DOPA decarboxylase and dopamine transporter, both detected by PET scan, raises an important question pertinent to genetics and neuroimaging. Is it possible that other partially active forms of HPRT, and perhaps other partially active forms of other genes, serve, in combination, to modify neurologic behaviors? Minor alteration of the levels of HPRT, DOPA decarboxylase, or the dopamine transporter may not lead to identifiable disorders, such as Lesch–Nyhan disease, but may still have some functional consequences in the brain. It is the detection and identification of these types of gene, called "susceptibility" or "vulnerability" genes, that is the realm of complex genetics.

Before addressing complex genetics, the contribution of two other genetic phenomena, expansion of trinucleotide repeat DNA sequences and imprinting, to the characteristics of the inheritance and course of a disorder will be mentioned briefly. These events can complicate the tracking of inheritance of a trait and point to the dynamic nature of the genome, something not widely appreciated prior to molecular analysis.

Trinucleotide repeat expansion and anticipation

Trinucleotide repeat expansion mutations cause several inherited neurodegenerative diseases, including Huntington's disease and several forms of spinocerebellar ataxia, often with significant neuropsychiatric symptoms. Expansion mutations have also been proposed to cause a number of other disorders, including bipolar affective disorder, schizophrenia, and autism. For as yet unknown reasons, some repeated sequences of three nucleotides (e.g., CGG or CAG, where C is cytosine, G is guanosine, and A is adenosine) are unstable and can increase in length (expand) during DNA replication. Repeats of a given length increase in size when transmitted from parents to offspring (intergenerational instability, "meiotic instability") and often show size variation within the tissues of an affected individual (somatic mosaicism, "mitotic instability"). Repeat instability is clinically important, because longer repeats result in earlier age of onset and more severe disease phenotype. Therefore, a molecular explanation for anticipation (increasing disease severity in successive affected generations) is given by the correlation of the length of a trinucleotide repeat to the severity of the phenotype.

Fragile X is an archetypal example of expansion of a trinucleotide repeat (de Vries et al., 1998). The mutation is caused by a repeat of the trinucleotide CGG in the promotor areas (DNA region that regulates the initiation and level of transcription of genes) of the *FMR-1* gene located on the X chromosome. An allele with a relatively small number of the trinucleotides (50–200 triplets or 150–600 base pairs) is termed a premutation because individuals carrying this size repeat are normal. Individuals with the full mutation show an expansion of 200–1000 trinucleotide repeats. Alleles become expanded primarily through female gamete formation (see imprinting phenomenon below), but expansion can also occur postzygotically. In this latter process, the sex of the embryo also appears to influence expansion (greater in male than female embryos). The full mutation causes the range of physical and behavioral symptoms associated with the fragile X syndrome. Huntington's disease is another typical example of trinucleotide expansion. In this disorder, lower cognitive performance has been correlated with longer trinucleotide repeats in at-risk gene carriers (Jason et al., 1997).

Imprinting

Another important aspect of genetic transmission of disease is that the sex of the parent can differentially affect the formation of repeats (imprinting phenomenon). Genomic imprinting is an epigenetic mechanism resulting in the preferential expression of the maternal or paternal alleles of a specific subset of genes. The basic mechanism of imprinting is methylation of DNA, in particular some cytosine residues when they are followed by a guanosine. Methylation is thought to regulate the ability of proteins in the nucleus of the cell to transcribe a gene in the general region of the methylated cytosine. Prader–Willi syndrome and Angelman syndrome are classical examples of the imprinting phenomenon (Feil and Kelsey, 1997). Patients with the former have neonatal hypotonia with failure to thrive, hyperphagia and severe obesity, hypogonadism, short stature, short hands and feet, mild mental retardation with learning disabilities, and obsessive-compulsive disorder. Symptomatology in Angelman syndrome includes ataxia, tremulousness, seizures, sleep disorder, hyperactivity, severe mental retardation with lack of speech, and a happy disposition with paroxysms of laughter. Both disorders are caused by the loss of function of imprinted genes (expressed from either maternal or paternal chromosome) in proximal 15q11-q13. However, deletions in Prader–Willi syndrome are of paternal origin whereas in Angelman syndrome they are of maternal origin. In approximately 2–4% of patients, a loss of function results from an imprinting defect. Molecular analysis of imprinting mutations that interfere with the appropriate establishment of the maternal and paternal epigenotypes has led to the identification of imprinted transcripts that could be involved in determining which gene is imprinted in the germline.

Complex genetics: interaction of multiple genes alter brain function

Severe diseases that are attributable to a single gene, such as Lesch–Nyhan disease, are rare. More common are disorders that are heritable in part but do not display a one-to-one correspondence between the disorder's presence and a single gene. These disorders are referred to as complex. Complex disorders may not be as severe as Lesch–Nyhan disease but are present in a large enough proportion of the population that the aggregate effect on society is large. In the case of complex disorders, several genes contribute to the disorder. Each of the altered genes alone is not *sufficient* or even *necessary* to cause the disorder, but the sum of multiple small effects from several altered genes leads to disease. Complex genetics are not limited to traits that we think of as diseases or disorders. Many traits demonstrate complex patterns of inheritance. Aspects of normal brain development are likely to be complex traits that depend on the action of multiple genes. For example, the volumes of specific brain nuclei can be inherited as complex traits. Complex traits can occur as a continuous (quantitative) characteristic, in which a normal distribution of values for the trait can be seen, or as a discontinuous (dichotomous) characteristic, in which a threshold value must be achieved to define the trait (for further description see Strachan and Read (1996) and Falconer (1989)).

A further level of complexity, in addition to the action of multiple genes, is the fact that a given constellation of altered genes (vulnerability or susceptibility genes) may only lead to a predisposition for the disease. This predisposition requires an interaction with environmental factors to produce the disease. Examples of disorders of this type that are actively investigated by neuroimaging methods are reading disorders (Grigorenko et al., 1997), attention-deficit hyperactivity disorder (ADHD) (Castellanos, 1997; Ernst et al., 1998), and substance abuse (Grant et al., 1996). Until recently these types of disorder were thought to be unapproachable by geneticists, because of, first, the inability to fit the disorders to traditional models of dominant or recessive inheritance, and, second, the recognition that a large number of genotypes would need to be examined.

Two major advances have occurred, or perhaps more accurately continue to occur, allowing the genetic analysis of complex disorders. The first advance was the application of the polymerase chain reaction (PCR) (Saiki et al., 1988) to human genetics. The application of PCR to genetics allows a short region of DNA containing a polymorphism to be amplified. The detection of the form, or forms, of the polymorphism present in the amplified DNA leads to a genotype in a much more rapid manner than achieved with the older methods. Two types of polymorphism are commonly detected. First, sites in which one nucleotide has been replaced by another are known as restriction fragment length polymorphisms (RFLPs) (Fig. 18.1). RFLPs were originally detected by Southern blot procedures that were costly, especially in the amount of DNA used, and time consuming. The second common polymorphism is a variable number of repeated nucleotides, known as a microsatellite (Fig. 18.2). (The most common such repeat is the dinucleotide CA, but a repeat can consist of three or more nucleotides and it is not unusual for 50 or more nucleotides to be the repeat unit.) PCR methods have led to the rapid identification of many regions of DNA containing polymorphisms scattered across the genome.

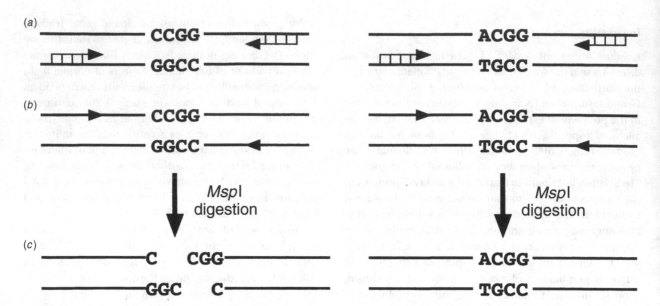

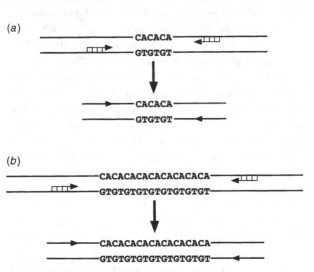

Fig. 18.1. Restriction fragment length polymorphisms can be detected with the use of the polymerase chain reaction (PCR) and a restriction enzyme. (*a*) Genomic DNA that differs by a single base, CCGG or ACGG, is amplified by PCR using primers designed to bind to DNA that flanks the altered sequence (small arrows). (*b*) This generates large numbers of the DNA product. The DNA is incubated with the restriction enzyme *Msp*I, which recognizes and cuts the sequence CCGG. (*c*) Two fragments of DNA are generated if the sequence CCGG is present (left-hand side), and one fragment if ACGG is present (right-hand side). These different DNA fragments can be detected by gel electrophoresis.

Fig. 18.2. Primers, shown as small arrows in (*a*) and (*b*), bind to two sites flanking a polymorphism. The polymorphism is a difference in the number of dinucleotide repeats, CA in this case, such that the allele in (*a*) contains three copies of CA and that in (*b*) contains nine copies. Multiple copies of the DNA are synthesized by the polymerase chain reaction and the difference in size between these products can be determined by gel electrophoresis.

In addition to identifying many new polymorphisms, PCR methods also increased the rate of acquisition of an individual's genotype at each polymorphic site. These sites are called genetic markers and, with PCR, many markers can be tested in a short period of time. The identification of candidate genes contributing to a complex trait requires the use of many genetic markers. These genetic markers may be anonymous pieces of DNA without a known function, but as long as their chromosomal location is known, it is possible to track the inheritance of the genetic marker and thus the DNA physically close to the marker on the chromosome. To date, about 19 000 markers have been identified throughout the human genome (Web site *www.gdb.org*; sadly this database is no longer being maintained, and the latest data are from 9 March 1998). Additional modifications of PCR, such as multiple reactions in a single tube, are causing further increases in the rate of acquisition of genotypes to the point that questions that were unanswerable prior to 1987, when PCR was invented, are now feasible with the resources of one or a few laboratories.

The second advance was the recognition that the identification of many genetic markers spaced closely along each chromosome would be more powerful for detection of the genes involved in complex diseases (Lander and Schork, 1994). The need for close spacing between markers is akin to driving down a dark road trying to find a barn by shining a flashlight outside the side window. If the flashlight is turned on once every mile, the chances of finding the barn are not great, but if the flashlight is turned on every 20 m the chances are much better. Additionally, it was recognized that the power to detect a gene's involvement in a disease would increase by analyzing two or more adjacent markers at a time, known as multipoint analysis. (If the genotypes are derived from a single chromosome they are called a haplotype.) Finally, new strategies were developed, such as the haplotype relative risk paradigm and the transmission disequilibrium test (TDT), which seek to maximize the information available by combining elements of traditional linkage (studying nuclear families) with elements of association tests (studying marker–phenotype relationship with, or without, requiring physical linkage). These methods are detailed below.

Study designs for complex traits in neuroimaging

Given that most traits measured in neuroimaging studies are genetically complex, how should one go about detecting the genes that underlie the trait? Psychiatric disorders are generally defined by behavioral characteristics that may not directly reveal biological function. Neuroimaging data from brain disorders provide quantitative measurements (continuous variables), which is the type of phenotypic information that is amenable to analysis by modern genetic methods. Indeed, a qualitative phenotype for a disorder (either having or not having the disorder, dichotomous variable) may not adequately describe the variability found in the disorder. Results of genetic studies may eventually aid in defining types and subtypes of disorder (nosology) (Leboyer et al., 1998), which in turn may aid in further refining genetic searches in a bootstrap approach. A greater understanding of the genetic component of these disorders will enable diagnosis of disease and open new therapeutic approaches. Finally, understanding the genetic component will allow for more accurate definition of the environmental factors that interact with genes to cause disease.

The recognition of the difficulty in finding multiple gene variants that contribute to complex disorders by traditional methods (analysis of pedigrees) has led geneticists to use new approaches that are generally termed nonparametric. These approaches fall into two categories: analysis of small nuclear families, or parts of families (e.g., sib-pairs), or analysis of cohorts of unrelated individuals (association studies). The approaches taken by these methods

are addressed briefly to give a rudimentary understanding of how the methods can be applied to neuroimaging data. For further details, the reader is referred to reviews by Risch (Risch and Merikangas, 1996; Risch, 1997) and Rao (1998).

Sample size is a serious issue in genetic studies and often constitutes the limiting factor in the completion of genetic investigations. The number of individuals needed varies with the neuroimaging question being asked, and the genetic method that is appropriate to the question. Most importantly, the sample size is dependent on three factors related to the neuroimaging study. The first critical factor is the error in measurement inherent in the neuroimaging technique. Because several genes may contribute to a small part of the data, the error in a neuroimaging measurement may be as large as, and mask, the effect of any one gene. An example, explained below, is dyslexia. Imaging studies might identify neurologic aspects of dyslexia that are genetic, but the imprecision in neuroimaging results, and the difficulty of defining a reading disability phenotype, will prevent easy detection of specific genes involved in the disorder. The second factor related to sample size is the fraction of the variance in measurement of the trait that is affected by genes, or more simply its degree of heritability. Many traits may have significant environmental components, making it difficult to detect the genetic components. Most frequently, heritability in humans is measured in studies that compare the frequency of a trait in pairs of monozygous and dizygous twins. A pair of twins is said to be concordant if the trait is present in both. For traits that have a heritable component, the concordance rate is expected to be higher in monozygous twins, who share all of their genes, than in dizygous twins, who share only half of their genes. A second measurement of heritability is the risk to relatives, in which one compares the incidence of a trait in family members of selected individuals with the incidence in the general population. An increased incidence in relatives suggests (but does not prove) a heritable component. An example of a heritable trait relevant to neuroimaging is dyslexia, certain forms of which were proposed to be hereditary (Hallgren, 1950), with genetics accounting for approximately half of the variability (DeFries et al., 1987; LaBuda et al., 1993). Single word reading and phonological decoding and awareness are measures of dyslexia that are currently being examined in genetic studies (Grigorenko et al., 1997; see also Chapter 15) as more narrowly defined traits, with the intent to minimize variability in phenotype classification. This study by Grigorenko et al. required approximately 100 individuals to identify two chromosomal regions as important for aspects of dyslexia. Third, and finally, it is also necessary that any single gene's contribution to the trait be large enough to be detected in the presence of the effect of other genes. With weak effects from several genes, more individuals will be needed in the study. In general, DNA collected from a single study may not provide a large enough sample. Data from several sites will need to be combined in a meta-analysis to generate sufficient power to detect genetic influences on neuroimaging phenotypes (Rao, 1998). This strategy also demands that data are reliable and comparable across the various imaging centers.

The following three sections describe different methods for detecting genes that contribute to a complex trait (Table 18.1). These methods do not rely on collecting the rare, large pedigrees typical of genetic studies of simple Mendelian genetic traits; instead, they focus on small nuclear families, siblings, or unrelated individuals.

Sib-pair designs

The genetic analysis of pairs of siblings examines the degree of similarity between affected siblings for a quantitative phenotype and compares it with the number of alleles shared by the siblings at a specific marker (Haseman and Elston, 1972). It is not necessary to know the state of the parents with respect to the trait under study for this analysis. Computer programs are available for the analysis of such data. A recent computer program, the MAP-MAKER/SIBS (Kruglyak and Lander, 1995) uses the genotype information for each sib-pair to estimate the "identical by descent" (IBD) status (see below) of each marker along the genome (parental information can be included to increase the power of the test). A major advantage of the sib-pair approach is that no prior assumption of the specific genetic model parameters is needed (nonparametric method). However, sib-pair analyses are not as powerful as family pedigree analyses and do not provide estimation of the strength of the linkage and the recombination fraction.

The analysis rests on the fact that, on average, siblings share one half of their genes (and genetic markers). At any single marker, the siblings may share 0, 1, or 2 alleles (for each of the pair of chromosomes that contains the marker), one being the average value. If each sibling inherited the same allele from one of their parents (the same ancestor), then the alleles are said to be IBD. Ideally, knowledge of the parents' genotype helps to assess the IBD status. For example, if each parent is heterozygous at a single genetic marker, and each of their alleles is different (i.e., paternal alleles are A1 and A2 and maternal alleles are A3 and A4), and both of their offspring have the A3 allele, then the offspring must have inherited A3 from their mother. In the event that parental information is not available, the likelihood of IBD status can be estimated from known population frequencies of the alleles. The IBD status predicts the covariance between the sibs for the phenotype; consequently, the higher the IBD status the higher the covariance for a linked trait (Fulker et al., 1995). In other words, if the number of siblings sharing the alleles IBD is significantly higher than expected by chance (50% of the time), then it is possible that a gene that accounts for variance in the trait is close to the marker being assessed.

Minimizing the number of sib-pairs may be possible by examining sib-pairs that are extremely dissimilar (discordant), and/or extremely similar (concordant) (Eaves and Meyer, 1994; Risch and Zhang, 1995). With these types of sampling from sib-pairs, traits for which heritability is in the range of 0.2 to 0.3 would require from 40 to 400 sib-pairs, depending on allele frequencies in the entire population and other parameters (Risch and Zhang, 1996).

Overall, sib-pair analysis is the most powerful approach for detecting linkage of a region of a chromosome to a quantitative trait. Once one is confident that these results can be replicated, determining which gene in that region is responsible for the trait becomes the next big task.

Transmission disequilibrium test

The TDT (Spielman et al., 1993) is a recently developed test that was designed to take advantage of small nuclear families (two parents and an offspring) as a way to avoid some of the pitfalls of detecting association (described below) and yet not require large pedigrees to detect linkage. The test requires that the offspring be classified in a qualitative fashion (affected/unaffected) but can be applied to quantitative traits by utilizing a cut-off value of the measured traits. The best cut-off point is one that is relevant to the biological underpinnings of the trait, but a relevant cut-off may not be easily selected if little is known about the biology of the trait.

The TDT is based on the fact that a parent donates a single chromosome of each pair and, thus, one allele of any particular genetic marker. The donation of one of the two chromosomes in a pair is random; therefore, each chromosome, detected by genetic markers on the chromosome, should appear in offspring 50% of the time (equilibrium). If transmission of a marker deviates from this expected frequency the marker is said to be in disequilibrium (hence the name of the test). The second chromosome of each pair is not transmitted, setting up a comparison of transmitted versus nontransmitted chromosomes by a chi-square test (see Table 18.2). For a marker to be informative, at least one parent must be heterozygous so that the two alleles can be distinguished. The advantage of this design is that both the

Table 18.1. Genetic tests and applications

Method	Sample types	Trait[a]	Advantages	Disadvantages	Reference
Linkage	Large pedigrees with many affected individuals	Qualitative	Gene linked within some distance of locus	Not appropriate for complex traits	Ott 1991
Sib-pair	Pairs of siblings	Quantitative	Detects linkage; easier to collect than pedigrees	Larger sample size than needed for linkage method	Haseman and Elston (1972) Fulker and Cherny (1996)
Affected family member	All combinations of family members	Quantitative	As in sib-pair detects linkage	Larger sample size than needed for linkage method	Weeks and Lange (1988)
Transmission disequilibrium test (TDT)	Parents-offspring trio with parents heterozygous	Qualitative	Minimizes population stratification	Must define a complex trait as dichotomous Detects linkage in presence of association	Spielman et al. (1993)
Sib-TDT	Affected/unaffected sibling pairs	Qualitative	Detects linkage in presence of association	Must define a complex trait as dichotomous	Spielman and Ewens (1998)
Haplotype-based haplotype relative risk	Parents-offspring trio	Qualitative	Minimizes population stratification	Tests for association but not linkage	Terwilliger and Ott (1992)
Population association	Unrelated individuals from one population (genetic)	Qualitative	Easy to perform	Generates false positives that are difficult to discern	

Note:

[a] A quantitative trait can be categorized into a qualitative trait by assigning individuals into two groups based on a cut-off value of the trait.

Table 18.2. *The transmission disequilibrium test[a]*

Transmitted	Nontransmitted	
	Allele 1	Allele 2
Allele 1	a	b
Allele 2	c	d

Note:
[a] The χ^2 test is $(b-c)^2/(b+c)$ with one degree of freedom.

transmitted and the nontransmitted alleles are coming from a single group (the parents), avoiding the possibility that comparing unrelated individuals will find allele frequency differences owing to ethnic background and not related to presence of disease. A further advantage is that the parents do not need to be phenotyped, which can result in significant cost savings for expensive neuroimaging procedures.

A recent extension of the TDT has been proposed using sibships when parental data do not exist (Spielman and Ewens, 1998). This sib-TDT may be very useful in studies collected over long periods of time, and for those in which parents are deceased or unavailable. This method, rather than comparing the transmission of an allele from parent to affected child, compares the genotypes of affected and unaffected siblings. Spielman and Ewens (1998) show that these data may be combined with data from families analyzed by the original TDT to further increase the available sample.

TDT utilizes samples of multiple small families. The number of families, or sib-pairs in the case of sib-TDT, is dependent on the heritability of the trait, with increasing heritability needing smaller samples. Risch and Merikangas (1996) provide tables of predicted sample sizes using genetic risk ratios of a trait (defined as the increased chance that an individual with a particular genotype has the trait) and the frequency of a disease allele in the population. For a genotypic risk ratio of 4, the number of families ranges from 48 to 235; a genotypic risk ratio of 2 requires 180–1970 families, and a genotypic risk ratio of 1.5 requires 484–7776 families. The range of families needed in the study is driven by the frequency of the disease allele (Risch and Merikangas, 1996). The TDT method works best with quantitative traits that have well-defined cut-off values that allow them to be analyzed as qualitative traits.

Population association design

The population association method is commonly used but has a serious caveat, which is the association test between two groups of unrelated individuals. This method is also termed a case-control method, although this term should be reserved for studies that actually select a control individual for each case (disease) individual, based on minimizing any relevant differences between the two individuals. The association test's attractiveness is the ease with which the study can be conducted. The genotypes are identified for two groups of subjects, individuals with a disorder or trait and individuals without the disorder. The frequency of alleles is compared between the two groups by a chi-square test. It is possible to determine genotypes from each group at many sites along the chromosome and make repeated comparisons, although a statistical Bonferroni correction for multiple tests should be made. The primary caveat of this type of study is that a positive association does not imply any relationship between the gene and disorder. It is equally possible that individuals with the disorder, and those without, may actually be genetically different subsets of a population; as a result, differences in allele frequency between the two groups would have nothing to do with the disorder but rather would reflect unanticipated ethnic differences (termed population stratification).

Population-based studies of this type have lost favor because of the difficulty in replicating published findings, probably because of population stratification. One example of an association that is frequently cited as being caused by stratification is the relationship between novelty seeking and the dopamine receptor D_4 (Benjamin et al., 1996; Ebstein et al., 1996; Malhotra et al., 1996; Vandenbergh et al., 1997b). True associations between a genetic marker and a trait can occur for only two reasons: (i) the marker may actually have some functional consequence that directly affects the phenotype being measured (functional allele), or (ii) if the marker does not alter function, then it must be extremely close to the polymorphic site of a gene that is the functional allele. These two sites on the chromosome, the marker and the functional polymorphism, must be so close that the two regions of DNA are always, or nearly always, co-inherited. This relationship of the co-inheritance of the two sites (loci) is known as linkage disequilibrium. There is very little information concerning the amount of linkage disequilibrium to expect between any two sites in large groups of people. It is clear that disequilibrium values will be high in regions of chromosomes that show high rates of recombination, or if two polymorphisms arose at evolutionarily ancient times allowing more time for recombination to occur between them. Recombination is the act of two sister chromosomes exchanging DNA (a normal part of meiosis) and results in segregation of markers that once were on a single chromo-

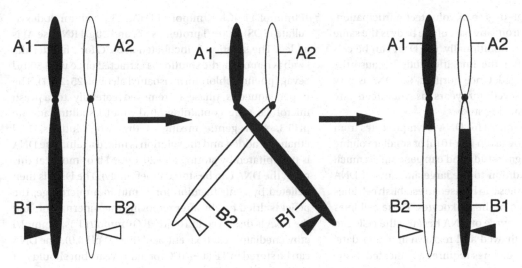

Fig. 18.3. An example of recombination is shown that results in exchange of the lower arms of sister chromosomes. A disease-related allele shown by the black triangle is co-inherited with both A1 and B1 markers in the alignment on the left. After recombination the disease-related allele remains associated with marker B1, but not with A1, as shown on the right.

some onto separate chromosomes (Fig. 18.3). The linkage disequilibrium also depends on population history, with more mixing of populations decreasing its value (Tishkoff, et al., 1996; Laan and Paabo, 1997; see also comments by Freimer et al., 1997). The lack of information concerning allele frequencies in ethnic groups makes the magnitude of the sample size difficult to predict and, therefore, association studies are of little value to neuroimaging phenotypes.

One exception to this general limitation of association studies is the case of functional alleles of genes: alleles that alter protein function, or concentration, in some way, as opposed to alleles at anonymous sites that have no known effect and are only markers. Functional alleles may allow for the inclusion of physiologic data to understand how a gene is related to the trait being studied. Several examples exist in the literature, such as alleles that alter the effect of the enzyme catecholamine-O-methyltransferase (metabolizes dopamine) on measures of substance abuse (Vandenbergh et al., 1997a), or alleles of the cytochrome P450 gene (*CYP2A6*, which metabolizes nicotine) on measures of cigarette smoking (Pianezza et al., 1998). The example of measuring DOPA decarboxylase activity in individuals with Lesch–Nyhan disease was driven by the possible relationship of dopamine to self-injurious behavior (Ernst et al., 1996).

Whole genome scans to detect genes that alter quantitative traits

The study designs described involve testing many genetic markers in a "whole genome scan". The results generated

define one, or more likely many, regions of the chromosomes in which different genes reside that contribute to the measured trait. Each region is known as quantitative trait locus (QTL). Generally, the QTLs described in these studies are large enough that many genes exist in the QTL, and those that are not related to the trait must be winnowed out. At this point, several different approaches may be necessary to narrow the selection process to find the relevant gene. Further genetic studies that focus on refining the position of the QTL may be necessary. Alternatively, searching for complementary DNA (cDNA) clones of the genes from the region, or genomic clones of the entire region, may be the next step before searching for allelic variants of the genes themselves. This process moves into a realm that combines molecular biology and genetics, and it is likely that this approach will grow and change rapidly in the next decade.

Genetic methods in neuroimaging studies: DNA collection

At its simplest, any genetic-neuroimaging study is the comparison of genotype status, determined from a research volunteer's DNA, with a particular phenotype, or trait, that may be derived from a neuroimaging study. In considering how to incorporate genetic analysis into a neuroimaging study, investigators need to plan very carefully the neuroimaging/genetic study design and not rely on the ease in collecting the DNA samples.

Indeed, collecting a sample of DNA from the research volunteers is a relatively easy addition to a study that already requires a high degree of volunteer participation. DNA that is collected from any part of the body is the same as that from the brain. Additionally, the DNA can be collected many years after the imaging study because the DNA remains unchanged. Once purified, the DNA is very stable and can be saved for years as volunteers are recruited to a neuroimaging study.

The most common source for DNA is lymphocytes from the blood, which can be taken in a 10 ml or smaller volume at the time of the imaging study and can generate as much as 500 μg DNA. In addition to the large amounts of DNA generated, blood samples can be used to establish cell lines by viral transformation of the leukocytes. These cell lines provide a permanent source of DNA because the cells can be stored frozen and thawed and regrown at a later date. The establishment of cell lines requires a dedicated tissue culture facility to infect, grow, and store the cells under liquid nitrogen, but it may be possible to find commercial sources to provide this service.

Another source of DNA is buccal cells taken by a cheek swab (Richards et al., 1993; Freeman et al., 1997). Buccal cells do not provide as much DNA as lymphocytes (up to 50 μg) but can be sent by mail, a particularly useful way to undertake genetic studies in individuals who already participated in neuroimaging investigations. Methods to grow buccal cells in culture as a means to increase the DNA yield are being explored in the author's laboratory (unpublished observations). Blood spotted on filter paper (McCabe, 1991), buccal cells from a saline mouth wash (Hayney et al., 1995), or cells from hair follicles (Higuchi et al., 1988) are additional sources of DNA, but the yield of DNA is so small that they are only practical for studies of very limited scope.

Well-established techniques for purifying DNA from eukaryotic cells are found in several molecular biology manuals (e.g., Sambrook et al., 1989; Ausubel et al., 1997). These techniques apply equally well to lymphocytes or buccal cells and use enzymatic digestion (proteinase K and RNAase A) in the presence of detergent followed by organic solvent (phenol/chloroform) extraction and ethanol precipitation. Several other techniques that use solvent extraction or resins or affinity gels have been described (Lahiri et al., 1993).

In ongoing experiments in the author's laboratory, the following method is being used for routine isolation of high-purity DNA from buccal swabs. Research volunteers swab the inside of their mouth for 1 min with a cotton swab and then swab again for 1 min with a second swab. Swabs with a plastic stick produce less residue than wooden sticks. The tip of the swab is cut off into a 1.5 ml microfuge tube, and 500 ml DNA lysis solution (10 mmol/l Tris, pH 8.0,

100 mmol/l NaCl, 10 mmol/l EDTA, 0.5% sodium dodexyl-sulfate (SDS), 200 g/l proteinase K, and 20 g/l RNAase A) is added. The solution is incubated at 55 °C for 2 h; after the swab is removed, the solution is extracted once with 500 μl Sevag (phenol/chloroform/isoamyl alcohol, 25:24:1). The upper, aqueous phase is removed carefully to a fresh microfuge tube containing 50 μl 3 mol/l sodium acetate pH 5.3. After gentle mixing of the two solutions, 1 ml ethanol is added and the solution is mixed again. The DNA is precipitated by storing at −20 °C for 1 h or more (at this point the DNA can be stored indefinitely). The DNA is then pelleted by centrifugation for 15 min in a microfuge; the pellet is dried briefly after removing the supernatant, and the DNA is dissolved in 100 μl TE (10 mmol/l Tris, 1 mmol/l ethylenediamine tetraacetic acid (EDTA) pH 8.0). The DNA can be stored in TE at −70 °C for many years but should not be thawed and refrozen repeatedly.

Summary and future directions

Although molecular genetics shows great promise in helping to break the genetic "codes" underlying complex disorders, still much hard work lies ahead. There should also be a note of caution in continuing work in this young field of complex genetics. Genetic results require replication and careful scrutiny with systematic approaches to ensure that the results are reliable. Advances in genetic methodology need to be paralleled with advances in the identification of phenotypes (see Chapter 19). Brain imaging findings are expected to help to define consistent phenotypes to be used in genetic studies. These brain-imaging findings need to be the direct consequences of the genetic characteristics and not secondary manifestations of neural adaptive changes. This requirement underlines the importance of studying childhood disorders early when adaptive changes have not yet taken place that may mask the primary deficits.

In addition, it is critical to refine the mathematical modeling of the contribution of genetics to psychiatric disorders. Indeed, the complexity of the task of identifying the functional relationships between genetic markers and phenotypes is highlighted by the fact that a given genetic marker may be associated with several different conditions, and a given phenotype with several genetic markers. As already mentioned, it is also unlikely that identified genes will be necessary and sufficient for the expression of a clinical phenotype. The understanding of the contribution of the genes will require one to dissect the clinical phenotype into elements that can be reliably and precisely quantified.

Ultimately, the interface of genetics and neuroimaging in the investigation of childhood psychiatric disorders is expected to further our understanding of basic neurobiologic mechanisms, which will help in the design of effective preventive and therapeutic interventions.

Appendix: glossary of genetic terms

Allele One of several alternative forms of a gene or any other DNA sequence. Alleles may be detected at the level of a gene product, usually as a protein (e.g., two or more forms of a receptor measured by differences in binding affinity) or at the level of DNA (e.g., a fragment of DNA that differs in length with no associated functional difference). An individual has only two alleles at any site (locus), one maternal and one paternal; however, many different alleles may exist at a site in a population.

Candidate gene Any gene whose characteristics suggest that it may be the trait-causing gene. The characteristic can be based on relevant function of its protein, or by physical proximity to markers that are tightly linked to a disease.

Complex genetics Patterns of inheritance suggesting that the sum of the effects of at least two, and usually more, genes are required to produce a trait. This pattern is sometimes referred to as nonMendelian.

Co-segregation Inheritance of two, or more, genetic factors together. These factors could be markers, genes, or traits.

Expression In the context of a particular gene, expression refers to the process of transcribing the gene into RNA so that a protein can be synthesized. In the context of a phenotype, it is the presence of the phenotype.

Genotype The two alleles of an individual at any site in the genome.

Haplotype A combination of two or more alleles that are found on a chromosome. For example, a haplotype A1B3 indicates a chromosome with allele A1 at site A and B3 at site B. Haplotype is sometimes used even if it is not known that both alleles are on one chromosome, or one on each sister chromosome.

Heterozygous Having two different alleles at a genetic marker (i.e., an individual's maternal and paternal alleles can be discerned).

Homozygous Having two alleles of the same type at a locus.

Linkage A measure of the tendency of two sites along a chromosome to be inherited as a unit.

LOD Log of odds, measure used to indicate the likelihood that a phenotype is located at a particular site. A LOD of 3 indicates odds of 1000/1.

Marker Any site (locus) on a chromosome at which a difference can be detected. The different forms of a marker are alleles and can be measured by differences in length of DNA, or differences in enzyme function for example.

Mendelian genetics Genetic patterns of inheritance that show characteristics of being caused by a mutation at a single gene. Mendelian traits show dominant or recessive characteristics.

Nonparametric A genetic test that does not require describing the mode of inheritance (dominant, recessive) is termed nonparametric.

p Symbol for the short (*petit*) arm of a chromosome, usually as part of a symbol for a specific site based on Giemsa stain banding of chromosomes (e.g., 5p15.3 is chromosome 5, short arm, band 15, sub-band 3) (*see also* q).

Parametric Genetic model with parameters describing the expected mode of inheritance, such as, dominant, recessive, sex-chromosome linked.

Penetrance A measure of how frequently a disease-causing mutation is inherited without expressing the disease. Complete penetrance, when the trait is always seen when the mutation is inherited, is contrasted with incomplete penetrance, when there is some dissociation of the trait and mutation.

Phenotype An observed characteristic of an individual (*see also* qualitative and quantitative phenotypes).

Polymerase chain reaction (PCR) A method of synthesizing multiple copies of a small region of DNA in a short period of time, usually less than 3 h. PCR is used to generate sufficient quantities of DNA containing a polymorphism to allow rapid analysis.

Polymorphic Having multiple forms.

Polymorphism An allele that is found with a frequency greater than or equal to 1%.

Positional cloning Identification and purification of a gene based on its position on a chromosome relative to genetic markers that have been mapped to nearby sites.

q Symbol for the long (not *petit*) arm of a chromosome (*see* p for more information).

Qualitative phenotypes Dichotomous, such as the presence or absence of a disease or presence or absence of an enzyme.

Quantitative phenotypes A normal distribution among a group of individuals, such as height. Neurotransmitter densities, patterns of cerebral blood flow activation, and brain nucleus volumes are likely to show quantitative characteristics.

Qualitative trait A trait defined as having only two possibilities (affected/unaffected, present/absent, above/below threshold value); also known as **discontinuous** or **dichotomous** traits.

Quantitative trait A trait that has a continuous range of possible values (e.g., receptor binding affinity, percentage change in blood oxygenation levels).

Quantitative trait locus (QTL) A region, or site, on a chromosome that accounts for some part of a quantitative trait.

Recombination Exchange of large fragments of DNA between sister chromosomes that serves to generate a new combination of alleles along a chromosome. The recombination fraction (θ) is the frequency with which recombination occurs between two sites; this increases with increasing distance between the sites.

Restriction fragment length polymorphism (RFLP) A marker detected by the presence or absence of the correct DNA sequence that allows the DNA to be cut by a restriction endonuclease. Absence of the correct sequence generates a larger fragment of DNA that can be detected by gel electrophoresis.

Trait See phenotype.

Variant Any allele detected, regardless of the frequency of the allele (*see* polymorphism).

References

Ausubel, F., Brent, R., Kingston, R. E. et al. (eds.) (1997). *Short Protocols in Molecular Biology*, 3rd edn. New York: Wiley.

Benjamin, J., Greenberg, B., Murphy, D. L., Lin, L., Patterson, C. and Hamer, D. H. (1996). Population and familial association between the D_4 dopamine receptor gene and measures of Novelty Seeking. *Nat. Genet.*, **12**, 81–4.

Castellanos, F. X. (1997). Toward a pathophysiology of attention-deficit/hyperactivity disorder. *Clin. Pediatr.*, **36**, 381–93.

DeFries, J. C., Fulker, D. W. and La Buda, M. C. (1987). Evidence for a genetic aetiology in reading disability in twins. *Nature*, **329**, 537–9.

de Vries, B. B., Halley, D. J., Oostra, B. A. and Niermeijer, M. F. (1998). The fragile X syndrome. *J. Med. Genet.*, **35**, 579–89.

Eaves, L. and Meyer, J. (1994). Locating human quantitative trait loci: guidelines for the selection of sibling pairs for genotyping. *Behav. Genet.*, **24**, 443–55.

Ebstein, R. P., Novick, O., Umansky, R. et al. (1996). Dopamine D_4 receptor (DRD4) exon III polymorphism associated with human personality trait of Novelty Seeking. *Nat. Genet.*, **12**, 78–80.

Ernst, M., Zametkin, A. J., Matochik, J. A. et al. (1996). Presynaptic dopaminergic deficits in Lesch–Nyhan Disease. *N. Engl. J. Med.*, **334**, 1568–1604.

Ernst, M., Zametkin, A. J., Matochik, J. A., Jons, P. H. and Cohen, R. M. (1998). Presynaptic dopaminergic activity in ADHD adults. A [fluorine-18]fluorodopa positron emission tomographic study. *J. Neurosci.*, **18**, 5901–7.

Falconer, D. S. (1989). *Introduction to Quantitative Genetics*, 3rd. edn. New York: Longman (Wiley).

Feil, R. and Kelsey, G. (1997). Insights from model systems. Genomic imprinting: a chromatin connection. *Am. J. Hum. Genet.*, **61**, 1213–19.

Freeman, B., Powell, J., Ball, D., Hill, L., Craig, I. and Plomin, R. (1997). DNA by mail: an inexpensive and noninvasive method for collecting DNA samples from widely dispersed populations. *Behav. Genet.*, **27**, 251–7.

Freimer, N. B., Service, S. K. and Slatkin, M. (1997). Expanding on population studies. (Comment on Laan and Paabo, 1997). *Nat. Genet.*, **17**, 371–3.

Fulker, D. W. and Cherny, S. S. (1996). An improved multipoint sib-pair analysis of quantitative traits. *Behav. Genet.*, **26**, 527–32.

Fulker, D. W., Cherny, S. S. and Cardon, L. R. (1995). Multipoint interval mapping of quantitative trait loci using sib pairs. *Am. J. Hum. Genet.*, **56**, 1224–33.

Gelerter, T. D., Collins, F. S. and Ginsburg, D. (1998). *Principles of Medical Genetics*, 2nd edn. Baltimore, MD: WIlliams & Wilkins.

Grant, S., London, E. D., Newlin, D. B. et al. (1996). Activation of memory circuits during cue-elicited cocaine craving. *Proc. Natl. Acad. Sci. USA*, **93**, 12040–5.

Grigorenko, E. L., Wood, F. B., Meyer, M. S. et al. (1997). Susceptibility loci for distinct components of developmental dyslexia on chromosomes 6 and 15. *Am. J. Hum. Genet.*, **60**, 27–39.

Hallgren, B. (1950). Specific dyslexia ('congenital word blindness'): a clinical and genetic study. *Acta Psychiatr. Neurol.*, **65**, 2–289.

Haseman, J. K. and Elston, R. C. (1972). The investigation of linkage between a quantitative trait and a marker locus. *Behav. Genet.*, **2**, 3–19.

Hayney, M. S., Dimlanlig, P., Lipsky, J. J. and Poland, G. A. (1995). Utility of a 'Swish and Spit' technique for the collection of buccal cells for TAP haplotype determination. *Mayo Clin. Proc.*, **70**, 951–4.

Higuchi, R., von Beroldingen, C. H., Sensabaugh, G. F. and Erlich, H. A. (1988). DNA typing from single hairs. *Nature*, **332**, 543–6.

Jason, G. W., Suchowersky, O., Pajurkova, E. M. et al. (1997). Cognitive manifestations of Huntington disease in relation to genetic structure and clinical onset. *Arch. Neurol.*, **54**, 1081–8.

Kruglyak, L. and Lander, E. (1995). Complete multipoint sib-pair analysis of qualitative and quantitative traits. *Am. J. Hum. Genet.*, **1**, 121–4.

Laan, M. and Paabo, S. (1997). Demographic history and linkage disequilibrium in human populations. *Nat. Genet.*, **17**, 435–8.

LaBuda, M. C., Gottesman, I. I. and Pauls, D. L. (1993). Usefulness of twin studies for exploring the etiology of childhood and adolescent psychiatric disorders. *Am. J. Med. Genet.*, **48**, 47–59.

Lahiri, D. K., Bye, S. and Nurnberger, J. I. Jr (1993). A non-organic and non-enzymatic extraction method gives higher yields of genomic DNA from whole-blood samples than do nine other methods tested. *J. Biochem. Biophys. Meth.*, **25**, 193–205.

Lander, E. S. and Schork, N. J. (1994). Genetic dissection of complex traits. *Science*, **265**, 2037–48.

Leboyer, M., Bellivier, F., Nosten-Bertrand, M., Jouvent, R., Pauls, D. and Mallet, J. (1998). Psychiatric genetics: search for phenotypes. *TINS*, **21**, 102–5.

Lewin, B. (1997). *Genes VI*. Cambridge, MA: MIT Press.

Malhotra, A. K., Virkkunen, M., Rooney, W., Eggert, M., Linnoila, M. and Goldman, D. (1996). The association between the dopamine D$_4$ receptor (DRD4) 16 amino acid repeat polymorphism and Novelty Seeking. *Mol. Psychiatry*, **1**, 388–91.

McCabe, E. R. B. (1991). Utility of PCR for DNA analysis from dried blood spots on filter paper blotters. *PCR Meth. Appl.*, **1**, 99–106.

McKusick, V. A. (1990). *Mendelian Inheritance in Man*, 9th edn. Baltimore, MD: Johns Hopkins University Press.

Ott, J. (1991). *Analysis of human genetic linkage*. Baltimore, MD: Johns Hopkins University Press.

Pianezza, M. L., Sellers, E. M. and Tyndale, R. F. (1998). Nicotine metabolism defect reduces smoking. *Nature*, **393**, 750.

Rao, D. C. (1998). CAT scans, PET scans, and genomic scans. *Genet. Epidemiol.*, **15**, 1–18.

Richards, B., Bkoletsky, J., Shuber, A. P. et al. (1993). Multiplex PCR amplification from the CFTR gene using DNA prepared from buccal brushes/swabs. *Hum. Mol. Genet.*, **2**, 159–63.

Risch, N. (1997). Evolving methods in genetic epidemiology. II. Genetic linkage from an epidemiologic perspective. *Epidemiol. Rev.*, **19**, 24–32.

Risch, N. and Merikangas, K. (1996). The future of genetic studies of complex human diseases. *Science*, **273**, 1516–17.

Risch, N. and Zhang, H. (1995). Extreme discordant sib pairs for mapping quantitative trait loci in humans. *Science*, **268**, 1584–9.

Risch, N. and Zhang, H. (1996). Mapping quantitative trait loci with extreme discordant sib pairs: sampling considerations. *Am. J. Hum. Genet.*, **58**, 836–43.

Saiki, R., Gelfand, D. J., Stoffel, S. et al. (1988). Primer-directed enzymatic amplification of DNA with a thermostable DNA polymerase. *Science*, **239**, 487–91.

Sambrook, J., Fritsch, E. F. and Maniatis, T. (1989). *Molecular Cloning, a Laboratory Manual*, 2nd edn. Cold Spring Harbor, NY: Cold Spring Harbor Laboratory Press.

Spielman, R. S. and Ewens, W. J. (1998). A sibship test for linkage in the presence of association: the sib transmission/disequilibrium test. *Am. J. Hum. Genet.*, **62**, 450–8.

Spielman, R. S., McGinnis, R. E. and Ewens, W. J. (1993). Transmission test for linkage disequilibrium: the insulin gene region and insulin-dependent diabetes mellitus (IDDM). *Am. J. Hum. Genet.*, **52**, 506–16.

Strachan, T. and Read, A. P. (1996). *Human Molecular Genetics*. New York: Wiley.

Terwilliger, J. D. and Ott, J. (1992). A haplotype-based 'haplotype relative risk' approach to detecting allelic association. *Hum. Hered.*, **42**, 337–46.

Tishkoff, S. A., Dietzsch, E., Speed, W. et al. (1996). Global patterns of linkage disequilibrium at the CD4 locus and modern human origins. *Science*, **271**, 1380–7.

Vandenbergh, D. J., Rodriguez, L. A., Miller, I., Uhl, G. R. and Lachman, H. M. (1997a). A high-activity catechol-O-methyltransferase allele is more prevalent in polysubstance abusers. *Am. J. Med. Genet.*, **74**, 439–42.

Vandenbergh, D. J., Zonderman, A. B., Huang, J., Uhl, G. R. and Costa, P. T. Jr (1997b). No association between Novelty Seeking and dopamine D$_4$ receptor (D4DR) exon III seven repeat alleles in Baltimore Longitudinal Study of Aging participants. *Mol. Psychiatry*, **2**, 417–19.

Weeks, D. E. and Lange, K. (1988). The affected-pedigree-member method of linkage analysis. *Am. J. Hum. Genet.*, **42**, 315–26.

Wong, D. F., Harris, J. C., Naidu, et al. (1996). Dopamine transporters are markedly reduced in Lesch–Nyhan disease *in vivo*. *Proc. Natl. Acad. Sci. USA*, **93**, 5539–43.

19

Issues in the genetic study of complex neurobehavioral conditions

David L. Pauls

Introduction

Several different methodologic approaches are useful to establish that genes are important for the development and manifestation of complex disorders. Historically, twin, adoption, and family studies have been the methods of choice. It is assumed that genetic factors are important in the expression of a disorder if (i) monozygotic twins have a higher concordance rate than do dizygotic twins, (ii) adopted children resembled their biological parents more often than they resemble their adoptive parents, or (iii) a particular condition is more likely to occur among biological relatives of the patient than would be expected by chance. If there is compelling evidence from these types of study, then genetic linkage studies can be initiated to identify regions of the genome that harbor susceptibility genes.

Genetic linkage has long been recognized as one of the most powerful methods for clarifying the role of genetics in the expression of human disorders. Historically, the method has had limited applicability because of the small number of sufficiently polymorphic genetic markers available for study in humans. This situation has changed dramatically. Advances in DNA technology have made it possible to detect many highly polymorphic genetic markers. These genetic markers, based on DNA sequence polymorphisms, have stimulated a renewed interest in linkage approaches to the study of human disorders. As a result, extensive linkage maps of all human chromosomes are available for use in genome wide scans (Gyapay et al., 1994). Theoretical and empirical work suggests that linkage studies can identify the location and thereby verify the existence of genetic loci important in the expression of complex human disorders (Lander and Kruglyak, 1995). However, there remain methodologic issues that need to be addressed so that linkage studies can be more effectively applied to the study of these conditions.

The focus of this volume is on functional neuroimaging in children. Methods are described that should help to delineate the structure and function of the human brain and how both might be related to variation in human behavior and it is expected that further methodologic development will allow finer description of the function and anatomy of the brain. Chapter 18 described the techniques of genetics that will facilitate the use of neuroimaging data in genetic studies. In this chapter, some of the issues that need to be considered in the genetic study of complex phenotypes are discussed and some examples are given of how neuroimaging data might be helpful in addressing some of these concerns.

Delineation of phenotype

Arguably, the most critical issue in any genetic study is the accurate delineation of the inherited phenotype. Before genes can be reliably identified, it is necessary to understand the range of expression of the phenotype under study. In most studies of neurobehavioral disorders done to date, the approach has been to use categorical diagnoses as the unit of analysis. Furthermore, in most instances, genetic studies begin with a narrow definition of affected status that is rigorously applied when probands are selected. However, when relatives are examined, wider and wider definitions are used in deciding whether relatives are affected. In most studies, considerable effort has been made to ensure that the probands are as clinically homogeneous as possible. However, when relatives are studied, most investigators have not applied the same strict classification to document who in the family is affected. It is essential to have additional assessments and evaluation criteria to help to decide which relatives will be considered to have the phenotype of interest.

As noted, to examine adequately hypotheses about the importance of genetic factors, it is necessary to know which individuals have the inherited phenotype. In genetic terms, we need to know something about the variable expressivity of the trait being studied. Variable expressivity is defined as the range of phenotypes resulting from a specific genotype (here genotype refers to the genetic makeup of the individual that is relevant to the expression of the condition being studied). Variable expressivity is not to be confused with comorbidity. To determine whether there is variable expressivity, it is essential to distinguish between comorbidity of two conditions and a spectrum of symptoms that may be part of the inherited trait. Data collected for genetic studies can be helpful in the examination of hypotheses about expression of the phenotype (see Pauls et al., 1993, 1994). If relatives of a proband with a narrowly defined phenotype are more likely to express other behaviors than would be expected by chance, this can be taken as evidence that those behaviors might be etiologically related to the phenotype of the proband. Furthermore, if twin studies suggest that monozygotic twins are more likely to exhibit those same behaviors as seen in relatives of probands, then it can be concluded that those behaviors are part of the inherited phenotype.

The issue of phenotypic classification is particularly critical in genetic linkage studies. In twin, family, and adoption studies, it is possible to demonstrate the importance of genetic factors even when the definition is not exactly correct. However, in genetic linkage studies, false-positive diagnoses can be fatal. The traditional approach in assigning affected status to relatives in a genetic linkage study has been to start with a very narrow rigorous definition of the phenotype and then progressively expand it. Another approach that has been applied in the study of specific reading disability (Grigorenko et al., 1997) is to examine component parts of the condition that might represent separately inherited phenotypes. (These components do not represent subtypes of reading disability, but rather processes that are important in learning to read (see Chapter 15).) In this study, the evidence for linkage was strongest with phenotypes that represented processes that put individuals at risk for reading problems (e.g., phonemic awareness and phonologic decoding).

Another example comes from work on obsessive-compulsive disorder (OCD). In several studies of OCD, it has been demonstrated that the wide array of symptoms observed among individuals can be reduced to a smaller number of factors that account for a significant proportion of the variance observed in a sample of patients (Baer, 1994; Leckman et al., 1997). These factors form different obsessive-compulsive behaviors. The factor that accounts for most of the variance in the OCD samples studied is characterized by aggressive, sexual, religious, and somatic obsessions and related checking compulsions. The behaviors that are included in the second factor are obsessions and compulsions related to symmetry, evening up, and having things feel and look just right. The third factor is characterized by concerns about dirt and germs and compulsions that include excessive washing and cleaning. The fourth factor includes obsessions and compulsions that have to do with hoarding. Furthermore, Alsobrook and colleagues (J. P. Alsobrook II et al., unpublished data) have shown that these factors appear to have separate genetic mechanisms. The results of complex segregation analyses suggest that there might be unique genes of major effect for the aggressive and symmetry factors, while the underlying genetic mechanisms for the other behaviors appear to be more complex. Both the reading and OCD work suggests that alternative strategies might be helpful in identifying phenotypes that are closer to the underlying biological mechanisms which are more likely to be under genetic control.

These two approaches represent ways in which the behavioral phenotype can be partitioned into more meaningful heritable components. Neuroimaging can also characterize individuals and identify different potential biological phenotypes that can be submitted to genetic analyses. By examining the specific functional and anatomic differences that might be associated with a specific neurobehavioral condition, it should be possible to delineate either subtypes of the disorder or components of the larger phenotype that might be under separate genetic control. If a relationship could be established between a behavioral phenotype and a specific region of the brain that is either structurally or functionally different, then that brain phenotype could become the phenotype of interest in subsequent genetic investigations, even in the absence of the behavioral phenotype. That is, it could be possible that brain changes could be observed in family members who did not show the behavioral phenotype. Those individuals might represent cases of "incomplete penetrance" for the behavioral phenotype but not the brain image.

Phenotypes of known genetic disorders

Another approach that is currently being used to understand the relationship between genes and behavior is to examine the so-called behavioral phenotypes of known genetic disorders. Nyhan (1972) first introduced the term "behavioral phenotype" to suggest that there might be specific clusters of symptoms that are associated with specific disorders known to have a specific genetic lesion. In fact, when Nyhan first proposed the notion of a behavioral phenotype, he proposed that the specific phenotype was chemically determined. At the present time, it is proposed that the genes responsible for the syndrome being studied determine the specific phenotype. Or, in the case of deletion syndromes, it is hypothesized that the behavioral phenotype results from one of the genes in the deleted segment of the chromosome that harbors the gene responsible for the specific genetic disorder being investigated. One of the best examples of a behavioral phenotype is the self-injurious behavior seen in patients with the Lesch–Nyhan syndrome. Another genetic syndrome that is being investigated in hopes of understanding part of the behavioral phenotype is Williams syndrome. Most individuals with Williams syndrome have a deletion in the short arm of chromosome 7. Hence, several genes are deleted and it is not yet known which one(s) is(are) responsible for the disorder.

Individuals with Williams syndrome are generally mildly to moderately retarded (IQ range 40–100, average 60) and usually have poor abilities in reading, writing, and arithmetic. Yet, despite these lower than average cognitive abilities, they often display remarkable strengths in several other domains. They often have language abilities far above what is expected given their IQs, a facility for recognizing faces, and unusual musical talent. They also tend to be sociable, loquacious, and empathetic. Researchers have been interested in Williams syndrome because it is expected that the unique abilities of these individuals may be related to the genes that are deleted in the region on chromosome 7 (see Lenhoff et al. (1997) for a review). The deleted piece of DNA can contain 15 genes or more. It is expected that as the deleted genes are identified, it will be possible to determine how their absence may be related to the profile of behaviors observed in typical individuals with Williams syndrome. For example, some of the genes involved in the deletion have been identified; these include those for elastin and LIM-kinase 1, and *FZD3*, *WSCR1*, and *RFC2*. The elastin gene is likely to be responsible for the physical characteristics of Williams syndrome (e.g., cardiac defects, hernias, premature wrinkling) but not for the cognitive aspects of the disorder. The gene for LIM-kinase 1 and *FZD3* and *WSCR1* are known to be expressed in the brain. LIM-kinase 1 is now thought to be involved in visuospatial processes. Concurrent to the search for responsible genes, functional neuroimaging can explore the functional neuroanatomy underlying the unique cognitive characteristics of the disorder and help to map the functional organization and adaptability of the normal brain. Ultimately, the linkage of genotype to behavioral phenotype in brain imaging studies can enhance our understanding of the neuroimaging phenotype. Several studies are currently underway to delineate the neuropsychology and neurobiology of this disorder, including brain imaging studies of patients. This approach, connecting gene function to neurobiology and finally to behavior, may become one way of identifying the effects of specific genes on the developing brain and subsequent behavior. It must be said, however, that while this approach may be useful in identifying the behavioral effects of genes that are deleted in specific genomic regions, it will most likely not be helpful in identifying genes of major effect for specific neurobehavioral syndromes.

Assessment of phenotype

Another critical issue in the search for genes important for the manifestation of behavior is the assessment of the phenotype. Most neurobehavioral genetic research (especially in psychiatric genetics) has been limited by reliance on categorical definitions of phenotype. Currently, much effort is directed to collecting data necessary to make diagnoses. In so doing, much of the richness of the information is lost when categories of illness are defined. This taxonomy has limited the power in many of the analyses and may have led to incomplete conclusions regarding transmission of traits within families. Given the variability in the manifestation of a neurobehavioral diagnosis, it might be useful to have assessments that would lead to continuous definitions or multidimensional definitions. Categorical definitions may be quite useful when considering treatment and outcome. However, for research purposes, it is helpful to have information about the range of symptom expression that might occur in "unaffected" relatives. Although some attempts have been made to include continuous assessment of phenotype, these have not been used extensively in genetic research.

Neuroimaging data could be very helpful in elucidating more quantitative biological aspects of the phenotype. Examining the variability in function or structure should allow a more comprehensive evaluation of the underlying genetic mechanism. A caveat needs to be mentioned. Most studies using quantitative phenotypes require sample sizes that are larger than the typical imaging study. If neuroimaging data are to be used in quantitative genetic studies, samples of at least 75–100 individuals will be necessary. This will require collaborative studies to collect sufficiently large samples to include in genetic studies. It should also be stated that imaging data would be required for all critical members of the family rather than just affected individuals. Therefore, for sib-pair studies it will be necessary to image at least both siblings and it would be preferable to get image data for both parents as well. For linkage studies of large multigenerational families, all members of the family for which DNA samples have been collected should be imaged. This will also add to the expense and complexity of the research.

Methodologic approaches

A third issue has to do with methodologic approaches. Until recently, there has been an almost exclusive commitment to one approach (i.e., genetic linkage studies of large multigenerational families and data analytic methods requiring specification of genetic model parameters, so-called parametric linkage studies). When it was not possible to replicate the initial genetic linkage findings for bipolar disorder and schizophrenia, those working in this field were faced with the question of whether this approach would really provide the desired results. In fact, there was considerable discussion in the literature expressing doubt about the possibility of finding any major genes responsible for the expression of any neurobehavioral disorder (see Pauls, 1994; Risch and Botstein, 1996). However, with continued development of methodologies (both laboratory and computational), it has been possible to use other genetic linkage paradigms to study more genetically complex disorders (see Chapter 18).

Considerable work has been done (and is ongoing) to clarify the limitations of the genetic linkage approach for the study of complex disorders. Current approaches include a variety of different kinds of family and analytic strategy that have been shown to be more appropriate for the study of complex conditions. Risch and Merikangas (1996) suggested that association studies might be the method of choice for identifying the actual susceptibility locus. Their argument was based on the assumption that a saturated map of the genome would be available. At the present time, such a map is not available and, even if it were, it would be too costly to undertake a genome-wide screen using this strategy. However, association studies can be used to assess the importance of specific candidate genes for specific traits. Genetic association studies are an efficient way to identify genotype/phenotype relationships, but in application, they are perilous. Association studies are highly susceptible to false-positive results (Gelernter et al., 1994). In general, false-positive results are most likely when marker polymorphisms, rather than coding region polymorphisms affecting structure, are used

and when selection of affected and unaffected groups does not control for ethnicity.

It is possible to reduce or eliminate these problems. First, by studying only polymorphisms in the coding region of a gene, the first problem is minimized. Second, by making allele frequency comparisons only between individuals in the same racial groups (unless it has been demonstrated that racial groups do not differ in allele frequency for a particular marker), it is possible essentially to eliminate the second problem. One way of perfectly matching for ethnicity is by applying the haplotype relative risk (HRR) method (Falk and Rubinstein, 1987; Terwilliger and Ott, 1992). This method controls for variation in allele frequency owing to ethnicity by constructing a control group of nontransmitted parental alleles (see Chapter 18). The nontransmitted parental alleles (determined by subtracting the set of the offspring's two alleles from the set of the parent's four alleles) are considered to be in the "control" group. Since the two parents each donate one allele to the "ill" group and one allele to the comparison group, it is clear that both groups are perfectly matched for ethnicity, as contributions to the two sets of alleles are completely balanced. The strength of the HRR method lies in the parental alleles that are not transmitted to the proband: these alleles form an independent control sample, thereby avoiding problems related to ascertaining control individuals appropriately matched for ethnicity. Neuroimaging studies could become increasingly important in future association studies. If specific regions of the brain are shown to be highly correlated with specific behavioral phenotypes, genes that are preferentially expressed in those regions would be candidate genes for the behavior being investigated. Of course, considerable work is needed first to demonstrate that specific genes are uniquely expressed in the brain region of interest. However, once it has been established which genes are preferentially expressed in the regions of the brain implicated by imaging studies for a particular trait, it is possible with association studies to determine if functional variants of genes are associated with differences in brain images. This could become a very powerful technique for future studies.

Risk factors other than genetic ones

A fourth issue in the study of the genetics of behavior, is the relative lack of attention to nongenetic risk factors. While most genetic investigators acknowledge the need to consider environmental factors in genetic studies, few studies have actually been able to measure environmental factors adequately. The same can be said for those studies focused on the impact of detrimental environments on the development of psychopathology. Researchers who focus on these effects also acknowledge the importance of genetic factors but most have failed to account for individual differences that might be a consequence of underlying genetic variability. There is a need for a concerted effort to combine strategies to identify all risk factors important for the expression of the phenotype. In fairness, it may not have been appropriate to include comprehensive assessment of the environment in the initial genetic studies of neurobehavioral conditions. In fact, it may not have been possible to the extent that it is today. At the present time, however, it is possible to combine the methods of neurobehavioral genetics with those from developmental psychology. If that were done, the investigator would have a better opportunity to learn more about the interaction of genes and environment. With appropriate experimental designs, it should be possible to document the role of both genetic and nongenetic factors in the development of abnormal behavior.

Developmental aspects

Finally, a fifth issue that needs to be considered is the lack of a developmental focus in genetic studies of behavior. For research focused on understanding the underlying genetics of neurobehavioral phenotypes, it is necessary to reshape our thinking in terms of human behavior across the lifespan. As is exemplified from the focus of this book, it is critical to learn more about the childhood manifestations that might lead to later adult behavior as a consequence of developmental and adaptive changes in the brain. In that regard, it is important to know about possible sensitive periods in development and their relationship to later normal/abnormal behavior. At the present time, the assumption is that some psychopathology is homotypic. That is, it is assumed that the phenotype for a specific disorder is invariant over time. For example, childhood depression is diagnosed with criteria for adults and is treated as the same condition in studies examining the familial transmission of major affective disorders. This is also true for OCD. While it may be possible that some disorders are homotypic, it is highly unlikely that childhood illness will mimic exactly what is seen in adult patients. New research designs are needed that will allow an examination of the possibility of a heterotypic phenotype. It is necessary to know how related behaviors are manifested over different stages of development.

Attention to development is particularly important if the ultimate goal is an understanding of the genetics of a specific condition. It is vital to know how genes function through all stages of development and what impact that function has on the ultimate expression of the phenotype throughout the lifespan. Gene function may be observed through specific behaviors, levels of neurochemicals, response to specific environmental stressors, interaction with family members or peers, specific brain structure or function, actual gene function at the cellular level, or some yet to be determined phenotype. New research paradigms will need to be developed that include assessments of a number of these domains.

It is imperative in future research directed at the elucidation of genetic factors that great care be taken to collect data so that it will be possible to examine both genetic and environmental contributions to the expression of neurobehavioral disorders. While it may be possible to find evidence that genes are important in the etiology of illness, it is unlikely that genetic factors will be both necessary and sufficient for the expression of any illness. It is also possible that it will only be possible to identify the genetic contribution to a specific condition when we have adequately documented the impact of nongenetic factors on the expression of the illness. It is also important that this work take place in a developmental context. Work in developmental psychology has demonstrated that early life experiences can have a significant impact on later mental health. For example, it has been clearly demonstrated that the quality of an infant's attachment to her or his mother has strong predictive power for later childhood behavior. While attachment theorists want to attribute much of deviant behavior to deviant attachments (Bowlby, 1988), it is becoming apparent that the genetic endowment of both parent and child may influence the attachment (Goldsmith and Alansky, 1987). Therefore, it is not unreasonable to deduce that the attachment of a child to the parent may influence how genetic factors may be manifested. This may be part of the unique environment that each child experiences and it may shape the phenotypic expression of the underlying genotype.

Work investigating the impact of environmental factors needs to be done in the context of a genetic design. Prospective longitudinal studies of children at risk need to be undertaken that take into account developmental stages throughout the lifespan. The goal of these studies should not just be to document early signs and symptoms of the syndrome (although this is a worthy goal). The studies should document the early experience of the individual. This experience is not just some global measure of the home and family life. Attempts should be made to document specific interactions within and outside the home (i.e., school experiences). In addition, biological assessments should be made including neurochemical measures and neuroimaging measures. Attention should also be given to diet, illness, and other "common" events in the child's life. While this sounds intrusive, research can be designed to obtain excellent data with minimal intrusion.

As suggested, these studies need to follow entire families, not just single children in families. Furthermore, the assessment of the individuals in these families needs to include various domains of behavior as well as other measures related to those behaviors (e.g., images of the brain). Furthermore, particular attention needs to be paid to critical developmental periods when these measures are obtained. It is important to document whether specific stressful events or neurochemical or neuroanatomic changes took place at a particularly critical time in development.

To facilitate this type of prospective longitudinal study, more descriptive studies of development should be initiated. It is necessary to know what normal development (both behavioral and neuroanatomic) is so that it will be possible to assess the impact of abnormal behavior on development (and vice versa) at each different stage. Behaviors are not invariant over time, certainly not from childhood to adulthood. So it is quite possible that the observed phenotype for a specific genotype will change over time; consequently, in cross-sectional studies it may not be possible to determine what the complete phenotype is. Furthermore, without longitudinal data, it may not be possible to determine exactly what the impact of specific genetic factors might be on an observed phenotype.

Finally, better studies of environmental risk factors are needed. They need to be designed so that the effects can be examined in the context of different genetic risk. Studies of environmental risk need to be carried out for all ages but, most importantly, we need to learn more about the work being done with very young people (infants). Attachment research has shown that the parental environment is critical for emotional development and the expression of emotions in young children. Some research also suggests that not all children respond in the same way to specific events. What is not known is whether this difference in response is in some way related to different genes. Certainly, it is not known whether it is in some way related to differences in brain structure and function. Consequently, it is important to incorporate more sensitive measurements of unique environments.

Summary and future directions

Genetic studies are done at the molecular level and, with the proposed use of neuroimaging techniques, some aspects of

the phenotype are being described in a more molecular way. It is important to examine the environment at the molecular level as well. Careful examination of parent–child dyads, sib–sib dyads, and peer–peer dyads is important so that the unique environment of individuals can be estimated. It is also important to measure the response to environment. This response should be evaluated in a number of ways: behaviorally, psychologically, neurochemically, and neuro-anatomically. These data combined with comprehensive quantitative phenotypic data and evaluated to determine if there is any relationship with genotypic data should help us to understand more fully the etiology of neurobehavioral disorders. The ability to utilize genotypic data and other aspects of genetic studies to design and carry out a study of nongenetic etiologic factors of a neurobehavioral trait is a significant methodological advancement that has not been possible heretofore. Data from prospective studies should make it possible to examine individuals with specific genotypes to determine which factors are important for the development of specific phenotypes.

References

Baer, L. (1994). Factor analysis of symptom subtypes of obsessive compulsive disorder and their relation to personality and tic disorders. *J. Clin. Psychiatry*, **55** (Suppl), 18–23.

Bowlby, J. (1988). Developmental psychiatry comes of age. *Am. J. Psychiatry*, **145**, 1–10.

Falk, C. T. and Rubinstein, P. (1987). Haplotype relative risks: an easy reliable way to construct a proper control sample for risk calculations. *Ann. Hum. Genet.*, **51**, 227–33.

Gelernter, J., Pauls, D.L., Leckman, J. et al. (1994). D$_2$ dopamine receptor (DRD2) alleles do not influence severity of Tourette's syndrome: results from four large kindreds. *Arch. Neurolog.*, **51**, 397–400.

Grigorenko, E. L., Wood, F. B., Meyer, M. S. et al. (1997). Susceptibility loci for distinct components of developmental dyslexia on chromosomes 6 and 15. *Am. J. Hum. Genet.*, **60**, 27–39.

Goldsmith, H. H. and Alansky, J. A. (1987). Maternal and infant temperamental predictors of attachment: a meta-analytic review. *J Consult. Clin. Psychol.*, **55**, 805–15.

Gyapay, G., Morissette, J., Vignal, A. et al. (1994). The 1993–94 Genethon human genetic linkage map. *J. Nat. Genet.*, **7**, 246–339.

Lander, E. S. and Kruglyak, L. (1995). Genetic dissection of complex traits: guidelines for interpreting and reporting linkage results. *Nat. Genet.*, **11**, 241–7.

Leckman, J. F., Grice, D. E., Boardman, J. et al. (1997). Symptoms of obsessive compulsive disorder. *Am. J. Psychiatry*, **154**, 911–17.

Lenhoff, H. M., Wand, P. P., Greenberg, F. and Bellugi, U. (1997). Williams syndrome and the brain. *Sci. Am.*, Dec., 68–73.

Nyhan, W. L. (1992). Behavioral phenotypes in organic genetic disease. *Pediatr. Res.*, **6**, 1–9.

Pauls, D. L. (1994). Genetic linkage studies in psychiatry: strengths and weaknesses. In *Einstein/Montefiore Monograph Series in Clinical and Experimental Psychiatry: Genetic Studies in Affective Disorders: Overview of Basic Methods, Current Directions and Critical Research Issues*, eds. D. F. Papolos and H. M. Lachman, pp. 91–104. New York: Brunner/Mazel.

Pauls, D. L., Leckman, J. F. and Cohen, D. J. (1993). The familial relationship between Gilles de la Tourette's syndrome, attention deficit disorder, learning disabilities, speech disorders and stuttering. *J Am. Acad. Child Adolesc. Psychiatry*, **32**, 1044–50.

Pauls, D. L., Leckman, J. F. and Cohen, D. J. (1994). Evidence against a genetic relationship between Gilles de la Tourette's syndrome and anxiety, depression, panic and phobic disorders. *Br. J. Psychiatry*, **164**, 215–21.

Risch, N. and Botstein, D. (1996). A manic depressive history. *Nat. Genet.*, **12**, 351–3.

Risch, N. and Merikangas, K. (1996). The future of genetic studies of complex human disorders. *Science*, **273**, 1516–17.

Terwilliger, J. D. and Ott, J. (1992). A haplotype-based 'haplotype relative risk' approach to detecting allelic associations. *Hum. Hered.*, **42**, 337–46.

20

The duplicity of plasticity: a conceptual approach to the study of early lesions and developmental disorders

Ralph-Axel Müller and Eric Courchesne

Introduction

Research on impairments of brain development has in the past been characterized by two empirical paradigms that examine developmental plasticity from very different perspectives. The early lesion paradigm, on the one hand, focuses on patients with gross structural brain damage acquired peri- or postnatally and investigates effects on cognitive, sensorimotor, and affective outcome. On the other hand, the study of developmental disorders, such as attention-deficit disorder, dyslexia, or autism, proceeds from a diagnostic profile of cognitive–behavioral symptoms to the exploration of underlying neurodevelopmental disturbances. The two approaches shed light on the malleability of the developing brain in opposite, yet complementary ways.

Research on the effects of early structural lesions has produced evidence for the brain's astounding capacity to compensate for loss of neural tissue. Extreme examples are studies of patients with resection or disconnection of a complete forebrain hemisphere. While extensive brain damage in *adults* results in severe and persistent region-specific deficits (as evidenced by aphasia following a left perisylvian lesion: Pedersen et al., 1995; Benson and Ardila, 1996), left hemispherectomy after an early lesion is often associated with good long-term language outcome if the right hemisphere is intact (Basser, 1962; Ogden, 1988; Vargha-Khadem and Polkey, 1992; Vargha-Khadem et al., 1997). The different meanings and implications of the broad term *early lesion* will be discussed later in this chapter. Roughly, this term will be used in the sense of acquired structural damage affecting one or several brain regions before these have fully matured.

Similar to early hemispherectomy, congenital unilateral brain damage is typically associated with general intellec-

tual outcome in the normal range, regardless of the side of lesion (Muter et al., 1997; Stiles et al., 1997; Bates et al., 1999).

In the study of developmental psychopathologies and learning disabilities, cognitive–behavioral disturbances are typically salient, while the underlying neurologic impairments remain mostly elusive. Even when neurologic abnormalities can be identified, they are typically microscopic, subtle, or variable across individuals. For example, a few autopsy studies on developmental dyslexia have shown neuronal ectopia and cortical microdysgenesis, especially in left perisylvian regions (Kemper, 1984; Galaburda, 1988). Yet it is unclear to what extent neuronal ectopia may occur even in *normal* ontogeny (Kaufmann and Galaburda, 1989). The histologic findings in dyslexia may be related to atypical morphologic asymmetry in the perisylvian region observed in some studies (for discussion, see below). Yet again, these morphologic findings in dyslexia are subtle, and sex or overall brain size appear to have a more robust effect on perisylvian morphology than diagnosis of dyslexia (Schultz et al., 1994).

Returning to the broader issue of theoretical approaches, the early acquired lesion paradigm predominantly illuminates *compensatory plasticity*, while the study of developmental disorders tends to emphasize the enhanced *vulnerability* associated with neurobiological impairments that occur at critical maturational stages. Accordingly, neuroimaging studies in patients with early acquired damage will primarily seek to identify enhanced activations in regions outside a structural lesion. Such activations are assumed to reflect functional compensation and recovery. By comparison, imaging studies in developmental disorders will typically look for an absence or abnormality of activation that is assumed to reflect a particular cognitive or affective impairment. This latter objective is reasonable because, in a prototypical developmental disorder, a discrete initial defect (owing to genetic mutation or a neurotoxin, for example) will tend to affect multiple systems, thus reducing the potential for compensatory reorganization across brain regions or neurofunctional circuits.

While the above framework undoubtedly captures a fundamental difference between early structural lesion effects and developmental disorders, it is intellectually unsatisfactory that the two paradigms and the empirical data they produce are often discussed in complete isolation. After all, both empirical paradigms deal with impairments of the developing brain, which suggests that some principles are shared. The comprehensive concept for these shared principles is *plasticity*. Traditionally, this concept has often been related only to those brain adaptations that are beneficial in terms of cognitive–behavioral outcome. For example, in the words of Gregory and Taylor (1987, p. 623) plasticity refers to an "ordered alteration of organization . . . that *makes some sort of sense biologically* or to the investigator" (our italics). We will argue that this view of plasticity is too narrow and that the concept should be understood as encompassing both beneficial *and detrimental* effects of developmental brain impairments. We will, therefore, attempt to approach early brain-behavioral disturbances from two complementary angles, considering a coexistence and interaction of effects of compensatory reorganization and vulnerability, and examine what these principles may imply for functional neuroimaging. We will begin with evidence indicating vulnerability effects in nonhuman animals and human patients with early structural lesions and will then discuss the interaction of vulnerability and compensatory events in developmental disorders, with exemplary focus on autism, developmental language impairment (DLI), and dyslexia. The discussion of early lesion studies will set the stage for another theme of this chapter, which is the distinction between *bottom-up* and *top-down* approaches, i.e., approaches that are predominantly informed by evidence on biological causes versus those informed by cognitive–behavioral outcome. Early lesion studies are characterized by relatively good knowledge of the neuroanatomic causes of outcome deficits. In fact, animal lesion studies, by definition, include bottom-up information and proceed from a known pathogenic event (for example, a surgical resection) to behavioral outcome. Finally, we will argue that an analogous bottom-up approach is essential for the elucidation of biological mechanisms underlying developmental disorders.

Effects of early structural lesion

Animal studies

A simple statement about maturational plasticity that is often referenced in the literature is the Kennard principle, epitomized in the phrase: "the earlier the lesion, the better the outcome" (all other things being equal; cf. Rudel et al., 1974; Teuber, 1974). This principle grossly refers to the work of Margaret Kennard on the effects of age at lesion onset in primates (Kennard, 1938, 1940) and, in particular, her finding "that cortical lesions made on young animals have less effect on behavior than have similar lesions in adults" (Kennard, 1938, p. 490). Many more recent animal studies provide overall support for the Kennard principle. For instance, Kolb and Tomie (1988) found that rats sustaining hemidecortication showed better recovery on visuospatial navigation and motor tasks when surgery was performed at postnatal day 1 than when performed on day 10. Focal resection of somatosensory cortex in neonatal rats results in reorganization of receptive barrel fields around the lesion, whereas such plasticity is not seen in rats undergoing surgery after postnatal day 10 (Seo and Ito, 1987). Removal of primary visual cortex (areas 17 and 18) in cats leads to enhanced development of intracortical connectivity (MacNeil et al., 1996) and of connections with the superior colliculus (Sun et al., 1994) at postnatal day 1 (and to a lesser degree at day 28), but not in adulthood. This anatomic plasticity is reflected in better behavioral outcome (in visual depth perception and orienting) following resection in the first days of life compared with later resection (Shupert et al., 1993).

However, there are drawbacks to maturational plasticity. Reviewing the effects of lesions in the superior colliculus of the neonatal hamster, Schneider (1979) showed that plastic reorganization of retinal afferents results in partial sparing of visually guided behavior but may also lead to severe deficits (for example, turning the head in the wrong direction in response to a visual stimulus). Schneider concludes that earlier damage is indeed related to greater reorganizational potential, but that "[c]hanges in brain structure occur as a result of the workings of developmental cellular mechanisms, *irrespective of whether the result is functionally adaptive*" (Schneider, 1979, p. 578).

The animal literature on cortical lesions has also made it clear that the Kennard principles applies only to gross comparisons between damage to the mature and to the developing brain, but not when different time windows *within* development are considered. Unfortunately, comparison of data from different species is complicated by the fact that neurodevelopmental stages occur at different

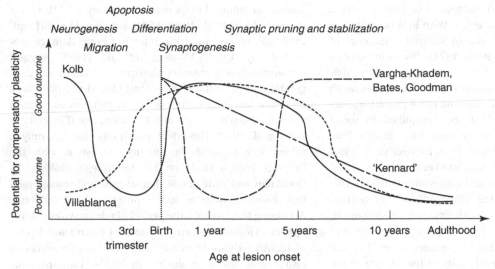

Fig. 20.1. Effect of age at lesion onset on the potential for compensatory reorganization. The position of neurodevelopmental stages at the top is approximate. Age at lesion onset refers to human developmental time. Findings from animal studies are converted to roughly equivalent human time. The line labeled 'Kennard' indicates a linear decrease in plasticity after birth until adulthood (— – —), which is a simple rendering of the Kennard principle (e.g., Teuber, 1974). Three alternative models are based on animal studies from different species (—; Kolb, 1995; Kolb et al., 1998), experiments in cats (- - - -; Villablanca et al., 1993a, b) and human lesion studies (— — —; Goodman and Yude, 1996; Bates et al., 1999; Vargha-Khadem et al., 1999).

conceptual and postnatal ages in different mammalian species (Villablanca et al., 1993b; Kolb, 1995). Rat and hamster brains are more immature at birth than is the cat brain, which is, in turn, slightly more immature than the brain of a human neonate. In rats, Kolb and colleagues found *less* functional sparing when bilateral frontal or parietal resections were performed at postnatal day 1 compared with day 10 (roughly corresponding to lesions at human gestational month 5 versus postnatal month 6: Kolb and Tomie, 1988; Kolb and Whishaw, 1989; Kolb, 1990; Kolb et al., 1996). Studying cats, Villablanca and colleagues (1993a,b) observed good recovery after left frontal cortical ablation at postnatal days 8–14, but severe sensorimotor impairments after similar ablation during the third gestational trimester. The anatomic correlates of lesion timing effects are generally concordant. Early postnatal focal resection in rats results in cortical thinning throughout the remaining hemisphere (Kolb et al., 1989). Prenatal unilateral frontal ablation in cats leads to hypoplasia of the entire lesioned hemisphere and bilateral abnormalities of gyral and sulcal formations (Villablanca et al., 1993a).

Kolb and colleagues conclude from a review of studies in rats, cats, and monkeys that there are two periods of optimal compensatory potential, one during neurogenesis and one during maximal synaptogenesis (Fig. 20.1). However, they find the cerebrum specifically *vulnerable* to insult during the periods of neuronal migration and

differentiation (Kolb, 1995; Kolb et al., 1998). In contrast, Villablanca et al. (1993b) propose that there is only a single "optimal developmental period" (when brain damage is associated with good recovery) occurring after neurogenesis is mostly achieved and while neuronal differentiation, synaptogenesis, and selective neuronal and synaptic loss are most pronounced. However, some caution is required with regard to the data illustrated in Fig. 20.1. It is hard to translate the above scenarios into human developmental time since species differences conceivably involve more than some unitary index of brain maturity. Instead, there are probably species-specific differences in the precise chronologic interaction of regionally differing maturational stages. These complex schedules will determine the nature of anatomic and functional recovery after brain damage at a given point in time. What the Kolb and the Villablanca scenarios have nonetheless in common is the finding that time-plasticity curves are nonmonotonic and that the Kennard principle requires modification.

Human neuropsychologic studies

This general conclusion from animal studies is reflected in human neuropsychologic studies of early lesion effects. Again, gross comparison of lesion-onset effects in childhood and in adulthood supports the Kennard principle of greater early plasticity. However, many studies suggest that the long-term outcome of congenital or early postnatal unilateral lesions is characterized both by a potential for compensatory restitution *and* by delayed emergence of latent deficits (cf. Rudel et al., 1974). The latter applies above all to damage in brain regions that normally participate in higher cognitive functions. Such lesions may result in deficits only detected at the time these cognitive functions are normally acquired, as exemplified in social deficits observed many years after early frontal lobe damage (Grattan and Eslinger, 1991; Eslinger et al., 1992; for related animal data, see Goldman et al., 1970). A cross-sectional study on children and adolescents with congenital hemiplegia by Banich et al. (1990) indeed suggested that intellectual deficit *increases* with time since lesion onset, presumably as a result of slowed cognitive development. However, these findings may have been skewed by the uncontrolled clinical heterogeneity of the sample (especially by the inclusion of patients with seizures) and were not replicated in a better-controlled longitudinal study (Muter et al., 1997). Nonetheless, several groups have reported that patients with unilateral lesions occurring before age 1 year showed worse intellectual outcome than patients sustaining lesions after age 1 year (Woods, 1980; Riva and Cazzaniga, 1986; Strauss et al., 1992). Aram and Eisele (1994), who also found lower verbal IQ (VIQ) and performance IQ (PIQ) in patients with unilateral lesion onset before age 1 year (compared with patients with lesions in childhood and adolescence), relate this finding to a "greater vulnerability of the immature brain" (p. 93). Findings from an extensive sample (1185) of patients with a history of intractable epilepsy presented by Strauss et al. (1995) further showed that seizure onset was a major predictor of long-term intellectual outcome. Onset before 1 year of age tended to be associated with low VIQ and PIQ (regardless of the side of lesion), and there was a positive correlation between age at onset and outcome on IQ measures. This finding was not confounded by seizure duration (the possible confounds of seizure type and frequency were not addressed in this study).

The above findings from human studies on early lesion effects are reminiscent of the chronologic schedule proposed by Kolb (1995), which suggests a window of vulnerability in humans around birth and extending into the first postnatal year (Fig. 20.1). However, it should be noted that in many of these earlier human studies, important clinical variables such as lesion site and size, type of lesion, or the occurrence of epilepsy could not be controlled. Some more recent studies with relatively large patient samples tell a slightly different story. Above all, the effects of congenital brain damage (especially when not accompanied by seizure disorder) on verbal and nonverbal intelligence have been reported to be overall relatively mild (Isaacs et al., 1996; Bates et al., 1999). Data on a sample of 161 children and adolescents with unilateral brain damage presented by Vargha-Khadem et al. (1999) suggest pronounced compensatory plasticity in children with congenital and perinatal lesions but reduced plasticity and, therefore, less long-term recovery in children with lesion onset between 6 months and 4 years of age (Fig. 20.1; cf. Bates et al., 1999). This effect, which was observed only in seizure-free patients, is roughly consistent with the findings from a study on 149 hemiplegic children by Goodman and Yude (1996) that suggest a U-shaped relation between time at lesion onset and IQ outcome. According to this study, the period of relative vulnerability applies to lesions occurring between 1 month and 5 years of age. An early study including 40 patients with unilateral lesion (and diverse etiologies) by McFie (1961) presents compatible data (i.e., lower full-scale IQ outcome after lesion onset from 1–4 years than after onset from 5–9 years). Potentially consistent findings also come from studies on cranial irradiation effects in children with leukemia that show greater long-term intellectual deficits when treatment occurred before 4 years of age than when treatment occurred later in childhood (Cousens et al., 1988).

An additional aspect of maturational vulnerability is reflected in so-called *crowding effects*, which may be observed after early left hemispherectomy and extensive left hemisphere lesion (Rudel et al., 1974; Strauss et al., 1990). Verbal sparing (i.e., higher VIQ than PIQ) in patients with early-onset lesion in either the right or the left hemisphere has been observed in some studies (e.g., Goodman and Yude, 1996; Riva and Cazzaniga, 1986; Carlsson et al., 1994; Nass and Stiles, 1996). Verbal sparing, however, was not found in a recent study by Glass et al. (1998), who report a double dissociation of language versus visuospatial deficits in children with pre- or perinatal left versus right hemisphere damage. These findings may be explained by mild lesions in most patients that presumably did not result in interhemispheric language reorganization. The phenomenon of verbal sparing may be partly (and trivially) explained by a greater sensitivity of PIQ measures to brain damage in general. The theoretically more interesting hypothesis of "crowding" pertains to a lesion-induced (re)organization of language in the right hemisphere *at the expense* of typical right-hemispheric functions (such as visuospatial processing). Strauss et al. (1995) observed a subtle but significant detrimental effect of atypical language laterality on PIQ in their extensive sample of patients whose hemispheric dominance was determined by means of the intracarotid amobarbital (amylobarbitone) procedure (Wada and Rasmussen, 1960).

In the terms introduced above, crowding effects reflect *compensatory reorganization* for language and concurrent selective *vulnerability* for nonverbal functions. This suggests that differential effects of vulnerability and compensation are domain specific (cf. Nass and Stiles, 1996). In this context, it is interesting that studies by Stiles and colleagues (1997) of children with congenital or perinatal right hemisphere lesion show persistent deficits in the visuospatial domain – an outcome that contrasts with the typically good language development following congenital *left* hemisphere lesion. Judging from neuropsychologic studies of children with early lesion, functions that predominantly involve the right hemisphere (such as visuospatial, prosodic, and affective processes) appear to be organized in similar ways in children and adults (Vicari et al., 1998; Stiles et al., 1999), whereas language organization may undergo fundamental changes in inter- and intra-hemispheric organization during the first years of life (Thal et al., 1991; Bates et al., 1997, 1999). For example, Thal et al. (1991) found that pre- or early postnatal right hemisphere lesion resulted in reduced lexical comprehension in toddlers. Since lexicosemantic processing strongly lateralizes to the left hemisphere in adults (Binder et al., 1997), this would indicate developmental changes in hemispheric organization. These changes may be related to an earlier maturation of the right hemisphere (as suggested by blood flow studies; cf. Chiron et al., 1997), possibly associated with an earlier establishment of a steady-state functional organization. Domain-specific differences in schedules of postlesional vulnerability and compensation could, therefore, be explained on the basis of the visuospatial domain reaching quasi-adult organization earlier than language (possibly analogous to its earlier emergence in phylogeny; Stiles and Thal, 1993).

All in all, while there are obvious differences between functional domains, the data from human lesion studies and animal models contradict a simple Kennard principle and instead indicate a nonmonotonic relationship between lesion onset and the potential for compensatory plasticity (Fig. 20.1). Inconsistencies regarding the precise timing of periods of compensation and vulnerability may be explained in several ways: (i) neurodevelopmental stages can be compared across species only indirectly, (ii) some animal studies apply symmetrical bilateral resections that do not correspond to naturally occurring lesions and the effects of which differ considerably from those of unilateral lesions (Kolb et al., 1989), (iii) resections in animal studies are performed in diverse locations and differ etiologically from lesions in humans, and (iv) tasks used to assess behavioral deficits in animal studies are qualitatively different from those used in

human studies. With regard to the last point, part of the reason why the plasticity curve for human patients appears to be shifted forward on the temporal axis (in comparison with animal findings) may lie in the fact that human studies assess higher cognitive functions subserved by association cortices that mature later than sensorimotor regions (Chugani et al., 1987; Huttenlocher and Dabholkar, 1997).

Neuroimaging studies

The message from animal studies on the effects of early structural brain damage is, therefore, more complex than the simple Kennard principle because of an interaction of effects that appear to work in opposite directions with regard to behavioral outcome. This duality of effects is reflected in functional neuroimaging studies in patients recovering from brain damage. At this point, it should be noted that compensatory plasticity is by no means an exclusive prerogative of the maturing brain. In fact, the first neuroimaging studies on functional remapping following brain lesion were performed in adult patients. Positron emission tomography (PET) studies using ^{15}O tracers have demonstrated enhanced right hemisphere activations during language performance in patients recovering from aphasia following left hemisphere insult (Price et al., 1993; Weiller et al., 1995; Belin et al., 1996). Analogously, reorganization of motor functions into regions that are normally not robustly involved in motor performance (such as the inferior parietal, insular and prefrontal cortices, and regions in the hemisphere ipsilateral to the movement) have been documented in adult patients suffering from stroke (Chollet et al., 1991; Seitz et al., 1998) and tumors (Sabatini et al, 1995; Seitz et al., 1995).

Neuroimaging studies examining postlesional functional reorganization in children and adolescents with early-onset lesion have been unavailable until recently (see review by Bookheimer and Dapretto, 1997). Using functional magnetic resonance imaging (fMRI), motor and language mapping was reported for a few pediatric patients with neoplasm (Chapman et al., 1995) and epilepsy (Benson et al., 1996; Hertz-Pannier et al., 1997; Zupanc, 1997). None of these patients showed clear evidence of lesion-induced regional or interhemispheric functional reorganization. Stapleton et al. (1997) examined the presurgical use of fMRI in 16 pediatric patients but did not address the question of postlesional or postsurgical reorganization.

In contrast, results from a series of $H_2^{15}O$ PET studies including patients with early- and late-onset unilateral lesions have overall supported the concept of greater reorganizational (presumably compensatory) plasticity in the developing compared with the mature brain. In a study of regional cerebral blood flow (rCBF) changes associated with unilateral finger movement (Müller et al., 1997c), enhanced interhemispheric reorganization (i.e., activation in regions ipsilateral to the side of movement) was found in patients with unilateral lesion occurring before age 4 years compared with patients with onset after age 10 years. These findings were robust for secondary motor cortices (premotor and supplementary motor areas), whereas a similar trend for the rolandic primary motor cortex was not significant (cf. Fig. 20.2, p. 242). In other studies (Müller et al., 1999c,b), stronger interhemispheric reorganization following early- rather than late-onset lesion was also found for the language domain, but here major interhemispheric reorganization was seen in the *primary* perisylvian language regions. This seems to indicate differences in interhemispheric reorganizational patterns between domains. While reorganization is predominantly homotopic for language (i.e., reduced activation in left perisylvian regions is accompanied by a gain in right perisylvian activation), homotopic interhemispheric reorganization for the primary motor cortex appears to be limited (Pascual-Leone et al., 1992; Caramia et al., 1996; Müller et al., 1997a, 1998b,d,e). As known from the study of congenital hemiplegia (or "cerebral palsy"), pre- or perinatal lesions affecting the motor system are frequently associated with persistent motor impairment (Rudel et al., 1974; Eicher and Batshaw, 1993). There is an interesting analogy here to the persistent visuospatial and visuoconstructive deficits following congenital right hemisphere lesion, as reported by Stiles and colleagues (1997, 1999; Vicari et al., 1998). This again underscores domain-specific differences in the effects of age at lesion onset on compensatory plasticity, which are not expressed in the simplified diagram of Fig. 20.1.

There are additional neuroimaging findings suggesting that developmental schedules of compensatory plasticity are more complex than assumed by the Kennard principle. Regarding language reorganization following early left hemisphere damage, for example, it has become clear that the loss of functional participation in the lesioned hemisphere typically exceeds the complementary gain in the contralesional hemisphere. Language-related activation in patients with early unilateral left hemisphere lesion was severely reduced in left perisylvian regions, whereas the complementary finding of enhanced activation in homotopic right hemisphere regions tended to be less pronounced (Müller et al., 1998c, 1999b,c). Analogous effects of loss in the lesioned hemisphere being greater than gain

in the contralesional hemisphere have been observed for motor activations in the primary motor cortex (Müller et al., 1997c). Such effects are, in part and rather trivially, explained by reduced activations in regions of structural brain damage. However, reduced activations were also observed in regions that appeared to be *unaffected* by structural damage. This phenomenon is akin to the classical finding of "diaschisis", i.e., impaired function in brain regions distal from the site of structural brain damage (von Monakow, 1914; Feeney and Baron, 1986). While diaschisis is typically transient, it may persist. PET studies have demonstrated reduced glucose metabolism and blood flow in regions far removed from the site of structural damage, such as crossed cerebellar diaschisis in patients with cerebral infarct (Pantano et al., 1986; Metter et al., 1987).

The $H_2^{15}O$ PET studies on the effects of early lesions included mostly epileptic patients and general conclusions should, therefore, be drawn with caution. Long-standing seizures are associated with reduced IQ (Vargha-Khadem et al., 1992; Goodman and Yude, 1996; Muter et al., 1997), even though this effect may be caused in part by larger lesions in patients with seizures (Levine et al., 1987). In patients with unilateral lesion, epilepsy and antiepileptic drugs can functionally impair the contralesional hemisphere (Jibiki et al., 1993; Sankar et al., 1995), which could have a dampening effect on interhemispheric reorganization. It may be that vulnerability effects after early structural lesion are less severe in the absence of seizure disorder.

In summary, functional neuroimaging is an important tool for the study of early structural lesion effects in at least two ways. First, it is uniquely suited to the identification of lesion-induced functional reorganization or atypical organization. Functional neuroimaging can detect hemodynamic correlates of events assumed to reflect functional compensation. Second, functional neuroimaging also sheds light on diaschisis effects, i.e., dampened function in regions distal from the site of a structural lesion. It, therefore, also serves as a tool for observing postlesional events that are assumed to be detrimental to cognitive behavioral outcome and that reflect maturational vulnerability.

What determines compensation and vulnerability?

So far, it has been argued that the effects of early structural lesions should be understood in terms of both compensatory reorganization *and* maturational vulnerability. Simple affirmation of a duality of effects per se is, of course, not truly enlightening because it leaves open the question of what variables determine the kind of effect at work in a

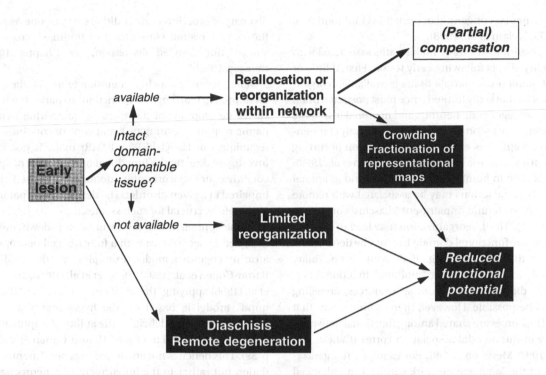

Fig. 20.3. Possible event paths determining compensation and vulnerability after prenatal or early postnatal lesion. White boxes indicate events reflecting compensation (i.e., events that benefit cognitive–behavioral outcome); black boxes indicate detrimental events that reflect vulnerability (see text for details).

given clinical case with a given type of lesion. Figure 20.3 is an attempt to sketch some of the most probable causal relationships that determine outcome after prenatal or early postnatal lesions. It acknowledges a considerable potential for functional reallocation. Realistically, what appears to be functional reallocation will usually be reorganization *within* a pre-existing network. For example, we have discussed neuroimaging studies showing that the premotor and supplementary motor areas may become more prominently involved in movement when the primary motor cortex is damaged (cf. Fig. 20.2*d,e*, p. 242). Language activations in patients with early lesion (and adult stroke) have been observed in right perisylvian regions that are probably involved in paralinguistic functions in the healthy brain (Ross, 1993) and that have been found to coactivate during language performance (Lassen et al., 1978; Just et al., 1996; Price et al., 1996; Cabeza and Nyberg, 1997).

While the precise modes of network reorganization undoubtedly depend on the functional domain (i.e., on the way the particular network was organized premorbidly, such reorganization may reflect a "reshuffling" of

functional responsibilities within a network. However as indicated in Fig. 20.3, the availability of intact *domain-compatible* tissue is a crucial variable that determines the degree to which reorganization is possible. This latter term conceptualizes the distinction between regions that are candidates for functional reallocation and those that are not. For example, there is no indication in the literature that early left perisylvian lesion could be compensated by reorganization of language functions into occipital or superior parietal cortices. These regions, therefore, do not appear to be domain compatible with language. Primary (and probably secondary) sensorimotor cortices exhibit very limited domain compatibility across modalities, even though there are exceptions. Cross-modal plasticity is possible when subcortical afferents are experimentally rewired or when tissue is transplanted within protocortex in the immature animal brain (Sur et al., 1990; Schlaggar and O'Leary, 1991; O'Leary et al., 1994). In humans, early loss of one sensory modality also permits cross-modal plasticity. The best documented example here is tactile and Braille reading-related processing in occipital cortex in blind subjects when blindness is congenital or occurs in childhood (Uhl et al., 1993; Sadato et al., 1998).

Figure 20.3 indicates three major paths associated with vulnerability effects following early lesion. First, if little or no intact domain-compatible tissue is available, reorganization will be markedly limited since most postnatal brain tissue cannot regenerate neurons and neuronal loss at the site of a structural lesion cannot therefore be fully compensated. An exception is early intrauterine lesion occurring before neuronal mitosis is terminated (cf. Kolb et al., 1998). Second, as seen in human imaging studies and in animal models, structural lesions may be associated with remote functional or structural impairment (diaschisis or remote degeneration). Third, reorganization may lead to (partial) recovery in one functional domain but may be detrimental to another through crowding. If domain compatibility existed only within discrete or "modular" functional networks that did not share neuronal resources, crowding would not be possible. However, there is little doubt that neuronal resources are shared among functional networks, especially in multimodal association cortex (Cabeza and Nyberg, 1997; Mesulam, 1998). For example, reorganization within the language network can lead to enhanced language involvement of parts of this network that are normally shared with some visuospatial functions, resulting in visuospatial impairment through crowding.

Neuroimaging and the study of developmental disorders

Turning to developmental disorders, we will now make a complementary argument. Our aim is to present developmental disorders both in terms of the obvious effects of maturational vulnerability *and* in terms of the typically more elusive effects of compensatory reorganization. The discussion will focus on autism and, to a lesser extent, on developmental disorders of language.

Autism and Asperger's syndrome

Until the mid-1990s, functional neuroimaging studies of autism were generally limited to single conditions. In many studies, subjects were scanned at rest, sometimes with eyes closed (Horwitz et al., 1988), sometimes with eyes open (Sherman et al., 1984; Schifter et al., 1994; Mountz et al., 1995) or during sedation (de Volder et al., 1987; Chiron et al., 1995). Other investigators have attempted to control mental states by continuous performance (Siegel et al., 1992) or verbal learning tasks (Haznedar et al., 1997). The

diversity of experimental conditions may be one reason for the lack of overall consistency of findings across these studies (for detailed discussion, see Chapter 10 and Rumsey, 1996b).

More recently, a few neuroimaging studies have attempted to map cognitive functions in patients with pervasive developmental disorders by comparing hemodynamic responses during task and control conditions. The techniques of $H_2^{15}O$ PET and fMRI make it possible to investigate directly the functional organization of specific cognitive or sensorimotor domains assumed to be impaired in a given disorder. The design of task paradigms is, therefore, crucial for such studies.

In one approach, which we will call top-down, tasks are designed in accordance with a fully fledged neuropsychiatric or cognitive model. Examples are the studies by Baron-Cohen et al. (1994), Fletcher et al. (1995), and Happé et al. (1996) applying "theory of mind" tasks. The "theory of mind" model is based on the hypothesis that autism involves a selective deficit in "the ability of impute mental states to oneself and to others" (Baron-Cohen et al., 1985: p. 39). This deficit is not attributed to *general* mental retardation but rather to the impairment of a neurocognitive module (Baron-Cohen et al., 1985; Baron-Cohen, 1991), i.e., a genetically specified and functionally autonomous cognitive subsystem (Fodor, 1983; Shallice, 1988).

A single photon emission computed tomography (SPECT) study by Baron-Cohen et al. (1994) and a PET study by Fletcher et al. (1995) showed activation in prefrontal cortex (Brodmann areas (BAs) 10 and 8, respectively) in healthy adults performing a "theory of mind" task. In the study by Happé and colleagues (1996), regional brain activations were studied using PET in a group of five adult men with a diagnosis of Asperger's syndrome, a pervasive developmental disorder similar to high-functioning autism but without major delay in language acquisition (American Psychiatric Association, 1994; Szatmari et al., 1995; Volkmar et al., 1996). The task condition – comprehension of a "theory of mind" story that involved understanding of the mental states of characters – was compared with comprehension of a story that solely involved "physical events". The strongest activation peak for the patient group was in a more inferior location (BA 9) than for a normal control group (BA 8). However, it is unclear whether the differences in stereotactic peak localization (20 mm on the superior-to-inferior z axis; much less on the x and y axes) are meaningful in view of the limited spatial resolution of the $H_2^{15}O$ PET technique. An obvious hypothesis for this study would have been *reduction or absence* of activation in the putative neurocognitive "theory of mind module" (presumed to be localized in prefrontal cortex; Fletcher et al., 1995) in subjects with Asperger's syndrome. Instead, the findings suggest *normal* magnitude of activation with differences in peak localizations that may well result from spatial normalization (see below), especially when performed in a small patient sample with potential neuroanatomic abnormalities (Minshew, 1994; Volkmar et al., 1996). According to the atlas by Talairach and Tournoux (1988), the peak activation in BA 8 reported by Fletcher et al. (1995) for *normal* adults is not cortical but is located in white matter in the depth of the frontal lobe. This illustrates the potentially problematic effects of spatial normalization. Changes identified in rCBF $H_2{}^{15}O$ PET are predominantly associated with synaptic function (Fox and Raichle, 1986; Jueptner and Weiller, 1995) and, therefore, occur almost exclusively in gray matter. Area 8 also incorporates the "frontal eye field" (e.g. Nieuwenhuys et al., 1988, p. 373) and the activation focus reported by Fletcher et al. (1995) is located in the vicinity of the supplementary eye field (Goldberg et al., 1991). Neither Fletcher et al. (1995) nor Happé et al. (1996) report recording of eye movements during task performance. Abnormalities of saccadic eye movements in autism have been reported (Kemner et al., 1998). While abnormalities of eye movements and gaze in autism (Baron-Cohen et al., 1997) are certainly of interest, it remains unclear whether the findings of the study by Happé and colleagues truly relate to "theory of mind" processing rather than to oculomotor phenomena.

Another $H_2{}^{15}O$ PET study of high-functioning verbal autistic adults (Müller et al., 1999a) explored possible hemodynamic reflections of abnormalities previously proposed in autism research: atypical functional asymmetries (e.g., Dawson et al., 1989; Chiron et al., 1995), disturbances of auditory perception, and cerebellar impairment (see below). Despite the equally small patient sample (five), some of the expected differences between autistic and age- and gender-matched control subjects (five) could be identified. For example, the leftward asymmetry of perisylvian activations during verbal auditory stimulation (listening to sentences compared with rest) found in normal adults (Müller et al., 1997b) was significantly reduced or reversed in autistic adults. In the four male patients, activation in a left frontal region (BA 46) and in the left thalamus was significantly reduced (Müller et al., 1998a) for this condition. Cerebellar activations were also reduced overall in autistic subjects during tonal stimulation. In addition, activation of the right-hemispheric deep cerebellar nuclei during verbal stimulation was found to be significantly reduced in autistic compared with normal men (Müller et al., 1998a). These results tentatively support the hypotheses of atypical functional asymmetry for language-related processing and of reduced cerebellar function in autism.

The studies by Happé et al. (1996) and Müller et al. (1999a) are exploratory and do not warrant any definitive conclusions. Their limitations highlight several general issues in the design of functional mapping in developmental disorders.

Sample size While it is difficult to collect functional imaging data from large samples of subjects with developmental disorders, in particular those typically associated with limited intelligence, hyperactivity, or hypersensitivity, a certain minimum size is required (probably on the order of eight subjects per group) for the detection of subtle group differences in regional activations (Kapur et al., 1995). However, the potentially conflicting need for homogeneity of clinical samples suggests different solutions for PET and fMRI because the latter technique allows more extensive data acquisition in fewer subjects (for example, single-trial designs (Dale and Buckner, 1997) or multiple runs comparing task and control conditions in each subject).

Undirected hypothesizing Even when significance thresholds are corrected for multiple comparisons, the risk of false-positive findings remains considerable in studies comparing patient and control groups with the "blind" hypothesis that *some* brain regional measure will show *some* kind of group difference. Psychiatric patients are likely to respond differently to given stimuli or tasks, and atypical patterns of hemodynamic response may simply reflect differences in cognitive strategies or in affective and physiologic states such as fear or arousal rather than true neurofunctional abnormalities. Preferable are hypothesis-driven designs that specify a limited number of brain regions of interest on an a priori basis (see below). This can be complemented by an additional exploratory and undirected analysis of hemodynamic changes in the entire brain (or the entire image volume acquired), which may in turn generate specific hypotheses for future studies.

Studying outcome rather than pathogenesis In principle, developmental disorders should be preferentially studied *during development*. Studies of younger patient groups and age-matched controls pose ethical problems when ionizing radiation is involved (as in PET or SPECT), even though there is little evidence for health hazards in studies limited to low-dose radiation (Ernst et al., 1998a). Functional mapping studies are, however, also feasible using fMRI. Even though task compliance and head motion artifacts are problematic in young subjects, children under the age of 10 years (Casey et al., 1997) and even as young as 4 years of age (Stapleton et al., 1997) have been successfully studied with fMRI. However, since crucial pathogenic events will occur even earlier in most developmental disorders, functional mapping studies remain inherently limited to the observation of outcome.

Spatial normalization Functional imaging data are most conveniently analyzed by first "warping" image volumes for each individual subject to a standard space, typically Talairach space (Talairach and Tournoux, 1988), and then performing group statistical analyses. In view of normal individual anatomic variability, this approach may be problematic in healthy adults (Steinmetz and Seitz, 1991; Rajkowska and Goldman-Rakic, 1995) and this is true a fortiori in *clinical* patients, who may show anatomic abnormalities (and possibly *systematic* divergence from the model brain of a 60-year-old Caucasian female selected by Talairach and Tournoux (1988)). Analyzing spatially normalized image volumes in combination with undirected hypotheses is especially precarious, since subtle differences in activation magnitude or peak stereotactic coordinates may be entirely the result of group differences in the effects of spatial normalization. An alternative is the identification of regions or volumes of interest based on specific hypotheses or regional brain abnormalities in a given clinical population. Volumes of interest can be identified on coregistered high-resolution MRI in each individual subject and the mean signal change or the number of activated voxels within the volume can be computed for statistical group comparisons.

Top-down and bottom-up approaches

As mentioned earlier, top-down approaches are defined as proceeding from a fully elaborated theoretical model of cognitive–behavioral outcome to the investigation of possible biological causes. Top-down functional neuroimaging designs, as in the study on Asperger's syndrome by Happé et al. (1996), are, therefore, critically dependent on the biological validity of the chosen theoretical model. While study designs will always be informed by preconceived theoretical ideas, and empirical data will, therefore, always be theory-laden to some extent (Kuhn, 1962), it is critically important whether a set of hypotheses remains falsifiable by empirical data produced within the given theoretical paradigm (Popper, 1965). Of course, top-down approaches may incorporate biological data or hypotheses about pathogenesis. The crucial characteristic of top-down approaches is, however, the attempt to *explain* available data in terms of a cognitive behavioral *outcome*. By comparison, while bottom-up approaches ideally incorporate

a maximum of behavioral outcome data, their objective will be to explain the latter in terms of biological *pathogenesis*.

With regard to the "theory of mind" model, it is not established that the prefrontal activations observed by Baron-Cohen et al. (1994) and Fletcher et al. (1995) truly reflect the function of a "theory of mind" module. The finding of a slightly atypical activation focus in patients with Asperger's syndrome by Happé et al. (1996) is, therefore, difficult to interpret. We believe that a "theory of mind" model captures typical *indirect outcomes* of neurodevelopmental disturbances in autism as opposed to elementary cognitive–behavioral impairments that may reflect pathogenesis. From a biological point of view, it is highly unlikely that a "theory of mind" module could be discretely "programmed" in the human genome and "hard-wired" into the brain during development (as seems to be suggested by Baron-Cohen (1992)). Most likely, the theoretical concept of "theory of mind" relates to a set of higher cognitive processes involving complex and *nonlocalizing* neural networks that gradually emerge during brain maturation as a result of learning in many different cognitive and perceptuomotor domains (cf. Mesulam, 1998).

The issue of a "theory of mind" module shows certain interesting parallels with the debate about the modularity of linguistic knowledge and the hypothesis of a genetically prespecified "universal grammar" (Fodor, 1983; Chomsky, 1988; Pinker, 1995; Stromswold, 1995), which will be presented later in this chapter. Baron-Cohen (1992) asserts that "theory of mind" meets all the criteria of a Fodorian module. (Modules are defined by Fodor (1983, p. 37, 47ff.) as domain-specific (i.e., they do not cross stimulus or content domains), innate (i.e., genetically programmed), computationally specific (i.e., they do not rely on general elementary subprocesses), possessing hardwired (i.e., that are nonequipotential) neural mechanisms computationally autonomous (i.e., they do not share resources, such as attention or memory, with other cognitive systems).) However, Baron-Cohen's assertion appears to be based on a misconception of Fodor's proposal. Even Fodor, who is perhaps the most outspoken proponent of the modularity concept in the cognitive sciences, limits his strong hypotheses to *perceptual* "input systems". More complex cognitive processing, in his view, is carried out by *holistic* (and thus nonmodular) "central systems". On a more general note, it is unfortunate that Fodor's treatise on the "modularity of mind", which incorporates neurobiological evidence only in a highly selective fashion and which Fodor himself (1985: p. 33) later called a "potboiler", should be chosen as a theoretical reference point for a neuropsychiatric model (cf.

Müller, 1992; Karmiloff-Smith, 1994). From an evolutionary, behavior genetic, and neurobiological perspective, complex multimodel cognitive domains (such as language or "theory of mind") can only be understood as products of prolonged epigenesis and are, therefore, unlikely to be neurally represented in terms of genetically prespecified modules (cf. O'Leary et al., 1994; Gottlieb, 1995; Müller, 1996; Quartz and Sejnowski, 1997). It appears more commendable – given our as yet limited knowledge of neurofunctional abnormalities in autism – to first address more elementary cognitive deficits in a bottom-up approach.

One example of such an approach concerns auditory processing. In a single-case autopsy study of an autistic woman, Rodier et al. (1996) found severe neuronal dysgenesis in two brainstem structures, the facial nucleus and the superior olive. Since the superior olive is involved in sound localization (van Adel and Kelly, 1998), dysgenesis of this structure would be expected to affect auditory function. There is indeed some evidence for auditory disturbances in autism, such as findings on abnormal listening preferences. For example, Klin (1991) found that a preference for maternal speech over multiple superimposed voices of strangers, as found in normal and nonautistic mentally retarded children, was absent in autistic children. (Another type of hearing abnormality in autism proposed by Rimland and Edelson (1995) is auditory hypersensitivity, which is less likely to be directly related to Rodier's finding in the superior olive.) While there appears to be some confound with peripheral hearing loss (Gordon, 1993; Klin, 1993), electrophysiologic studies also indicate auditory processing abnormalities of the CNS in some patients with autism. Abnormal auditory event-related potentials have been related to generators in the brainstem (Tanguay and Edwards, 1982; Thivierge et al., 1990; Wong and Wong, 1991; but cf. Courchesne et al., 1985) and in cerebral cortex (Lincoln et al., 1995). Electrophysiologic indications of auditory abnormalities in autism may be related to findings of a recent PET study reporting bilateral hypoperfusion in auditory cortex in autistic children under sedation (Zilbovicius et al., 1998; cf. also Bruneau et al., 1992). As mentioned above, Müller et al. (1999a) found significantly reduced activations in the bilateral cerebellar hemispheres and the vermis during nonverbal auditory stimulation in a small sample of autistic adults. Reduced activation for this condition was also observed in lateral temporal cortex, including primary auditory cortex.

Our discussion is not meant to imply that the findings on auditory potentials in brainstem and cortex are specific to autism or apply to all variants of autism (Dunn, 1994), nor do we wish to claim that there is any established etiologic link between auditory deficits and the multiple clinical symptoms in autism (cf. Gordon, 1993 versus Gillberg and Steffenburg, 1993). What is of interest here are the conceptual merits of a bottom-up approach, that is, an attempt to explain multiple neurofunctionally distributed deficits in the adult autistic brain in terms of discrete critical maturational events and identified neuropathologic substrates. While the empirical validity of auditory abnormalities in autism is not fully established, this line of research has a bottom-up character in two ways: first, by considering the possibility of primary impairments in brainstem that may lead to secondary misdifferentiation in forebrain and, second, by examining the role of elementary sensory processes in the development of sociocommunicative impairment (Tanguay and Edwards, 1982; Wong and Wong, 1991; Rodier et al., 1996).

Another, in our view empirically more consistent, example of a bottom-up approach to autism relates to attentional functions. Studies of event-related potentials showing reduced amplitude of endogenous potentials (N_c and auditory P3b) indicate attentional impairment in autism (Courchesne, 1987; Courchesne et al., 1989). Several convergent lines of evidence suggest that certain attentional deficits are linked to anatomic findings in the cerebellum and the parietal lobes. The cerebellum is a rather consistent locus of structural involvement in autism, both in terms of Purkinje cell loss, as documented in autopsy studies (Williams et al., 1980; Bauman and Kemper, 1985, 1994; Ritvo et al., 1986; Bailey et al., 1998), and in terms of macroscopic hypoplasia, reported in several MRI studies (e.g., Courchesne et al., 1994b; Hashimoto et al., 1995; Ciesielski et al., 1997). These structural findings have more recently been related to behavioral data indicating selective deficits in the ability to shift attention in autism. For example, autistic patients with cerebellar abnormalities showed deficits when required to shift attention quickly from the visual to the auditory domain and vice versa, whereas they performed normally when required to focus attention within the auditory or visual domain, or when given more time (> 2.5 s) for attention shifts between sensory modalities (Courchesne et al., 1994c). The rationale for relating these deficits to cerebellar impairments is twofold. First, patients with acquired cerebellar lesions show attentional deficits similar to those found in autistic subjects (Akshoomoff and Courchesne, 1992; Courchesne et al., 1994c). Second, fMRI studies in healthy adults have demonstrated cerebellar involvement in nonmotor attentional processes (Allen et al., 1997) and specifically in shifts of attention within the visual domain (for example, between color and shape; Le et al., 1998). It appears that in autism reduced numbers of Purkinje cells result from early disturbances in prenatal development

(Courchesne, 1997). Attentional deficits could play a role in autistic ontogeny from very early on and contribute to an impairment of joint attention that interferes with normal mother–infant interaction (Courchesne et al., 1994c; Voeller, 1996; Baron-Cohen and Hammer, 1997).

In addition to cerebellar anatomic and functional defects in autism, abnormalities in other brain systems are likely. However, as evidenced by the diversity of findings from structural imaging studies (for reviews, see Minshew, 1994; Rumsey, 1996b; Courchesne, 1997), involvement of noncerebellar structures is probably more variable within the autistic spectrum. Volume loss in the parietal lobes has been found in a sizable subset of autistic subjects (Courchesne et al., 1993). Similar to patients with acquired parietal lesions (Posner et al., 1984), autistic subjects with parietal volume loss (but not those without) show deficits in redirecting attention in visual space, manifesting an abnormally narrow "spotlight" of attention (Townsend and Courchesne, 1994; Townsend et al., 1996). This suggests that attentional deficits are not exclusively a consequence of cerebellar malfunction, but rather of disturbances in cerebro-cerebellar networks (cf. Schmahmann, 1996).

A final example of a bottom-up approach in autism research concerns the motor domain. In view of the evidence of structural and functional impairment of the cerebellum in autism, it is interesting to note that some motor functions activate the cerebellum in seemingly normal ways in autism. In the $H_2^{15}O$ PET studies mentioned above, cerebellar activations were reduced for all nonverbal and verbal auditory and expressive language conditions but *not* for motor speech functions (i.e., repeating sentences compared with listening; Müller et al., 1998a, 1999a). According to a series of PET studies in normal adults by Jueptner and Weiller (1998), cerebellar activity – apart from its known role in motor learning (Jenkins et al., 1994) – reflects the processing of proprioceptive feedback during movement (rather than motor execution per se). In a recent fMRI study, robust activation for finger movement was found in the anterior cerebellum of male autistic subjects (Allen et al., 1998). In fact, anterior cerebellar activation was more pronounced and bilateral in autistic compared with normal subjects. This finding is intriguing in view of the motor coordination impairments (such as clumsiness and abnormalities of gait) that are often observed in autism, which resemble impairments observed in some patients with cerebellar lesion (Hallett et al., 1993; Haas et al., 1996).

An example of cerebellar activations for finger movement in an autistic subject with such motor deficits is shown in Fig. 20.4. While cerebellar activation during movement is normally restricted to the ipsilateral anterior cerebellum and vermis (Desmond et al., 1997), in this autistic subject activations are widespread throughout the bilateral cerebellum. Purkinje cell loss, as observed in autopsy studies (Williams et al., 1980; Bauman and Kemper, 1985; Ritvo et al., 1986; Bailey et al., 1998), could account for these findings in the sense that a partial loss of processing units in the ipsilateral anterior cerebellum could result in atypical spreading and fractionation of activations throughout the cerebellum in autism. This spreading would reflect a compensatory reorganization not unlike the functional reallocations within the forebrain observed in patients with early lesions. However, cerebellar reorganization (or atypical organization) appears to be more microscopic, affecting multiple cerebellar foci recruited for motor function from regions normally involved in higher cognitive processes (Leiner et al., 1995; Schmahmann, 1996; Courchesne and Allen, 1997). This reorganization may, therefore, be analogous to the "crowding effects" discussed above in the context of early-lesion studies. Though speculative, it could be hypothesized that an unusually wide distribution of motor processing throughout the cerebellum would render neocerebellar regions less available for cognitive processing and, thus, contribute to reduced intelligence in autism.

This hypothetical scenario implies that the pathogenesis of autism is not exclusively characterized by vulnerability effects but also involves compensatory plasticity. Differences in compensatory reorganization could explain some of the surprising variability in cognitive and neuro-anatomic measures observed in autism studies on monozygotic twins, who are in fact sometimes discordant for autism (Le Couteur et al., 1996; Kates et al., 1998). Minor genetically or epigenetically based neurodevelopmental differences may lead to different reorganizational paths and different cognitive–affective profiles within a given developmental disorder. These issues will be discussed in detail in the final sections of this chapter.

The causal links established between the findings of auditory, attentional, or motor abnormalities and characteristic social, language, cognitive, and behavioral impairments in autism remain speculative. At early stages of research, bottom-up approaches may be insufficient to bridge the gap fully between biological and cognitive–behavioral findings. Nonetheless, bottom-up approaches provide a biologically solid platform for experimental design in the study of developmental disorders, in particular in neuroimaging studies. This contrasts with top-down approaches, which present with a complementary weakness (unestablished links between well-described phenotypic profiles and biological parameters)

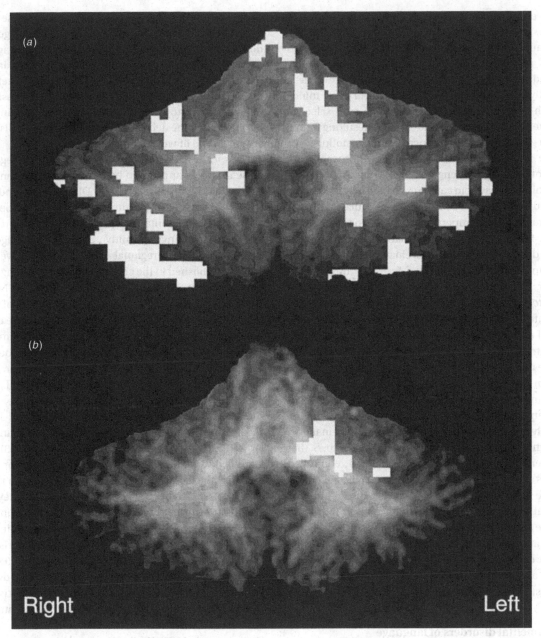

Fig. 20.4. Coronal slices through the cerebellum showing activations (superimposed in white onto structural MRI) for repetitive thumb movements of the dominant left hand in a 21-year-old autistic subject (*a*) who demonstrated motor deficit on neurologic examination typically observed in patients with cerebellar damage (impairment of fine motor coordination and gait; Haas et al., 1996; Hallett et al., 1993). While an age-, sex-, and handedness-matched normal control subject (*b*) shows circumscribed activation in the ipsilateral anterior cerebellum, activations are scattered across the cerebellum bilaterally in the autistic subject (*a*). The statistical map is based on a correlational analysis of the time course for each voxel compared with a hemodynamic model (Bandettini et al., 1993), a statistic with relatively low risk of type I errors owing to movement artifacts. (Adapted from Allen et al., 1998 and G. Allen, R.-A. Müller and E. Courchesne, unpublished data.)

with fewer complementary strengths (cf. Rodier et al., 1997). In spite of this, top-down approaches can be appealing because they appear "elegant", i.e., they seem to "explain" a multitude of phenomena within a well-delineated and coherent theoretical framework. For example, a maximally elegant version of the "theory of mind" approach "explains" autism by reference to a selective impairment of a "theory of mind" module resulting from a defect in genes that normally encode for this module.

In the cognitive sciences, top-down approaches are often motivated by an "engineering" logic, according to which a biological system can be explained in terms of how one could best *construct a machine* that simulates relevant behavioral or output properties of the system (Jacob, 1977; Gardner, 1987; Müller, 1992). Translated into the problem space of developmental neuropsychiatry, this engineering logic implies that an optimal *description* of outcome behavior (or impairment) is construed as an optimal *explanatory* model. Biological mechanisms are, therefore, investigated only *after* the outcome model has been fully designed and are understood as mere "implementations" or "substrates" of conceptual elements of the cognitive outcome model (e.g., Fodor and Pylyshyn, 1988).

Bottom-up approaches, by comparison, are more directly informed by biological and cognitive–behavioral data (even if these appear inconsistent) and can, therefore, ultimately provide more powerful etiological explanations. The animal literature on early-lesion effects shows that even when critical variables are experimentally controlled (which is much less possible in human studies), conclusions are hard to draw, most likely because additional neuromaturational and other unrecognized variables influence outcome through epigenetic mechanisms. These considerations apply even more to developmental disorders that cannot usually be defined in terms of a circumscribed anatomic lesion (for further discussion, see Courchesne et al., 1999).

Developmental disorders of language

Even though our discussion focuses on pervasive developmental disorders, the conceptual and empirical divergence between bottom-up and top-down approaches can also be observed in the study of other developmental disorders. In this section, we will discuss some aspects of the debate about developmental disorders of spoken language and those of written language, which we will refer to as DLI (we prefer this term rather than the more commonly used term specific language impairment, because the latter may imply unjustified theoretical assumptions of linguistic specificity and (developmental) dyslexia, respectively.

There are fundamental differences between these disorders. DLI affects receptive and expressive language functions that develop much earlier than written language. The degree of continuity between dysphasia and dyslexia is not fully established (Aram, 1993; Catts, 1993). Nonetheless, in the context of our present conceptual discussion of bottom-up and top-down approaches, there are interesting parallels in the debates about developmental disorders of spoken and of written language.

The spectrum of neuroanatomic hypotheses regarding these disorders appears to be more restricted than is the case for autism (see reviews on DLI in Rapin and Allen (1988) and on dyslexia in Rumsey (1996a)). This is because, in part, developmental disorders of language predominantly affect a single cognitive domain ("language") for which adult brain regional specializations have been grossly established in the clinical and neuroimaging literature (e.g., Benson and Ardila, 1996; Cabeza and Nyberg, 1997). It is, therefore, not surprising that, in spite of a considerable diversity of findings, there is some degree of convergence in the neuroimaging literature. Autopsy and MRI studies of normal adults have shown associations between asymmetries in posterior (Witelson and Kigar, 1992; Foundas et al., 1994) and anterior (Foundas et al., 1996) perisylvian anatomy and language dominance. Many studies on DLI (Plante et al., 1991; Jackson and Plante, 1996; Gauger et al., 1997; Clark and Plante, 1998) and dyslexia (Kusch et al., 1993; Leonard et al., 1993) have identified some pattern of atypical morphology or asymmetry in (the vicinity of) perisylvian regions, even though some dyslexia studies are nonconfirmatory (Rumsey et al., 1997a) and suggest that age and sex may be major confounds (Schultz et al., 1994). Rare functional neuroimaging studies in children with DLI tentatively suggest perisylvian abnormalities (Lou et al., 1990; Tzourio et al., 1994). The more numerous studies in adults with a history of dyslexia have also mostly detected abnormalities in perisylvian regions (Flowers et al., 1991; Rumsey et al., 1992; Paulesu et al., 1996; Salmelin et al., 1996; Rumsey et al., 1997b; Shaywitz et al., 1998). While functional impairment of posterior perisylvian cortex in phonologic and orthographic tasks appears to be a rather consistent finding, inferior frontal blood flow changes were normal (Rumsey et al., 1994b, 1997b) or even greater than normal (Shaywitz et al., 1998) in some dyslexia studies. However, Horwitz et al. (1998) recently reported reduced correlations of activation in the left angular gyrus with activations in frontotemporal language areas (including inferior frontal cortex) and in visual association cortex, suggesting functional disconnection within a reading network in dyslexia. Detailed critical review of the imaging findings on dyslexia is beyond the scope of this chapter (see Chapter 15). Instead, we will focus on certain conceptual characteristics of the research on developmental disorders of language that span an interesting spectrum of approaches primarily informed by linguistic theory, on the one hand, and by neurobiological evidence, on the other.

When "specific language impairment" is approached from a theoretical linguistic perspective that assumes the genetically specified modularity of language knowledge (Chomsky, 1988; Pinker, 1995; Stromswold, 1995), the obvious question of a discrete deficit affecting only one or a limited number of linguistic "modules" arises (for relevant discussions, see Clahsen, 1989; Curtiss et al., 1992; Rice, 1994). An analogous debate in the research on developmental dyslexia concerns the question of an underlying *specifically linguistic* deficit (such as impaired phonological awareness; Shankweiler et al., 1995; Lyon and Chhabra, 1996) versus an underlying *nonlinguistic* sensory or perceptual impairment (Tallal et al., 1993). In the context of evidence for familial aggregation of "specific language impairment", Gopnik and colleagues suggested a highly specific and modular deficit of certain syntactic and semantic features (such as tense or number; Gopnik, 1990) possibly caused by a single gene defect (Gopnik and Crago, 1991). At first glance, the attempt to relate DLI to gene defects may appear as a prime example of bottom-up theorizing. There is indeed irrefutable evidence from several research groups for the importance of genetic factors in DLI (Tallal et al., 1989; Tomblin and Buckwalter, 1994; Bishop et al., 1995) and dyslexia (Pennington, 1995; DeFries and Alarcón, 1996). However, the readiness to link an apparently "modular" language deficit to gene defects is motivated by a theoretical approach to the cognitive organization of language (Chomsky, 1981; Fodor, 1983), which is itself little concerned with the empirical evidence on the linkage between genes and cognitive–behavioral variables (for discussion, see Bates, 1994; Müller, 1992).

Leaving aside programmatic statements from linguists regarding the genetic prespecification of "universal grammar", it is unlikely that a complex and phylogenetically recent cognitive domain such as language could be "hard-wired" into the brain on the basis of a small and discrete set of genes. Instead, the typical scenario linking genome and higher cognitive function is *polygenic* and *pleiotropic*, which means that numerous genes, each influencing many phenotypic outcomes (pleiotropy), interact in the epigenesis of a cognitive domain (Pennington and Smith, 1983; Hay, 1985; Gottlieb, 1995). Polygenic inheritance is by no means contradicted by the fact that in some instances single gene defects can lead to

gross and specific abnormalities of phenotype. For instance, phenylketonuria, a single gene defect associated with a severe disorder of amino acid metabolism and toxic accumulation of phenylalanine, is phenotypically characterized not only by mental retardation but also by social behavioral deficits, seizures, stunted bodily growth and microcephaly, and dermatologic symptoms (Blau, 1979; Hay, 1985). Likewise, mutations of the gene for the L1 cell adhesion molecule (CAM), which is involved in neuronal migration as well as axonal growth and myelination, are associated with a wide range of deficits (mental retardation, aphasia, gait abnormalities, spasticity) and neuroanatomic defects (callosal hypoplasia, hydrocephalus) in humans (Fransen et al., 1995). Pleiotropic effects of *L1CAM* mutation or knock-out have been confirmed in animal models (Fransen et al., 1998). Note that even though these mutations affect only a single gene, phenotypic manifestations are not focal but rather affect multiple, seemingly unrelated biological systems. Even these examples of well-established linkages between genetic and phenotypic defects, therefore, suggest that genetic influences are shared between neurocognitive and nonneural systems (Courchesne et al., 1999). Interestingly, with respect to the findings of familial aggregation of DLI mentioned above, Gopnik has recently acknowledged that these do not imply the discovery of a "gene for grammar" (Gopnik et al., 1996).

The studies on syntactic–semantic "feature blindness" by Gopnik and colleagues (Gopnik, 1990; Gopnik et al., 1996), which were described above, highlight a further characteristic of the top-down approach: empirical selectivity. Simply speaking, the chances of identifying a modular deficit in a patient are inversely related to the breadth of neuropsychologic and neurologic examinations. The presentation of DLI-affected members of the family studied by Gopnik and colleagues suggested a highly selective linguistic deficit restricted to certain aspects of grammar, compatible with the notion of an autonomous neurofunctional organization of language vis-à-vis other cognitive domains (Fodor, 1983) and a modular organization of linguistic subsystems (Chomsky, 1981; Pinker, 1991). Yet broader testing of the same family members by a different group (Vargha-Khadem et al., 1995) subsequently showed that the deficits were by no means selective and discrete. Not only did affected family members have significantly lower *performance* IQ scores than unaffected members, but Vargha-Khadem et al. (1995) also found evidence of orofacial apraxia, further significantly distinguishing affected from unaffected members. Studying a different sample, Hill (1998) recently reported that children with specific language impairment had deficits in the production and imitation of meaningful gestures, similar to children with developmental dyspraxia (or "developmental coordination disorder"; American Psychiatric Association, 1994). These findings suggest that linguistic deficits in some variants of DLI may be linked to underlying motor or praxic impairment (for related data on acquired aphasia, see Kimura and Watson, 1989). However, the notion that perceptuomotor functions could be instrumental in the ontogenesis of grammatical capacities is anathema to the linguistic theorizing of the Chomskian school (Chomsky, 1965; cf. Piattelli-Palmarini, 1980), which may explain why impairments in these domains were neglected in reports by Gopnik and coworkers and, more generally, why studies of specific language impairment often fail to include measures of extralinguistic function (for discussion, see Johnston, 1994).

The innatist and modularist approach to DLI (or "intelligence without language", as it is labeled by Pinker (1995, p. 273)) appears to be an extreme example of theory-driven top-down modeling and does not occupy a majority position in research of developmental disorders of language. At the other end of the spectrum of theoretical approaches, these disorders have been related to basic (i.e., nonlanguage-specific) perceptuomotor deficits. In a study of 15 dyslexic men, Rumsey et al. (1994a) found impaired performance on a nonverbal tone discrimination and short-term memory task that was associated with reduced right superior temporal and inferior frontal activations. Eden et al. (1996) studied six dyslexic men who showed normal activations in response to a stationary high-contrast visual pattern but impaired stimulus *velocity* judgments and a failure to activate area V5/MT in bilateral occipitotemporal extrastriate cortex in response to a low-contrast, moving stimulus. Correlational PET activation analyses (Horwitz et al., 1998) suggest a disruption of normal connectivity between this visual area and the left temporoparietal cortex (known to be importantly involved in reading; Bavelier et al., 1997). These findings may suggest that underlying deficits in dyslexia are not specifically linguistic but affect more basic sensory processing in the visual (Cornelissen et al., 1991) or auditory domains (Kraft, 1993; Nicolson and Fawcett, 1993; for review, see Bishop, 1992). In particular, dyslexia has been related to disorders in the processing of rapidly changing stimuli in visual (May et al., 1988; Gross-Glenn et al., 1995) and auditory perception (Ribary et al., 1997), with possible analogous motor impairment (Wolff, 1993; Heilman et al., 1996). Some studies in children with DLI (Wright et al., 1997) and developmental dyslexia (McAnally and Stein, 1996) suggest that, in addition to impaired perception of rapid auditory sequences, these disorders also affect the ability to distinguish subtle frequency differences between auditory stimuli.

The studies by Tallal and colleagues (1993, 1996), which are based on the assumption of a developmental continuity between DLI and dyslexia, support the notion of underlying auditory deficit, understood in the context of a general supramodal impairment in rapid perception (and possibly speech production). The findings of this group may be related to autopsy data from a small sample of subjects with history of developmental dyslexia reported by Galaburda and Livingstone (1993). These authors found evidence for anomalies (reduced cell size and abnormally shaped cells) in the magnocellular layers of the lateral geniculate nucleus, with sparing of the parvocellular layers. The magnocellular system is known to be important for the rapid processing of moving and low-contrast visual stimuli (Livingstone and Hubel, 1988). fMRI findings by Eden et al. (1996), which were described above, and by Demb and colleagues (1997, 1998) are consistent with a selective impairment of the magnocellular system in dyslexia. Demb et al. (1997) found reduced activation in extrastriate area MT+ during low-luminance visual stimulation in dyslexic subjects: an area that is involved in motion perception and believed to receive strong input from magnocellular pathways. Galaburda et al. (1994) also report histologic findings for the *medial* geniculate nucleus analogous to those for the lateral geniculate nucleus (reduced number of large neurons, increased number of small neurons) in their autopsy dyslexia sample, which could suggest that the auditory domain is affected in similar ways.

At the present time, there appears to be no consensus regarding the empirical evidence for specific hypotheses of the magnocellular theory (McAnally et al., 1997) and the efficacy of therapeutic interventions based on it (Tallal et al., 1996; for a recent review, see Stein and Walsh, 1997). For example, Borsting et al. (1996) report psychophysical data suggesting that magnocellular defect in the visual domain applies only to a subgroup of dyslexics (i.e., those with impaired grapheme–phoneme correspondence rules ("dysphoneidetics"), but not those with deficits in visual word gestalt perception ("dyseidetics")). Other studies altogether refute the notion of an underlying auditory temporal processing (as opposed to phonologic) deficit (Mody et al., 1997). What is of sole interest here is the conceptual conflict between the linguistically informed top-down models that explain developmental disorders of language in terms of specific disruption of language modules and the bottom-up approaches that account for such disorders in terms of more elementary sensorimotor disturbances and suspected neuropathology. This conflict is analogous to our earlier discussion of pervasive developmental disorders and the conflict between the "theory of mind" model and bottom-up approaches pertaining to more elementary impairments in auditory, attentional, visuospatial, and motor domains.

Verbal sparing or verbal vulnerability?

Our discussion of developmental disorders indicates an interesting apparent conflict with findings from early lesion studies. If developmental brain impairments share the principles of compensation and vulnerability, then why would early structural lesions be often associated with verbal sparing (at the expense of nonverbal functions), whereas language appears to be selectively vulnerable in developmental disorders – so much so that some researchers present language deficit as a central impairment in autism (e.g., Fay and Mermelstein, 1982; Baltaxe and Simmons, 1992) or view autism and the semantic-pragmatic subtype of DLI as located on a single continuum of disorders (Bishop, 1989)? One explanation for this apparent paradox would relate to the fact that language involves multiple sensorimotor modalities and cognitive domains and, therefore, a great number of brain regions. This could account for enhanced vulnerability in the sense that a distributed system can be disrupted at more numerous neurofunctional loci than a focally organized system.

However, in the context of early structural lesions, this distributive organization appears to *enhance* rather than diminish the compensatory potential for language. An alternative explanation relates to the anatomically more diffuse nature of neuropathologies thought to underlie developmental disorders. Whereas, for instance, structural lesions caused by stroke are usually unilateral, developmental disorders are much less likely to be confined to one brain hemisphere. This is related to pleiotropic principles, which will be discussed in the following section. While neurofunctional disturbances in developmental disorders may be subtle, they tend to be widespread. The potential for language reorganization may, therefore, be reduced in developmental disorders owing to a lack of intact domain-compatible tissue. Interestingly, language prognosis is equally poor when early *structural* lesion affects both hemispheres. For example, when hemispherectomy is performed within the first decade of life, cognitive and linguistic outcome tends to be good if the pre-existing lesion is confined to one hemisphere (Vargha-Khadem et al., 1997; Zupanc, 1997), as is often the case in Rasmussen's encephalitis or Sturge–Weber disease (Ogunmekan et al., 1989; Vining et al., 1993). Conversely, hemispherectomy performed in patients with hemimegalencephaly is usually

associated with less positive outcome, most likely as a result of pre-existing impairment in the unresected hemisphere (Rintahaka et al., 1993).

Perspectives

Pleiotropy results in multiple brain-behavior impairments

Our discussion of bottom-up approaches in the study of developmental disorders does not imply that we believe primary causes or elementary impairments can be studied directly with behavioral, electrophysiologic, neuroimaging, or other techniques. In a trivial sense, this is so because affected subjects are not available for study when pathogenic events first occur. (This limitation can be potentially circumvented in genetic linkage studies (Cook et al., 1998; Schroer et al., 1998) and animal genetic knock-out models (Fransen et al., 1998; Lipp and Wolfer, 1998).) Figure 20.5 is an attempt to illustrate possible epigenetic paths connecting biological etiologies with classes of developmental disorder. Initial pathogenic events will typically affect multiple brain regions but may be in some cases limited to a single region. When a brain region is affected (for example, by reduced neurogenesis or early loss of neurons, as hypothesized for cerebellar Purkinje cells in autism), this may or may not have detrimental effects on the differentiation of other brain regions. For instance, recent volumetric evidence of inverse correlations between the sizes of the cerebellar vermis and the frontal lobes in autism (Carper and Courchesne, 1999) might be explained by reduced inhibitory function of Purkinje cells, leading to remote overexcitation of the frontal lobes via dentato–thalamo–cortical pathways (Middleton and Strick, 1994) and to misdifferentiation of frontal cortex. Another region well known for its differentiating role in brain development is the thalamus. Thalamo-cortical afferents are crucial for the functional differentiation of cerebral cortex (Shatz, 1992; O'Leary et al., 1994). In Fig. 20.5, such regions that are important for the functional differentiation of other regions are characterized by the label "remote differentiation". When such regions are affected in a developmental disorder, the etiological course will result in *misconstruction* (for example, abnormalities of neuronal differentiation and connectivity or of gross morphologic organization) in many regions besides the one originally affected by pathogenic events.

A developmental disorder can, therefore, involve multiple neurofunctional systems at various hierarchical levels of brain organization (neocortical, subcortical, brainstem,

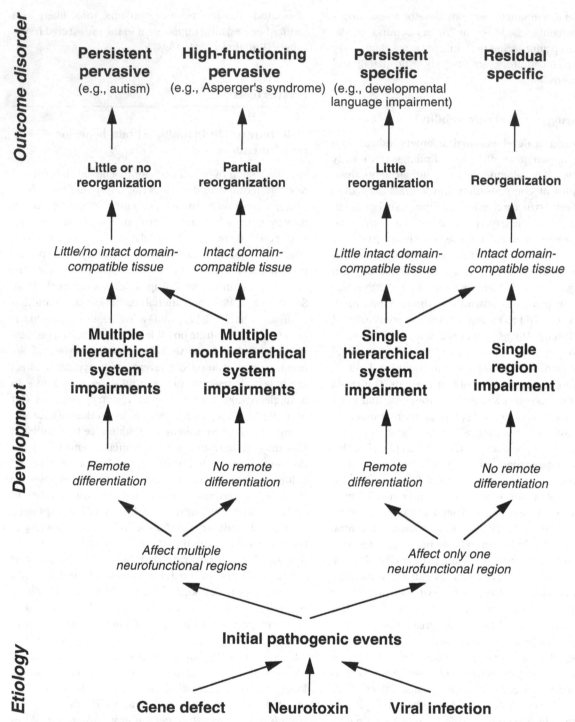

Fig. 20.5. Possible neurodevelopmental paths determining vulnerability and compensation in developmental disorders. For explanation of terms such as "remote differentiation" and "domain compatibility", see main text. The linearity of events indicated by the arrows constitutes a simplification. For example, a genetic deficit may cause persistent pathogenic states (rather than only one initial pathogenic event) and will, therefore, be associated, with persistent vulnerability, reducing the potential for compensatory reorganization. A further limitation of the figure is its emphasis of structure–function relationships. *Qualitative* differences between diffuse disturbances of different neurotransmitter systems – for instance, of serotonin in autism (McDougle et al., 1996) or of dopamine in attention-deficit hyperactivity disorder (Ernst et al., 1998b) – are not taken into account.

cerebellar). Alternatively, it is theoretically possible that it remains confined to more circumscribed regions throughout development. The upper part of Fig. 20.5 maps paths of potential compensatory reorganization in ways similar to those conceptualized in Fig. 20.3 for early structural lesions. In multiple hierarchical system impairments, intact domain-compatible tissue will typically be unavailable, thus limiting the potential for reorganization. In the most severe case, a pervasive disorder such as autism will persist throughout development (i.e., show little cognitive–behavioral improvement). If there is more sparing or if partial reorganization is possible, high-functioning variants of a pervasive developmental disorder, such as Asperger's syndrome, may develop. With more confined impairments, affecting only a single region or only regions connected by a circumscribed cortico-subcortical pathway ("single hierarchical system impairments"), domain-compatible tissue may be available to varying degrees. Accordingly, there will be varying degrees of cognitive–behavioral improvement over time and outcome may range from a persistent specific developmental disorder (such as DLI) to a residual and mild form of impairment that may be continuous with the normal spectrum. For example, as argued by Shaywitz et al. (1992), developmental dyslexia often resolves into very mild forms of the deficit that blend with the lower tail of the normal distribution of reading abilities.

The above considerations focus on pleiotropic effects in the pathogenesis of developmental disorders. (Our use of the term pleiotropy is broader than its definition in behavior genetics and includes the spreading of detrimental effects over multiple biological subsystems following nongenetic pathogenic events (such as viral infection or neurotoxic exposure).) With regard to spectrum disorders such as autism however, it is likely that different etiological pathways can lead to a phenotype that will meet diagnostic criteria (Yeung-Courchesne and Courchesne, 1997). This insight highlights the fundamental limitations of pure top-down approaches because an outcome disorder is equivocal with regard to multiple potential etiologies. Therefore, regardless of the empirical validity of findings on "theory of mind" deficit in autism, such findings cannot elucidate the pathogenesis of autism *unless* there is *independent biological* evidence supporting the model (see Courchesne et al., 1999, for further discussion).

As Fig. 20.5 indicates, developmental disorders will likely affect multiple brain regions. For instance, in our exemplary discussion of autism we do not assume that cerebellum-based attentional deficits represent a singular impairment underlying all other abnormalities observed within the autistic spectrum. This would be unexpected in view of our understanding that gene defects (which play a major role in autism; Bailey et al., 1995) act *pleiotropically* (i.e., result in widespread disturbances throughout the brain; Yeung-Courchesne and Courchesne, 1997; Courchesne et al., 1999). We, therefore, hypothesize that certain attentional functions are *specifically vulnerable* to the type of neurodevelopmental disturbance and misconstruction found in autism. Attentional impairment is not expected to be modality or stimulus specific nor is it expected to be tied to the exclusive dysfunction of a single anatomic structure. In view of its widely distributed connectivity and its potential participation in numerous cortico–subcortical networks (Schmahmann, 1996) and in view of the evidence for dysgenesis or early loss of Purkinje neurons (Courchesne, 1997; Bailey et al., 1998), the cerebellum could play a pivotal role as "mediator of neurogenetic misconstruction" in multiple neocortical, limbic, and subcortical regions. We have discussed evidence for parietal lobe dysfunction above, but involvement of other brain regions can also be expected in autism, though possibly in more subtle ways or only in portions of the autistic population. This expectation is supported by the multitude of brain structures for which some degree of abnormality has been found in previously studied samples (see reviews: Minshew, 1994; Bailey et al., 1996; Rumsey, 1996b; Courchesne, 1997).

One example concerns the frontal lobes. Involvement of the frontal lobes has been suggested in earlier studies based on clinical symptomatology (Damasio and Maurer, 1978) and event-related potentials associated with attentional functions (Courchesne et al., 1984; Ciesielski et al., 1990), as well as in developmental studies on CBF (Zilbovicius et al., 1995) and serotonin synthesis capacity (Chugani et al., 1997; see Chapter 10). As mentioned above, Carper and Courchesne (1999) found that the size of vermal lobules VI and VII (frequently hypoplastic in autism) was inversely correlated with frontal lobe volume, possibly suggesting a pathogenic link between cerebellar and frontal findings. Deficits on putative "frontal-lobe tests" of executive function and problem solving have been identified in autism (Prior and Hoffman, 1990; McEvoy et al., 1993). According to Ciesielski and Harris (1997), high-functioning autistic subjects appear to be "stuck-in-set", i.e., impaired in switching between problem-solving strategies. This is reminiscent of the attention-shifting deficits discussed above; however an executive-shifting deficit suggests predominantly prefrontal involvement (Alexander et al., 1989). Evidence for cerebellar participation in multiple neurocognitive networks (Leiner et al., 1995; Schmahmann, 1996; Courchesne and Allen, 1997) and for massive connectivity between deep cerebellar output nuclei and the dorsolateral prefrontal cortex (Middleton and Strick, 1994; Schmahmann, 1996) suggests that the cerebellum may be additionally involved to an unknown degree in these executive-shifting functions (cf. Hallett and Grafman, 1997).

Studies combining neuropsychologic, structural imaging, electrophysiologic, and functional mapping techniques can be used to investigate brain–behavior relationships in an analogous manner to those demonstrated for the parietal lobe and the cerebellum (Akshoomoff and Courchesne, 1992; Townsend and Courchesne, 1994; Townsend et al., 1996). A catalogue of brain–behavior links for cognitive networks involving various cortical–hemispheric, subcortical, and cerebellar systems that may be impaired in autism could help to identify neurofunctionally based variants within the autistic spectrum from an outcome perspective. Analogous considerations apply to other forms of developmental psychopathology (cf. Weinberg et al., 1995). However, brain–behavior relationships in developmental disorders cannot be based on the literature of lesions acquired by adults since it is unlikely that lesion locality and outcome impairment are linked by the same rules in the developing as in the mature brain. Brain–behavior links, therefore, need to be independently established for each developmental disorder in affected populations.

In a further step, such taxonomies may be linked to genetically defined variants of each developmental disorder. While a direct mapping from genetically to brain-behaviorally defined variants is unlikely, only a bidirectional approach, integrating ontogenetic with outcome data, promises an eventual biological understanding of autistic and other psychopathologic spectra and the development of therapies adequate for given variants of each disorder.

Is there compensation in developmental disorders?

As argued above, functional neuroimaging can be an empirical tool for addressing vulnerability and compensation in the study of developmental disorders and the effects of early structural lesions. As a first approximation and assuming a simple dichotomy, developmental disorders may be viewed as predominantly characterized by vulnerability. Neuroimaging can, therefore, serve to identify the multitude of anatomically and functionally distributed outcome impairments (indicated by a "V" in Fig. 20.6) caused by some putative genetic defect or early pathogenic event. From this perspective, pleiotropic effects of gene defects reduce the potential for compensatory reorganization because these effects may not respect the boundaries of neurofunctional organization (and may in the worst case affect the entirety of neurofunctional circuits). Conversely, in patients with early structural lesion, functional imaging can focus on loci of compensatory reorganization (indicated by a "C" in Fig. 20.6). The potential for compensatory reorganization may be pronounced because a structural lesion may be confined to one or a few brain regions and, therefore, may leave other domain-compatible tissue intact.

These fundamental differences between the effects of early structural lesions and developmental disorders are related to the fact that initial pathogenic events tend to occur earlier in developmental disorders (in which genetic factors have been established or are suspected). The time-plasticity curves in Fig. 20.1 may be misunderstood as reflecting a purely quantitative effect of time at lesion onset. However, as discussed earlier, findings in animals can be applied only with difficulty to the human species because conceptual and postnatal ages and corresponding maturational states cannot be linearly translated across species. Since ontogenetic time is linked to certain sets of neurodevelopmental events, it is inherently qualitative (Rodier, 1980; Kolb, 1995). For example, an intrauterine infarct occurring before neuronal migration and destroying neuroblasts in the germinal matrix will have qualitatively different effects from an infarct destroying an area of cortex postmigration (cf. Kolb et al., 1996). The first type of structural lesion shares some pleiotropic features with developmental disorders in that a focal insult in the germinal matrix may have widespread effects on developing cortex (Walsh and Cepko, 1992).

As discussed in the previous sections, a simple and discrete dichotomy between developmental disorders and early structural lesion effects, even though plausible as a first approach, represents an oversimplification. This is well documented for early structural lesions, which often result in compensatory reorganization accompanied by functional diaschisis in remote regions and that appear to be extremely detrimental at some stages of early development. Regarding developmental disorders, there is an obvious rationale for neuroimaging studies that examine multiple neurofunctional impairments (i.e., functionally and spatially distributed effects of vulnerability). Conversely, it is less obvious how compensatory reorganization may be identified. It may well be that some variants of developmental disorders exclusively reflect vulnerability, in the sense that a singular early disturbance (e.g., gene defect) leads to widespread misconstruction of brain circuits without significant potential for functional compensation (cf. the path on the left in Fig. 20.5). A case in point might be autism with severe mental retardation.

Nonetheless, autistic patients often show obsessive

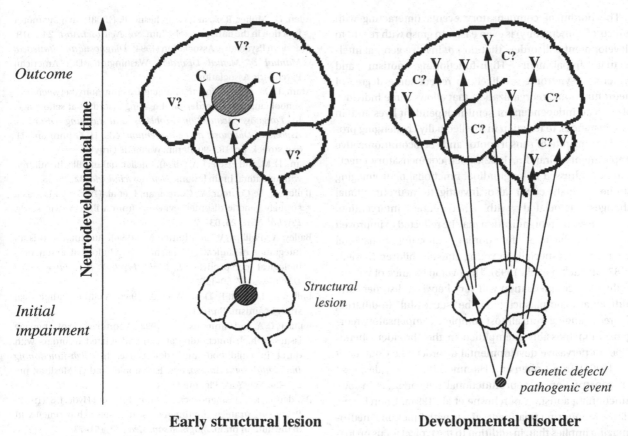

Fig. 20.6. Contrasting effects of developmental disorders and early structural lesions across neurodevelopmental time. The location of symbols is arbitrary and does not refer to actual brain regions. The prototypical early structural lesion results in an area of dysfunctional brain tissue (or encephalomalacia) at the outcome stage. Some of the functions typically assumed by the lesioned area will be reallocated to other areas, for example to surrounding brain regions that perform compensatory functions (C). However, structural damage may also trigger vulnerability effects (V), such as functional diaschisis or remote degeneration. The prototypical developmental disorder is characterized by a focal early defect that has pleiotropic effects on various distributed neurofunctional circuits over time. Depending on the availability of domain-compatible tissue, these multiple impairments caused by vulnerability (V) may be accompanied by compensatory reorganization (C).

activity limited to certain kinds of object or event, which in its extreme form may develop into so-called savantism (Treffert, 1988). As a further example, Williams syndrome (a genetic disorder of calcium metabolism) is characterized by a very uneven cognitive profile of low overall intelligence and severely impaired visuospatial and visuoconstructive functions but some highly developed sociocommunicative functions (including some components of language; Udwin and Yule, 1991; Bellugi et al., 1994; Tager-Flusberg et al., 1998). Consequently, when asked about elephants, a patient with Williams syndrome will be able to provide an elaborate verbal description but will be unable to produce a coherent drawing (Bellugi et al., 1992). The obsessive specializations in savants or the overdeveloped sociocommunicative functions in patients with Williams syndrome can

be conceptualized as reflections of compensatory neuro-functional reorganization, with cognitive processing being rechannelled into domains of relative sparing. While such reorganization has yet to be definitively demonstrated in neuroimaging studies, it is likely that narrow specializations in the context of general intellectual deficit will be reflected by recruitment of atypical brain circuits. In Williams syndrome, for example, the cerebellar tonsils (Wang et al., 1992) and lobules VI and VII of the cerebellar vermis (Jernigan and Bellugi, 1990), as well as temporal limbic regions (Jernigan and Bellugi, 1994), have been found to be of normal size or hyperplastic in the context of overall cerebral hypoplasia. Such regions could conceivably participate in neurofunctional circuits involved in these subjects' hypercommunicative behavior.

The notion of compensatory events (interacting with effects of vulnerability) is even easier to grasp with regard to developmental disorders that do *not* involve general intellectual impairment. High-functioning autism and Asperger's syndrome are likely to reflect some degree of neurofunctional reorganization that allows some individuals to lead independent or semi-independent lives and, in rare instances, to function in intellectually challenging professions in spite of sensorimotor and sociocommunicative impairments (Grandin, 1992). Such compensatory effects can be addressed in longitudinal functional neuroimaging studies, which could also investigate neurofunctional changes associated with therapeutic intervention. Compensatory reorganization may be reflected in improved cognitive–behavioral functioning following behavioral intervention, especially in young autistic children (Lovaas, 1987; McEachin et al., 1993). The overall balance of vulnerability and compensation will vary between disorders and individuals, and plasticity may be "successful" to differing degrees, ranging from almost complete compensatory reorganization (possibly exemplified in the "broader phenotype" of pervasive developmental disorders; Le Couteur et al., 1996; Baron-Cohen and Hammer, 1997) to widespread misconstruction of neurofunctional networks (as in low-functioning autism; Courchesne et al., 1994a; Courchesne, 1997). Monitoring treatment effects with functional neuroimaging implies that, in addition to the typical focus on loss and anomaly of activations, imaging studies could attempt to identify the neural bases of *spared* functions in a given developmental disorder and thus explore optimal windows for therapeutic intervention.

Acknowledgments

We would like to thank Elizabeth Bates, Faraneh Vargha-Khadem, and Pamela Moses for comments on an earlier draft of this chapter and to Mark Harwood for technical help.

References

Akshoomoff, N. A. and Courchesne, E. (1992). A new role for the cerebellum in cognitive operations. *Behav Neurosci*, 106, 731–8.

Alexander, M. P., Benson, D. F. and Stuss, D. T. (1989). Frontal lobes and language. *Brain Lang.*, 37, 656–91.

Allen, G., Buxton, R. B., Wong, E. C. and Courchesne, E. (1997). Attentional activation of the cerebellum independent of motor involvement. *Science*, 275, 1940–3.

Allen, G., Müller, R.-A. and Courchesne, E. (1998). Imaging motor function in the autistic cerebellum. *Soc. Neurosci. Abst.*, 24, 1519.

American Psychiatric Association (1994). *Diagnostic and Statistical Manual of Mental Disorders*. Washington, DC: American Psychiatric Association.

Aram, D. M. (1993). How to characterize continuity between pre-school language disorders and reading disorders at school age. In *Language Acquisition Problems and Reading Disorders: Aspects of Diagnosis and Intervention*, eds. H. Grimm and H. Skowronek, pp. 183–90. Berlin: Walter de Gruyter.

Aram, D. M. and Eisele, J. A. (1994). Intellectual stability in children with unilateral brain lesions. *Neuropsychologia*, 32, 85–95.

Bailey, A., Le Couteur, A., Gottesman, I. et al. (1995). Autism as a strongly genetic disorder: evidence from a British twin study. *Psychol. Med.*, 25, 63–77.

Bailey, A., Phillips, W. and Rutter, M. (1996). Autism: towards an integration of clinical, genetic, neuropsychological, and neuro-biological perspectives. *J. Child Psychol. Psychiatry Allied Disciplines*, 37, 89–126.

Bailey, A., Luthert, P., Dean, A. et al. (1998). A clinicopathological study of autism. *Brain*, 121, 889–905.

Baltaxe, C. A. and Simmons, J. Q. (1992). A comparison of language issues in high-functioning autism and related disorders with onset in childhood and adolescence. In *High-functioning Individuals with Autism*, eds. E. Schopler and G. Mesibov, pp. 201–24. New York: Plenum Press.

Bandettini, P. A., Jesmanowicz, A., Wong, E. C. and Hyde, J. S. (1993). Processing strategies for time-course data sets in functional MRI of the human brain. *Magn. Reson. Med.*, 30, 161–73.

Banich, M., Levine, S., Kim, H. and Huttenlocher, P. (1990). The effects of developmental factors on IQ in hemiplegic children. *Neuropsychologia*, 28, 35–47.

Baron-Cohen, S. (1991). The development of a theory of mind in autism: deviance and delay? *Psychiatr. Clin. North Am.*, 14, 33–51.

Baron-Cohen, S. (1992). Debate and argument: on modularity and development in autism: a reply to Burack. *J. Child Psychol. Psychiatry Allied Disciplines*, 33, 623–9.

Baron-Cohen, S. and Hammer, J. (1997). Parents of children with Asperger syndrome: what is the cognitive phenotype? *J. Cogn. Neurosci.*, 9, 548–54.

Baron-Cohen, S., Leslie, A. M. and Frith, U. (1985). Does the autistic child have a "theory of mind?" *Cognition*, 21, 37–46.

Baron-Cohen, S., Ring, H., Moriarty, J., Schmitz, B., Costa, D. and Ell, P. (1994). Recognition of mental state terms. Clinical findings in children with autism and a functional neuroimaging study of normal adults. *Br. J. Psychiatry*, 165, 640–9.

Basser, L. S. (1962). Hemiplegia of early onset and the faculty of speech with special reference to the effects of hemispherectomy. *Brain*, 85, 427–60.

Bates, E. (1994). Modularity, domain specificity and the development of language. *Discuss. Neurosci.*, 10, 136–49.

Bates, E., Thal, D., Trauner, D. et al. (1997). From first words to grammar in children with focal brain injury. *Dev. Neuropsychol.*, 13, 275–343.

Bates, E., Vicari, S. and Trauner, D. (1999). Neural mediation of language development. In *Neurodevelopmental Disorders: Contributions to a New Framework from the Cognitive Neurosciences*, Vol. 13, ed. H. Tager-Flusberg, pp. 533–81. Cambridge, MA: MIT Press.

Bauman, M. and Kemper, T. L. (1985). Histoanatomic observations of the brain in early infantile autism. *Neurology*, 35, 866–75.

Bauman, M. L. and Kemper, T. L. (1994). Neuroanatomic observations of the brain in autism. In *The Neurobiology of Autism*, eds. M. L. Bauman and T. L. Kemper, pp. 119–45. Baltimore: Johns Hopkins University Press.

Bavelier, D., Corina, D., Jezzard, P. et al. (1997). Sentence reading: a functional MRI study at 4 Tesla. *J. Cogn. Neurosci.*, 9, 664–86.

Belin, P., van Eeckhout, P., Zilbovicius, M. et al. (1996). Recovery from nonfluent aphasia after melodic intonation therapy: a PET study. *Neurology*, 47, 1504–11.

Bellugi, U., Bihrle, A., Neville, H., Doherty, S. and Jernigan, T. (1992). Language, cognition, and brain organization in a neurodevelopmental disorder. In *Developmental Behavioral Neuroscience. The Minnesota Symposia on Child Psychology*, Vol. 24, ed. C. A. N. Megan and R. Gunnar, pp. xiii, 249. Hillsdale, NJ: Lawrence Erlbaum.

Bellugi, U., Wang, P. P. and Jernigan, T. L. (1994). Williams syndrome: an unusual neuropsychological profile. In *Atypical Cognitive Deficits in Developmental Disorders*, eds. S. H. Broman and J. Grafman, pp. 23–56. Hillsdale, NY: Lawrence Erlbaum.

Benson, D. F. and Ardila, A. (1996). *Aphasia*. New York: Oxford University Press.

Benson, R. R., Logan, W. J., Cosgrove, G. R. et al. (1996). Functional MRI localization of language in a 9-year-old child. *Can. J. Neurol. Sci.*, 23, 213–19.

Binder, J. R., Frost, J. A., Hammeke, T. A., Cox, R. W., Rao, S. M. and Prieto, T. (1997). Human brain language areas identified by functional magnetic resonance imaging. *J. Neurosci.*, 17, 353–62.

Bishop, D. V. (1989). Autism, Asperger's syndrome and semantic-pragmatic disorder: where are the boundaries? *Br. J. Disord. Communication*, 24, 107–21.

Bishop, D. V. M. (1992). The underlying nature of specific language impairment. *J. Child Psychol. Psychiatry*, 33, 3–66.

Bishop, D. V. M., North, T. and Donlan, C. (1995). Genetic basis of specific language impairment: evidence from a twin study. *Dev. Med. Child Neurol.*, 37, 56–71.

Blau, K. (1979). Phenylalanine hydroxylase deficiency: biochemical, physiological, and clinical aspects of phenylketonuria and related phenylalaninemias. In *Aromatic Amino Acid Hydroxylases and Mental Disease*, ed. M. B. H. Youdim, pp. 77–139. New York: Wiley.

Bookheimer, S. Y. and Dapretto, M. (1997). Functional neuroimaging of language in children: current directions and future challenges. In *Developmental Neuroimaging*, eds. R. W. Thatcher, G. R. Lyon, J. Rumsey et al., pp. 143–55. San Diego: Academic Press.

Borsting, E., Ridder III, W. H., Dudeck, K., Kelley, C., Matsui, L. and Motoyama, J. (1996). The presence of a magnocellular defect depends on the type of dyslexia. *Vision Res.*, 36, 1047–53.

Bruneau, N., Dourneau, M. C., Garreau, B., Pourcelot, L. and

Lelord, G. (1992). Blood flow response to auditory stimulations in normal, mentally retarded, and autistic children: a preliminary transcranial Doppler ultrasonographic study of the middle cerebral arteries. *Biol. Psychiatry*, 32, 691–9.

Cabeza, R. and Nyberg, L. (1997). Imaging cognition: an empirical review of PET studies with normal subjects. *J. Cogn. Neurosci.*, 9, 1–26.

Caramia, M. D., Iani, C. and Bernardi, G. (1996). Cerebral plasticity after stroke as revealed by ipsilateral responses to magnetic stimulation. *Neuroreport*, 7, 1756–60.

Carlsson, G., Uvebrant, P., Hugdahl, K., Arvidsson, J., Wiklund, L.-M. and von Wendt, L. (1994). Verbal and non-verbal function of children with right- versus left-hemiplegic cerebral palsy of pre- and perinatal origin. *Dev. Med. Child Neurol.*, 36, 503–12.

Carper, R. A. and Courchesne, E. (1999). Frontal lobe volume in children with autism. *Brain*, in press.

Casey, B. J., Trainor, R. J., Orendi, J. L. et al. (1997). A developmental functional MRI study of prefrontal activation during performance of a go-no-go task. *J. Cogn. Neurosci.*, 9, 835–47.

Catts, H. W. (1993). The relationship between speech-language impairments and reading disabilities. In *Language Acquisition Problems and Reading Disorders: Aspects of Diagnosis and Intervention*, eds. H. Grimm and H. Skowronek, pp. 167–81. Berlin: Walter de Gruyter.

Chapman, P. H., Buchbinder, B. R., Cosgrove, G. R. and Jiang, H. J. (1995). Functional magnetic resonance imaging for cortical mapping in pediatric neurosurgery. *Pediatr. Neurosurg.*, 23, 122–6.

Chiron, C., Leboyer, M., Leon, F., Jambaqué, I., Nuttin, C. and Syrota, A. (1995). SPECT of the brain in childhood autism: evidence for a lack of normal hemispheric asymmetry. *Dev. Med. Child Neurol.*, 37, 849–60.

Chiron, C., Jambaqué, I., Nabbout, R., Lounes, R., Syrota, A. and Dulac, O. (1997). The right brain hemisphere is dominant in human infants. *Brain*, 120, 1057–65.

Chollet, F., Di Piero, V., Wise, R. J. S., Dolan, R. J. and Frackowiak, R. S. J. (1991). The functional anatomy of motor recovery after stroke in humans: a study with positron emission tomography. *Ann. Neurol.*, 29, 63–71.

Chomsky, N. (1965). *Aspects of the Theory of Grammar*. Cambridge, MA: MIT Press.

Chomsky, N. (1981). *Lectures on Government and Binding*. Dordrecht: Foris.

Chomsky, N. (1988). *Language and Problems of Knowledge*. Cambridge MA: MIT Press.

Chugani, H. T., Phelps, M. E. and Mazziotta, J. C. (1987). Positron emission tomography study of human brain functional development. *Ann. Neurol.*, 22, 487–97.

Chugani, D. C., Muzik, O., Rothermel, R. D. et al. (1997). Altered serotonin synthesis in the dentato-thalamo-cortical pathway in autistic boys. *Ann. Neurol.*, 14, 666–9.

Ciesielski, K. T. and Harris, R. J. (1997). Factors related to performance failure on executive tasks in autism. *Child Neuropsychology*, 3, 1–12.

Ciesielski, K. T., Courchesne, E. and Elmasian, R. (1990). Effects of focused selective attention tasks on event-related potentials in autistic and normal individuals. *Electroencephalogr. Clin. Neurophysiol.*, 75, 207–20.

Ciesielski, K. T., Harris, R. J., Hart, B. L. and Pabst, H. F. (1997). Cerebellar hypoplasia and frontal lobe cognitive deficits in disorders of early childhood. *Neuropsychologia*, 35, 643–55.

Clahsen, H. (1989). The grammatical characterization of developmental dysphasia. *Linguistics*, 27, 897–920.

Clark, M. M. and Plante, E. (1998). Morphology of the inferior frontal gyrus in developmentally language-disordered adults. *Brain Lang.*, 61, 288–303.

Cook, E. H., Jr, Courchesne, R. Y., Cox, N. J. et al. (1998). Linkage-disequilibrium mapping of autistic disorder, with 15q11–13 markers. *Am. J. Hum. Genet.*, 62, 1077–83.

Cornelissen, P., Bradley, L., Fowler, S. and Stein, J. (1991). What children see affects how they read. *Dev. Med. Child*, 33, 755–62.

Courchesne, E. (1987). A neurophysiological view of autism. In *Neurobiological Issues in Autism*, eds. E. Scopler and G. B. Mesibov, pp. 285–324. New York: Plenum Press.

Courchesne, E. (1997). Brainstem, cerebellar and limbic neuroanatomical abnormalities in autism. *Curr. Opin. Neurobiol.*, 7, 269–78.

Courchesne, E. and Allen, G. (1997). Prediction and preparation, fundamental functions of the cerebellum. *Learning Memory*, 4, 1–35.

Courchesne, E., Kilman, B. A., Galambos, R. and Lincoln, A. J. (1984). Autism: processing of novel auditory information assessed by event-related brain potentials. *Electroencephalogr. Clin. Neurophysiol.*, 59, 238–48.

Courchesne, E., Courchesne, R. Y., Hicks, G. and Lincoln, A. J. (1985). Functioning of the brain-stem auditory pathway in nonretarded autistic individuals. *Electroencephalogr. Clin. Neurophysiol.*, 61, 491–501.

Courchesne, E., Lincoln, A. J., Yeung-Courchesne, R., Elmasian, R. and Grillon, C. (1989). Pathophysiologic findings in nonretarded autism and receptive developmental language disorder. *J. Autism Dev. Disord.*, 19, 1–7.

Courchesne, E., Press, G. A. and Yeung-Courchesne, R. (1993). Parietal lobe abnormalities detected with MR in patients with infantile autism. *Am. J. Roentgen.*, 160, 387–93.

Courchesne, E., Chisum, H. and Townsend, J. (1994a). Neural activity-dependent brain changes in development: implications for psychopathology. *Dev. Psychopathol.*, 6, 697–722.

Courchesne, E., Saitoh, O., Townsend, J. et al. (1994b). The brain in infantile autism: posterior fossa structures are abnormal. *Neurology*, 44, 214–23.

Courchesne, E., Townsend, J., Akshoomoff, N. A. et al. (1994c). Impairment in shifting attention in autistic and cerebellar patients. *Behav. Neurosci.*, 108, 848–65.

Courchesne, E., Yeung-Courchesne, R. and Pierce, K. (1999). Biological and behavioral heterogeneity in autism: role of pleiotropy and epigenesis. In *The Changing Nervous System: Neurobehavioral Consequences of Early Brain Disorders*, eds. S. H. Broman and J. M. Fletcher. New York: Oxford University Press, in press.

Cousens, P., Waters, B., Said, J. and Stevens, M. (1988). Cognitive effects of cranial irradiation in leukaemia: A survey and meta-analysis. *J. Child Psychol. Psychiatry Allied Disciplines*, 29, 839–52.

Curtiss, S., Katz, W. and Tallal, P. (1992). Delay versus deviance in the language acquisition of language-impaired children. *J. Speech Hearing Res.*, 35, 373–83.

Dale, A. M. and Buckner, R. L. (1997). Selective averaging of rapidly presented individual trials using fMRI. *Hum. Brain Map.*, 5, 329–40.

Damasio, A. R. and Maurer, R. G. (1978). A neurological model for childhood autism. *Arch. Neurol.*, 35, 777–86.

Dawson, G., Finley, C., Phillips, S. and Lewy, A. (1989). A comparison of hemispheric asymmetries in speech-related brain potentials of autistic and dysphasic children. *Brain Lang.*, 37, 26–41.

de Volder, A. G., Bol, A., Michel, C., Cogneau, M. and Goffinet, A. M. (1987). Brain glucose metabolism in children with the autistic syndrome: positron emission analysis. *Brain Dev.*, 9, 581–7.

DeFries, J. C. and Alarcón, M. (1996). Genetics of specific reading disability. *Mental Retard. Dev. Disabil. Res. Rev.*, 2, 39–47.

Demb, J. B., Boynton, G. M. and Heeger, D. J. (1997). Brain activity in visual cortex predicts individual differences in reading performance. *Proc. Natl. Acad. Sci. USA*, 94, 13363–6.

Demb, J. B., Boynton, G. M. and Heeger, D. J. (1998). Functional magnetic resonance imaging of early visual pathways in dyslexia. *J. Neurosci.*, 18, 6939–51.

Desmond, J. E., Gabrieli, J. D., Wagner, A. D., Ginier, B. L. and Glover, G. H. (1997). Lobular patterns of cerebellar activation in verbal working-memory and finger-tapping tasks as revealed by functional MRI. *J. Neurosci.*, 17, 9675–85.

Dunn, M. (1994). Neurophysiological observations in autism and implications for neurologic dysfunction. In *The Neurobiology of Autism*, eds. M. L. Bauman and T. L. Kemper, pp. 45–65. Baltimore: Johns Hopkins University Press.

Eden, G. F., van Meter, J. W., Rumsey, J. M., Maisog, J. M., Woods, R. P. and Zeffiro, T. A. (1996). Abnormal processing of visual motion in dyslexia revealed by functional brain imaging. *Nature*, 382, 66–9.

Eicher, P. S. and Batshaw, M. L. (1993). Cerebral palsy. *Child Dev. Disabil.*, 40, 537–51.

Ernst, M., Freed, M. E. and Zametkin, A. J. (1998a). Review of health hazards of radiation exposure in the context of brain imaging research: special consideration for children. *J. Nucl. Med.*, 39, 689–98.

Ernst, M., Zametkin, A. J., Matochik, J. A., Jons, P. H. and Cohen, R. M. (1998b). DOPA decarboxylase activity in attention deficit hyperactivity disorder adults. A [fluorine-18]fluorodopa positron emission tomography study. *J. Neurosci.*, 18, 5901–7.

Eslinger, P. J., Grattan, L. M., Damasio, H. and Damasio, A. R. (1992). Developmental consequences of childhood frontal lobe damage. *Arch. Neurol.*, 49, 764–9.

Fay, D. and Mermelstein, R. (1982). Language in infantile autism. In *Handbook of Applied Psycholinguistics*, ed. S. Rosenberg, pp. 393–428. Hillsdale, NJ: Lawrence Erlbaum.

Feeney, D. M. and Baron, J.-C. (1986). Diaschisis. *Stroke*, 17, 817–30.

Fletcher, P. C., Happé, F., Frith, U. et al. (1995). Other minds in the brain: a functional imaging study of "theory of mind" in story comprehension. *Cognition*, 57, 109–28.

Flowers, L. D., Wood, F. B. and Naylor, C. E. (1991). Regional cerebral blood flow correlates of language processing in reading disability. *Arch. Neurol.*, 48, 637–43.

Fodor, J. A. (1983). *The modularity of mind*. Cambridge, MA: MIT Press.

Fodor, J. A. (1985). Précis of "The Modularity of Mind". *Behav. Brain. Sci.*, 8, 1–42.

Fodor, J. A. and Pylyshyn, Z.W. (1988). Connectionism and cognitive architecture: a critical analysis. Special Issue: Connectionism and symbol systems. *Cognition*, 28, 3–71.

Foundas, A. L., Leonard, C. M., Gilmore, R., Fennell, E. and Heilman, K. M. (1994). Planum temporale asymmetry and language dominance. *Neuropsychologia*, 32, 1225–31.

Foundas, A. L., Leonard, C. M., Gilmore, R. L., Fennell, E. B. and Heilman, K. M. (1996). Pars triangularis asymmetry and language dominance. *Proc. Natl. Acad. Sci. USA*, 93, 719–22.

Fox, P. T. and Raichle, M. E. (1986). Focal physiological uncoupling of cerebral blood flow and oxidative metabolism during somatosensory stimulation in human subjects. *Proc. Natl. Acad. Sci. USA*, 83, 1140–4.

Fransen, E., Lemmon, V., van Camp, G., Vits, L., Coucke, P. and Willems, P. J. (1995). CRASH syndrome: clinical spectrum of corpus callosum hypoplasia, retardation, adducted thumbs, spastic paraparesis and hydrocephalus due to mutations in one single gene, L1. *Eur. J. Hum. Genet.*, 3, 273–84.

Fransen, E., D'Hooge, R., van Camp, G. et al. (1998). L1 knockout mice show dilated ventricles, vermis hypoplasia and impaired exploration patterns. *Hum. Mol. Genet.*, 7, 999–1009.

Galaburda, A. M. (1988). The pathogenesis of childhood dyslexia. In *Language, Communication, and the Brain*, ed. F. Plum, pp. 127–37. New York: Raven Press.

Galaburda, A. and Livingstone, M. (1993). Evidence for a magnocellular defect in developmental dyslexia. *Ann. N. Y. Acad. Sci.*, 682, 70–82.

Galaburda, A. M., Menard, M. T. and Rosen, G. D. (1994). Evidence for aberrant auditory anatomy in developmental dyslexia. *Proc. Natl. Acad. Sci. USA*, 91, 8010–13.

Gardner, H. (1987). *The Mind's New Science*. New York: Basic Books.

Gauger, L. M., Lombardino, L. J. and Leonard, C. M. (1997). Brain morphology in children with specific language impairment. *J. Speech, Lang. Hearing Res.*, 40, 1272–84.

Gillberg, C. and Steffenburg, S. (1993). The evidence for pathogenetic role of peripheral hearing deficits in autism is extremely limited. *J. Child Psychol. Psychiatry Allied Disciplines*, 34, 593–6.

Glass, P., Bulas, D. I., Wagner, A. E., Rajasingham, S. R., Civtello, L. A. and Coffman, C. E. (1998). Pattern of neuropsychological deficit at age five years following neonatal unilateral brain injury. *Brain Lang.*, 63, 346–56.

Goldberg, M. E., Eggers, H. M. and Gouras, P. (1991). The ocular motor system. In *Principles of Neural Science*, 3rd edn, eds. E. R. Kandel, J. H. Schwartz and T. M. Jessell, pp. 660–77. New York: Elsevier.

Goldman, P. S., Rosvold, H. E. and Mishkin, M. (1970). Evidence for behavioral impairment following prefrontal lobectomy in the infant monkey. *J. Comp. Physiol. Psychol.*, 70, 454–63.

Goodman, R. and Yude, C. (1996). IQ and its predictors in hemiplegia. *Dev. Med. Child Neurol.*, 38, 881–90.

Gopnik, M. (1990). Feature blindness: a case study. *Lang Acquisit.: J. Dev. Linguistics*, 1, 139–64.

Gopnik, M. and Crago, M. B. (1991). Familial aggregation of a developmental language disorder. *Cognition*, 39, 1–50.

Gopnik, M., Dalalakis, J., Fukuda, S. E., Fukuda, S. and Kehayia, E. (1996). Genetic language impairment: unruly grammars. In *Proceedings of the British Academy*, Vol. 88, *Evolution of Social Behaviour Patterns in Primates and Man*, eds. W. G. Runciman, J. M. Smith and R. I. M. Dunbar, pp. 223–49. Oxford, UK: Oxford University Press.

Gordon, A. G. (1993). Debate and argument: interpretation of auditory impairment and markers for brain damage in autism. *J. Child Psychol. Psychiatry Allied Disciplines*, 34, 587–92.

Gottlieb, G. (1995). Some conceptual deficiencies in "developmental" behavior genetics. *Hum. Dev.*, 38, 131–41.

Grandin, T. (1992). An inside view of autism. In *High-functioning Individuals with Autism*, eds. E. Schopler and G. Mesibov, pp. 105–26. New York: Plenum Press.

Grattan, L. M. and Eslinger, P. J. (1991). Frontal lobe damage in children and adults: a comparative review. *Dev. Neuropsychol.*, 7, 283–326.

Gregory, R. M. and Taylor, J. S. H. (1987). Plasticity in the nervous system. In *The Oxford Companion to the Mind*, eds. R. L. Gregory and O. L. Zangwill, pp. 623–8. Oxford: Oxford University Press.

Gross-Glenn, K., Skottun, B. C., Glenn, W. et al. (1995). Contrast sensitivity in dyslexia. *Visual Neurosci.*, 12, 153–63.

Haas, R. H., Townsend, J., Courchesne, E., Lincoln, A. J., Schreibman, L. and Yeung-Courchesne, R. (1996). Neurologic abnormalities in infantile autism. *J. Child Neurol.*, 11, 84–92.

Hallett, M. and Grafman, J. (1997). Executive function and motor skill learning. In *The Cerebellum and Cognition*, ed. J. D. Schmahmann, pp. 297–323. San Diego, CA: Academic Press.

Hallett, M., Lebiedowska, M. K., Thomas, S. L., Stanhope, S. J., Denckla, M. B. and Rumsey, J. (1993). Locomotion of autistic adults. *Arch. Neurol.*, 50, 1304–8.

Happé, F., Ehlers, S., Fletcher, P. C. et al. (1996). "Theory of mind" in the brain. Evidence from a PET scan study of Asperger syndrome. *Neuroreport*, 8, 197–201.

Hashimoto, T., Tayama, M., Murakawa, K. et al. (1995). Development of the brainstem and cerebellum in autistic patients. *J. Autism Dev. Disord.*, 25, 1–18.

Hay, D. A. (1985). *Essentials of Behavior Genetics*. Melbourne: Blackwell.

Haznedar, M. M., Buchsbaum, M. S., Metzger, M., Solimando, A., Spiegel-Cohen, J. and Hollander, E. (1997). Anterior cingulate gyrus volume and glucose metabolism in autistic disorder. *Am. J. Psychiatry*, 154, 1047–50.

Heilman, K. M., Voeller, K. and Alexander, A. W. (1996). Developmental dyslexia: a motor-articulatory feedback hypothesis. *Ann. Neurol.*, 39, 407–12.

Hertz-Pannier, L., Gaillard, W. D., Mott, S. H. et al. (1997). Noninvasive assessment of language dominance in children and adolescents with functional MRI: a preliminary study. *Neurology*, **48**, 1003–12.

Hill, E. L. (1998). A dyspraxic deficit in specific language impairment and developmental coordination disorder? Evidence from hand and arm movement. *Dev. Med. Child Neurol.*, **40**, 388–95.

Horwitz, B., Rumsey, J. M., Grady, C. L. and Rapoport, S. I. (1988). The cerebral metabolic landscape in autism: intercorrelations of regional glucose utilization. *Arch. Neurol.*, **45**, 749–55.

Horwitz, B., Rumsey, J. M. and Donohue, B. C. (1998). Functional connectivity of the angular gyrus in normal reading and dyslexia. *Proc. Natl. Acad. Sci. USA*, **95**, 8939–44.

Huttenlocher, P. R. and Dabholkar, A. S. (1997). Regional differences in synaptogenesis in human cerebral cortex. *J. Comp. Neurol.*, **387**, 167–78.

Isaacs, E., Christie, D., Vargha-Khadem, F. and Mishkin, M. (1996). Effects of hemispheric side of injury, age at injury, and presence of seizure disorder on functional ear and hand asymmetries in hemiplegic children. *Neuropsychologia*, **34**, 127–37.

Jackson, T. and Plante, E. (1996). Gyral morphology in the posterior sylvian region in families affected by developmental language disorder. *Neuropsychol. Rev.*, **6**, 81–94.

Jacob, F. (1977). Evolution and tinkering. *Science*, **196**, 1161–6.

Jenkins, I. H., Brooks, D. J., Nixon, P. D., Frackowiak, R. S. and Passingham, R. E. (1994). Motor sequence learning: a study with positron emission tomography. *J. Neurosci.*, **14**, 3775–90.

Jernigan, T. L. and Bellugi, U. (1990). Anomalous brain morphology on magnetic resonance images in Williams syndrome and Down syndrome. *Arch. Neurol.*, **47**, 529–33.

Jernigan, T. L. and Bellugi, U. (1994). Neuroanatomical distinctions between Williams and Down syndromes. In *Atypical Cognitive Deficits in Developmental Disorders*, eds. S. H. Broman and J. Grafman, pp. 57–66. Hillsdale: Erlbaum.

Jibiki, I., Kido, H., Matsuda, H., Yamaguchi, N. and Hisada, K. (1993). Diffuse cerebral hypoperfusion in epileptic patients observed from quantitative assessment with single photon emission computed tomography using *N*-isopropyl-(iodine-123)-*p*-iodoamphetamine. *Eur. Neurol.*, **33**, 366–72.

Johnston, J. R. (1994). Cognitive abilities of children with language impairment. In *Specific Language Impairments in Children*, eds. R. V. Watkins and M. L. Rice, pp. 107–21. Baltimore, MD: Paul H. Brookes.

Jueptner, M. and Weiller, C. (1995). Does measurement of regional cerebral blood flow reflect synaptic activity? Implications for PET and fMRI. *Neuroimage*, **2**, 148–56.

Jueptner, M. and Weiller, C. (1998). A review of differences between basal ganglia and cerebellar control of movements as revealed by functional imaging studies. *Brain*, **121**, 1437–49.

Just, M. A., Carpenter, P. A., Keller, T. A., Eddy, W. F. and Thulborn, K. R. (1996). Brain activation modulated by sentence comprehension. *Science*, **274**, 114–16.

Kapur, S., Hussey, D., Wilson, D. and Houle, S. (1995). The statistical power of [^{15}O]-water PET activation studies of cognitive processes. *Nucl. Med. Commun.*, **16**, 779–84.

Karmiloff-Smith, A. (1994). Précis of Beyond Modularity. *Behav. Brain Sci.*, **17**, 693–745.

Kates, W. R., Mostofsky, S. H., Zimmerman, A. W. et al. (1998). Neuroanatomical and neurocognitive differences in a pair of monozygous twins discordant for strictly defined autism. *Ann. Neurol.*, **43**, 782–91.

Kaufmann, W. E. and Galaburda, A. M. (1989). Cerebrocortical microdysgenesis in neurologically normal subjects: a histopathologic study. *Neurology*, **39**, 238–44.

Kemner, C., Verbaten, M. N., Cuperus, J. M., Camfferman, G. and van Engeland, H. (1998). Abnormal saccadic eye movements in autistic children. *J. Autism Dev. Disord.*, **28**, 61–7.

Kemper, T. L. (1984). Asymmetrical lesions in dyslexia. In *Cerebral Dominance: The Biological Foundations*, eds. N. Geschwind and A. M. Galaburda, pp. 75–89. Cambridge, MA: Harvard University Press.

Kennard, M. A. (1938). Reorganization of motor function in the cerebral cortex of monkeys deprived of motor and premotor areas in infancy. *J. Neurophysiol.*, **1**, 477–96.

Kennard, M. A. (1940). Relation of age to motor impairment in man and in subhuman primates. *Arch. Neurol. Psychiatry*, **44**, 377–97.

Kimura, D. and Watson, N. V. (1989). The relation between oral movement control and speech. *Brain Lang.*, **37**, 565–90.

Klin, A. (1991). Young autistic children's listening preferences in regard to speech: a possible characterization of the symptom of social withdrawal. *J. Autism Dev. Disord.*, **21**, 29–42.

Klin, A. (1993). Auditory brainstem responses in autism: brainstem dysfunction or peripheral hearing loss? *J. Autism Dev. Disord.*, **23**, 15–35.

Kolb, B. (1990). Sparing and recovery of function. In *The Cerebral Cortex of the Rat*, eds. B. Kolb and R. C. Tees, pp. 537–61. Cambridge, MA: MIT Press.

Kolb, B. (1995). *Brain Plasticity and Behavior*. Mahwah, NJ: Lawrence Erlbaum.

Kolb, B. and Tomie, J.-A. (1988). Recovery from early cortical damage in rats. IV. Effects of hemidecortication at 1, 5 or 10 days of age on cerebral anatomy and behavior. *Behav. Brain Res.*, **28**, 259–74.

Kolb, B. and Whishaw, I. Q. (1989). Plasticity in the neocortex: mechanisms underlying recovery from early brain damage. *Prog. Neurobiol.*, **32**, 235–76.

Kolb, B., Zaborowski, J. and Whishaw, I. Q. (1989). Recovery from early cortical damage in rats. V. Unilateral lesions have different behavioral and anatomical effects than bilateral lesions. *Psychobiology*, **17**, 363–9.

Kolb, B., Petrie, B. and Cioe, J. (1996). Recovery from early cortical damage in rats. VII. Comparison of the behavioral and anatomical effects of medial prefrontal lesions at different ages of neural maturation. *Behav. Brain Res.*, **79**, 1–13.

Kolb, B., Cioe, J. and Muirhead, D. (1998). Cerebral morphology and functional sparing after prenatal frontal cortex lesions in rats. *Behav. Brain Res.*, **91**, 143–55.

Kraft, R. H. (1993). Deficits in auditory sequential processing found for both gifted and average IQ reading-impaired boys. *Ann. N.Y. Acad. Sci.*, **682**, 366–8.

Kuhn, T. (1962). *The Structure of Scientific Revolutions*. Chicago: University of Chicago Press.

Kushch, A., Gross-Glenn, K., Jallad, B. et al. (1993). Temporal lobe surface area measurements on MRI in normal and dyslexic readers. *Neuropsychologia*, 31, 811–21.

Lassen, N., Ingvar, D. and Skinhøj, E. (1978). Brain function and blood flow. *Sci. Am.*, 239, 50–9.

Le, H. T., Pardo, J. V. and Hu, X. (1998). 4 T-fMRI study of nonspatial shifting of selective attention: cerebellar and parietal contributions. *J. Neurophysiol.*, 79, 1535–48.

Le Couteur, A., Bailey, A. Goode, S. et al. (1996). A broader phenotype of autism: the clinical spectrum in twins. *J. Child Psychol. Psychiatry Allied Disciplines*, 37, 785–801.

Leiner, H. C., Leiner, A. L. and Dow, R. S. (1995). The underestimated cerebellum. *Hum. Brain Map.*, 2, 244–54.

Leonard, C. M., Voeller, K. K. S., Lombardino, L. J. et al. (1993). Anomalous cerebral structure in dyslexia revealed with magnetic resonance imaging. *Neurology*. 50, 461–9.

Levine, S., Huttenlocher, P., Banich, M. and Duda, E. (1987). Factors affecting cognitive functioning in hemiplegic children. *Dev. Med. Child Neurol.*, 29, 27–35.

Lincoln, A. J., Courchesne, E., Harms, L. and Allen, M. (1995). Sensory modulation of auditory stimuli in children with autism and receptive developmental language disorder: event-related brain potential evidence. *J. Autism Dev. Disord.*, 25, 521–39.

Lipp, H.-P. and Wolfer, D. P. (1998). Genetically modified mice and cognition. *Curr. Opin. Neurobiol.*, 8, 272–80.

Livingstone, M. and Hubel, D. (1988). Segregation of form, color, movement, and depth: anatomy, physiology, and perception. *Science*, 240, 741–9.

Lou, H. C., Henriksen, L. and Bruhn, P. (1990). Focal cerebral dysfunction in developmental learning disabilities. *Lancet*, 335, 8–11.

Lovaas, O. I. (1987). Behavioral treatment and normal educational and intellectual functioning in young autistic children. *J. Consult. Clin. Psychol.*, 55, 3–9.

Lyon, G. R. and Chhabra, V. (1996). The current state of science and future of specific reading disability. *Mental Retard. Dev. Disab. Res. Rev.*, 2, 2–9.

MacNeil, M. A., Lomber, S. G. and Payne, B. R. (1996). Rewiring of transcortical projections to middle suprasylvian cortex following early removal of cat areas 17 and 18. *Cerebr. Cortex*, 6, 362–76.

May, J. G., Williams, M. C. and Dunlap, W. P. (1988). Temporal order judgments in good and poor readers. *Neuropsychologia*, 26, 917–24.

McAnally, K. I. and Stein, J. F. (1996). Auditory temporal coding in dyslexia. *Proc. R. Soc. Lond. Series B*, 263, 961–5.

McAnally, K. I., Hansen, P. C., Cornelissen, P. L. and Stein, J. F. (1997). Effect of time and frequency manipulation on syllable perception in developmental dyslexics. *Journal of Speech, Language, and Hearing Research*, 40, 912–24.

McDougle, C. J., Naylor, S. T., Cohen, D. J., Volkmar, F. R., Heninger, G. R. and Price, L. H. (1996). A double-blind, placebo-controlled study of fluvoxamine in adults with autistic disorder. *Arch. Gen. Psychiatry*, 53, 1001–8.

McEachin, J. J., Smith, T. and Lovaas, O. I. (1993). Long-term outcome for children with autism who received early intensive behavioral treatment. *Am. J. Mental Retardation*, 97, 359–72; discussion 73–91.

McEvoy, R. E., Rogers, S. J. and Pennington, B. F. (1993). Executive function and social communication deficits in young autistic children. *J. Child Psychol. Psychiatry Allied Disciplines*, 34, 563–78.

McFie, J. (1961). Intellectual impairment in children with localized post-infantile cerebral lesions. *J. Neurol. Neurosurg. Psychiatry*, 24, 361–5.

Mesulam, M.-M. (1998). From sensation to cognition. *Brain*, 121, 1013–52.

Metter, E. J., Kempler, D., Jackson, C. A. et al. (1987). Cerebellar glucose metabolism in chronic aphasia. *Neurology*, 37, 1599–606.

Middleton, F. A. and Strick, P. L. (1994). Anatomical evidence for cerebellar and basal ganglia involvement in higher cognitive function. *Science*, 266, 458–61.

Minshew, N. J. (1994). In vivo neuroanatomy of autism: neuroimaging studies. In *The Neurobiology of Autism*, eds. M. L. Bauman and T. L. Kemper, pp. 66–85. Baltimore: Johns Hopkins University Press.

Mody, M., Studdert-Kennedy, M. and Brady, S. (1997). Speech perception deficits in poor readers. Auditory processing or phonological coding? *J. Exp. Child Psychol.*, 64, 199–231.

Mountz, J. M., Tolbert, L. C., Lill, D. W., Katholi, C. R. and Liu, H. G. (1995). Functional deficits in autistic disorder: characterization by technetium-99m-HMPAO and SPECT. *J. Nucl. Med.*, 36, 1156–62.

Müller, R.-A. (1992). Modularity, holism, connectionism: old conflicts and new perspectives in aphasiology and neuropsychology. *Aphasiology*, 6, 443–75.

Müller, R.-A. (1996). Innateness, autonomy, universality? Neurobiological approaches to language. *Behav. Brain Sci.*, 19, 611–75.

Müller, R.-A., Chugani, H. T., Muzik, O., Rothermel, R. D. and Chakraborty, P. K. (1997a). Language and motor functions activate calcified hemisphere in patients with Sturge-Weber syndrome: a positron emission tomography study. *J. Child Neurol.*, 12, 431–7.

Müller, R.-A., Rothermel, R. D., Behen, M. E. et al. (1997b). Receptive and expressive language activations for sentences: a PET study. *Neuroreport*, 8, 3767–70.

Müller, R.-A., Rothermel, R. D., Muzik, O., Behen, M. E., Chakraborty, P. K. and Chugani, H. T. (1997c). Plasticity of motor organization in children and adults. *Neuroreport*, 8, 3103–8.

Müller, R.-A., Chugani, D. C., Behen, M. E. et al. (1998a). Impairment of dentato-thalamo-cortical pathway in autistic men. Language activation data from positron emission tomography. *Neurosci. Lett.*, 245, 1–4.

Müller, R.-A., Chugani, H. T., Muzik, O. and Mangner, T. J. (1998b). Brain organization of motor and language functions following hemispherectomy: a [^{15}O]-water PET study. *J. Child Neurol.*, 13, 16–22.

Müller, R.-A., Rothermel, R. D., Behen, M. E. et al. (1998c). Brain organization of language after early unilateral lesion. *Brain Lang.*, 62, 422–51.

Müller, R.-A., Rothermel, R. D., Behen, M. E., Muzik, O., Mangner, T. J. and Chugani, H. T. (1998d). Differential patterns of language and motor reorganization following left-hemisphere lesion. *Arch. Neurol.*, **55**, 1113–19.

Müller, R.-A., Watson, C. E., Muzik, O., Chakraborty, P. K. and Chugani, H. T. (1998e). Motor organization following intrauterine middle cerebral artery stroke: a single-case PET study. *Pediatr. Neurol.*, **19**, 294–8.

Müller, R.-A., Behen, M. E., Rothermel, R. D. et al. (1999a). Brain mapping of language and auditory perception in high-functioning autistic adults: a PET study. *J. Autism Dev. Disord.*, **29**, 19–31.

Müller, R.-A., Behen, M. E., Rothermel, R. D., Muzik, O., Chakraborty, P. K. and Chugani, H. T. (1999b). Brain organization for language in children, adolescents, and adults with left hemisphere lesion. *Progr. Neuropsychopharmacol. Biol. Psychiatry*, **23**, 657–68.

Müller, R.-A., Behen, M. E., Rothermel, R. D., Muzik, O., Chakraborty, P. K. and Chugani, H. T. (1999c). Language organization in pediatric and adult patients with left hemisphere lesion. *Neuropsychologia*, **37**, 547–57.

Muter, V., Taylor, S. and Vargha-Khadem, F. (1997). A longitudinal study of early intellectual development in hemiplegic children. *Neuropsychologia*, **35**, 289–98.

Nass, R. and Stiles, J. (1996). Neurobehavioral consequences of congenital focal lesions. In *Pediatric Behavioral Neurology*, ed. Y. Frank, pp. 149–78. Boca Raton, FL: CRC Press.

Nicolson, R. I. and Fawcett, A. J. (1993). Children with dyslexia automatize temporal skills more slowly. *Ann. N.Y. Acad. Sci.*, **682**, 390–2.

Nieuwenhuys, R., Voogd, J. and van Huijzen, C. (1988). *The Human Central Nervous System*. Berlin: Springer.

O'Leary, D. D. M., Schlaggar, B. L. and Tuttle, R. (1994). Specification of neocortical areas and thalamocortical connections. *Annu. Rev. Neurosci.*, **17**, 419–39.

Ogden, J. A. (1988). Language and memory functions after long recovery periods in left-hemispherectomized subjects. *Neuropsychologia*, **26**, 645–59.

Ogunmekan, O. A., Hwang, P. A. and Hoffman, H. J. (1989). Sturge–Weber–Dimitri disease: role of hemispherectomy in prognosis. *Can. J. Neurol. Sci.*, **16**, 78–80.

Pantano, P., Baron, J. C., Samson, Y., Bousser, M. G., Desrouesne, C. and Comar, D. (1986). Crossed cerebellar diaschisis. *Brain*, **109**, 677–94.

Pascual-Leone, A., Chugani, H. T., Cohen, L. G. et al. (1992). Reorganization of human motor pathways following hemispherectomy. *Ann. Neurol.*, **32**, 261.

Paulesu, E., Frith, U., Snowling, M. et al. (1996). Is developmental dyslexia a disconnection syndrome? Evidence from PET scanning. *Brain*, **119**, 143–57.

Pedersen, P. M., Jørgensen, H. S., Nakayama, H., Raaschou, H. O. and Olsen, T. S. (1995). Aphasia in acute stroke: incidence, determinants, and recovery. *Ann. Neurol.*, **38**, 659–66.

Pennington, B. F. (1995). Genetics of learning disabilities. *J. Child Neurol.*, **10** (Suppl. 1), S69–77.

Pennington, B. F. and Smith, S. D. (1983). Genetic influences on learning disabilities and speech and language disorders. *Child Dev.*, **54**, 369–87.

Piattelli-Palmarini, M. (ed.) (1980). *Language and Learning*. Cambridge (Mass.): Harvard University Press.

Pinker, S. (1991). Rules of language. *Science*, **253**, 530–5.

Pinker, S. (1995). Facts about human language relevant to its evolution. In *Origins of the Human Brain*, eds. J.-P. Changeux and J. Chavaillon, pp. 262–83. New York: Clarendon Press.

Plante, E., Swisher, L., Vance, R. and Rapcsak, S. (1991). MRI findings in parents and siblings of specifically language-impaired boys. *Brain Lang.*, **40**, 52–66.

Popper, K. R. (1965). *Conjectures and Refutations: The Growth of Scientific Knowledge*. New York: Routledge & Kegan Paul.

Posner, M. I., Walker, J. A., Friedrich, F. J. and Rafal, R. D. (1984). Effects of parietal injury on covert orientating of attention. *J. Neurosci.*, **4**, 1863–74.

Price, C. J., Wise, R. J. S., Howard, D., Warburton, E. and Frackowiak, R. S. J. (1993). The role of the right hemisphere in the recovery of language after stroke. *J. Cereb. Blood Flow Metabol.*, **13** (Suppl. 1), S520.

Price, C. J., Wise, R. J. S., Warburton, E. et al. (1996). Hearing and saying: the functional neuroanatomy of auditory word processing. *Brain*, **119**, 919–31.

Prior, M. and Hoffman, W. (1990). Neuropsychological testing of autistic children through an exploration with frontal lobe tests. *J. Autism Dev. Disord.*, **20**, 581–90.

Quartz, S. R. and Sejnowski, T. J. (1997). The neural basis of cognitive development: a constructivist manifesto. *Behav. Brain Sci.*, **20**, 537–96.

Rajkowska, G. and Goldman-Rakic, P. S. (1995). Cytoarchitectonic definition of prefrontal areas in normal human cortex. II. Variability in locations of areas 9 and 46 and relationship to the Talairach coordinate system. *Cereb. Cortex*, **5**, 323–37.

Rapin, I. and Allen, D. A. (1988). Syndromes in developmental dysphasia and adult aphasia. In *Language, Communication, and the Brain*, ed. F. Plum, pp. 57–75. New York: Raven.

Ribary, U., Miller, S. L., Joliot, M. et al. (1997). Early auditory temporal processing and alteration during language-based learning disability. *Neuroimage*, **5**, S95.

Rice, M. L. (1994). Grammatical categories of children with specific language impairment. In *Specific Language Impairments in Children*, eds. R. V. Watkins and M. L. Rice, pp. 69–89. Baltimore, MD: Paul H. Brookes.

Rimland, B. and Edelson, S. M. (1995). Brief report: a pilot study of auditory integration training in autism. *J. Autism Dev. Disord.*, **25**, 61–70.

Rintahaka, P. J., Chugani, H. T., Messa, C. and Phelps, M. E. (1993). Hemimegalencephaly: evaluation with positron emission tomography. *Pediatr. Neurol.*, **9**, 21–8.

Ritvo, E. R., Freeman, B. J., Scheibel, A. B. et al. (1986). Lower Purkinje cell counts in the cerebella of four autistic subjects: initial findings of the UCLA–NSAC autopsy research report. *Am. J. Psychiatry*, **143**, 862–6.

Riva, D. and Cazzaniga, L. (1986). Late effects of unilateral brain lesions sustained before and after age one. *Neuropsychologia*, 24, 423–8.

Rodier, P. M. (1980). Chronology of neuron development: animal studies and their clinical implications. *Dev. Med. Child Neurol.*, 22, 525–45.

Rodier, P. M., Ingram, J. L., Tisdale, B., Nelson, S. and Romano, J. (1996). Embryological origin for autism: developmental anomalies of the cranial nerve motor nuclei. *J. Comp. Neurol.*, 370, 247–61.

Rodier, P. M., Ingram, J. L., Tisdale, B. and Croog, V. J. (1997). Linking etiologies in humans and animal models: studies of autism. *Reprod. Toxicol.*, 11, 417–22.

Ross, E. D. (1993). Nonverbal aspects of language. *Neurol. Clin.*, 11, 9–23.

Rudel, R. G., Teuber, H. L. and Twitchell, T. E. (1974). Levels of impairment of sensori-motor functions in children with early brain damage. *Neuropsychologia*, 12, 95–108.

Rumsey, J. M. (1996a). Developmental dyslexia: anatomic and functional neuroimaging. *Mental Retard. Dev. Disab. Res. Rev.*, 2, 28–38.

Rumsey, J. M. (1996b). Neuroimaging studies of autism. In *Neuroimaging. A Window to the Neurological Foundations of Learning and Behavior in Children*, eds. G. R. Lyon and J. M. Rumsey, pp. 119–46. Baltimore, MD: Paul H. Brookes.

Rumsey, J. M., Andreason, P., Zametkin, A. J. et al. (1992). Failure to activate the left temporoparietal cortex in dyslexia. *Arch. Neurol.*, 49, 527–34.

Rumsey, J. M., Andreason, P., Zametkin, A. J. et al. (1994a). Right frontotemporal activation by tonal memory in dyslexia, an ^{15}O PET Study. *Biol. Psychiatry*, 36, 171–80.

Rumsey, J. M., Zametkin, A. J., Andreason, P. et al. (1994b). Normal activation of frontotemporal language cortex in dyslexia, as measured with oxygen 15 positron emission tomography. *Arch. Neurol.*, 51, 27–38.

Rumsey, J. M., Donohue, B. C., Brady, D. R., Nace, K., Giedd, J. N. and Andreason, P. (1997a). A magnetic resonance imaging study of planum temporale asymmetry in men with developmental dyslexia. *Arch. Neurol.*, 54, 1481–9.

Rumsey, J. M., Nace, K., Donohue, B., Wise, D., Maisog, J. M. and Andreason, P. (1997b). A positron emission tomographic study of impaired word recognition and phonological processing in dyslexic men. *Arch. Neurol.*, 54, 562–73.

Sabatini, U., Pantano, P., Brughitta, G. et al. (1995). Presurgical integrated MRI/SPECT localization of the sensorimotor cortex in a patient with a low-grade astrocytoma in the rolandic area. *Neuroreport*, 7, 105–8.

Sadato, N., Pascual-Leone, A., Grafman, J., Deiber, M., Ibanez, V. and Hallett, M. (1998). Neural networks for Braille reading by the blind. *Brain*, 121, 1213–29.

Salmelin, R., Service, E., Kiesilea, P., Uutela, K. and Salonen, O. (1996). Impaired visual word processing in dyslexia revealed with magnetoencephalography. *Ann. Neurol.*, 40, 157–62.

Sankar, R., Wasterlain, C. G. and Sperber, E. S. (1995). Seizure-induced changes in the immature brain. In *Brain Development and Epilepsy*, ed. P. A. Schwartzkroin, pp. 268–88. New York: Oxford University Press.

Schifter, T., Hoffman, J. M., Hatten, H. P. et al. (1994). Neuroimaging in infantile autism. *J. Child Neurol.*, 9, 155–61.

Schlaggar, B. and O'Leary, D. (1991). Potential of visual cortex to develop an array of functional units unique to somatosensory cortex. *Science*, 252, 1556–60.

Schmahmann, J. D. (1996). From movement to thought: anatomic substrates of the cerebellar contribution to cognitive processing. *Hum. Brain Map.*, 4, 174–98.

Schneider, G. E. (1979). Is it really better to have your brain lesion early? A revision of the "Kennard principle". *Neuropsychologia*, 17, 557–83.

Schroer, R. J., Phelan, M. C., Michaelis, R. C. et al. (1998). Autism and maternally derived aberrations of chromosome 15q. *Am. J. Med. Genet.*, 76, 327–36.

Schultz, R. T., Cho, N. K., Staib, L. H. et al. (1994). Brain morphology in normal and dyslexic children: the influence of sex and age. *Ann. Neurol.*, 35, 732–42.

Seitz, R. J., Huang, Y., Knorr, U., Tellmann, L., Herzog, H. and Freund, H. J. (1995). Large-scale plasticity of the human motor cortex. *Neuroreport*, 6, 742–4.

Seitz, R. J., Höflich, P., Binkofski, P., Tellmann, L., Herzog, H. and Freund, H. J. (1998). Role of premotor cortex in recovery from middle cerebral artery infarction. *Arch. Neurol.*, 55, 1081–8.

Seo, M. L. and Ito, M. (1987). Reorganization of rat vibrissa barrelfield as studied by cortical lesioning on different postnatal days. *Exp. Brain Res.*, 65, 251–60.

Shallice, T. (1988). *From Neuropsychology to Mental Structure*. Cambridge, UK: Cambridge University Press.

Shankweiler, D., Crain, S., Katz, L. et al. (1995). Cognitive profiles of reading-disabled children: comparison of language skills in phonology, morphology, and syntax. *Psychol. Sci.*, 6, 149–56.

Shatz, C. J. (1992). How are specific connections formed between thalamus and cortex? *Curr. Opin. Neurobiol.*, 2, 78–82.

Shaywitz, S. E., Escobar, M. D., Shaywitz, B. A., Fletcher, J. M. and Makuch, R. (1992). Evidence that dyslexia may represent the lower tail of a normal distribution of reading ability. *N. Engl. J. Med.*, 326, 145–50.

Shaywitz, S. E., Shaywitz, B. A., Pugh, K. R. et al. (1998). Functional disruption in the organization of the brain for reading in dyslexia. *Proc. Natl. Acad. Sci. USA*, 95, 2636–41.

Sherman, M., Nass, R. and Shapiro, T. (1984). Brief report: regional cerebral blood flow in autism. *J. Autism Dev. Disord.*, 14, 439–46.

Shupert, C., Cornwell, P. and Payne, B. (1993). Differential sparing of depth perception, orienting, and optokinetic nystagmus after neonatal versus adult lesions of cortical areas 17, 18 and 19 in the cat. *Behav. Neurosci.*, 107, 633–50.

Siegel, B. V. Jr, Asarnow, R., Tanguay, P. et al. (1992). Regional cerebral glucose metabolism and attention in adults with a history of childhood autism. *Journal of Neuropsychiatry and Clinical Neurosciences*, 4, 406–14.

Stapleton, S. R., Kiriakopoulos, E., Mikulis, D. et al. (1997). Combined utility of functional MRI, cortical mapping, and frameless stereotaxy in the resection of lesions in eloquent areas of brain in children. *Pediatr. Neurosurg.*, 26, 68–82.

Stein, J. and Walsh, V. (1997). To see but not to read; the magnocellular theory of dyslexia. *Trends Neurosci.*, **20**, 147–52.

Steinmetz, H. and Seitz, R. J. (1991). Functional anatomy of language processing: neuroimaging and the problem of individual variability. *Neuropsychologia*, **29**, 1149–61.

Stiles, J. and Thal, D. (1993). Linguistic and spatial cognitive development following early focal brain injury: patterns of deficit and recovery. In *Brain Development and Cognition*, ed. M. J. Johnson, pp. 641–64. Cambridge, MA: Blackwell.

Stiles, J., Trauner, D., Engel, M. and Nass, R. (1997). The development of drawing in children with congenital focal brain injury. *Neuropsychologia*, **35**, 299–312.

Stiles, J., Bates, E., Thal, D., Trauner, D. and Reilly, J. (1999). Linguistic, cognitive and affective development following early focal brain injury: a ten-year overview from the San Diego Longitudinal Project. In *Advances in Infancy Research*, ed. C. Rovee-Collier, pp. 641–64. Norwood, NJ: Ablex.

Strauss, E., Satz, P. and Wada, J. (1990). An examination of the crowding hypothesis in epileptic patients who have undergone the carotid amytal test. *Neuropsychologia*, **28**, 1221–7.

Strauss, E., Wada, J. and Hunter, M. (1992). Sex-related differences in the cognitive consequences of early left-hemisphere lesions. *J. Clin. Exp. Neuropsychol.*, **14**, 738–48.

Strauss, E., Loring, D., Chelune, G. et al. (1995). Predicting cognitive impairment in epilepsy. Findings from the Bozeman Epilepsy Consortium. *J. Clin. Exp. Neuropsychol.*, **17**, 909–17.

Stromswold, K. (1995). The cognitive and neural bases of language acquisition. In *The Cognitive Neurosciences*, ed. M. S. Gazzaniga, pp. 855–70. Boston, MA: MIT Press.

Sun, J. S., Lomber, S. G. and Payne, B. R. (1994). Expansion of suprasylvian cortex projection in the superficial layers of the superior colliculus following damage of areas 17 and 18 in developing cats. *Visual Neurosci.*, **11**, 13–22.

Sur, M., Pallas, S. L. and Roe, A. W. (1990). Cross-modal plasticity in cortical development: differentiation and specification of sensory neocortex. *Trends Neurosci.*, **13**, 227–33.

Szatmari, P., Archer, L., Fisman, S., Streiner, D. L. and Wilson, F. (1995). Asperger's syndrome and autism: differences in behavior, cognition, and adaptive functionings. *J. Am. Acad. Child Adolesc. Psychiatry*, **34**, 1662–71.

Tager-Flusberg, H., Boshart, J. and Baron-Cohen, S. (1998). Reading the windows to the soul: evidence of domain-specific sparing in Williams syndrome. *J. Cogn. Neurosci.*, **10**, 631–9.

Talairach, J. and Tournoux, P. (1988). *Co-Planar Stereotaxic Atlas of the Human Brain*. Stuttgart: Georg Thieme.

Tallal, P., Ross, R. and Curtiss, S. (1989). Familial aggregation in specific language impairment. *J. Speech Hearing Disord.*, **54**, 167–73.

Tallal, P., Miller, S. and Fitch, R. H. (1993). Neurobiological basis of speech. *Ann. N.Y. Acad. Sci.*, **682**, 27–47.

Tallal, P., Miller, S. L., Bedi, G. et al. (1996). Language comprehension in language-learning impaired children improved with acoustically modified speech. *Science*, **271**, 81–4.

Tanguay, P. E. and Edwards, R. M. (1982). Electrophysiological studies of autism: the whisper of the bang. *J. Autism Dev. Disord.*, **12**, 177–84.

Teuber, H. L. (1974). Functional recovery after lesions of the nervous system. II. Recovery of function after lesions of the central nervous system: history and prospects. *Neurosci. Res. Program Bull.*, **12**, 197–211.

Thal, D., Marchman, V., Stiles, J. et al. (1991). Early lexical development in children with focal brain injury. *Brain Lang.*, **40**, 491–527.

Thivierge, J., Baedard, C., Caotae, R. and Maziade, M. (1990). Brainstem auditory evoked response and subcortical abnormalities in autism. *Am. J. Psychiatry*, **147**, 1609–13.

Tomblin, J. B. and Buckwalter, P. R. (1994). Studies of genetics of specific language impairment. In *Specific Language Impairments in Children*, eds. R. V. Watkins and M. L. Rice, pp. 17–34. Baltimore, MD: Paul H. Brookes.

Townsend, J. and Courchesne, E. (1994). Parietal damage and narrow "spotlight" spatial attention. *J. Cogn. Neurosci.*, **6**, 220–32.

Townsend, J., Courchesne, E. and Egaas, B. (1996). Slowed orienting of covert visual-spatial attention in autism: specific deficits associated with cerebellar and parietal abnormality. *Dev. Psychopathol.*, **8**, 563–84.

Treffert, D. A. (1988). The idiot savant: a review of the syndrome. *Am. J. Psychiatry*, **145**, 563–72.

Tzourio, N., Heim, A., Zilbovicius, M., Gerard, C. and Mazoyer, B. (1994). Abnormal regional cerebral blood flow in dysphasic children during a language task. *Pediatr. Neurol.*, **10**, 20–6.

Udwin, O. and Yule, W. (1991). A cognitive and behavioral phenotype in Williams syndrome. *J. Clin. Exp. Neuropsychol.*, **13**, 232–44.

Uhl, F., Franzen, P., Podreka, I., Steiner, M. and Deecke, L. (1993). Increased regional cerebral blood flow in inferior occipital cortex and cerebellum of early blind humans. *Neurosci. Lett.*, **150**, 162–4.

van Adel, B. A. and Kelly, J. B. (1998). Kainic acid lesions of the superior olivary complex: effects on sound localization by the albino rat. *Behav. Neurosci.*, **112**, 432–46.

Vargha-Khadem, F. and Polkey, C. E. (1992). A review of cognitive outcome after hemidecortication in humans. In *Recovery from Brain Damage*, eds. F. D. Rose and D. A. Johnson, pp. 137–51. New York: Plenum Press.

Vargha-Khadem, F., Isaacs, E., van der Werf, S., Robb, S. and Wilson, J. (1992). Development of intelligence and memory in children with hemiplegic cerebral palsy. The deleterious consequences of early seizures. *Brain*, **115**, 315–29.

Vargha-Khadem, F., Watkins, K., Alcock, K., Fletcher, P. and Passingham, R. (1995). Praxic and nonverbal cognitive deficits in a large family with a genetically transmitted speech and language disorder. *Proc. Natl. Acad. Sci. USA*, **92**, 930–3.

Varghar Khadem, F., Carr, L. C., Isaacs, E., Bretl, E., Adams, C. and Mishkin, M. (1997). Onset of speech after left hemispherectomy in a nine-year-old boy. *Brain*, **120**, 159–82.

Vargha-Khadem, F., Isaacs, E., Watkins, K. E. and Mishkin, M. (1999). Neuropsychological deficits in children with extensive hemispheric pathology. In *Intractable Focal Epilepsy: Medical and Surgical Treatment*, eds. J. M. Oxbury, C. E. Polkey and M. Duchowny. London: Saunders.

Vicari, S., Stiles, J., Stern, C. and Resca, A. (1998). Spatial grouping activity in children with early cortical and subcortical lesions. *Dev. Med. Child Neurol.*, **40**, 90–4.

Villablanca, J. R., Hovda, D. A., Jackson, G. F. and Gayek, R. (1993a). Neurological and behavioral effects of a unilateral frontal cortical lesion in fetal kittens. I. Brain morphology, movement, posture, and sensorimotor tests. *Behav. Brain Res.*, **57**, 63–77.

Villablanca, J. R., Hovda, D. A., Jackson, G. F. and Infante, C. (1993b). Neurological and behavioral effects of a unilateral frontal cortical lesion in fetal kittens. II. Visual system tests, and proposing an 'optimal developmental period' for lesion effects. *Behav. Brain Res.*, **57**, 79–92.

Vining, E. P., Freeman, J. M., Brandt, J., Carson, B. S. and Uematsu, S. (1993). Progressive unilateral encephalopathy of childhood (Rasmussen's syndrome): a reappraisal. *Epilepsia*, **34**, 639–50.

Voeller, K. K. S. (1996). Developmental neurobiological aspects of autism. *J. Autism Dev. Disord.*, **26**, 189–93.

Volkmar, F. R., Klin, A., Schultz, R. et al. (1996). Asperger's syndrome. [Clinical conference] *J. Am. Acad. Child Adolesc. Psychiatry*, **35**, 118–23.

von Monakow, C. (1914). *Die Lokalisation im Grosshirn und der Abbau der Funktion durch Kortikale Herde.* Wiesbaden: Bergmann.

Wada, J. and Rasmussen, T. (1960). Intracarotid injection of sodium amytal for the lateralization of cerebral speech dominance. *J. Neurosurg.*, **17**, 266–82.

Walsh, C. and Cepko, C. L. (1992). Widespread dispersion of neuronal clones across functional regions of the cerebral cortex. *Science*, **255**, 434–40.

Wang, P. P., Hesselink, J. R., Jernigan, T. L., Doherty, S. and Bellugi, U. (1992). Specific neurobehavioral profile of William's syndrome is associated with neocerebellar hemispheric preservation. *Neurology*, **42**, 1999–2002.

Weiller, C., Isensee, C., Rijntjes, M. et al. (1995). Recovery from Wernicke's aphasia: a positron emission tomographic study. *Ann. Neurol.*, **37**, 723–32.

Weinberg, W. A., Harper, C. R. and Brumback, R. A. (1995). Neuroanatomic substrate of developmental specific learning disabilities and select behavioral syndromes. *J. Child Neurol.*, 10 (Suppl. 1), S78–80.

Williams, R. S., Hauser, S. I., Purpura, D., De Long, R. and Swisher, C. N. (1980). Autism and mental retardation. *Arch. Neurol.*, **37**, 749–53.

Witelson, S. F. and Kigar, D. L. (1992). Sylvian fissure morphology and asymmetry in men and women: bilateral differences in relation to handedness in men. *J. Comp. Neurol.*, **323**, 326–40.

Wolff, P. H. (1993). Impaired temporal resolution in developmental dyslexia. *Ann. N.Y. Acad. Sci.*, **682**, 87–103.

Wong, V. and Wong, S. N. (1991). Brainstem auditory evoked potential study in children with autistic disorder. *J. Autism Dev. Disord.*, **21**, 329–40.

Woods, B. (1980). The restricted effects of right-hemisphere lesions after age one: Wechsler test data. *Neuropsychologia*, **18**, 65–70.

Wright, B. A., Lombardino, L. J., King, W. M., Puranik, C. S., Leonard, C. M. and Merzenich, M. M. (1997). Deficits in auditory temporal and spectral resolution in language-impaired children. [See comments] *Nature*, **387**, 176–8.

Yeung-Courchesne, R. and Courchesne, E. (1997). From impasse to insight in autism research: from behavioral symptoms to biological explanations. *Dev. Psychopathol.*, **9**, 389–419.

Zilbovicius, M., Garreau, B., Samson, Y. et al. (1995). Delayed maturation of the frontal cortex in childhood autism. *Am. J. Psychiatry*, **152**, 248–52.

Zilbovicius, M., Barthelemy, C., Belin, P. et al. (1998). Bitemporal hypoperfusion in childhood autism. *Neuroimage*, 7, S503.

Zupanc, M. L. (1997). Neuroimaging in the evaluation of children and adolescents with intractable epilepsy: II. Neuroimaging and pediatric epilepsy surgery. *Pediatr. Neurol.*, **17**, 111–21.

21

Utility of CANTAB in functional neuroimaging

Andy C. H. Lee, Adrian M. Owen, Robert D. Rogers,
Barbara J. Sahakian and Trevor W. Robbins

Introduction

The design, theoretical rationale, and validation of the Cambridge Neuropsychological Test Automated Battery (CANTAB) are described in this chapter. The utility of the battery for functional neuroimaging studies is examined, based on its links with animal neuropsychological research, its decomposition of complex tests of cognition into their constituent parts, and its validation in patient groups with defined brain lesions. The use of selected tests from the battery is then surveyed, including the Tower of London test of planning, tests of spatial span and self-ordered working memory, a rapid visual information processing test of sustained attention, a delayed-matching-to-sample test of visual recognition, and a test of attentional set shifting. Each paradigm is shown to be associated with distinct neural networks of elevated regional cerebral blood flow (rCBF) using positron emission tomography (PET) based on $H_2^{15}O$. The use of these paradigms to delineate impaired neural networks in depression and other neuropsychiatric disorders is described. The final discussion assesses the prospects of future applications, including the use of other neuroimaging paradigms, such as functional magnetic resonance imaging (fMRI) and the PET ligand-displacement method.

The CANTAB was originally devised to assess cognitive function in elderly and dementing subjects (Robbins et al., 1994a). However, in the 1990s, it has also been used in the analysis of cognitive function in a range of adult neuropsychiatric syndromes, following drug treatments in healthy adult volunteers, and also in a neurodevelopmental context. The CANTAB comprises a set of computerized tests administered with the aid of a touch-sensitive screen. The two main guiding principles have been to use some tests that can be related to the extensive neuropsychologic literature in animals and to employ tests that can be broken down into their discrete cognitive components in order to define more readily which functions are impaired and which are spared, and thus the overall specificity of any deficits. Some examples of these principles can be gleaned from a brief survey of the main tests contained within the battery, which itself is divided into smaller batteries of tests of "visual memory", "spatial working memory and planning" and "attention" (Table 21.1). For example, the delayed-matching-to-sample (DMTS) test of visual recognition memory is derived from an analogous paradigm used with monkeys (Mishkin, 1982) and the test of attentional-set shifting is in fact a simplified and decomposed version of the Wisconsin Card Sorting Test (WCST), which is frequently used to assess frontal lobe function (Milner, 1964). The CANTAB version of the attentional set-shifting task is based on tests of visual discrimination learning and reversal, as well as specific transfer tests termed "intra" and "extra"-dimensional shifts, the latter capturing the essential qualities of the WCST. Moreover, the self-ordered test of spatial working memory is based on similar procedures used in experimental animals that derive from foraging paradigms (Olton, 1982; Passingham, 1985; Owen et al., 1990). These tests are further described in Chapter 22.

However, it is worth emphasizing that the CANTAB is not solely preoccupied with extrapolation from animals to humans and vice versa. One of the most prominent tests from the working memory and planning battery is an adaptation of the Tower of London test of planning, which derives from cognitive psychology more than from the animal literature (Shallice, 1982). This test, however, does exemplify the decompositional principle: as measures of thinking time are derived from a yoked control procedure in which the sequence of moves actually used by the subjects is played back to them, move by move, in order to quantify the time taken in visuomotor execution, thus

Table 21.1. *Main sub-batteries of CANTAB and constituent tests*

Test battery	Constituent tests[a]
Visual memory	Pattern and spatial recognition memory Simultaneous and delayed matching-to-sample Paired visuospatial associates learning
Spatial working memory and planning	Spatial span Self-ordered spatial working memory (spatial search) Tower of London (Stockings of Cambridge)
Attention	Serial choice reaction time Visual search, matching-to-sample Attentional set-formation and shifting Rapid visual information processing

Note:

[a] The motor screening test is common to all three batteries. These batteries are identical for use in children or adults.

assessing sensorimotor components of the latency measures. This sensorimotor component is then subtracted from the overall response latency to estimate the residual "thinking time", this being done both for the initial latency before the subject implements the solution and also for the subsequent "thinking time" during problem completion (see Owen et al., 1990).

The CANTAB has now been used quite extensively in the testing of patients with Alzheimer's disease and other forms of dementia (Sahakian et al., 1988, 1990; Sahgal et al., 1991, 1992; Fowler et al., 1997), patients with basal ganglia disorders such as Parkinson's (Downes et al., 1989; Owen et al., 1992, 1993) and Huntington's diseases (Lange et al., 1995; Lawrence et al., 1996), and those with Korsakoff's syndrome (Joyce and Robbins, 1991), depression (Abas et al., 1990; Beats et al., 1996; Elliott et al., 1996) and schizophrenia (Pantelis et al., 1997; Elliott et al., 1998; Hutton et al., 1998).

Like most cognitive test batteries initially designed for use in adult subjects, the CANTAB has not yet been employed often in developmental neuropsychology, although the ability of the battery to draw parallels with the animal neuropsychologic literature and its limited dependence on language abilities makes it attractive as a means of testing hypotheses about the neural substrates of cognition in children. One of our studies did use some of the tests from CANTAB to assess children with either learning disabilities or autism (Hughes et al., 1994). This study was successful in showing that autistic children had selective difficulties with two of the main CANTAB tests sensitive to frontal lobe dysfunction: extradimensional set-shifting

and Tower of London planning performance. This study has been theoretically significant in recent debates about the "theory of mind" and "executive" hypotheses of the core cognitive deficit in autism. Many of the CANTAB tests have been used recently in a large cross-sectional study that has made inferences about cognitive development in the context of cortical maturation (Luciana and Nelson, 1998; see Chapter 22).

Two main issues in the use of CANTAB in a clinical neuropsychologic context relate to its standardization and validation. These issues have been dealt with in other publications and will not be discussed in great detail here, except to point out that the tests have been standardized on large populations of healthy normal subjects across a wide age span (Robbins et al., 1994a, 1996, 1998). Questions such as test–retest reliability are currently being addressed. The validation of the tests depends, in part, on their sensitivity relative to other clinical instruments and their ability to discriminate deficits in marginal cases of brain dysfunction or in early stages of disease processes, for example in asymptomatic HIV (Sahakian et al., 1995), gene-positive Huntington's disease (Lawrence et al., 1998a), or early in the course of dementia of the Alzheimer type (Fowler et al., 1997). The precise clinical utility of computerized tests is still under debate, although advantages in terms of the standardized presentation of tests and objective and accurate recording of the data are obvious. The automatized nature of the tests makes them suitable for adaptation to functional neuroimaging designs. Their componential nature, which allows complex performance to be broken down into constituent parts, also lends itself well to the functional imaging approach, as will be made clear later in this chapter. The goal of functional neuroimaging is to elucidate neural networks that underlie different cognitive processes, as well as the effects of defined brain lesions on performance on the different tests. Such information can be extrapolated in part from the effects of lesions in experimental animals, particularly nonhuman primates. For example, we now have extensive knowledge of the neural substrates of delayed nonmatching-to-sample (DNMTS) task in macaque monkeys, which bears on the design of the human analog DNMTS task that is included in the CANTAB. These include deleterious effects of lesions to different regions of the temporal lobes, the midline thalamic nuclei, and the ventromedial prefrontal cortex (see Murray (1992) for review). Similar analyses might be applied to the CANTAB tests of self-ordered working memory and attentional set-shifting, which depend on different regions of the prefrontal cortex (Petrides et al., 1993a; Petrides, 1996; Dias et al., 1996).

The validation process is strengthened by the study of patients with defined brain lesions, such as neurosurgical excisions of the frontal or temporal lobes (e.g., Owen et al., 1995a; Robbins et al., 1997). Some of the CANTAB tests are sensitive to frontal lobe and others to temporal lobe damage or to amygdalo-hippocampectomy (Owen et al., 1991, 1995a). However, this approach is limited in determining the nature of the neural networks engaged by the various cognitive processes because of the arbitrary and essentially ill-defined nature of brain lesions in humans. An appropriate paradigm for determining neural activity, therefore, is that of functional neuroimaging, whether using PET or fMRI. The knowledge to be gained from the combination of studies of brain lesions and functional imaging in normal subjects is attractive, because the evidence from the lesion studies helps to establish the causal (direct and indirect) nature of any apparent involvement of a particular structure. The logic involved here is quite clear. If an activation is detected in a particular structure from a neuroimaging study and yet performance of the task remains normal when that area is absent or damaged, questions can be asked about whether the structure in question is, in fact, necessary for efficient task performance. If, however, there is a deficit following a lesion to a structure that is activated in the normal brain during task performance, this provides quite strong evidence for the causal involvement of that structure in performance. If there is no activation in the structure, then a deficit following a lesion could conceivably reflect an indirect impairment caused by a compensatory change in other brain regions. Alternatively, the lack of activation in the normal brain might reflect inadequacies or insensitivity in the neuroimaging technique employed.

The CANTAB tasks used clinically often have to be modified for the purposes of neuroimaging, not only because of the intrinsic requirements of the PET or fMRI protocols but more particularly to avoid ceiling effects that can occur in younger and more intelligent normal adult volunteers. The following review examines, in turn, results from some of the main CANTAB tests employed in functional imaging, usually PET studies with $H_2{}^{15}O$. Defining appropriate neural networks for particular tasks is not an end in itself, but it may be an essential preliminary step in investigating the neural substrates of altered performance in neuropsychiatric disorders with no obvious structural damage (e.g., depression or schizophrenia). Therefore, several studies have examined the neural substrates of impaired task performance in patients with neuropsychiatric disorders such as depression or schizophrenia having previously focused on normal subjects, who can then serve as a suitable control group.

Use of CANTAB in functional imaging paradigms

To date, of the CANTAB tests, variants of the Tower of London task have been the most frequently employed in functional neuroimaging studies, although more recently, several other tasks from the battery have also been investigated, mainly in PET studies of rCBF using $H_2{}^{15}O$.

Planning ability (Tower of London/Stockings of Cambridge)

Planning is the ability to think ahead and is necessary in situations where a goal must be reached through a series of intermediate steps, each of which does not necessarily lead directly toward that goal (Owen, 1997a). Research into the fundamental neural mechanisms of planning has been carried out in studies of lesions in nonhuman primates (e.g., Petrides, 1994), and in neuropsychologic studies of human patients (e.g., Klosowska, 1976; Shallice, 1982, Owen et al., 1990). Both types of study have implicated the frontal lobe as being essential in planning behavior (for review see Owen, 1997a). However, it is only with the emergence of functional neuroimaging techniques such as single photon emission computed tomography (SPECT), PET and fMRI during the 1990s that the precise anatomic substrates of planning have been investigated in healthy human subjects. Typically, changes in rCBF measured by these techniques while subjects are engaged in specific tasks serve as an indirect index of neuronal activity during cognitive, motor, and/or sensory processing.

Using a three-dimensional computerized version of the Tower of London task presented on a touch-sensitive screen, Morris et al. (1993) employed SPECT to investigate the neural correlates of planning in normal adults. In comparison with a control task that did not require planning but was matched for motor movements and visual stimulation, a significant increase in rCBF was observed in the left prefrontal cortex during the Tower of London task. This result had some similarities to those reported by Rezai et al. (1993) and supports the general role of the frontal lobe in planning behavior. However, given the relatively low spatial resolution of SPECT, this technique is inadequate for investigating the precise functional specialization of the distinct cytoarchitectonic areas within the prefrontal cortex.

In comparison with SPECT, and depending on the particular scanner used, PET possesses greater spatial resolution, which when combined with structural MRI can provide more precise localization of function. Several more recent studies have used PET to measure rCBF during the Tower of London task. Using this technique, 6–12 scans are conducted and for each, a radioactive tracer is introduced into the vascular system, usually ^{15}O in the form of $H_2{}^{15}O$. The PET scanner measures the spatial distribution of the tracer over a 60–120 s period, during which the subject carries out an experimental or control task. The experimental task involves the cognitive, motor, or sensory process of interest while the control task is designed to require many, but not all, of the same processes. A common approach to statistical analysis is via subtraction whereby scans from different conditions are "subtracted" from one another (e.g., experimental task – control task) to isolate regions activated by the processes of interest involved in the experimental task but not in the control task. A basic comparison is of the task with a "rest" condition (e.g., "eyes closed") in which there are no specific task requirements. From our perspective, the closer the cognitive requirements of the experimental and control tasks, the greater is the chance of isolating activations specific to a particular cognitive function. The subtractions can then be coregistered with a normalized structural MRI scan, enabling the precise location of significant regions of activation. Local maxima of activation are usually reported in terms of stereotaxic coordinates (x, y, z; Talairach and Tournoux, 1988) and/or the cytoarchitectonic region in which they lie (e.g., Brodmann area (BA)).

Owen et al. (1996a) used PET to investigate the role of distinct frontal cortical areas in planning behavior using the computerized Tower of London (or Stockings of Cambridge) task from the CANTAB in healthy adult male volunteers. The subjects were scanned during easy (two or three move) and difficult (four or five move) Tower of London problems of the task and also during a control condition. By subtracting the control condition from the easy and difficult planning conditions and also the easy and difficult planning conditions from each other, the network of cortical and subcortical areas involved in the planning aspect of the Tower of London task can be isolated.

Subtraction of the control condition from the difficult planning condition yielded a significant increase in rCBF in the left mid-dorsolateral frontal cortex, which comprises mainly BA 9 and BA 46 and lies within the superior and middle frontal gyri. There was also a trend for increase in rCBF in slightly more anterior regions of the same area in the opposite hemisphere, but this failed to reach statistical significance. That only the left prefrontal activation reached significance does not necessarily indicate that the process of planning is strongly lateralized to the left hemisphere. In fact, this observation is more likely to have been an artifact of the subtraction technique employed (Owen, 1997a). Since both the planning and control conditions involve visuospatial processes that are believed to be mediated largely by the right hemisphere (Milner, 1971, 1974), subtracting the control condition from the planning condition would inevitably remove or, at least reduce, any right hemisphere activation in the comparison. This interpretation is supported by Owen et al. (1996a), who observed significant right dorsolateral prefrontal cortex activation compared with a resting condition in the difficult planning condition prior to the subtraction of the specific task control condition. Furthermore, planning deficits are evident in patients with either right or left prefrontal cortical damage (Shallice, 1982; Owen et al., 1990, 1995b).

Subtractions of the control condition from the easy planning condition did not, however, yield a significant increase in rCBF in the prefrontal cortex, although a significant increase in rCBF was observed in the right premotor cortex and in bilateral regions of the parietal and occipital lobes. This probably reflects the fact that the easier two/three move problems can be solved simply by matching each ball in the sample configuration with its corresponding ball in the target configuration, with little need for thinking ahead (i.e., comparable with a visual matching-to-sample). Consequently, the need for planning is minimized or even absent, resulting in a decreased involvement of the prefrontal cortex. In contrast, a visual matching-to-sample strategy may place a greater load on posterior visual and attentional systems, while activation of the premotor cortex may reflect more basic processes of motor planning (Owen, 1997a).

The difference in activation observed between difficult and easy Tower of London problems in the study by Owen et al. (1996a) could conceivably reflect the difference in movement demands; while difficult problems require over four movements, simple problems can be solved within three moves. To account for this, a modified version of the task developed previously (Owen et al., 1995b) was used during PET by Baker et al. (1996). This version, known as the "one-touch" Tower of London (Fig. 21.1), requires the subjects to indicate their answers to problems at all levels of difficulty by executing a single movement. In brief, for each problem the subjects are required to plan the minimum number of moves that are required to reach the goal position from the initial position without actually physically making any of the moves. They indicate their answer instead by touching the appropriate number (standing for the number of moves required to solve the problem) on a response panel at the bottom of the touch-screen monitor. As a control condition, the subjects are presented with identical upper and lower arrays. Following a delay matched to the latency of their response in the corresponding test trial, one of the balls "blinks" and the subject responds by touching the number 3.

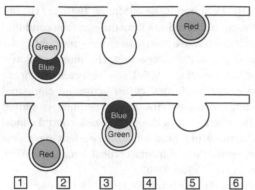

Fig. 21.1. The display on the touch-screen monitor for the "one-touch" Tower of London test of planning, as it appears to the subject. The subject is required to select (by simply touching it) one of the numbered boxes at the bottom of the display according to the number of moves the subject estimates for the solution to the problem of mentally matching or converting the bottom arrangement of "balls" to the top "goal" arrangement (three for the problem shown above). The instruction is that this should be done in the minimum number of mental "moves", as constrained by the hanging arrangement of the "pool balls" lodged in "pockets" or "socks". Illegal moves, such as trying to remove a ball when there was another ball sitting above it in the same pocket, were carefully explained to the subject; if attempted, such moves evoked no response from the computer. Only when subjects were entirely familiar with these "rules" were they allowed to proceed to test problems. Further details are provided in Owen et al. (1995b).

Baker et al. (1996) scanned subjects while they solved easy and difficult "one touch" Tower of London problems as well as during the corresponding yoked control task. It was found that both easy and difficult planning problems activated the premotor cortex bilaterally as well as the more posterior occipitoparietal cortical areas. In contrast to the results described by Owen et al. (1996a), the prefrontal cortex was significantly activated in *both* the easy and difficult conditions. However, the distribution of this activation differed between these two conditions: both conditions activated the dorsolateral prefrontal cortex bilaterally but, in addition, the difficult planning condition activated an extensive region of the right rostrolateral prefrontal cortex (notably BA 10 and BA 9/46). The predominant right hemisphere activation relative to the study by Owen et al. (1996a) may reflect the greater demands placed by the "one touch" Tower of London on visual imagery (Owen, 1997a).

A more recent study has used PET with a modified "one-touch" Tower of London task to investigate differences in the neural response to negative and positive feedback in healthy subjects during planning (Elliott et al., 1997a). Slight modifications were made to the task in that the sub-jects were required to respond within 10 s of the problem being presented. Furthermore, there were three feedback conditions, namely, *no feedback, positive feedback,* and *negative feedback.* In the positive condition, 100% of trials were followed by a "YOU ARE RIGHT" message regardless of whether the responses made were actually correct. In contrast, in the negative condition, only 20% of trials were followed by this positive message; the other 80% were followed by a "YOU ARE WRONG" message regardless of whether the responses were actually wrong. The same feedback conditions were presented for a guessing task that also acted as a control task for the planning task. In that task, the subjects were presented with two identical arrays of colored balls that would disappear after a short delay. The subjects were required to "guess" by touching one of six response buttons. Prior to the task, they were informed that three of these buttons were randomly assigned as correct on each trial.

On comparing the planning task with the guessing task without regard to the use of feedback or its absence, it was found that similar, though less extensive, regions were activated relative to those reported by Baker et al. (1996). It is possible that the guessing task was a more demanding control than that employed by Baker et al. (1996) and, therefore, led to a significant proportion of the activations being "subtracted out" in the comparison. In the presence of feedback relative to the no-feedback condition, a significant increase in rCBF was observed in the medial caudate nucleus and the ventromedial orbitofrontal cortex. Examining negative and positive feedback separately showed an increase in rCBF in the same areas during the guessing task, although there was no such increase for the planning task. This may reflect the possibility that neural processing of feedback is greater in tasks in which the outcome is unpredictable and beyond control.

Planning, as measured by the Tower of London task, has been shown to be impaired in depressed patients (e.g. Elliott et al., 1996), as well as in patients with Parkinson's disease (Morris et al., 1988; Owen et al., 1992, 1995b) and other neurodegenerative conditions (Robbins et al., 1994b; Lange et al., 1995). In an attempt to understand the relation between cognitive dysfunction in these conditions and the underlying neurophysiologic abnormalities, several patient groups have been studied using the Tower of London task. Using the $H_2^{15}O$ PET technique, Elliott et al. (1997b) scanned a group of unipolar depressed patients on the "one touch" Tower of London task and compared the results with those of the normal subjects reported in Baker et al. (1996). Relative to controls, the depressed patients exhibited a significant attenuation of bilateral rCBF activation of the cortical and subcortical regions that are involved in the Tower of London task. Those regions included the anterior cingulate cortex, caudate nucleus, thalamus, and cerebellum, as well as the more posterior cortical areas. In addition, there were significant attenuations in the right dorsolateral and rostrolateral prefrontal cortex of the depressed patients.

Recently, PET has been used by Owen et al. (1998) to investigate striatal and prefrontal cortical blood flow in patients with Parkinson's disease during planning and spatial working memory tasks. For the planning aspect, patients with moderate disease were scanned while performing easy and difficult CANTAB Tower of London problems and rCBF changes were compared with those of age-matched control subjects performing the same task. During a control condition, subjects were required to carry out a visuomotor task in which they attended to the lower half of the Tower of London test display and touched a series of locations that were highlighted with yellow rings. The moves that were required corresponded to the moves produced by the same subject during the difficult planning condition; furthermore, the subjects' responses were paced according to their own response latencies in the previous condition.

When the visuomotor control condition was subtracted from the difficult planning condition, a significant increase in rCBF was observed in the age-matched control subjects in the dorsolateral, ventrolateral, and premotor areas of the left frontal lobe: in the ventral frontal, premotor, posterior, parietal, and prestriate cortices of the right hemisphere; and in the striate cortex at the midline. The same subtraction for the patients with Parkinson's disease patients yielded a significant increase in rCBF in the ventrolateral and premotor regions of the right frontal lobe and in the left prestriate cortex. An increase in rCBF was also observed in the right dorsolateral frontal cortex and in the left mid-dorsolateral frontal region, but both of these failed to reach statistical significance according to conventional statistical criteria.

However, a highly significant difference was observed between the two subject groups in the region of the right globus pallidus. Specifically, the planning task was associated with an increase in rCBF in the internal segment of the globus pallidus in the control subjects, whereas in the patients with Parkinson's disease, the tasks were associated with a decrease in rCBF in the same region. In the same study, very similar findings were observed when the subjects were scanned during a spatial working memory condition, also known to place significant demands on frontal lobe systems. From these results, it was suggested that striatal dopamine depletion in patients with Parkinson's disease disrupts the normal pattern of basal ganglia outflow, which, in turn, disrupts the various cognitive functions of the frontal lobe by interrupting normal transmission of information through frontostriatal circuitry. One such circuit is the fronto-cortico–striatal loop, which consists of efferent projections from the internal segment of the globus pallidus to discrete frontal regions and afferent projections from the same frontal regions to the neostriatum of the basal ganglia.

Spatial working memory

Whereas the Tower of London task is primarily conceptualized as a planning task, it undoubtedly involves many other discrete cognitive components that combine to produce an efficient plan of action. One of these is working memory, which is recognized to be closely related to planning behavior in both neural and neurophysiologic terms (for full review see Owen, 1997a). In brief the term "working memory" was first introduced by Baddeley (1986) and refers to the temporary storage and on-line manipulation of information that may occur while carrying out a wide range of tasks.

Two CANTAB tests specifically target spatial working memory functions, the spatial span and the self-ordered spatial working memory tasks (referred to below as "spatial search"). Both have been used in the context of PET scanning to resolve a number of theoretical issues concerning the organization of working memory within the frontal lobe. Research in this area has been carried out via lesion and electrophysiologic studies in nonhuman primates (for review see Goldman-Rakic, 1987; Petrides, 1994), neuropsychologic studies of patients with frontal lobe damage or excisions (e.g. Petrides and Milner, 1982; Owen et al., 1990, 1995a,b, 1996c), and functional neuroimaging studies in humans (e.g., Jonides et al., 1993; Petrides et al., 1993a,b; Courtney et al., 1996; Owen et al., 1996a,b; for full review see Owen, 1997b). Two contrasting theories have arisen out of this research, both of which describe a functional difference between the ventrolateral prefrontal cortex, or BA 45 and BA 47, and the dorsolateral prefrontal cortex, or BA 9 and BA 46. The first theory suggests that these two areas subserve the same function of working memory storage and retrieval but differ in terms of the modality of information processed according to their connections to modality-specific posterior cortical regions. Thus, while the dorsolateral prefrontal cortex has been suggested to be specific for spatial information, the ventrolateral prefrontal cortex has been suggested to be specific for object-based information such as shape and color (Goldman-Rakic, 1996). While the delayed response task in nonhuman primates may map onto some of the

CANTAB tests of spatial memory (e.g., spatial recognition memory, or spatial span), it is less clear how the object-based tasks map directly onto tests sensitive to frontal lobe dysfunction in humans, whether from the CANTAB or from the wider neuropsychologic literature. In contrast, the second theory does not suggest that the dorsolateral and ventrolateral prefrontal cortices differ in terms of information modality per se, but rather that they are involved in different working memory processing systems. At a lower level, the ventrolateral prefrontal cortex has been suggested to be concerned primarily with working memory storage and retrieval while at a higher level, the dorsolateral prefrontal cortex has been suggested to be concerned primarily with the implementation of executive functions on information in working memory, for example the use of strategies needed to carry out a task and the manipulation and monitoring of information (Petrides, 1996).

A recent PET study has used the spatial span and the self-ordered spatial search tasks to provide evidence for two working memory processing systems within the lateral prefrontal cortex (Owen et al., 1996b). In this study, normal subjects were scanned while performing five different spatial working memory tasks on a touch-sensitive monitor, including variants of the CANTAB spatial search and spatial span tasks. On subtracting a matched visual control task from the two versions of the search tasks (involving eight or ten search boxes), a significant increase in rCBF was observed in the right mid-dorsolateral prefrontal cortex. A significant increase in rCBF was also observed in the ventrolateral prefrontal cortex during these tasks relative to the visuomotor control task. In contrast, when the control task was subtracted from the spatial span task, there was a similarly significant increase in rCBF in the right midventrolateral prefrontal cortex but no change in the dorsolateral prefrontal region. From these findings, it was suggested that the mid-dorsolateral frontal cortex is only recruited when spatial working memory tasks, such as the CANTAB self-ordered spatial search task, require the active monitoring and manipulation of information within working memory. However, in less complex tasks, such as the CANTAB spatial span task, which simply requires the explicit retrieval of information from working memory, only the ventrolateral prefrontal cortex is required. Further support for this position has been obtained in a recent study using forward and backward spatial span and digit span tasks. Recalling spatial/digit sequences backwards requires the manipulation of information in working memory. Therefore, relative to forward spatial and digit span, backward spatial and digit span tasks require the dorsolateral prefrontal cortex (see Owen, 1997b).

Rapid visual information processing

Sustained attention, or vigilance, is the ability to maintain attention on a series of stimuli over a period of time and is closely related to working memory. The CANTAB rapid visual information processing task (RVIP) is a test of sustained attention that also requires working memory; it has been used in neuropsychologic studies of different patient groups, for example those with dementia implicating the frontal lobe rather than typical Alzheimer's disease (e.g., Coull et al., 1996a).

To investigate the neural network underlying the RVIP task and, thus, sustained attention and working memory, Coull et al. (1996b) used PET to scan a group of four left- and four right-handed healthy male adult subjects during performance of variations of the RVIP task and a control task. For the RVIP task, the subjects were required to monitor a sequence of pseudo-random digits presented on a computer screen at a standard or fast rate and were required to detect prespecified consecutive sequences of two (e.g., 2–4, 6–8) or three digits (e.g., 4–6–8, 3–5–7) by using a simple computer mouse-press response. For the control task, the subjects were similarly presented with pseudo-random digits but were simply required to respond to the occurrence of 0. A rest condition was also used in which the subjects were scanned while keeping their eyes closed. In comparison with the rest condition, the RVIP task caused significant increases in rCBF bilaterally in the inferior frontal gyrus, parietal cortex, and fusiform gyrus, and also in the right rostral superior frontal gyrus. By subtracting the control condition from the RVIP, a similar pattern of activation was observed, except that the increase in rCBF in the right rostral superior frontal gyrus was less significant. Increasing the digit presentation speed was found to increase rCBF bilaterally in the more posterior occipital cortex and fusiform gyrus, whereas changing the working memory load of the task (two sequence versus three sequence detection) had no significant effect on rCBF in any region. No significant effects of handedness were seen.

From their observations, Coull et al. (1996b) suggested that the right rostral superior frontal gyrus may interact with specific areas of the parietal cortex in mediating sustained attention. By comparison, the left inferior frontal gyrus may be involved with specific areas of the parietal cortex in mediating certain components of auditory working memory. One such component is the phonologic loop, a common mechanism of memory rehearsal whereby presented auditory stimuli are repeated continuously in a "loop" to facilitate memory encoding. Other PET studies appear to support the notion that specific areas of the left prefrontal cortex (notably Broca's area) are responsible for subserving the phonologic loop (e.g., Paulesu et al., 1993).

Attentional set-formation and shifting

The CANTAB suite of visual discrimination learning and shifting tests constitutes a decomposition of the WCST and has been shown to be sensitive to effects of frontal lobe excisions in humans, as well as basal ganglia disorders such as Parkinson's and Huntington's diseases and progressive supranuclear palsy (see Owen and Robbins, 1993; Lawrence et al., 1998a). Its suitability for research with nonhuman primates has meant that it has been possible to relate different aspects of visual discrimination learning, including reversal learning (where the reinforcement between two invariant stimuli is switched, e.g., between one shape that is reinforced and another shape that is not) and extradimensional shifting (from a previously relevant perceptual dimension to a previously irrelevant dimension, e.g., from "nonsense" lines to complex shapes), on the basis of shifting reinforcing feedback, as in the WCST (Downes et al., 1989) to different portions of the monkey prefrontal cortex. In the study by Dias et al. (1996), lesions of the orbitofrontal cortex in monkeys disrupted reversal learning but not extradimensional shifting, and lesions of the lateral prefrontal cortex had the reverse pattern of effects. There were no effects of either lesion on intradimensional shifting, where a subject has to shift responses to novel stimuli of the same perceptual dimension. This intradimensional shift condition acts as a control for both of the other forms of shifting. As different regions of the prefrontal cortex project to different areas within the striatum, the results obtained by Dias et al. (1996) could potentially explain the greater susceptibility of patients with Huntington's disease to difficulties with extradimensional shifting early in the course of the disease and to deficits in reversal learning late in the disease process (because of the dorsal to ventral spread of the disease throughout the striatum; Lawrence et al., 1998a).

We have recently completed a $H_2^{15}O$ PET imaging study with an adapted version of the CANTAB attentional set-shifting paradigm in order to test some of the predictions about the neural substrates for the task in healthy male, adult volunteers (Rogers et al., 2000). Subjects were scanned while completing discrimination learning or performance in four main conditions: (i) compound discrimination (i.e., visual discrimination between exemplars varying in at least two perceptual dimensions) where subjects continued to respond on a visual discrimination task learned prior to scanning, (ii) intradimensional shift, (iii) extradimensional shift, and (iv) reversal learning. The four

conditions were repeated three times each (12 scans in all). The design of the stimuli was modified from those used in the original paradigm because of the above-average IQ levels of our volunteer sample. Specifically, stimuli could be derived from three, rather than two, perceptual dimensions. The design allowed several types of comparison: (i) all three conditions with the baseline discrimination task, (ii) comparison of each of reversal and extradimensional shifting with intradimensional shifting and, (iii) the contrast of extradimensional shifting directly with reversal.

The results are complex; some predictions were upheld and others were not. For example, the extradimensional shift did appear to activate the frontal pole (BA 10) on the left side and BA 9/46 on the right. However, no caudate activation was discernible, as might have been predicted from neuropsychologic studies of Huntington's disease. Reversal learning predictably engaged a different circuitry, which, as expected, did include subcortical structures functionally associated with the ventromedial prefrontal cortex, specifically the ventral striatum and (on the first scan only, when the task was novel) the amygdala. However, there was no strong evidence for an activation of the orbitofrontal cortex itself. It is possible that this apparent failure reflects the relatively rapid nature of shifts in reversal learning paradigms. The temporal resolution of PET is approximately 30–90 s and, therefore, PET is limited in its ability to detect instantaneous activation changes associated with shifts in response. We are investigating the above hypothesis further using more difficult reversal tasks where the shift may occur over several trials, which might bring a small orbitofrontal activation suprathreshold; alternatively, the present paradigm may be more successful with imaging modalities with finer temporal resolution, such as fMRI. This experiment, however, does exemplify the importance of cross-validation between different types of neuroimaging modality, as well as with neuropsychologic studies in humans and nonhuman primates, to identify critical neural circuitry.

Visual recognition memory: delayed-matching-to-sample

In the CANTAB, short-term visual recognition memory is assessed using the DMTS task. Performance on this task is particularly affected by temporal lobe excisions (Owen et al., 1995b) and by Alzheimer's disease (Sahakian et al., 1988), which affects posterior cortical regions. Unlike the tests described above, there is relatively little evidence that performance on this test requires the integrity of frontal cortical function, although there is evidence that

DNMTS task performance in monkeys depends on intact ventromedial prefrontal function (see Murray, 1992).

A variation of this task has been used in a PET study by Elliott and Dolan (1998) in an effort to investigate the neural network underlying short-term visual memory. The underlying experimental paradigm was that subjects were presented with a test stimulus composed of four subelements and then, after a short delay of a few seconds, four choice stimuli made of similar subelements. Depending on the condition, the subelements of the choice stimulus were either the same shape as those of the test stimulus but of a different color (*color-only* condition), the same color as those of the test stimulus but of a different shape (*shape-only* condition) or, a mixture of these two (*conjunction* condition). The subjects had to remember and recall the test stimulus on the basis of either the colors of the subelements, the shape, or both the color and the shape of the subelements. The control task was designed to match the perceptual and motor demands of the experimental tasks but lacked a visual memory component. Subjects were presented with four choice stimuli, which were also made up of four subelements but did not bear any resemblance to the preceding test stimuli. The subjects were explicitly instructed not to remember the test stimuli and to respond to the four choice stimuli by simply pressing a prespecified response button.

By subtracting the perceptuomotor control from all of the memory conditions combined, Elliott and Dolan (1998) were able to isolate regions specific to short-term visual memory. These regions included the extrastriate cortex, medial and lateral parietal cortex, anterior cingulate cortex, inferior frontal cortex, and the thalamus. In contrast to many of the tests reviewed above, the DMTS paradigm did not produce a widespread pattern of activation in the prefrontal cortex, congruent with the relative lack of effects of frontal lobe excisions on this task (Owen et al., 1995a). Subtracting the color-only and shape-only conditions from each other showed that these conditions were associated with subtly different activation patterns. However, the conjunction condition was found not to activate any regions that were not already active in the color-only or shape-only condition. This finding suggests that, at least in short-term visual memory, there are no specific cortical regions that are responsible for remembering perceptual conjunctions between features. Rather, there may be specific posterior areas that are responsible for remembering specific types of feature. From their observations, Elliott and Dolan (1998) suggest that the left lingual gyrus may be involved in the memory of color whereas the medial occipital gyrus, right inferior parietal cortex and

precuneus may be specifically associated with memory for shape.

Summary and future directions

The use of functional neuroimaging has greatly increased the power of the CANTAB by enabling the definition of specific neural networks that are necessary for the adequate performance of the different tasks (Fig. 21.2). These data help to validate the neural assumptions of the battery, which are based on studies of humans or monkeys with brain lesions, and also help to isolate discrete cognitive components of the tests, with consequent implications for theories of their underlying cognitive processes. We have also illustrated the use of the tests for analyzing further the nature of the cognitive deficits exhibited in disorders such as depression or Parkinson's disease, a list we can expect to grow longer and to include neurodevelopmental disorders. The particular attractions of CANTAB for this purpose includes (i) its relationship to the existing animal neuropsychologic literature; (ii) its lack of dependence on language functions; and (iii) its componential nature, which is just as well suited to the gradual development of cognitive function as its gradual decline (as occurs in the dementias, which provided the initial impetus for the construction of the battery).

Whereas the $H_2^{15}O$ PET method is powerful, it is likely that it will be supplanted, or at any rate augmented, by alternative neuroimaging methods with greater temporal or chemical specificity. Reference was made to the possibility of using fMRI to resolve some interesting issues for the attentional set-shifting task. So far, this method with its improved temporal resolution has not often been used with the CANTAB; however we expect this to change in the near future in cognitive activation studies, especially with the better prospects offered for imaging children using fMRI than PET (because of the ethical constraints imposed by the latter, see Chapter 2). It is useful to note that there has been a recent study of the "one touch" Tower of London task using fMRI that largely confirmed the results obtained using PET reviewed above (Baker et al., 1996). The "easy" and "difficult" conditions both produced a significant activation of the dorsolateral prefrontal cortex. Dorso–ventral and anterior–posterior extensions of these activations were associated with the increased working memory load involved in planning more difficult solutions (Granon et al., 1998).

It has also proved possible recently to correlate the performance of several of the CANTAB tests, including the Tower of London and spatial span, with levels of dopamine

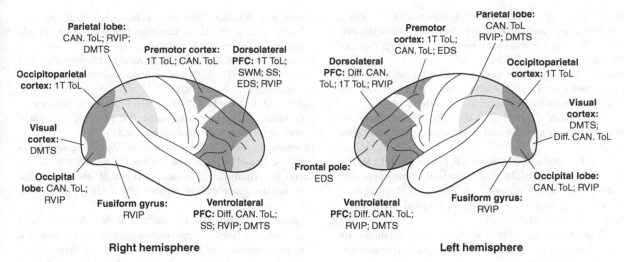

Fig. 21.2. Summary of the cerebral cortical locations of the main activations described for the CANTAB tests described in this chapter. RVIP, rapid visual information processing; SWM, spatial working memory; SS, spatial span; DMTS, delayed-matching-to-sample; CAN. ToL, CANTAB version of the Tower of London; Diff. CAN. ToL, difficult problems (four or more moves) of CAN. ToL; IT ToL, one-touch Tower of London; EDS, extradimensional shift on the attentional set-shifting paradigm; PFC, prefrontal cortex (see text for further details).

D_1 and D_2 receptor ligands in the caudate and putamen of patients with Huntington's disease (Lawrence et al., 1998b), suggesting an approach to understanding the neurochemical basis of performance on some of the tasks. The approach here was one of straightforward correlation of performances on several neuropsychologic tests, including those from CANTAB, measured outside the scanner with indices of ligand binding obtained via PET. This might be expanded still further in light of the exciting recent demonstration of displacement of a dopamine D_2 receptor ligand from binding sites in the ventral striatum by performance of a video game by healthy men (Koepp et al., 1998). A complementary approach is suggested by the results of several recent psychopharmacologic investigations of tests from CANTAB, including effects of adrenergic (clonidine; Coull et al., 1995), cholinergic (scopolamine (hyoscine); Robbins et al., 1997), and dopaminergic agents (methylphenidate, Elliott et al., 1997c). It would obviously be of interest to locate the specific sites at which these drugs are exerting their effects by observing changes in rCBF that correlate with the drug effect. With the availability of specific ligands, including for these drugs themselves, the question of neuroanatomic localization of drug effects can be addressed more directly than has previously been feasible. This will obviously be of considerable significance for our attempts to localize the neural sites of action of compounds, such as methylphenidate, that have special significance for developmental cognitive and behavioral disorders.

Acknowledgements

We acknowledge support from the Wellcome Trust. A. Lee holds a BBSRC studentship. CANTAB is commercially available from CeNeS Cognition, Compass House, Vision Park, Chivers Way, Histon, CB4 4ZR, UK (FAX (0)1223 266467).

References

Abas, M. A., Sahakian, B. J. and Levy, R. (1990). Neuropsychological deficits and CT scan changes in elderly depressives. *Psychol. Med.*, **20**, 507–20.

Baddeley, A. D. (1986). *Working Memory*. New York: Oxford University Press.

Baker, S. C., Rogers, R. D., Owen, A. M. et al. (1996). Neural systems engaged by planning: a PET study of the Tower of London task. *Neuropsychologia*, **34**, 515–26.

Beats, B. C., Sahakian, B. J. and Levy, R. (1996). Cognitive performance in tests sensitive to frontal lobe dysfunction in the elderly depressed. *Psychol. Med.*, **26**, 591–603.

Coull, J. T., Middleton, H. C., Robbins, T. W. and Sahakian, B. J. (1995). Contrasting effects of clonidine and diazepam on tests of working memory and planning. *Psychopharmacology*, **120**, 311–21.

Coull, J. T., Sahakian, B. J. and Hodges, J. R. (1996a). The (α-2 antagonist, idazoxan, remediates certain attentional and executive dysfunction in patients with dementia of frontal type. *Psychopharmacology*, **123**, 239–49.

Coull, J. T., Frith, C. D., Frackowiak, R. S. J. and Grasby, P. M. (1996b). A fronto-parietal network for rapid visual information processing: a PET study of sustained attention and working memory. *Neuropsychologia*, **35**, 515–26.

Courtney, S. M., Ungerleider, L. G., Keil, K. and Haxby, J. V. (1996). Object and spatial visual working memory activate separate neural systems in human cortex. *Cereb. Cortex*, **6**, 39–49.

Dias, R., Roberts, A. and Robbins, T. W. (1996). Dissociation in prefrontal cortex of affective and attentional shifts. *Nature*, **380**, 69–72.

Downes, J. J., Roberts, A. C., Sahakian, B. J., Evenden, J. L., Morris, R. G. and Robbins, T. W. (1989). Impaired extra-dimensional shift performance in medicated and unmedicated Parkinson's disease: evidence for a specific attentional dysfunction. *Neuropsychologia*, **27**, 1329–43.

Elliott, R. and Dolan, R. J. (1998). The neural response in short-term visual recognition memory for perceptual conjunctions. *Neuroimage*, **7**, 14–22.

Elliott, R., Sahakian, B. J., McKay, A. P., Herrod, J. J., Robbins, T. W. and Paykel, E. S. (1996). Neuropsychological impairments in unipolar depression: the influence of perceived failure on subsequent performance. *Psychol. Med.*, **26**, 975–89.

Elliott, R., Frith, C. D. and Dolan, R. J. (1997a). Differential neural response to positive and negative feedback in planning and guessing tasks. *Neuropsychologia*, **35**, 1395–1404.

Elliott, R., Baker, S. C., Rogers, R. D. et al. (1997b). Prefrontal dysfunction in depressed patients performing a complex planning task: a study using positron emission tomography. *Psychol. Med.*, **27**, 931–42.

Elliott, R., Sahakian, B. J., Matthews, K., Bannerjea, A., Rimmer, J. and Robbins, T. W. (1997c). Effects of methylphenidate on spatial working memory and planning in healthy young adults. *Psychopharmacology*, **131**, 196–206.

Elliott, R., McKenna, P. J., Robbins, T. W. and Sahakian, B. J. (1998). Specific neuropsychological deficits in schizophrenic patients with preserved intellectual function. *Cogn. Neuropsychiatry*, **3**, 45–70.

Fowler, K. S., Saling, M. M., Conway, E. L., Semple, J. M. and Louis, W. J. (1997). Computerized neuropsychological tests in the early detection of dementia: prospective findings. *J. Int. Neuropsychol. Soc.*, **3**, 139–46.

Goldman-Rakic, P. S. (1987). Circuitry of primate prefrontal cortex and the regulation of behaviour by representational memory. In *Handbook of Physiology*, Sect. 1, Vol. 5, *The Nervous System*, eds. F. Plum and V. Mountcastle, pp. 373–417. Bethesda, MD: American Physiological Society.

Goldman-Rakic, P. S. (1996). The prefrontal cortex landscape: implications of functional architecture for understanding human mentation and the central executive. *Philos. Trans. R. Soc. Lond. Ser. B.*, **351**, 1445–53.

Granon, S., Anton, J. L., Dauchot, K. et al. (1998). Human prefrontal cortex activity in planning and working memory using functional MRI. In *Proceedings of the 1st FENS Meeting*, Berlin, Germany.

Hughes, C., Russell, J. and Robbins, T. W. (1994). Evidence for executive dysfunction in autism. *Neuropsychologia*, **32**, 477–92.

Hutton, S. B., Puri, B. K., Duncan, L.-J., Robbins, T. W., Barnes, T. R. E. and Joyce, E. M. (1998). Executive function in first-episode schizophrenia. *Psychol. Med.*, **28**, 463–73.

Jonides, J., Smith, E. E., Koeppe, R. A., Awh, E., Minoshima, S. and Mintun, M. A. (1993). Spatial working memory in humans as revealed by PET. *Nature*, **363**, 623–5.

Joyce, E. M. and Robbins, T. W. (1991). Frontal lobe function in Korsakoff and non-Korsakoff alcoholics: planning and spatial working memory. *Neuropsychologia*, **29**, 709–23.

Klosowska, D. (1976). Relation between ability to program actions and location of brain damage. *Pol. Psychol. Bull.*, **7**, 245–55.

Koepp, M. J., Gunn, R. N., Lawrence, A. D. et al. (1998). Evidence for striatal dopamine release during a video game. *Nature*, **393**, 266–8.

Lange, K. W., Sahakian, B. J., Quinn, N. P., Marsden, C. D. and Robbins, T. W. (1995). Comparison of executive and visuospatial memory function in Huntington's disease and dementia of Alzheimer type matched for degree of dementia. *J. Neurol. Neurosurg. Psychiatry*, **58**, 598–606.

Lawrence, A. D., Sahakian, B. J., Hodges, J. R., Rosser, A. E., Lange, K. W. and Robbins, T. W. (1996). Executive and mnemonic functions in early Huntington's disease. *Brain*, **119**, 1633–45.

Lawrence, A., Sahakian, B. J. and Robbins, T. W. (1998a). Cognitive functions and corticostriatal circuits: insights from Huntington's disease. *Trends Cogn. Sci.*, **2**, 379–88.

Lawrence, A. D., Weeks, R. A., Brooks, et al., 1998b). The relationship between striatal dopamine receptor status and cognitive performance in Huntington's disease. *Brain*, **121**, 1343–55.

Luciana, M. and Nelson, C. A. (1998). The functional emergence of prefrontally-guided working memory systems in four-to-eight year old children. *Neuropsychologia*, **36**, 273–93.

Milner, B. (1964). Some effects of frontal lobectomy in man. In *The Frontal Granular Cortex and Behaviour*, ed. J. M. Warren and K. Akert, pp. 313–31. New York: McGraw Hill.

Milner, B. (1971). Interhemispheric difference and psychological processes. *Br. Med. Bull.*, **27**, 272–7.

Milner, B. (1974). Hemispheric specialization: scope and limitations. In *The Neurosciences: Third Study Program*, eds. F. O. Schmitt and F. G. Worden, pp. 75–89. Cambridge, MA: MIT Press.

Mishkin, M. (1982). A memory system in the monkey. *Philos. Trans. R. Soc. Lond. Ser. B.*, **298**, 85–95.

Morris, R. G., Downes, J. J., Evenden, J. L., Sahakian, B. J., Heald, A. and Robbins, T. W. (1988). Planning and spatial working memory in Parkinson's disease. *J. Neurol. Neurosurg. Psychiatry*, **51**, 757–66.

Morris, R. G., Ahmed, S., Syed, G. M. and Toone, B. K. (1993). Neural correlates of planning ability: frontal lobe activation during the Tower of London test. *Neuropsychologia*, **31**, 1367–78.

Murray, E. (1992). What have ablation studies told us about the neural substrates of stimulus memory? *Semin. Neurosci.*, **8**, 13–22.

Olton, D. S. (1982). Spatially organised behaviours of animals: behavioural and neurological studies. In *Spatial Abilities*, ed. M. Potegal, pp. 325–60. New York: Academic Press.

Owen, A. M. (1997a). Cognitive planning in humans: neuropsychological, neuroanatomical and neuropharmacological perspectives. *Prog. Neurobiol.*, **59**, 4321–450.

Owen, A. M. (1997b). The functional organisation of working memory processes within human lateral frontal cortex: The contribution of functional imaging. *Eur. J. Neurosci.*, **9**, 1329–39.

Owen, A. M. and Robbins, T. W. (1993). Comparative neuropsychology of Parkinsonian syndromes. In *Mental Dysfunction in Parkinson's Disease*, eds. P. Wolters and E. C. Scheltens, pp. 221–42. Amsterdam: Vrieje University Press.

Owen, A. M., Downes, J. D., Sahakian, B. J., Polkey, C. E. and Robbins, T. W. (1990). Planning and spatial working memory following frontal lobe lesions in man. *Neuropsychologia*, **28**, 1021–34.

Owen, A. M., Roberts, A. C., Polkey, C. E., Sahakian, B. J. and Robbins, T. W. (1991). Extra-dimensional versus intra-dimensional set-shifting performance following frontal lobe excisions, temporal lobe excisions or amygdalo-hippocampectomy in man. *Neuropsychologia*, **29**, 993–1006.

Owen, A. M., James, M., Leigh, P. N. et al. (1992). Fronto-striatal cognitive deficits at different stages of Parkinson's disease. *Brain*, **115**, 1727–51.

Owen, A. M., Beksinska, M., James, M. et al. (1993). Visuospatial memory deficits at different stages of Parkinson's disease *Neuropsychologia*, **31**, 627–44.

Owen, A. M., Sahakian, B. J., Semple, J., Polkey, C. E. and Robbins, T. W. (1995a). Visual-spatial short term recognition memory and learning after temporal lobe excisions, frontal lobe excisions or amygdalo-hippocampectomy in man. *Neuropsychologia*, **33**, 1–24.

Owen, A. M., Sahakian, B. J., Hodges, J. R., Summers, B. A., Polkey, C. E. and Robbins, T. W. (1995b). Dopamine-dependent fronto-striatal planning deficits in early Parkinson's disease. *Neuropsychology*, **9**, 126–40.

Owen, A. M., Doyon, J., Petrides, M. and Evans, A. C. (1996a). Planning and spatial working memory: a positron emission tomography study in humans. *Eur. J. Neurosci.*, **8**, 353–64.

Owen, A. M., Evans, A. C. and Petrides, M. (1996b). Evidence for a two-stage model of spatial working memory processing within the lateral frontal cortex: a positron emission tomography study. *Cereb. Cortex*, **6**, 31–8.

Owen, A. M., Morris, R. G., Sahakian, B. J., Polkey, C. E. and Robbins, T. W. (1996c). Double dissociations of memory and executive functions in working memory tasks following frontal lobe excisions, temporal lobe excisions or amygdalo-hippocampectomy in man. *Brain*, **119**, 1597–1615.

Owen, A. M., Doyon, J., Dagher, A., Sadikot, A. and Evans, A. C. (1998). Abnormal basal ganglia outflow in Parkinson's disease identified with PET: implications for higher cortical functions. *Brain*, **121**, 949–65.

Pantelis, C., Barnes, T. R. E., Nelson, H. E. et al. (1997). Frontal-striatal cognitive deficits in patients with chronic schizophrenia. *Brain*, **120**, 1823–43.

Passingham, R. E. (1985). Memory of monkeys (*Macaca mulatta*) with lesions in the prefrontal cortex. *Behav. Neurosci.*, **99**, 3–21.

Paulesu, E., Frith, C. D. and Frackowiak, K. S. (1993). The neural correlates of the verbal component of working memory. *Nature*, **362**, 342–5.

Petrides, M. (1994). Frontal lobes and working memory: evidence from investigations of the effects of cortical excisions in non-human primates. In *Handbook of Neuropsychology*, Vol. 9, eds. F. Boller and J. Grafman, pp. 59–82. Amsterdam: Elsevier.

Petrides, M. (1996). Specialized systems for the processing of mnemonic information within the primate frontal cortex. *Philos. Trans. R. Soc. Lond. Ser. B.*, **351**, 1455–61.

Petrides, M. and Milner, B. (1982). Deficits on subject-ordered tasks after frontal and temporal lobe lesions in man. *Neuropsychologia*, **20**, 249–62.

Petrides, M., Alivisatos, B., Evans, A. C. and Meyer, E. (1993a). Dissociations of human mid-dorsolateral from posterior dorsolateral frontal cortex in memory processing. *Proc. Natl. Acad. Sci. USA*, **90**, 873–7.

Petrides, M., Alivisatos, B., Evans, A. C. and Meyer, E. (1993b). Functional activation of the human prefrontal cortex during the performance of verbal working memory tasks. *Proc. Natl. Acad. Sci. USA*, **90**, 878–82.

Rezai, K., Andreasen, N. C., Allinger, R., Cohen, G., Swaze, V. and O'Leary, D. S. (1993). The neuropsychology of the prefrontal cortex. *Arch. Neurol.*, **50**, 636–42.

Robbins, T. W., James, M., Owen, A. M. et al. (1994a). Cognitive deficits in progressive supranuclear palsy, Parkinson's disease and multiple system atrophy in tests sensitive to frontal lobe dysfunction. *J. Neurol., Neurosurg. Psychiatry*, **57**, 79–88.

Robbins, T. W., James, M., Owen, A. M., Sahakian, B. J., McInnes, L. and Rabbitt, P. M. (1994b). The Cambridge Neuropsychological Test Automated Battery CANTAB; a factor analytical study in a large number of normal elderly volunteers. *Dementia*, **5**, 266–81.

Robbins, T. W., James, M., Owen, A. M., Sahakian, B. J., McInnes, L. and Rabbitt, P. M. (1996). A neural systems approach to the cognitive psychology of aging: studies with CANTAB on a large sample of the normal elderly population. In *Methodology of Frontal and Executive Function*, ed. P. M. Rabbit, pp. 215–38. Hove, UK: Lawrence Erlbaum.

Robbins, T. W., Semple, J., Kumar, R. et al. (1997). Effects of scopolamine on delayed-matching-to-sample and paired associates tests of visual memory and learning in human subjects: comparison with diazepam and implications for dementia. *Psychopharmacology*, **134**, 95–106.

Robbins, T. W., James, M., Owen, A. M. et al. (1998). A study of performance on tests from the CANTAB battery sensitive to frontal lobe dysfunction in a large sample of normal volunteers: implications for theories of executive functioning and cognitive aging. *J. Int. Neuropsychol. Soc.*, **4**, 474–90.

Rogers, R. D., Andrews, T. C., Grasby, P. M., Brooks, D. and Robbins, T. W. (2000). Contrasting cortical and sub-cortical PET activations produced by reversal learning and attentional-set-shifting in humans. *J. Cogn. Neurosci.*, **12**, 142–62.

Sahakian, B. M., Morris, R. G., Evenden, J. L. et al. (1988). A comparative study of visuospatial memory and learning in Alzheimer-type dementia and Parkinson's disease. *Brain*, **111**, 695–718.

Sahakian, B. J., Downes, J. J., Eager, S. et al. (1990). Sparing of attentional relative to mnemonic function in a subgroup of patients with dementia of the Alzheimer type. *Neuropsychologia*, **28**, 1197–213.

Sahakian, B. J., Elliott, R., Low, N., Mehta, M., Clark, R. T. and Pozniak, A. L. (1995). Neuropsychological deficits in tests of executive function in asymptomatic and symptomatic HIV-1 seropositive men. *Psychol. Med.*, **25**, 1233–46.

Sahgal, A., Sahakian, B. J., Robbins, T. W. et al. (1991). Detection of visual memory and learning deficits in Alzheimer's disease using the Cambridge Neuropsychological Test Automated Battery. *Dementia*, **2**, 150–8.

Sahgal, A., Galloway, P. H., McKeith, I. G., Edwardson, J. A. and Lloyd, S. (1992). A comparative study of attentional deficits in senile dementias of the Alzheimer and Lewy body types. *Dementia*, **3**, 350–4.

Shallice, T. (1982). Specific impairments of planning. *Philos. Trans. R. Soc. Lond. Ser. B*, **298**, 199–209.

Talairach, J. and Tournoux, P. (1988). *Co-planar Stereotactic Atlas of the Human Brain: 3-Dimensional Proportional System: An Approach to Cerebral Imaging*. Stuttgart: Georg. Thieme Verlag.

22

Neurodevelopmental assessment of cognitive function using CANTAB: validation and future goals

Monica Luciana and Charles A. Nelson

Introduction

Despite the existence of test batteries designed to assess general levels of intellectual ability (e.g., the Wechsler Intelligence Scale for Children (WISC)), well-validated assessments for the study of brain–behavior relations in children are lacking. The establishment of such relations has proven difficult, because it has not been feasible to establish links between brain functioning and overt behavior without the use of invasive strategies that cannot typically be justified for use in healthy children. The discipline of developmental neuropsychology has entered a new era with the advent of brain imaging techniques that are increasingly less invasive from a methodologic standpoint and aimed at elucidating specific structure–function relations (Casey et al., 1995). It is now possible not only to examine the development of specific cognitive behaviors but also to do so within a framework that allows direct observation of brain activity in the course of behavior. What is needed within this context is a battery of tests that reliably reflects localized patterns of neural activity in individuals throughout the lifespan. While instruments have been developed for use with age-specific populations, there are few, if any, instruments that can be used without changes in task presentation, items, or format to test individuals across a broad range of ages. Hence, comparability of findings across age groups is questionable, and the ability to identify developmentally driven changes in functional brain development using such instruments has not been methodologically feasible. The field of experimental neuropsychology provides an exception to this general rule in the form of a recently developed neurobehavioral test battery that has been used successfully to pattern trajectories of normal cognitive development in individuals from ages 4 to 90 years. This battery of tests, the Cambridge Neuropsychological Testing Automated Battery (CANTAB),

was developed at the University of Cambridge, UK by Barbara Sahakian, Trevor Robbins, and their colleagues (see Chapter 21).

CANTAB

Chapter 21 describes the theoretical rationale and validation of CANTAB. It consists of subtasks that index three behavioral domains: working memory/planning, visual memory, and visual attention. Each task is administered through the use of a touch-screen computer and supervised by clinicians trained in neuropsychologic assessment to measure simple reaction time, discrimination learning, recognition memory for patterns and objects, and working memory skills involving self-guided visual search and planning. All CANTAB subtasks are visually guided and require little, if any, verbal mediation and no verbal responses. While the emphasis on nonverbal processes potentially limits the generalizability of findings, it ensures that CANTAB can be used in populations that vary in verbal expertise and/or literacy (Robbins and Sahakian, 1994). Although the CANTAB is currently being used to test individuals with varying levels of language proficiency, the precise limits of language proficiency that are needed to produce valid results have not been determined. Hughes et al. (1994) used selected CANTAB subtasks to study children with autism and mental retardation. Language impairments were present in both populations. In our developmental studies, we have found that healthy children below the age of 4 years are not consistently able to understand task instructions, although this pattern appears to be a consequence of a combination of cognitive immaturity and immature language development. This conclusion is partly based on the observation that older children whom we have tested who are not English

Table 22.1. Pediatric CANTAB studies: number of participants

Age group (years)	Normative sample	Children treated in the neonatal intensive care unit (NICU)	Probands with phenylketonuria (PKU)	Early deprivation (foreign-born adoptees)	Temporal lobe lesion
4	47				
5	41			1	
6	64			1	
7	65	11		3	
8	68	21			
9	34	8		1	
10	6			1	
11	14				1
12	10				
13–19	7		12		
20–29	11		6		
Total group	368 (189M, 179F)	40 (19M, 21F)	18 (9M, 9F)	7 (3M, 4F)	1 (0M, 1F)

Note: M, male; F female.

proficient are able to acquire task instructions nonverbally, through visual observation of the task.

Where CANTAB is unique among experimental test batteries is that, in addition to a rigorous theoretical framework that was used to guide subtest selection, its developers have undertaken a comprehensive effort to validate its neural correlates in adult humans. This validation process has centered around several lines of inquiry: (i) normative studies of behavioral performance in elderly adults, (ii) studies of adults with focal brain lesions, (iii) studies of adults with specific neuropathologies, (iv) the effects of pharmacologic manipulations on task performance, and (v) assessment of brain–behavior correlates using both functional magnetic resonance imaging (fMRI) and positron emission tomography (PET) neuroimaging techniques. These efforts, which have yielded approximately 80 published reports in the period 1990–99, strongly support the CANTAB as a valid measure for the assessment of frontal, temporal, and/or subcortical/striatal functions in adults. While specific aspects of CANTAB performance appear to be affected by dysfunction in these brain regions, use of the CANTAB in neuroimaging contexts permits not only an examination of the brain regions that mediate specific cognitive processes but also an examination of the large-scale neural networks that support cognition (Chapter 21).

Use of the CANTAB in pediatric populations

In contrast to its increasingly widespread use in adult samples, the use of CANTAB with pediatric populations has been quite limited. Prior to 1995, only a single study reported on the use of the CANTAB in impaired children

(Hughes et al., 1994). In 1995, the MacArthur Research Network on Psychopathology and Development began a systematic validation of the CANTAB as an assessment tool for children. As part of this project, we are in the process of collecting normative data from healthy children between the ages of 4 and 18 years (see Luciana and Nelson, 1998), as well as data from several clinical populations (Luciana et al., 1999; M. Luciana, J. Sullivan and C. A. Nelson, unpublished data). Table 22.1 summarizes our sample characteristics to date. Our aim, through this research endeavor, is to generate data on tyically and atypically developing children using a behavioral battery with increasingly well-established neural correlates in adults to determine whether these same correlates exist in children.

The CANTAB appears to be particularly amenable to the study of children. Although the use of computerized assessment in clinical evaluation has been controversial, the computerized format readily lends itself to rapport building, even among atypically developing children. The method of test administration is highly standardized, and variations in findings owing to experimenter error are negligible. Although children must possess enough verbal skill to understand task instructions, there are no additional demands for verbally mediated information processing in the course of testing.

CANTAB and the developmental assessment of frontal lobe function

Because of its role in mediating high-level cognition including working memory and planning functions, the prefrontal cortex is being widely studied from a developmental stand-point (Diamond and Goldman-Rakic, 1989; Diamond, 1990; Welsh et al., 1991; Huttenlocher and Dabhholker, 1997). Based on neurophysiologic studies in humans and primates, it has been suggested that the prefrontal cortex is not physiologically mature in the human until some time point between adolescence and early adulthood. For instance, PET studies have demonstrated that while metabolic activity in the temporal lobes increases within the first 3 postnatal months, similar rates of glucose utilization in the prefrontal cortex are not reached until several months later (Chugani, 1994; Chugani and Phelps, 1986). The process of myelination does not appear to be complete until adolescence, as indicated by autopsy studies (Huttenlocher, 1994; Huttenlocher and Dabhholker, 1997). While synaptogenesis, the formation of functional connections between cells, peaks in the frontal cortex during early childhood, the selective pruning of unnecessary connections follows a more protracted course; synaptic density within the frontal cortex appears to decline well into early adulthood (Huttenlocher, 1994; Huttenlocher and Dabhholker, 1997).

Whether these neural changes are directly correlated with the functional development of the frontal lobe has not been studied in humans. What has been done is to identify behavioral functions that are disrupted by frontal lobe lesions and, hence, mediated by intact frontal functioning. The most consistently employed measure of prefrontal function in experimental studies has been the delayed response task (Jacobsen, 1936), formally similar to Piaget's A-not-B task. Goldman-Rakic and colleagues (Goldman-Rakic, 1987) have convincingly demonstrated that spatial delayed response performance (also referred to as spatial working memory) is mediated by the dorsolateral region of the prefrontal cortex in nonhuman primates. Additionally, there is a correspondence between the development of spatial working memory skills in the monkey and the ontogenetic development of the same abilities in human infants (Diamond and Goldman-Rakic, 1989). That the prefrontal cortex mediates aspects of working memory performance in adults is supported by a plethora of studies (see Damasio and Anderson (1994) and Goldman-Rakic (1987) for reviews). The accurate sensorimotor integration of representational traces linking past events with future goals is core to definitions of working memory (Goldman-Rakic, 1987; Fuster, 1995). Hence, empirical measures that have been used to assess working memory functions in adult humans are relatively complicated in nature and include not only the delayed response task but also temporal judgments (Smith and Milner, 1988), self-ordered searching tasks (Petrides and Milner, 1982), and look-ahead planning tasks (Shallice, 1982). While young chil-

dren, like adults with frontal lobe lesions, might demonstrate the component processes necessary for working memory – that is, intact recognition memory, sensory perception, and motor skills – they may lack the cognitive resources to organize, monitor, and/or strategize their behavioral actions to integrate the present environmental context with future outcomes (Damasio, 1994; Damasio and Anderson, 1994; Luciana and Nelson, 1998). Indeed, it may not be until the age of at least 12 years that children exemplify adult levels of "metacognition": the type of attentional monitoring that permits self-evaluation of ongoing sequences of behavior in an executive manner (Flavell et al., 1966; Passler et al., 1985).

Our research is aimed at examining the emergence of executive functions in normal children between the ages of 4 and 18 years and validating the utility of CANTAB as a measure of frontal lobe function in children. The primary measures of frontal lobe function within the CANTAB battery are (i) spatial working memory, a self-guided search task; (ii) the Tower of London, a test of planning and behavioral inhibition; and (iii) the intradimensional/extradimensional set-shifting task, which measures the ability to shift cognitive response sets both within and across categories. CANTAB measures temporal lobe recognition memory functions through delayed-match-to-sample (DMTS) recognition memory tasks. Functional imaging using PET and fMRI in adults have revealed the neural circuitry underlying performance on variations of these tasks.

CANTAB assessment of frontal lobe function

Spatial working memory

The spatial working memory test is a self-ordered searching task (Petrides and Milner, 1982) that measures working memory for spatial stimuli and requires the subject to use mnemonic information to work toward a goal. On each trial of this task, a number of colored squares are displayed on the screen (Fig. 22.1). The child is told that tokens are hidden inside the colored squares. To find a token, the child must touch the colored squares one at a time to "open" them. If a square contains a token, the child must move it to another area of the screen to "put it away". Each colored square will contain only one token at some point in the course of a trial. Hence, the rule for the task is that once a token is found inside a colored square, there will never be another token inside that same square. In order to perform the task most efficiently without searching repeatedly in previously targeted locations, the child must remember where s/he has *searched and found* a token. Returning to

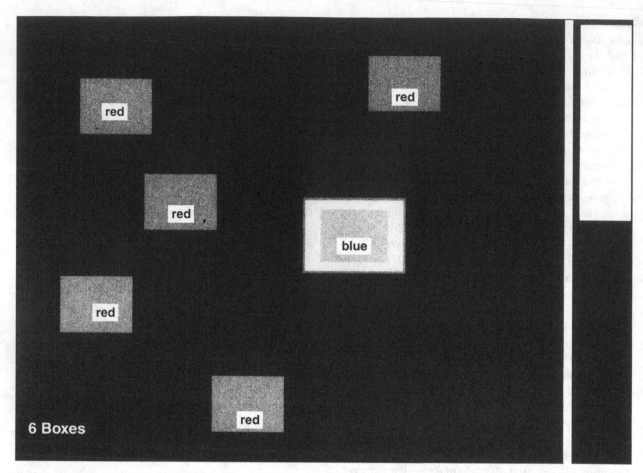

Fig. 22.1. The spatial working memory task. Color names are presented for clarity but are not part of the actual stimulus display. On each trial, colored squares are presented on the screen. The subject must touch a colored square to "open" it. When a blue token is found inside a square, the subject must place it in the black column at the right of the screen. The square then "closes" (i.e., returns to its original color). When the subject begins to search for other tokens, s/he must ignore squares where tokens have been found. If the subject returns to search a location where a token has been found, s/he has made a "forgetting error".

an "empty" box where a token has already been found during a particular search constitutes a "forgetting" error.

The order in which the subject searches the colored squares is self-determined. The number of colored squares starts at two. The subject ultimately completes four trials each with 2, 3, 4, 6, and 8 items.

It is possible to reduce the memory load for a given trial by searching strategically for the tokens. One strategy that has been defined as effective is to follow a predetermined search sequence, beginning with a particular square and then, once a token is found, returning to that same starting point when initiating the next search (Owen et al., 1990; Fray et al., 1996). The extent to which this repetitive search strategy is used is estimated from the number of searches that start with the same location, within each of the 6-item and 8-item searches. A high score (many searches starting with different locations) indicates low use of this strategy, whereas a low score (many searches starting with the same location) indicates more consistent use of this strategy.

Based on PET data, this task appears to activate both the dorsal and ventral prefrontal regions (Owen et al., 1996a). Additionally, adult neurosurgical patients with frontal lobe lesions demonstrate distinct patterns of performance, namely high numbers of mnemonic errors as well as deficient use of strategy in guiding their performance (Owen et al., 1990, 1996c). These errors occur at all levels of task difficulty and appear to be restricted to working memory within the spatial (versus verbal) domain (Owen et al., 1996c). In contrast, patients with damage to the temporal lobe demonstrate a high number of mnemonic errors but in the context of normal strategy use. Their mnemonic errors appear to occur only at the most difficult levels of the

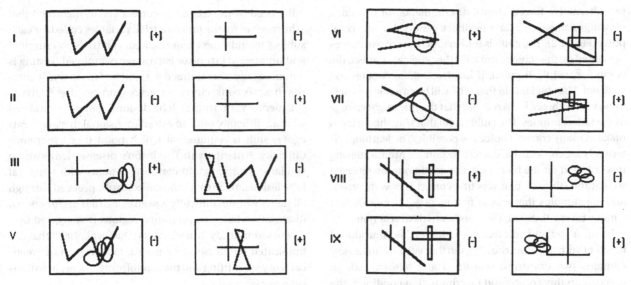

Fig. 22.2. The intradimensional/extradimensional set-shifting task. The subject views two patterns on the screen and must select the one that is "correct". If the subject selects the correct pattern, it turns green, providing positive reinforcement to the subject. The first two stages of the task involve (I) discriminating between two lined patterns and then (II) reversing one's response to the other pattern when selection of the first one is no longer reinforced. On subsequent stages of the task (III, IV, and V), a second shaped pattern is added to the lined patterns. The subject is reinforced for continuing to respond to lined patterns while ignoring the "shape" dimension. The first demand for a shift occurs at stage VI. The subject views new exemplars of lines and shaped figures but is still reinforced for responding to lines at stages VI and VII (intradimensional shift and reversal, respectively). At stages VIII and IX, the subject is reinforced for switching his/her responses from "line" to "shape" (the extradimensional shift and reversal). Note, stage IV is intentionally omitted from the figure because it does not add significant graphical information.

task (Owen et al., 1996c). Using a modified version of the spatial working memory task, Owen and colleagues (1996a) have demonstrated that when normal control subjects perform the most difficult task items in the course of PET neuroimaging, significant changes in regional cerebral blood flow (rCBF) are evident in the right mid-dorsolateral prefrontal cortex as well as bilaterally in the ventrolateral frontal region. Additionally, the right hippocampus is activated. These findings have led Owen and colleagues (1996a, p. 1611) to conclude that "spatial working memory involves a network of interconnected and functionally related cortical and subcortical areas including, at the very least, the prefrontal cortex and the hippocampus", a viewpoint that is consistent with what has been found in nonhuman primates (Goldman-Rakic, 1987).

Intradimensional/extradimensional set-shifting

One of the most popularly used measures for the assessment of frontal lobe dysfunction is the Wisconsin Card Sort Test (WCST; Milner, 1964). It is a well-established phenomenon that patients with frontal lobe dysfunction, as well as patients with schizophrenia, demonstrate a high number of

errors on this test, and perseverative errors in particular. Since the WCST requires the examinee to shift response set among three dimensions (color, shape, and number) in response to verbal feedback (correct or incorrect), deficient performance has been attributed to the inability to shift response set between conceptual categories. However, the precise nature of the cognitive deficit underlying task failure has yet to be determined, because the task actually requires several abilities, including the ability to discriminate relative stimulus cues perceptually, the ability to respond to feedback about correct versus incorrect performance, the ability to attend selectively to one response set when another is present, and the ability to shift between sets. Through the intradimensional/extradimensional set-shift task, the CANTAB provides a method to assess these separate components of cognitive function within the same task.

This task measures discrimination and reversal learning under conditions in which the subject is required to shift attention to changing patterns of visual stimuli. A full description can be found in Downes et al. (1989). Briefly, this task progresses along a series of stages of increasing difficulty (Fig. 22.2). In the first stage (termed the "simple discrimination" stage), the child is required to learn a two-alternative forced-choice discrimination of two lined drawings using immediate feedback provided by the computer (Fig. 22.2). The child is told to touch one of two figures presented on the screen, and if his/her choice is correct, the computer will flash green; if incorrect, the computer will flash red. The child is told that s/he will learn a rule to determine which choice is correct but that the rule might change as the task continues. The child is told that s/he should try to make as many correct choices as possible. The learning criterion is six consecutive correct responses. After achieving this criterion on the first stage, the conditions are reversed so that the stimulus that was first correct is now incorrect, and the stimulus that was at first incorrect is now correct (simple reversal). Again, there are six trials to criterion.

Next, a second dimension (shapes) is introduced together with the lined drawings so that each stimulus now contains two drawings: one lined and one shaped. To succeed on this compound discrimination condition, the subject must continue to respond to the previously relevant dimension ("respond to lines") while ignoring the presence of the new irrelevant dimension (shapes). Two compound discrimination conditions (stage III and stage IV) are administered, one where the lined and shaped drawings are presented separately (e.g., side by side) and one where the stimuli are superimposed upon each other. Following successful completion of these two conditions, there is a compound discrimination reversal (i.e., the correct stimulus becomes incorrect and vice versa).

The next (VIth) stage involves the first demand for an attentional shift using novel stimuli. Termed the intradimensional shift stage, novel or never-seen exemplars of each of the two dimensions (line and shape) are introduced without further instructions, and the subject's responses to the previously relevant dimension (lined drawings) are correct. Success on this stage requires that the subject generalize the rule from previous learning (e.g., "lined drawings are correct") to new stimuli. Following another intradimensional reversal, a demand for a second type of attentional shift is imposed. This stage is termed the extradimensional shift. Once again, novel exemplars of each stimulus dimension are presented without further instructions. To succeed at the extradimensional shift stage, the subject must shift response set from the previously relevant dimension (lines) to the previously irrelevant dimension (shapes). This shift requires that the subject learn and respond to a new rule (e.g., "lines are no longer correct; shapes are correct"). This stage is presumably analogous to the types of category shift that are required by more difficult tests of set-shifting ability such as the WCST. The final task stage is a reversal of the extradimensional shift.

Each response made by the subject is presumably influenced by the feedback (correct versus incorrect) that s/he receives on the previous trial. Variables coded for each subject include the stage reached, the trials to criterion, and number of errors for each stage completed. Testing is automatically discontinued if a subject fails to reach criterion (i.e., six consecutive correct responses) after 50 trials.

Patients with frontal lobe lesions generally proceed without difficulty until an extradimensional (between-category) shift is required, at which point they experience difficulty. Patients with Parkinson's disease demonstrate similar impairments. In contrast, patients with temporal lobe lesions, relative to normal controls, proceed through all stages without difficulty (Owen et al., 1991). A functional dissociation between prefrontal regions is suggested by a recent lesion study in marmosets (Dias et al., 1996) that has implicated the dorsolateral prefrontal cortex in between-category set shifting and the orbitofrontal cortex in within-category reversal shifts.

Planning and behavioral inhibition: the Tower of London

The Tower of London task was first described by Shallice (1982) and measures planning and behavioral inhibition. It is described in detail in Chapter 21 and illustrated in Fig. 21.1. The task has a minimum number of moves in which it can be completed successfully, and the solution can be reached after a minimum of two, three, four, or five moves. For each trial, the number of moves to complete the trial, as well as execution times, are recorded.

Additionally, the child completes a "yoked control" condition in order to provide baseline measures of motor initiation and execution times. On each trial of the control condition, the computer executes a series of moves using the stimuli on the top half of the screen. The subject is required to imitate this sequence of movements using his/her balls on the bottom half of the screen. The movements are designed to require visuomotor integration and to occur one ball at a time; that is, the computer moves one ball, following which the child copies the computer's move. This task is yoked to the first half of the test in that for each trial of the yoked condition, the movements of the balls are exact replicas of moves made by the child in the corresponding test trials. The measurement of the selection and execution latencies in the yoked condition provides baseline estimates of motor initiation and execution times (Veale et al., 1996). These movement times are then used to derive measures of planning or "thinking" times in the experimental task. In each problem, the initial thinking time is the time between the initial presentation of the problem and the first touch minus the corresponding motor initiation time as calculated from the yoked control task. The subsequent thinking time is the time between the first move and the completion of the problem minus the total motor execution time derived from the control task.

In all, the following variables are computed for each problem set representing four levels of problem difficulty (2-, 3-, 4-, and 5-move problems): average number of moves to complete each set, initial thinking time, and subsequent thinking time. For the purpose of data analysis, two variables are of primary interest: the average number of moves to complete each problem set and initial thinking (i.e., planning) times.

Adults with either unilateral or bilateral frontal lobe lesions require more moves to solve Tower of London problems than do normal controls (Owen et al., 1990). Their initial planning times (the time before starting a given problem) do not differ from those of normal control subjects but their subsequent thinking times are increased. Owen et al. (1990) interprets this pattern as evidence that patients with frontal lesions, unlike patients with temporal lobe lesions, frequently initiate a response before fully thinking it through.

This task has been modified for use in a neuroimaging environment. Briefly, subjects are required to solve the problems mentally and then report the number of moves required. PET imaging has been conducted in normal adults during the problem-solving phase of the task. A distributed network of cortical areas including bilateral prefrontal, cingulate, and parietal cortices was activated (Baker et al., 1996). Of significance is the fact that increased problem difficulty was associated with activation in right rostral prefrontal cortex. Concordantly, Morris et al. (1993), using single photon emission computed tomography (SPECT), reported increased regional cerebral blood flow in the left prefrontal cortex during planning compared with that in a motor control task. This lateralized activation was particularly associated with increased planning time, as well as increased efficiency of task performance.

Other abilities measured by CANTAB

Although the strength of the CANTAB lies in its use as a tool for the assessment of frontostriatal dysfunction, several other tasks included in the battery rely on other neural circuitry underlying basic neuropsychologic functions. Among these functions are psychomotor speed and accuracy, memory-storage capacity, and recognition memory. In our normative studies, we have included three other CANTAB tasks as controls for the frontal lobe-mediated behavioral functions that are of primary interest.

Motor screening task

The motor screening task measures psychomotor speed and accuracy. The child's task is to touch visual targets that are presented one at a time on the computer screen quickly and accurately. Accuracy and response latency are recorded.

Spatial span task

The spatial span task is based on the Corsi block task (Milner, 1971) and measures memory for a spatial sequence. Briefly, on each trial, the child views an array of 10 white boxes displayed on the computer screen. At the start of the task, two boxes change color one at a time, in a sequence. After completion of the sequence, the child hears a beep that signals him/her to reproduce the sequence (e.g., touch the box that changed color first, then the box that changed color second, and so on). If the child reproduces the two-item sequence correctly by touching the boxes in the correct order, the computer advances to the next trial, which includes a sequence of three boxes. The maximum sequence length (which defines the length of the child's memory span) that can be achieved is nine. The child has three attempts at each difficulty level to pass that level. If the child fails all three attempts at a difficulty level, the test is terminated. Prior to the start of test trials, the child is given two practice trials to assure his/her understanding of the task.

The verbal counterpart to this test is the digit span test of the Wechsler Intelligence Scales and/or the Wechsler Memory Scale.

This task differs from the spatial working memory task described above in that it yields a measure of nonverbal memory capacity rather than the extent to which memory can be utilized to reach a self-directed goal. Typically, we have found that an individual's memory span is negatively correlated with the number of forgetting errors on the spatial working memory task (Luciana and Nelson, 1998). However, the spatial working memory task uniquely measures executive skills that are nonmnemonic in nature. For example, the spatial working memory strategy score is not necessarily related to memory span but is dependent upon behavioral organization.

Pattern recognition

Pattern recognition employs a DMTS paradigm to measure recognition memory for visual patterns. (CANTAB also includes a more-complicated DMTS task that was not used in our normative study because of its increased time demands.) For each of two blocks, the subject is told to

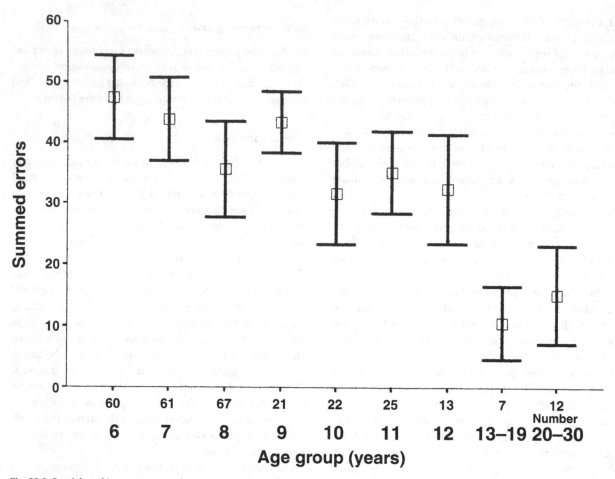

Fig. 22.3. Spatial working memory performance. The means and 95% confidence intervals for the number of forgetting errors summed across searches of 6 and 8 items are represented by age group. As described in the text, performance has not reached adult levels by the age of 12 years.

attend to the computer screen. At the center of the screen, a series of geometric patterns is presented one after the other for a 3 s viewing interval. Following the presentation of the pattern series, the screen "pauses" for a duration of 5 s, after which the subject is presented with two geometric patterns. One of the two designs is from the previously viewed list. The other is a completely novel stimulus. The two designs differ in shape but not in color. The child is told to touch the design that s/he remembers having seen. Twelve trials, one containing each of the 12 target stimuli, are presented in each of the two blocks for a total of 24 trials. Accuracy and response latency are recorded. The percentage of correct responses across both blocks is used to represent the subject's pattern recognition score. Notably, performance on this task is highly sensitive to posterior brain lesions in adult patients and appears to be unaffected by frontal lobe pathology (B. J. Sahakian, personal communication 1998).

In addition to the specific brain–behavior correlates described above for these subtasks, the CANTAB appears to be sensitive to fluctuations in ascending cholinergic and monoaminergic neurotransmitter levels, as is apparent from several recent treatment studies in patients with dementia and in acute pharmacologic challenges with normal volunteers (Robbins et al., 1994; Robbins, 1996).

Developmental findings

Our data consistently indicate that planning and working memory skills have not reached adult levels by the age of 12 years. This conclusion is illustrated based on analysis of two CANTAB tasks that are reliable correlates of frontal lobe function in adults: the Tower of London and the spatial working memory task. As can be seen in Fig. 22.3, the number of total forgetting errors on the spatial working memory task is con-

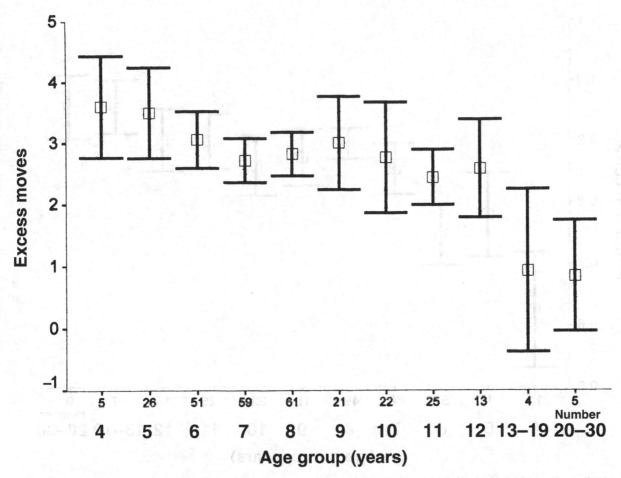

Fig. 22.4. Tower of London performance by age group. The average number of excess moves (means and 95% confidence intervals) to complete the most difficult 5-move problems are displayed as a function of age group. A score of "0" represents perfect performance.

sistently high from 5 to 12 years of age. Although sample sizes are small (13) for children above the age of 11, it appears that forgetting errors have declined significantly by 20 years of age. Additionally, when performance on the most difficult problems of the Tower of London is examined, a similar profile is evident (Fig. 22.4). Figure 22.4 indicates the average number of moves used to solve the most difficult 5-move problems by children between the ages of 5 and 18 years. As can be seen, 12-year-old children are still making a number of "excess" moves to solve the problems relative to young adults, indicating that their "look ahead planning skills" are not fully developed. These findings are consistent with the literature demonstrating a protracted course of neurodevelopment of prefrontal, relative to other, brain regions through early adolescence (Huttenlocher, 1994; Huttenlocher and Dabhholker, 1997).

In contrast, abilities that rely on posterior brain regions, including pattern recognition memory (Fig. 22.5), appear

to plateau by the age of 8. Although the pattern recognition memory test requires a forced response to one of two choices, leading to the possibility that these findings may indicate a ceiling effect on performance in older children, these findings are consistent with a large body of literature indicating early maturity of the temporal lobe hippocampal system that supports visual recognition memory (see Nelson (1995) for a review). Conversely, abilities that involve interactions between posterior brain regions and the frontal lobe, such as spatial memory span, show an intermediate developmental pattern, whereby there appear to be linear increments in memory span from 4 years of age (Fig. 22.6).

It is unclear how performance on the CANTAB relates to more general measures of intellectual function (e.g., IQ) in normally developing children. To estimate verbal and performance IQ, respectively, we have included two subtests from the Wechsler Intelligence Scale for Children-third

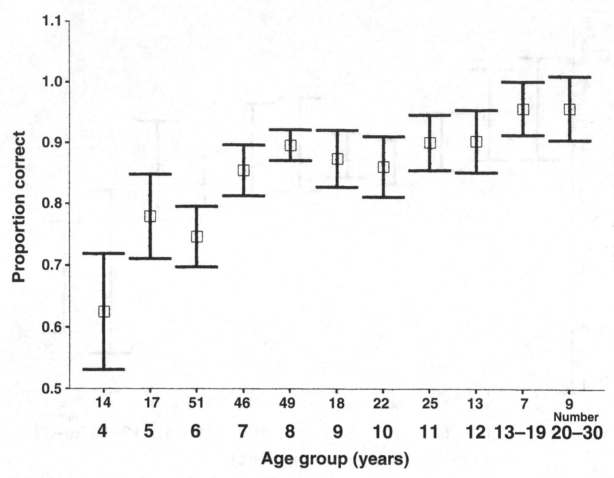

Fig.22.5. Pattern recognition scores as a function of age group. Boxes represent the means and bars represent the 95% confidence interval for the proportion of correct responses out of a total of 24 trials.

edition (WISC-III). These are the vocabulary and the block design subtests, both of which are highly representative of full-scale IQ scores (Sattler, 1992). Preliminary data indicate that there are not significant correlations between Wechsler vocabulary scores and CANTAB performance in school-aged children (see Table 22.2). However, correlations between Wechsler block design scores and CANTAB performance are moderate with respect to several subtasks. These data further validate the CANTAB as primarily a measure of nonverbal information processing skill.

Having developed a normative database from which to infer the natural trajectory of functional development of memory and problem-solving skills in children, two goals remain. The first is to assess whether CANTAB is a useful tool for identifying neuropsychologic impairments in pediatric populations and whether differential patterns of performance will be reliably observed in distinct clinical subsamples relative to normal controls. The second goal is to link both the normative and clinical performance para-

meters to brain functioning using electrophysiology, psychopharmacologic manipulations, and functional brain imaging.

Clinical validation of CANTAB in children with neurologic disorders

Adolescents with phenylketonuria

Phenylketonuria (PKU) is an inborn disorder of metabolism whereby an individual cannot metabolize phenylalanine. Because phenylalanine is present in a typical diet, toxic levels build up in the bodies and nervous systems of affected individuals, resulting in mental retardation and other disturbances. Successful treatment requires early identification of the disorder and dietary restriction of phenylalanine. Although restriction of phenylalanine appears to prevent mental retardation, there have been

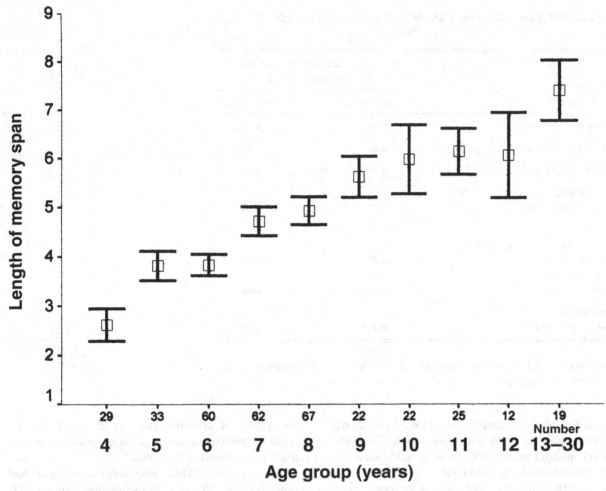

Fig. 22.6. Spatial memory span as a function of age group. Maximum memory span that can be achieved is nine; the minimum span possible is zero. Boxes represent means and bars represent the 95% confidence intervals for performance within each age group.

several reports of deficits in executive functions in individuals treated early and continuously for PKU. These deficits may be a consequence of decreased dopaminergic activity in frontal cortex resulting from low tyrosine levels. Tyrosine is a necessary precursor for dopamine synthesis and may be decreased when phenylalanine levels are high (see Diamond et al. (1997) for a review). In a study directed at cognitive outcomes in adolescents and young adults with PKU (M. Luciana, J. Sullivan and C. A. Nelson, unpublished data), the CANTAB was administered to 18 individuals who had been treated since birth at the PKU clinic at the University of Minnesota Hospital, and the data were compared with those of several groups of age-matched controls. This study is unique in that only individuals with IQ values in the normal range were selected for study. Additionally, it is one of the few studies of long-term cognitive outcome in PKU. Data from young children treated

from birth for PKU have suggested deficits in executive functions (Diamond et al., 1997), raising the concern of significant cognitive deficit even in individuals without impaired general intelligence.

Our data indicate that it is not necessarily the case that young adults with PKU show stable (i.e., trait) deficits on tests of executive function relative to age-matched controls. Rather, performance on the Tower of London, spatial working memory, and set-shifting tasks appears to be moderated by phenylalanine levels, even after controlling for IQ levels. Those PKU probands with high phenylalanine levels, presumably resulting from inadequately controlled diets, demonstrate impaired executive function, while those with lower phenylalanine levels achieve scores that are comparable to those of normal controls. In contrast, performance on the pattern recognition memory, motor screening, and spatial memory span tasks appears to be

Table 22.2. *Correlations between CANTAB performance and Wechsler IQ subtests*

CANTAB variable	Correlation coefficients[a] for Wechsler subtest scaled scores	
	Block design	Vocabulary
Motor response accuracy	−0.09	−0.09
Motor response latency	−0.09	−0.05
Spatial memory span	0.41*	0.14
Spatial working memory		
Total forgetting errors	−0.07	0.06
Strategy score	−0.08	−0.03
Tower of London moves to complete		
3-move problems	−0.19	−0.28*
4-move problems	0.03	−0.15
5-move problems	0.04	0.03
Pattern recognition		
Proportion correct responses	0.42*	0.51*

Notes:
[a] Correlation coefficients are partial correlations for 105 children in the normative sample, ages 6 to 9 years, with age partialled out.
* $p < 0.01$.

unrelated to phenylalanine levels and does not diverge from that observed in the normative sample. These preliminary findings using CANTAB support the view that subtle alterations in neurotransmission to the frontal cortex (see Diamond et al., 1997) may be present in young adults who have been treated early for PKU, and that these alterations exert subtle, but measurable, effects on frontal lobe-mediated working memory and planning skills (M. Luciana, J. Sullivan and C. A. Nelson, unpublished data).

Children with histories of neonatal neurologic injury

Cognitive deficits are believed to be common sequelae of high-risk births (Volpe, 1995; Ross et al., 1996). Yet the impact of early adverse neurologic events on school-aged children who are placed in mainstream classrooms has not been widely studied. To investigate these effects, the CANTAB was administered to school-aged children (age 7–9 years) who were preterm infants treated at birth in the neonatal intensive care unit (NICU) at the University of Minnesota Children's Hospital. Perinatal events that place infants at risk for neurocognitive sequelae were quantified by chart review and included degree of prematurity, hypoxia, the presence of intraventricular hemorrhage, intrauterine growth retardation (birth weight z-scores < 2),

development of bronchopulmonary dysplasia (supplemental oxygen requirement at 28 days), apnea, and neonatal seizures (Luciana et al., 1999).

Findings for the NICU survivors, relative to age-matched normal controls differ from those obtained from the PKU sample. In addition to demonstrating slower and less-accurate responses on the motor screening task, as well as more errors in pattern recognition memory and decreased length of memory span (which would suggest subcortical and/or temporal lobe pathology), NICU survivors showed strikingly deficient spatial working memory performance, making approximately 25% more forgetting errors than age-matched subjects in the normative sample (Fig. 22.7).

Additionally, the NICU group had a higher mean strategy score (indicating lower use of organized searching) than the normative group (Fig. 22.7). With respect to planning skills, NICU and normative groups did not differ in their total number of moves made to complete Tower of London problems, but the average planning time across problem sets was longer in NICU survivors. Motor initiation times did not differ between groups for yoked control problems, indicating that these latency differences are not a result of group differences in simple motor initiation processes in response to Tower of London task stimuli.

Several factors were considered as potential moderators

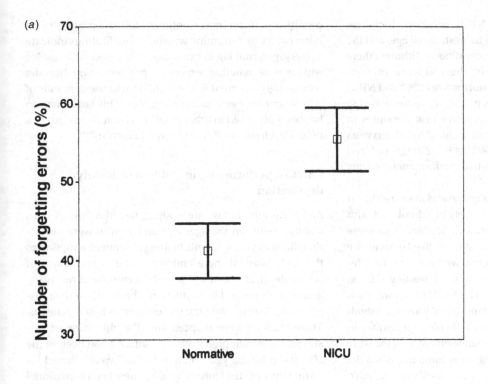

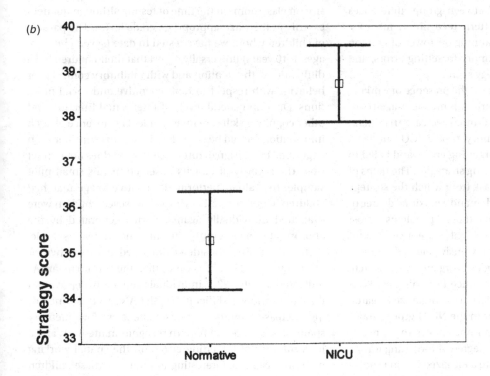

Fig. 22.7. Spatial working memory performance at 7–9 years of age in children requiring treatment at birth in a neonatal intensive care unit (NICU). Relative to children in the normative sample ($n = 86$), NICU survivors ($n = 39$) make more forgetting errors (*a*) and have higher strategy scores, indicating decreased use of strategic searching (*b*), suggesting that they are experiencing impairments in organizational skills mediated by the prefrontal cortex.

of the deficits found in the NICU survivors, including gender, handedness, birth weight, gestational age, and the presence of specific neurologic conditions. Although there was a significant difference in the incidence of non-righthandedness between the normative (17%) and NICU (28%) groups, handedness was not significantly related to performance on any of the cognitive task measures in either group. Additionally, classification of NICU survivors by birth weight (<1500, 1500–2499, 2500 g) did not significantly distinguish cognitive performance on any task.

All but one child in the NICU group was placed either at or above their expected grade levels in school, but with some parental reports of academic difficulties. Since these difficulties were not assessed in a standardized manner, we conservatively identified each child with a reported academic problem (typically in the domain of reading skill) as "potentially learning disabled". The NICU group was then divided into those children with potential learning disabilities and those without reported difficulty. No significant differences in cognitive performance on any task measure were found between these subgroups. Similarly, when the group with potential learning disabilities was excluded from the overall analyses comparing the NICU and normative groups, significant between-group differences remained with respect to pattern recognition memory, spatial memory span, slow planning on Tower of London problems, spatial working memory forgetting errors, and spatial working memory strategy score.

The results of this study suggest the presence of working and recognition memory impairments in school-aged children with histories of neonatal intensive care treatment. On the spatial working memory task, NICU survivors exhibited a high number of forgetting errors and failed to organize efficient problem-solving strategies. The items of the spatial working memory task from which the strategy score is derived are those that demand a maximal degree of "multi-tasking". To perform these problems most efficiently, one must remain highly attentive, recruit memory skills to remember previously selected and targeted locations, develop strategies to organize each search, and maintain use of a strategy once it is initiated. With increased task difficulty, initiation of organized search strategies is less likely to occur in the NICU group, and if strategies are initiated, they do not appear to be maintained, as indicated by a high degree of forgetting errors. These findings may not indicate a localized lesion process in NICU survivors but rather may indicate that the entire brain performs less efficiently under high demand. This interpretation would appear to be most consistent with our inability to associate any one neonatal risk factor with

cognitive performance. Continued follow-up assessment is necessary to determine whether these findings indicate a developmental lag in brain maturation that will resolve with age or whether executive problems will become increasingly apparent in these children as the demands of school and life become more rigorous. This latter pattern has been observed in other conditions that demonstrate a neurodevelopmental course (Weinberger, 1988).

CANTAB performance in children with early deprivation

Another group that we are studying includes foreign-born children between the ages of 4 and 10 who were institutionalized as young infants before subsequent adoption to the USA. Most of these children endured conditions of severe deprivation, in terms both of emotional nurturing and of environmental stimulation. The details of their histories are diverse, and their presentation is heterogeneous. Three children were adopted from the Philippine Islands and four were adopted from Romania. All had been in the USA for at least a year when tested and were referred for testing through the University of Minnesota's International Adoption Clinic. All adoptees were functioning in mainstream classrooms at the time of testing although not necessarily at their age-appropriate grade levels. The parents of children whom we have tested to date (seven children, ages 4–10 years) universally report that their children have difficulties with attention and with inhibitory control over behavior with respect to both cognitive and social functions. Data on general levels of intellectual function and other cognitive skills are unavailable. The absence of such information should be considered a serious consideration in guiding the design of future studies but does not detract from the severity of deficits observed in this small pilot sample. To evaluate performance relative to age-matched children in our normative sample, the seven children were evaluated individually against norms generated by the appropriate age group in the normative sample. Performance was considered impaired if it was two or more standard deviations worse than the control mean. As indicated in Table 22.3, individuals with early deprivation display a variety of difficulties with CANTAB tasks, including increased motor response latencies, low memory spans, low accuracy of pattern recognition memory, and a high number of forgetting errors on the spatial working memory task. It is interesting to note that these children are similar in their performance to the children with neonatal neurologic injuries. Unfortunately, the adoptive parents rarely knew details of the birth and prenatal histories of their children, so the relative contributions of pre-

Table 22.3. Cognitive impairments in children with neurodevelopmental neurologic disorders

CANTAB measure	Children with phenylketonuria	Children treated in the neonatal intensive care unit	Children with early deprivation (adoptees)	Temporal lobe lesion
Number	18	40	7	1
Motor accuracy		X		
Motor latency			X	X
Memory span		X	X	X
Spatial working memory errors over 6–8 item searches	X	X	X	
Spatial working memory strategy		X	X	
Tower of London average moves	X		X[a]	
Tower of London planning time		X	X[a]	
Attentional set-shifting			X	X
Pattern recognition		X	X	
Locus of dysfunction	Frontal	Diffuse	Diffuse	Temporal

Notes:

[a] The difficulties that this population appears to have with the Tower of London are unique for their age group(s). Of seven children tested, only three understood the task requirements well enough to complete at least one block of items. This pattern is characteristic of 4 year olds whom we have tested in our normative sample and was not a result of simple language impairment per se, but rather of an inability to grasp conceptually what was being required by the task.

and perinatal complications verus early postnatal deprivation cannot be determined. However, we hope to be able to obtain this information in the form of a more comprehensive neurologic assessment as our study progresses.

Focal brain lesions

A body of literature has demonstrated that adults with focal lesions display distinctive patterns of performance on the CANTAB (Owen et al., 1990, 1991, 1995, 1996b,c). Whether CANTAB can be used to identify similar problems in children is unknown, as a comparable literature does not exist for children with acquired focal lesions. To begin to investigate such relationships, we have repeatedly tested one child, an 11-year-old girl, during the course of treatment for temporal lobe epilepsy that began after an episode of status epilepticus when she was 18 months old.

This patient was tested at three intervals: at age 11 years, several days prior to neurosurgery; 2 weeks following a right temporal lobe excision; and 1 year postsurgery. Functional and structural MRI and a complete neuropsychologic workup were also done. In adult patients with temporal lobe lesions, deficits in visual memory are apparent (Owen et al., 1995). Relative to other children in her age group prior to surgery, this patient had a spatial memory span of five items (corresponding to the 50th percentile

relative to others (n = 23) in her age group). She performed at the 85th percentile with respect to spatial working memory error scores. Her performance on the Tower of London planning task was generally within the normal range. On the set-shifting task, she successfully completed all stages of the task but made a high number of errors when there was a demand for the first within-category attentional shift. Her pattern recognition performance was at the 60–75th percentile.

Immediately postsurgery, several functions were noted to have markedly improved, while there were transient decrements in selective frontal lobe functions, namely in spatial working memory (where she demonstrated a high number of forgetting errors and decreased strategy use). Her spatial memory span increased from 5 to 7 items (70–90th percentile). Her pattern recognition memory performance was 100% correct, unchanged from her performance prior to surgery. Tower of London performance was unchanged. On the set-shifting task (where different items were used from the original test session), she made negligible errors when demands in set-shifting were required. One year later, this patient was completely seizure free for the first time since infancy. Memory span had dramatically increased to eight items, comparable with the 95th percentile for her age. Spatial working memory errors dropped by 45% (relative to immediate postsurgery values), and a

10% improvement in her use of strategy was noted. Tower of London performance remained unaltered. Set-shifting and recognition memory skills remained identical to those measured immediately postsurgery.

To summarize, the most dramatic gain observed from before surgery to 1 year postsurgery was in the length of her memory span, which increased from five to eight items. While test–retest reliability studies of CANTAB performance in children have not been conducted, this magnitude of gain would not be expected within a single year of normal development based on cross-sectional normative data. Her spatial recognition memory performance had also improved from 65 to 80% correct. Spatial working memory errors demonstrated a transient increase immediately postsurgery, suggesting a temporary disorganization in the brain network mediating this behavior, but stabilized 1 year later, showing a 30% improvement over initial testing.

Other clinical groups

CANTAB has been used to assess the patterns of impairment observed in several distinct populations of children with neurologic and/or neurodevelopmental impairments. The results are summarized in Table 22.3.

In addition to the work described above conducted in our laboratories, several other sites affiliated with the MacArthur Research Network on Psychopathology and Development are using the CANTAB to study children, including those with attention-deficit hyperactivity disorder (Dr Ellen Lipman at McMaster University), autism (Dr Geraldine Dawson at the University of Washington), anxiety disorders (Dr Kathleen Merikangas at Yale University), children of depressed mothers (Dr Geraldine Dawson), and adolescents with histories of violent offenses (Drs Laurence Steinberg and Elizabeth Cauffman at Temple University and Stanford University, respectively). Through these endeavors, the discriminative validity of specific CANTAB tasks for identifying individuals with specific disorders affecting cognitive function will be further assessed.

In summary, the CANTAB is a useful tool for the study of cognitive development in children. While the CANTAB appears to be a sensitive instrument for the assessment of neurobehavioral injury in children, its specificity with respect to localized brain impairment has yet to be demonstrated (linkage to discrete brain regions cannot be determined at this time). Nonetheless, because its neural correlates have been established in adult populations, informed hypotheses about localized brain dysfunction in children, such as those involved in our studies of PKU and

neonatal neurologic injury, are available. Although the clinical samples that we have tested involve cases with heterogeneous presentations (e.g., the NICU children), we believe that they are representative of the types of case that present for assessment and treatment at pediatric neuropsychology clinics.

Strategies for further validation of CANTAB in childhood assessment

Although additional behavioral studies of children with focal brain abnormalities would be a useful parallel to the adult data that has been gathered from neurosurgical patients, continued study of normative populations is also needed. Such studies have the goal of establishing that the brain–behavior correlates observed in adult populations are present in children. For instance, although it is apparent from several studies that CANTAB's spatial working memory task is sensitive to frontal lobe impairment in adults (cf., Owen et al., 1996c), a definitive link to frontal lobe function in children or adolescents has yet to be established. However, work has been initiated to develop neuroimaging protocols for use with children, utilizing CANTAB subtasks to address this issue (C. A. Nelson et al., unpublished data). This endeavor has been initiated through the use of a DMTS recognition memory task. This CANTAB subtest has been omitted from our normative studies because of its time demands. Briefly, a geometric pattern (the "sample") is displayed in the center of the computer screen for a brief interval. Following delays of 0, 4, 8 or 12 s, four patterns are displayed on-screen, one of which is the sample pattern. The child must correctly recall, and respond by touching, the sample pattern.

For use in fMRI, this task has been redesigned as a delayed nonmatch-to-sample (DNMTS). DNMTS task was selected because it has been extensively studied in nonhuman primates to determine its neural correlates and is widely considered to be the prototypical task for measuring visual recognition memory (e.g., Mishkin and Delacour, 1975). In DNMTS, the subject (generally a monkey) is first presented with several training trials in which a stimulus object is baited with a reward. Following training, the subject is presented with the original object and a novel object. If the subject reaches for the novel object, s/he is again rewarded. This task requires formulating a memory from a visual perception of the first object and creating a motoric response based on the memory. Lesion studies with monkeys have shown that this task is highly dependent on the hippocampus and underlying perirhinal cortex (Meunier et al., 1993; Alvarez et al., 1994), as well as on the ventromedial prefrontal cortex (Kowalska et al., 1991).

For use with fMRI, the stimuli consist of the same abstract colored visual patterns that are used in CANTAB's DMTS task. On each trial, subjects are first presented with a single target stimulus for a 3 s duration, after which the screen is blank for a 12 s delay interval. After this delay, the target stimulus and a novel stimulus appear together on screen for 3 s. Subjects are instructed to press a button that corresponds to the screen side of the novel stimulus. As in the monkey studies, this task requires that the subjects create a visual memory and form a motoric action based on the memory. In a perceptual control condition, the task is exactly the same except that there are no memory demands. Specifically, the stimulus is presented on the screen for the 3 s familiarization period and remains on the screen throughout the 12 s delay and the response period. As a result, rather than relying on memory to determine which button to press, the subject can determine the correct answer perceptually. Then, following standard fMRI methodology (e.g., Cohen et al., 1993), the functional brain activation from the perceptual control task is subtacted from the memory task to identify the brain structures that are involved in the visual memory component of the task. In our initial work with four adult subjects (ages 22–30 years), a network of neural structures was activated. Specifically, similar to the monkey studies, the medial temporal lobe (including the hippocampus and parahippocampal gyrus, along with the underlying perirhinal cortex) and the dorsolateral prefrontal cortex were activated.

Once past the pilot stage, studies will be conducted to determine if these findings can be extended to children. Behavioral studies with CANTAB's DMTS task, using stimuli identical to the ones used in the fMRI DNMTS task protocol, have found that adult-like performance on this task is not reached until 7 years of age (Fig. 20.5; Luciana and Nelson, 1998). Therefore, this study will examine the covariance between behavioral performance and patterns of neural activity in children between the ages of 6 years and adolescence (we currently lack Institutional Review Board permission to test healthy children below 6 years of age in fMRI studies). Of interest are the brain structures that subserve task performance in children. One might speculate that relatively mature structures, such as those within the medial temporal lobe, would be relatively more activated in children than in adults and would permit successful performance for children. Moreover, it may be possible to understand better how the lack of maturity of other structures (e.g., regions of the prefrontal cortex) alters the characteristics of the task-relevant neural network in children.

Summary

The CANTAB is useful for the evaluation of frontal and temporal lobe dysfunction in adults with acquired lesions. Whether these same neural correlates hold in the course of normal development has not been investigated. Neuroanatomic data suggest a protracted course of frontal lobe development through childhood, a finding that is consistent with our observation that children have not reached adult levels of performance on frontal lobe tasks before the age of 12 years (Luciana and Nelson, 1998). Although several studies of neurologically impaired pediatric samples suggest that CANTAB is able to discriminate between groups of children with and without neurologic impairment, its specificity as a diagnostic tool has yet to be determined. However, the use of a well-validated battery of tests, like the CANTAB, within a multimethod approach that includes neuroimaging, may lead to more refined assessments of brain–behavior relations in children.

References

Alvarez, P., Zola-Morgan, S. and Squire, L. R. (1994). The animal model of human amnesia: long term memory impaired and short term memory intact. *Proc. Natl. Acad. Sci. USA*, **91**, 5637–41.

Baker, S. C., Rogers, R. D., Owen, A. M. et al. (1996). Neural systems engaged by planning: a PET study of the Tower of London task. *Neuropsychologia*, **34**, 515–26.

Casey, B. J., Cohen, J. D., Jezzard, P. et al. (1995). Activation of prefrontal cortex in children during a nonspatial working memory task with functional MRI. *Neuroimaging*, **2**, 221–9.

Chugani, H. T. (1994). Development of regional brain glucose metabolism in relation to behavior and plasticity. In *Human Behavior and the Developing Brain*, eds. G. Dawson and K. Fischer, pp. 153–75. New York: Guilford Press.

Chugani, H. T. and Phelps, M. E. (1986). Maturational changes in cerebral function in infants determined by [^{18}O]FDG positron emission tomography. *Science*, **231**, 840–3.

Cohen, J. D., Noll, D. C. and Schneider, W. (1993). Functional magnetic resonance imaging: overview and methods for psychological research. *Behav. Res. Meth. Instruments Computers*, **25**, 101–13.

Damasio, A. (1994). *Descartes Error*. New York: Plenum Press.

Damasio, A. and Anderson, S. W. (1994). The frontal lobes. In *Clinical Neuropsychology*, 3rd edn, eds. K. M. Heilman and E. Valenstein, pp. 409–60. New York: Oxford University Press.

Diamond, A. (1990). The development and neural bases of memory formation as indexed by the AB and delayed response tasks in human infants and infant monkeys. *Ann. N. Y. Acad. Sci.*, **761**, 267–317.

Diamond, A. and Goldman-Rakic, P. S. (1989). Comparison of human infants and rhesus monkeys on Piaget's AB task: evidence for dependence on dorsolateral prefrontal cortex. *Exp. Brain Res.*, **74**, 24–40.

Diamond, A., Prevor, M. B., Callendar, G. and Druin, D. P. (1997). Prefrontal cortex cognitive deficits in children treated early and continuously for PKU. *Monogr. Soc. Res. Child Dev.*, **62**, 1–207.

Dias, R., Robbins, T. W. and Roberts, A. C. (1996). Dissociation in prefrontal cortex of attentional and affective shifts. *Nature*, **380**, 69–72.

Downes, J. J., Roberts, A. C., Sahakian, B. J., Evenden, J. L., Morris, R. G. and Robbins, T. W. (1989). Impaired extra-dimensional shift performance in medicated and unmedicated Parkinson's disease: evidence for a specific attentional dysfunction. *Neuropsychologia*, **27**, 1329–43.

Flavell, J. H., Beach, D. R. and Chinsky, J. M. (1966). Spontaneous verbal rehearsal in a memory task as a function of age. *Child Dev.*, **37**, 283–99.

Fray, P. J., Robbins, T. Wl. and Sahakian, B. J. (1996). Neuropsychiatric applications of CANTAB. *Int. J. Geriat. Psychiatry*, **11**, 329–36.

Fuster, J. M. (1995). Temporal processing. *Ann. N. Y. Acad. Sci.*, **769**, 173–83.

Goldman-Rakic, P. S. (1987). Circuitry of primate prefrontal cortex and the regulation of behavior by representational memory. In *Handbook of Physiology, the Nervous System, Higher Functions of the Brain*, Vol. 1, ed. F. Plum, pp. 373–417. Bethesda, MD: American Physiological Society.

Hughes, C., Russell, J. and Robbins, T. W. (1994). Evidence for executive dysfunction in autism. *Neuropsychologia*, **32**, 477–92.

Huttenlocher, P. R. (1994). Synaptogenesis, synapse elimination, and neural plasticity in human cerebral cortex. In Minnesota Symposium on Child Psychology, Vol. 27, *Threats to Optimal Development: Integrating Biological, Psychological, and Social Risk Factors*, ed. C. A. Nelson, pp. 35–54. Hillsdale, NJ: Lawrence Erlbaum.

Huttenlocher, P. R. and Dabhholkar, A. S. (1997). Regional differences in synaptogenesis in human cerebral cortex. *J. Comp. Neurol.*, **387**, 167–78.

Jacobsen, C. F. (1936). Studies of cerebral function in primates. *Comp. Psychol. Monogr.*, **13**, 1–68.

Kowalska, D. M., Bachevalier, J. and Mishkin, M. (1991). The role of the inferior prefrontal convexity in performance of delayed non-matching to sample. *Neuropsychologia*, **29**, 583–600.

Luciana, M., Lindeke, L., Georgieff, M., Mills, M. and Nelson, C. A. (1999). Neurobehavioral evidence for working memory deficits in school-age children with histories of prematurity. *Devel. Med. Child Neurol.*, **41**, 521–33.

Luciana, M. and Nelson, C. A. (1998). The functional emergence of prefrontally-guided working memory systems in four-to-eight year-old children. *Neuropsychologia*, **36**, 273–93.

Meunier, M., Bachevalier, J., Mishkin, M. and Murray, E. A. (1993). Effects on visual recognition of combined and separate ablations of the entorhinal and perirhinal cortices in rhesus monkeys. *J. Neurosci.*, **13**, 5418–32.

Milner, B. (1964). Some effects of frontal lobectomy in man. In *The Frontal Granular Cortex and Behavior*, eds. J. M. Warren and K. Akert, pp. 313–34. McGraw-Hill: New York.

Milner, B. (1971). Interhemispheric differences and psychological processes. *Br. Med. Bull.*, **27**, 272–7.

Mishkin, M. and Delacour, J. (1975). An analysis of short-term visual memory in the monkey. *J. Exp. Psychol. Anim. Behav. Process.*, **1**, 326–34.

Morris, R. G., Ahmed, S., Syed, G. M. and Toone, B. K. (1993). Neural correlates of planning ability: frontal lobe activation during the Tower of London test. *Neuropsychologia*, **31**, 1367–78.

Nelson, C. A. (1995). The ontogeny of human memory: a cognitive neuroscience perspective. *Dev. Psychol.*, **31**, 723–38.

Owen, A. M., Downes, J. J., Sahakian, B. J., Polkey, C. E. and Robbins, T. W. (1990). Planning and spatial working memory deficits following frontal lobe lesions in man. *Neuropsychologia*, **28**, 1021–34.

Owen, A. M., Roberts, A. C., Pokley, C. E., Sahakian, B. J. and Robbins, T. W. (1991). Extra-dimensional versus intra-dimensional set-shifting performance following frontal lobe excisions, temporal lobe excisions, or amygdalo-hippocampectomy in man. *Neuropsychologia*, **29**, 993–1006.

Owen, A. M., Sahakian, B. J., Semple, J., Polkey, C. E. and Robbins, T. W. (1995). Visuospatial short-term recognition memory and learning after temporal lobe excision, frontal lobe excision, or amygdalo-hippocampectomy in man. *Neuropsychologia*, **33**, 1–24.

Owen, A. M., Doyon, J., Petrides, M. and Evans, A. C. (1996a). Planning and spatial working memory: a positron emission tomography study in humans. *Eur. J. Neurosci.*, **8**, 353–64.

Owen, A. M., Evans, A. C. and Petrides, M. (1996b). Evidence for a two-stage model of spatial working memory processing within the lateral frontal cortex: a positron emission tomography study. *Cereb. Cortex*, **6**, 31–8.

Owen, A. M., Morris, R. G., Sahakian, B. J., Polkey, C. E. and Robbins, T. W. (1996c). Double-dissociation of memory and executive functions in working memory tasks following frontal-lobe excisions, temporal lobe excisions or amygdalo-hippocampectomy in man. *Brain*, **119**, 1597–615.

Passler, M. A., Isaac, W. and Hynd, G. (1985). Neuropsychological development of behavior attributed to frontal lobe functioning in children. *Dev. Neuropsychol.*, **1**, 349–70.

Petrides, M. and Milner, B. (1982). Deficits on subject-ordered tasks after frontal and temporal lobe lesions in man. *Neuropsychologia*, **20**, 249–62.

Robbins, T. W. (1996). Dissociating executive functions of the prefrontal cortex. *Proc. R. Soc. Lond. Ser. B*, in press.

Robbins, T. W. and Sahakian, B. J. (1994). Computer methods of assessment of cognitive function. In *Principles and Practice of Geriatric Psychiatry*, eds. J. R. M. Copeland, M. T. Abou-Saleh and D. G. Blazer, pp. 205–9. Chichester, UK: Wiley.

Robbins, T. W., Roberts, A. C., Owen, A. M. et al. (1994). Monoaminergic-dependent cognitive functions of the prefrontal cortex in monkey and man. In *Motor and Cognitive Functions of the Prefrontal Cortex*, ed. A. M. Thierry, pp. 93–111. New York: Springer-Verlag.

Ross, G., Boatright, S., Auld, P. A. and Nass, R. (1996). Specific cognitive abilities in two year-old children with subependymal and mild intraventricular hemorrhage. *Brain Cognit.*, **32**, 1–13.

Sattler, J. M. (1992). *Assessment of Children*, 3rd edn. San Diego: Jerome M. Sattler.

Shallice, T. (1982). Specific impairments in planning. *Philos. Trans. R. Soc. Lond. Ser. B*, **298**, 199–209.

Smith, M. L. and Milner, B. (1988). Estimation of frequency of occurrence of abstract designs after frontal or temporal lobectomy. *Neuropsychologia*, **26**, 297–306.

Veale, D. M., Sahakian, B. J., Owen, A. M. and Marks, I. M. (1996). Specific cognitive deficits in tests sensitive to frontal lobe dysfunction in obsessive compulsive disorder. *Psychol. Med.*, **26**, 1261–9.

Volpe, J. (1995). *Neurology of the Newborn*, 3rd edn. Philadelphia, PA: Saunders.

Weinberger, D. L. (1988). Evidence for dorsolateral prefrontal involvement in the pathogenesis of schizophrenia. *Arch. Gen. Psychiatry*, **45**, 609–15.

Welsh, M. C., Pennington, B. F. and Grossier, D. B. (1991). A normative development study of executive function: a window on prefrontal function in children. *Dev. Neuropsychol.*, **7**, 131–49.

23

Functional neuroimaging in child psychiatry: future directions

Monique Ernst and Judith M. Rumsey[1]

Introduction

The future of functional neuroimaging in child psychiatry is bound not only to technologic progress but also to the refinement of our skills in exploiting these techniques to answer the ultimate questions of why and how symptoms occur. These skills require a clear understanding of the physiologic meaning of the signals recorded by the various neuroimaging techniques, the formulation of rational models of normal and deviant processes that can be evaluated systematically in a logical and stepwise fashion, and the intimately interactive and synergistic collaboration with other disciplines. Indeed, clinical taxonomy, psychopharmacology, molecular genetics, and basic neuroscience all provide critical clues for understanding the mechanisms underlying psychiatric disorders.

Ultimately, hypothesis generation and the interpretation of functional neuroimaging findings in child psychiatry will rely heavily upon the synthesis of scientific evidence originating from neuroscience and clinical research. The impact of brain maturation and brain plasticity lies at the forefront of the understanding of brain imaging findings in children and adolescents. How one approaches questions depends on one's theoretical assumptions concerning the extent of the brain's capacity for plasticity, the regional convergence and divergence of inputs, and the degree of equipotency of brain regions for adaptation. Functional neuroimaging can serve to bridge clinical science and basic neuroscience and, in doing so, realize its potential for translating advances in neuroscience into clinical applications.

After highlighting findings and hypotheses emerging from recent functional neuroimaging studies in both chil-

dren and adults, this chapter will examine some of the critical needs that still need to be addressed to move the field of pediatric neuroimaging forward. The second part of the chapter will delineate recent advances in technology (progress in widely used modalities and new techniques) as well as in methodology (study design and data analysis). Finally, the authors will outline future directions in neuroimaging research in child psychiatry.

Selected contributions of functional neuroimaging in child psychiatry

With respect to its potential for addressing questions of pathophysiology in psychiatry, functional neuroimaging research has and continues to be met with some skepticism. Often, findings seem only to confirm hypotheses concerning human brain function previously demonstrated in animal studies or supported by clinical reports, rather than substantively extending our knowledge base. The validation of models in humans is, however, critical for the formulation of new hypotheses directly applied to humans. In addition, because new knowledge overlaps with familiar theories, its import tends to be lost. Although it is still too early to appreciate fully the gains of functional neuroimaging in child psychiatry, studies of adult and adolescent patients have begun to suggest important developmental differences and similarities across age groups in the pathophysiology of psychiatric disorders, as well as to elucidate the neural bases of the therapeutic effects of medications.

Attention-deficit hyperactivity disorder (ADHD) is recognized as a highly prevalent and potentially lifelong disorder and is probably the childhood psychiatric disorder most studied in children and adolescents using functional neuroimaging to date. Symptom patterns of ADHD are

---

[1] The order of authorship does not reflect on the relative contributions of the coauthors; both contributed equally to this work.

known to change across the lifespan, from childhood into adolescence into adulthood. Accordingly, positron emission tomography (PET) studies now offer provocative evidence suggesting an evolution of neural deficits with age, both supporting and extending a priori hypotheses of the neuropathophysiology of this disorder. While attentionally challenged, adolescents show discrete reductions in glucose metabolism relative to controls, particularly in the left anterior prefrontal cortex (Zametkin et al., 1993; Ernst et al., 1994). Adults show widespread cerebral hypometabolism, which, however, affects predominantly the left anterior prefrontal cortex (Zametkin et al., 1990). Together, these findings suggest that the global reduction in synaptic activity in adults may be secondary to an initial causal deficit, whereas dysfunction in the left anterior prefrontal cortex may reflect a more primary defect. The most likely mechanism underlying the observed reductions in brain metabolism is a dampening of modulatory synaptic activity that originates in subcortical structures and predominantly affects the prefrontal cortex.

PET studies using [^{18}F]-fluorodopa (FDOPA) also suggest age-related differences in the pathophysiology of ADHD (Ernst et al., 1999a). Adults with ADHD have shown an abnormally low FDOPA signal in the anterior prefrontal cortex (Ernst et al. 1998). In contrast, although also showing an emerging reduction of the FDOPA signal in the anterior medial frontal cortex, adolescents with ADHD have demonstrated an elevated FDOPA signal in the midbrain (substantia nigra and ventral tegmentum complex) (Ernst et al., 1999a). These findings provide the most direct evidence to date in support of the dopaminergic hypothesis of ADHD (Solanto, 1984; Levy, 1991; Castellanos, 1997; Ernst, 1998) and suggest a need for additional studies probing systematically the presynaptic and postsynaptic dopaminergic systems.

In schizophrenia, age-related similarities in neuroimaging findings support a common pathophysiology for the adult-onset and much rarer childhood-onset forms. As detailed earlier in this volume, studies using magnetic resonance spectroscopy (MRS) have revealed regionally specific reductions of N-acetylaspartate, suggestive of neuronal involvement, in the mesial temporo-limbic and prefrontal cortices in both childhood-onset and adult-onset schizophrenia. Abnormally low frontal activity (hypofrontality), one of the most consistent findings in PET/SPECT (single photon emission computed tomography) research in adult-onset schizophrenia, has also been reported in adolescents with early-onset schizophrenia.

Preliminary studies of anorexia nervosa using PET and SPECT suggest a role of the temporal lobe in both adults (Herholz et al., 1987) and adolescents (Gordon et al., 1997),

a role already proposed in the 1950s (Anand and Brobeck, 1951). Temporal lobe dysfunction is hypothesized to reflect a functional imbalance in the limbic system, leading to a disturbance in the hypothalamic–pituitary axis directly responsible for the clinical presentation of anorexia nervosa. However, neuroimaging findings also suggest that adult pathology involves additional structures including the caudate nucleus (Herholz et al., 1987) and parietal cortex (Delvenne et al., 1997).

In Tourette's disorder, metabolic, blood flow, and, to a lesser extent, radioligand studies have implicated the basal ganglia portions of the cortico–striato–thalamo–cortical circuitry in the pathophysiology of this disorder. These findings may, in part, reflect secondary compensatory function (i.e., attentional processing associated with tic suppression) and require further investigation. While a study of the dopaminergic system of adult patients has failed to identify abnormalities (Turjanski et al., 1994), adolescents with Tourette's disorder have shown elevated accumulations of FDOPA in the left caudate and right midbrain (Ernst et al., 1999b). Together, these studies suggest the possibility of important developmental changes, again reinforcing the need for further studies that include children.

Other emerging findings have begun to localize the effects of therapeutic medications in child psychiatry. Blood flow studies suggest that stimulants may normalize prefrontal activity in ADHD (Teicher et al., 1996; Vaidya et al., 1998) but fail to normalize brain activity in other regions (i.e., striatum; Vaidya et al., 1998). Such paradigms offer opportunities for localizing the sites of the therapeutic impact of pharmacologic and other treatments. In addition, this approach opens possibilities for exploring the neural substrates of age-related differences in drug response, such as differences in the efficacy of antidepressant treatments of adolescent versus adult depression.

Critical needs in pediatric neuroimaging

In most domains of inquiry, research in children has lagged behind research in adults. This chapter proposes several areas of need specific to the investigation of children that are fundamental to the successful application of neuroimaging in child psychiatry. These areas include the collection of age-related normative data relevant to indices of brain function at rest and during task performance, the development of age-appropriate brain atlases, and the prioritization of research questions in this extraordinary burgeoning field. Finally, integrative models capable of bridging the gap between basic neuroscience and clinical science are needed for hypothesis generation, data interpretation and theory building.

Normative models of structural, functional, and biochemical brain development

The analysis and interpretation of functional brain imaging data relies on its integration with structural data. The use of a common algorithm for stereotaxic normalization in functional imaging studies assumes that brain anatomy is comparable across individuals and groups. Systematic changes with age or disease introduce error in mapping function to structure and in averaging normalized data across subjects for group comparisons. Because existing atlases are derived from a single or at best a few individual brains, anatomic variability is largely ignored. Therefore, such atlases are more accurate for brain regions with low intersubject variability and for sites close to the landmarks of the reference system than for more variable regions (e.g., neocortex, asymmetrical perisylvian regions). To address these limitations, efforts are underway to develop digital and probabilistic brain atlases. These atlases use data from large populations, which provide probabilistic information on variability in brain architecture, and base their landmarks on intersubject stability (Mazziotta et al., 1995; Thompson et al., 1996, 1997). Such atlases will provide a means of detecting, mapping and distinguishing age- and disease-related deviations in brain anatomy and a framework for integrating functional and anatomic data across subjects and imaging modalities.

Also needed is a better understanding of normal functional brain development. To date, few functional neuroimaging studies have directly examined the effects of maturation in pediatric samples. Not only is it critical to understand how the brain develops in humans to elucidate pathology, but such data can also foster the development of mathematical models to apply in the analysis of brain imaging data from children. Such mathematical models can be used to correct for age-related differences, which can confound the effects of variables under study, and help to reduce the number of subjects required for a given study. In fact, mathematical models of maturational changes, such as those in glucose metabolism, are under development (Muzik et al., 1999), but data needed to make these models fully operant are lacking.

Adequate normative models of functional brain development underlying specific neurobehavioral abilities of relevance to child psychiatric disorders are lacking. While activation studies have assumed a prominent role in defining the neural circuitry involved in a host of neurocognitive and neurobehavioral functions in adults,

studies seeking to delineate their development in children are just emerging. For example, Luna et al. (1999) have begun to map the neural circuitry subserving response inhibition in children (ages 8 to 13 years), adolescents (ages 14 to 17 years), and adults using an antisaccade task. Preliminary results suggest that maturational improvements in voluntary inhibition are subserved by striato–thalamic and cerebello–thalamic modulation of higher-order fronto–parietal cortical networks.

Brain neurochemical development can also be modeled using functional neuroimaging and may help to elucidate the underlying biology of abnormalities identified using activation paradigms. However, neurochemical investigations are lagging behind activation studies because, so far, neurotransmitter studies can be conducted only with PET and SPECT technology. While the ethical issue of radiation exposure with these techniques remains a concern in studies of children, such studies are critical for the understanding of the neural mechanisms responsible for aberrant behavior and the subsequent development of rational therapeutic interventions.

Setting priorities in research questions

Which psychologic functions, neurotransmitter systems, and neural circuitry represent priorities for human brain mapping in child psychiatry? What role do they play in these disorders? Which of the available study designs are best suited to addressing them? These are all important questions that must be addressed.

Child psychiatric disorders are multifaceted, involving emotional and behavioral dysregulation and cognitive deficits as well as underlying neurotransmitter and neuroendocrine disturbances. Therefore, their study can be approached from a variety of perspectives, using both activation paradigms and neurochemical methods. Challenges include the choice of the appropriate affective, attentional, cognitive, or pharmacological probes. This choice depends on the nature of the processes hypothesized to be critically involved in a given disorder and the presumed primary or secondary role of the function under scrutiny. The investigation of relatively unexplored areas such as emotions and their role in learning (a manifestation of brain plasticity) may also represent a priority for neuroimaging research in child psychiatry. Neural models of emotional development and its interaction with cognitive development have the potential to revolutionize the field of psychopathology.

Nature of the process under study

Deficits in executive functions, attention, and working memory are broadly implicated in child psychiatric disorders, and, therefore, these domains constitute priorities for neuroimaging in child psychiatry. These processes are involved in emotional, cognitive, and behavioral self-regulation. Each of them is multifactorial and subsumes a variety of elemental functions, which presumably engage somewhat different neural networks or impose differential demands on them. While impairments within these domains have been noted across a wide range of developmental neuropsychiatric disorders, their specific nature within and across disorders and their developmental precursors require further elucidation. For example, whereas deficits in executive function characterize both autism and ADHD, their nature differs between these disorders. Deficits in vigilance and response inhibition are prominent in ADHD but not in autism, which instead is characterized by deficits in the disengagement and shifting of attention (Pennington and Ozonoff, 1996). Behavioral studies elucidating core deficits associated with specific disorders thus provide for the rational selection of activation tasks for use in neuroimaging studies. While executive functions, attention, and working memory are thought to rely on fronto–subcortical brain circuits throughout human development, this remains a working hypothesis in need of testing in normally developing children and in those with psychiatric disorders. Circuit-specific probes capable of distinguishing disorders will help to further our knowledge of the diversity of ways in which key fronto–subcortical circuits are affected in child psychiatric disorders.

Primary versus secondary role of deficits

The choice of study tasks and conditions depends heavily on assumptions concerning the primary (causal) or secondary (resultant) role of identified deficits in child psychiatric disorders. For example, whereas deficits in the ability to understand other's intentions ("theory of mind" deficits) characterize autism, these may be secondary and develop as a result of early deficits in conjoint (social) attention, which in turn may stem from deficits in the ability to shift attention rapidly and flexibly from one object to another (e.g., from mother to objects in the environment). If this is the case, the identification of the neural substrates of such secondary deficits will be of limited value in elucidating the primary underlying neurobiology.

Forays into new areas

To date, neuroimaging has been used less in studies of emotional processing than in studies of cognitive functions, even though emotional disturbances are part of the clinical picture of most psychiatric disorders. Activation paradigms for examining the neural bases of emotion and

limbic function are, however, emerging. Functional imaging has not only confirmed the role of limbic structures in human emotions but is also providing new evidence of deficient habituation as a potential mechanism underlying psychopathology. For example, the passive viewing of facial expressions has been shown to elicit amygdalar activation in adult volunteers (Breiter et al., 1996). These responses, elicited in healthy individuals, show rapid habituation relative to nonlimbic brain regions involved in facial recognition (e.g., fusiform gyrus), thus providing a potentially useful index of physiologic adaptability. Abnormalities of resting amygdalar blood flow in depression (Drevets, 1998) and task-related amygdalar blood flow in anxiety disorders (Rauch et al., 1998) suggest the involvement of this limbic structure in psychiatric disorders. Hyper-reactivity or an inability to habituate to threat stimuli may characterize anxiety disorders, whereas dysfunction affecting the ability to assess emotional stimuli may characterize depressive disorders or autism. Studies in children can clarify whether neural abnormalities involving limbic responsivity and habituation constitute strong predictors or early signs of disorder or whether they evolve over the course of illness.

Important relationships between cognitive and emotional development can be examined using paradigms assessing emotionally based learning. For example, imaging paradigms have begun to examine the role of the amygdala in conditioned fear acquisition and extinction in adults (LaBar et al., 1998). The circuitry underlying emotional learning has been elaborated in an event-related functional magnetic resonance imaging (fMRI) study in which faces were conditioned through pairing with an aversive tone (Buchel et al., 1998), eliciting responses in the amygdalae, anterior cingulate, and anterior insula, regions involved in emotional processing. The use of passive paradigms (e.g., facial expression paradigms) with young children may help to assess the integrity of primary emotional brain systems, whereas the use of conditioning paradigms may help to assess the impact of these systems (or lack thereof) on learning.

Integrative models

There is a need for the development of theoretical models of systems-level and large-scale neural networks that mediate and link the emotional/behavioral dysregulation and the cognitive deficits concurrently present in child psychiatric disorders. One such model is that proposed by Damasio (1994), who views emotion and cognition as intimately linked in the brain and partners in the regulation of behavior. Within this model, primary emotions, which are wired in at birth, are processed and categorized by the early sensory cortices and detected by limbic structures, including the amygdala and anterior cingulate. Secondary emotions develop as connections between neural representations of categories, objects, and situations are formed. These processes are supported by widely distributed neural networks, which include the prefrontal and somatosensory cortices. Therefore, emotions and "feelings of emotion" (which include both primary emotional and cognitive elements) are represented at many different neural levels, including the neocortical level.

Damasio (1994) highlights the unique and privileged role of the prefrontal cortices in the integration of emotion and cognition. Receiving signals from all the sensory systems and from bioregulatory systems (e.g., brainstem neurotransmitter nuclei, basal forebrain, amygdala, anterior cingulate, hypothalamus), the prefrontal cortices have available to them knowledge of the external world, of innate biological regulatory preferences, and of prior and current body states. The prefrontal cortices mediate categorizations of the contingencies of personal life experiences and, thus, provide a basis for the projecting scenarios of future outcomes required for predictions and planning. Finally, the prefrontal cortices can directly affect cerebral output (e.g., motor and chemical responses). The integrated functioning of these prefrontal systems allows humans to think ahead, predict outcomes, preemptively avoid danger, generalize, and respond flexibly based on personal experience. Clearly, such a model can help to organize the different phases of a research plan aimed at elucidating the origin and evolution of a particular disorder. However, such research can occur only if it is supported by reliable and sensitive technologies and methodologies.

Technologic advances

Enhancements of existing technology

Technologic progress entails the enhancement of the sensitivity and specificity of the physiologic signals, the implementation of the combined use of available complementary techniques, and the minimization of health hazards. Improvements of spatial and temporal resolution and developments in methodology continue to be at the forefront of technical efforts in neuroimaging research. Current fMRI techniques provide spatial resolution as good as 2–5 mm and temporal resolution of less than 1 s. The ultimate limits of temporal resolution are not yet known and depend on the signal-to-noise ratio of imaging

measurements and on the underlying variance in hemodynamic latencies. Variance in the delay and shape of the hemodynamic curve observed across brain regions and subjects may, in part, reflect delayed neuronal processing, opening possibilities for further improvements in temporal resolution (see Rosen et al., 1998). Higher magnetic field strengths, improvements in radiofrequency receiver coil technology, and greater sophistication in data analytic methods offer the hope of further improvements in sensitivity and spatiotemporal resolution.

In addition, the combined use of different functional neuroimaging techniques can facilitate the dissection in time and space of the neural processes that mediate behavior and cognition. For example, both fMRI and PET maps related to specific tasks can be further analyzed using event-related potential and magnetoencephalographic techniques to define the underlying temporal dynamics of distinct regional activations more exactly (George et al., 1995; Thatcher, 1996; Rosen et al., 1998). However, multimodal neuroimaging is difficult to implement because of the constraints imposed by cost, time, technical feasibility, and instrument availability; consequently its use to date is limited. Nonetheless, the development of methods for integrating imaging modalities is expected to contribute to coherent models of the neural systems underlying normal and aberrant emotional and behavioral development.

Advances in fMRI are emphasized because of the paucity of use of new PET or SPECT techniques with children. The development of MRI as a functional imaging tool presents minimal health hazards when appropriate caution is exercised. Its lack of ionizing radiation allows the repeated study of both adults and children. Practical considerations imposed by comfort and movement, rather than radiation dose, have now become the most relevant limiting factors for subjects when using fMRI.

However, it is also important to note that the development of increasingly sensitive PET and SPECT scanners is reducing the doses of radioactive tracer necessary to obtain reliable images. These doses, which are already minimal, may eventually reach a level that will cease to raise health concerns. In addition, alterations of experimental design can minimize the dosages required for studies of children (Zametkin et al., 1993). As already mentioned, PET and SPECT are the only techniques to date that can provide reliable measures of neurobiochemical systems, particularly neurotransmitter activities. The development of ligands and of mathematical models to extract the physiological information of the behavior of these ligands constitutes the major efforts in PET and SPECT research.

Although fMRI presents critical advantages over PET and SPECT in activation studies, fMRI has two relative disadvantages. While motion artifacts pose a major problem in fMRI studies of children, they are less of an issue with PET or SPECT. The other relative disadvantage of fMRI is the inability to measure neural activity associated with behavior outside of the scanner, in contrast to PET or SPECT where the uptake of the tracer can often occur outside of the scanner. This may present a significant advantage for subjects who cannot easily be trained to remain still and to tolerate the confines of fMRI magnets. This also makes it possible to sedate severely impaired children for scanning only after tracer uptake.

New techniques

The range of functional imaging modalities and the tools available for use in conjunction with functional neuroimaging continue to expand. One promising new modality with exquisite temporal resolution is optical imaging (Frostig et al., 1990). Optical imaging makes use of the transmission of infrared light through the head and brain to measure localized scattering and absorption changes in optical reflectance. These changes in optical reflectance are influenced by the concentrations of oxygenated and deoxygenated hemoglobin, which are dependent on local neural activity (Malonek and Grinvald, 1997). The temporal resolution of this technique reaches the picosecond range; yet the spatial resolution can exceed 1 cm. In addition, measures are limited to superficial cortical regions.

Of particular interest is the potential use of this technique in association with electrical recordings to clarify relationships between neuronal activity and hemodynamic changes. Optical imaging has been used in humans to detect visual evoked activity in the occipital cortex. Gratton et al. (1997) found that event-related optical signals elicited in occipital cortex (with latencies of approximately 100 ms) colocalized with the signals obtained with fMRI. The temporal and spatial resolution of the optical imaging signal makes it a promising technique for assessing the time course of activity in localized superficial cortical brain areas.

Another relatively new tool that can enhance the capabilities of functional neuroimaging is transcranial magnetic stimulation (TMS). TMS can be used in combination with functional neuroimaging to map the substrates of simple to complex behaviors and neuronal connections. This tool permits the stimulation of discrete brain areas and can be employed to disrupt function, to enhance cortical excitability and (potentially) function, and to determine the functional connectivity between brain regions (Pascual-Leone et al., 1999). The disruption of task performance through focal TMS stimulation can provide evidence that a stimulated region is critical for performance. However, future applications of this new tool in studies of children will require additional evaluation of safety.

Recent applications of this technology to the study of plasticity have included the effects of practice on cortical network representations (Classen et al., 1998) and the cortical reorganization of visual cortex in blind subjects (Cohen et al., 1997). In the latter application, midoccipital TMS interfered with Braille reading but not with speech in early-blind subjects, thus indicating the intimate involvement of this region in their reading. Stimulation of somatosensory cortex, but not occipital cortex, disrupted the ability of sighted subjects to identify embossed letters tactilely, whereas the opposite pattern (a double dissociation) was seen in blind subjects, further suggesting cross-modal plasticity as a mechanism of functional compensation.

The combined use of TMS with PET offers a novel approach to mapping functional connections in humans. To determine patterns of functional connectivity without requiring the subject to engage in a specific task, Paus et al. (1997) stimulated selected cortical regions while simultaneously measuring local and remote changes in resting regional cerebral blood flow. Stimulation of the left frontal eye field provided significant correlations between the number of TMS pulse trains and blood flow in the visual cortex of the superior and medial parieto-occipital regions, consistent with the known anatomic connectivity of the monkey frontal eye field. Because no task was involved, potential confounds associated with task parameters and performance variables were avoided. Given the importance of plasticity in brain maturation, the use of this tool may be particularly well suited for studying connectivity in developmental neuropsychiatric disorders.

Clinical therapeutic applications of TMS in psychiatry are being investigated. Brain regions that are hypometabolic in a psychiatric disorder may be stimulated to enhance cortical excitability with potentially therapeutic results. Particularly promising is a role for TMS in the treatment of depression (Kirkcaldie et al., 1997; George et al., 1999). Recent work by Keenan et al. (1999) has demonstrated enhancement of the ability to recognize one's own face (one aspect of self-awareness) by repetitive TMS delivered to the right prefrontal cortex of normal adults. While it is too early to evaluate realistically the range of potential therapeutic applications, such findings raise the possibility of future clinical applications within child psychiatry.

Developments in research design and image analysis

The review of neuroimaging studies raises issues of specificity and sensitivity with respect to findings of relevance to psychiatric disorders. Small sample sizes, limited statistical methods available for analyzing multiple variables, difficulty in controlling all experimental variables, and limited compatibility of some research designs with current models of brain function all present limitations for the interpretation of results. Advances in research design and image analysis have begun to address these problems. Progress in design strategies and data analysis are expected to enhance the capabilities of neuroimaging further.

The large number of statistical comparisons involved in imaging multiple brain regions using either voxel-based or regions-of-interest approaches, together with small samples sizes, significantly limits statistical power in most functional neuroimaging studies. The type of correction that should be used for multiple comparisons in the analysis of brain imaging findings continues to be debated. However, for the most effective exploitation of neuroimaging in exploratory studies, the risk of accepting a false finding (type I error) must be balanced against that of dismissing important new findings (type II error). Indeed, exploratory studies are critical to pave the way for hypothesis-driven investigations using neuroimaging and other methods for independent confirmation of findings. Noteworthy, molecular genetics, in which the number of comparisons is frequently disproportionately large relative to sample size and the variability of the measures, faces similar considerations. Statistical developments in genetics may prove helpful to the brain imaging field as well. Solutions attempted in neuroimaging studies include the use of large samples (an expensive undertaking), the strategy of splitting data sets and reporting only results that replicate within samples, and the replication of results in independent samples (the most acceptable standard for research in general).

Another avenue for demonstrating the replicability of results rests with individual data analysis made possible by the advent of fMRI and improvements in PET technology. While sample sizes must be large enough to offset the effects of variability in the measures and of multiple comparisons, the reporting of both individual and group results may help to offset the need for inordinately large samples. Treating individual data from homogeneous samples as single-case studies may increase confidence in the replicability of results. Conversely, interindividual variability may yield important clues for understanding clinical heterogeneity.

Hemodynamic-based techniques permit the examination of discrete neural circuits and psychologic functions known or hypothesized to play a critical role in child psychiatric disorders. The refinements in PET technology and the emergence of fMRI have decreased the reliance on single-state, particularly resting-state, studies, which prevailed in early work, in favor of activation studies. Attempts to isolate the neural correlates of discrete cognitive operations have most frequently employed subtraction designs, in which an experimental task is compared with a control task that differs only on the single cognitive variable of interest. Patterns of neural activity associated with the performance of experimental and control tasks are compared, generally on a pixel-by-pixel basis, using traditional statistical tests such as the Student t-test. For example, to identify brain regions involved in processing facial affect, the matching of faces based on their identity might serve as a control task.

While representing an advance over prior single-state designs, subtraction designs are nonetheless limited in their ability to control adequately all the processing steps associated with task performance. Implied in the subtraction approach is the assumption that the elemental processes under scrutiny are independent and additive, an assumption unlikely to be valid for higher-level psychologic functions (e.g., Sergent et al., 1992; Demonet et al., 1993). Furthermore, whereas this approach is well suited to the study of regional specialization, it is limited in its ability to delineate the integrated activity of the neural circuitry involved in complex mental activity.

The dilemma presented by multiple statistical comparisons and the limitations of the subtraction approach are being addressed, in part through the increasing availability of diverse statistical approaches. These strategies are designed to examine both the functional segregation (regional specialization) and the functional integration (based on distributed neural networks) of brain activity (see Friston, 1996). Functional specialization is probed using either regions of interest or pixel-based approaches to image analysis (e.g., statistical parametric mapping) not only with subtraction but also with other newly emerging techniques. Issues of multiple univariate tests are being addressed, in part, with methods that take into account the spatial extent of observed activations (e.g., the contiguity of activated pixels, which decreases the probability of pixels being activated by chance). As an alternative to subtraction designs, parametric designs that systematically vary a single parameter (i.e., stimulus presentation rate, number of practice trials, difficulty level) permit the examination of linear and nonlinear relationships between physiology and sensory, perceptual, and cognitive parameters (Braver et al., 1997; Buchel et al., 1998). Such designs hold promise for the delineation of developmental effects. In addition, factorial designs can now be used for assessing interaction effects in brain imaging data (e.g., modulatory drug effects on task-dependent physiologic responses, Friston, (1996)).

Given the increasing recognition of the dependence of cerebral activity on networks of interacting brain regions, mathematical methods designed to capture neural connectivity have been developed and continue to evolve. These techniques have primarily been developed using PET to complement other data analytic approaches but are now being extended to fMRI (Buchel and Friston, 1997). Covariance approaches, using such methods as correlations, regression, and principal components analysis (Friston et al., 1993; Horwitz, 1994) are being used to characterize whole-brain patterns of correlated activity, or functional connectivity. To test specific hypotheses based on animal, lesion, or other clinical data, neural modeling approaches (e.g., structural equation modeling) are being developed and applied to map the strengths of the functional interactions between the critical nodes (i.e., brain regions) of the networks under study, providing maps of effective connectivity (McIntosh et al., 1994; Fletcher et al., 1999; Horwitz et al., 1999).

Furthermore, fMRI has stimulated the development of a number of novel strategies capable of further enhancing temporal resolution and dissecting the neural signals associated with various behaviors or aspects of cognitive processing. Data analytic paradigms now allow better temporal differentiation of stages of learning and information processing in normal and aberrant development. Event-related fMRI methods (Buckner, 1998) permit individual trial events to be presented rapidly, in randomly intermixed order, and the associated hemodynamic responses to be mapped essentially in realtime. Following the completion of a scanning session, trials may be sorted by the subject performance or the occurrence of symptoms (e.g., tics) and averaged to ascertain differences in neural responses accompanying specific behaviors.

Future directions

Neuroimaging findings in adolescents have begun to suggest developmental differences as well as similarities in brain function associated with psychiatric disorders. Cross-sectional studies that directly compare patients of different age groups, controlling for relevant variables such as severity and age of onset, are needed to confirm and refine these findings further. Even more promising for

future work is the undertaking of longitudinal studies of patients near (or even prior to) the onset of symptoms. Such longitudinal within-subject designs will permit a more accurate assessment of primary pathophysiology and improve sensitivity to age-related changes. In addition, single-subject data analysis can help to bridge the gap between research and clinical applications and to identify individual differences and potentially valid subtypes for further confirmatory testing.

The rational selection of appropriate study designs and imaging modalities can optimize the search for the neural substrates of psychiatric disorders. For example, activation studies, using predominantly fMRI, will provide sensitive probes for identifying brain regions and circuits that are dysfunctional or potentially compensatory in relationship to aberrant behavior. Within these circuits, altered connectivity may be explored with the use of covariance techniques applied to PET and fMRI datasets, as well as through the combined use of TMS with neuroimaging. Neural modeling can be used to integrate the diverse array of data obtained through neuroimaging with that obtained from other approaches (e.g., animal, lesion, autopsy findings). Finally, neurochemical correlates of alterations in synaptic activity can be established using PET to help to guide rational approaches to pharmacologic therapies. Another much needed application is the evaluation of therapeutic and long-term effects of medication and other interventions for their impact on brain function across development.

Genetic vulnerabilities and other biological risk factors may also be studied with an eye toward the development of prevention strategies. One important application of this latter type of research falls within the area of substance abuse. Children and adolescents, particularly those with disorders that place them at risk for substance abuse, may be studied prior to the development of substance abuse and followed throughout or past the vulnerable developmental period.

The time is ripe for exploiting the research opportunities afforded by functional neuroimaging to enhance our understanding of the underlying neurobiology of child psychiatric disorders and for using this knowledge to improve clinical diagnosis, treatment, and prevention. Many challenges accompany these vast opportunities – some technological, some practical, and some ethical. As we stand at the threshold of an era of new discoveries, we must judiciously balance the need to protect individuals in their capacity as research subjects against the need to advance the potential benefits to be derived from clinical research. As with other areas of clinical research (Vitiello and Jensen, 1997), the exclusion of children from research prevents the gain of potential health benefits and increases the health risks associated with extrapolating from research in adults when diagnosing and treating children.

References

Anand, B. K. and Brobeck, J. R. (1951). Localisation of a "feeding centre" in hypothalamus of the rat. *Proc. Soc. Exp. Biol. Med.*, **77**, 323–4.

Braver, T. S., Cohen, J. D., Nystrom, L. E., Jonides, J., Smith, E. E. and Noll, D. C. (1997). A parametric study of prefrontal cortex involvement in human working memory. *Neuroimage*, **5**, 49–62.

Breiter, H. C., Etcoff, N. L., Whalen, P. J. et al. (1996). Response and habituation of the human amygdala during visual processing of facial expression. *Neuron*, **17**, 873–87.

Buchel, C., Holmes, A. P., Rees, G. and Friston, K. J. (1998). Characterizing stimulus-response functions using nonlinear regressors in parametric fMRI experiments. *Neuroimage*, **8**, 140–8.

Buchel, C. and Friston, K. J. (1997). Modulation of connectivity in visual pathways by attention: cortical interactions evaluated with structural equation modeling and fMRI. *Cereb. Cortex*, **7**, 768–78.

Buckner, R. L. (1998). Event-related fMRI and the hemodynamic response. *Hum. Brain Map.*, **6**, 373–7.

Castellanos, F. X. (1997). Toward a pathophysiology of attention-deficit/hyperactivity disorder. *Clin. Pediatr.*, **36**, 381–93.

Classen, J., Liepert, J., Wise, S. P., Hallett, M. and Cohen, L. G. (1998). Rapid plasticity of human cortical movement representation induced by practice. *J. Neurophysiol.*, **79**, 1117–23.

Cohen, L. G., Celnick, P., Pascual-Leone, A. et al. (1997). Functional relevance of cross-modal plasticity in blind humans. *Nature*, **389**, 180–3.

Damasio, A. R. (1994). *Descartes' Error: Emotion, Reason, and the Human Brain.* New York: Avon Books.

Delvenne, V., Goldmann, S., de Maertelaer, V., Wikler, D., Damhaut, P. and Lotstra, F. (1997). Brain glucose metabolism in anorexia nervosa and affective disorders: influence of weight loss or depressive symptomatology. *Psychiatr. Res.*, **74**, 83–92.

Demonet, J. F., Wise, R. and Frackowiak, R. S. K. (1993). Language functions explored in normal subjects by positron emission tomography: a critical review. *Hum. Brain Map.*, **1**, 39–47.

Drevets, W. C. (1998). Functional neuroimaging studies of depression: the anatomy of melancholia. *Annu. Rev. Med.*, **49**, 341–61.

Ernst, M. (1998). Dopaminergic function in ADHD. In *Proceedings of the IBC International Symposium on Dopaminergic Disorders*, pp. 235–60.

Ernst, M., Liebenauer, L., Fitzgerald, G., Cohen, R. and Zametkin, A. J. (1994). Reduced brain metabolism in hyperactive girls. *J. Am. Acad. Child Adolesc. Psychiatry*, **33**, 858–68.

Ernst, M., Zametkin, A. J., Matochik, J. A., Jons, P. H. and Cohen, R. M. (1998). Presynaptic dopaminergic activity in ADHD adults. A [fluorine-18]fluorodopa positron emission tomographic study. *J. Neurosci.*, **18**, 5901–7.

Ernst, M., Zametkin, A. J., Matochik, J. A., Pascualvaca, D., Jons, P. and Cohen, R. M. (1999a). High midbrain DOPA decarboxylase activity in children with ADHD. *Am. J. Psychiatr.*, **156**, 1209–15.

Ernst, M., Zametkin, A. J., Jons, M. A., Matochik, J. A., Pascualvaca, D. and Cohen, R. M. (1999b). High presynaptic dopaminergic activity in children with Tourette's disorder. *J. Am. Acad. Child Adolesc. Psychiatry*, **38**, 86–94.

Fletcher, P., McKenna, P. J., Friston, K. J., Frith, C. D. and Dolan, R. J. (1999). Abnormal cingulate modulation of fronto-temporal connectivity in schizophrenia. *Neuroimage*, **9**, 337–42.

Friston, K. J. (1996). Functional specialization and integration in the brain: an example from schizophrenia research. In *Developmental Neuroimaging: Mapping the Development of Brain and Behavior*, eds. R. W. Thatcher, G. R. Lyon, J. Rumsey and N. Krasnegor. San Diego, CA: Academic Press.

Friston, K. J., Frith, C. D., Liddle, P. F. and Frackowiak, R. S. J. (1993). Functional connectivity: the principal-component analysis of large (PET) data sets. *J. Cereb. Blood Flow Metab.*, **13**, 5–14.

Frostig, R. D., Lieke, E. E., Ts'o, D. Y. and Grinvald, A. (1990). Cortical functional architecture and local coupling between neuronal activity and the microcirculation revealed by in vivo high-resolution optical imaging of intrinsic signals. *Proc. Natl. Acad. Sci. USA*, **87**, 6082–6.

George, J. S., Aine, C. J., Mosher, J. C. et al. (1995). Mapping function in the human brain with magnetoencephalography, anatomical magnetic resonance imaging, and functional magnetic resonance imaging. *J. Clin. Neurophysiol.*, **12**, 406–31.

George, M. S., Lisanby, S. H. and Sackeim, H. A. (1999). Transcranial magnetic stimulation: applications in neuropsychiatry. *Arch. Gen. Psychiatry*, **56**, 300–11.

Gordon, I., Lask, B., Bryant-Waugh, R., Christie, D. and Timimi, S. (1997). Childhood-onset anorexia nervosa: towards identifying a biological substrate. *Int. J. Eating Disord.*, **22**, 159–65.

Gratton, G., Fabiani, M., Corballis, P. M. et al. (1997). Fast and localized event-related optical signals (EROS) in the human occipital cortex: comparisons with the visual evoked potential and fMRI. *Neuroimage*, **6**, 168–80.

Herholz, K., Krieg, J., Emrich, H. M. et al. (1987). Regional cerebral glucose metabolism in anorexia nervosa measured by positron emission tomography. *Biol. Psychiatry*, **22**, 43–51.

Horwitz, B. (1994). Data analysis paradigms for metabolic-flow data: combining neural modeling and functional neuroimaging. *Hum. Brain Map.*, **2**, 112–22.

Horwitz, B., Tagamets, M. A. and McIntosh, A. R. (1999). Neural modeling, functional brain imaging, and cognition. *Trends Cogn. Sci.*, **3**, 91–8.

Keenan, J. P., Hamilton, R., Freund, S. and Pascual-Leone, A. (1999). Self-face identification is increased by repetitive transcranial magnetic stimulation delivered to the right prefrontal cortex. (Cognitive Neuroscience Society Annual Meeting Program 1999) *J. Cogn Neurosci., Suppl.*, p. 83.

Kirkcaldie, M., Pridmore, S. and Reid, P. (1997). Bridging the skull: electroconvulsive therapy (ECT) and repetitive transcranial magnetic stimulation (rTMS) in psychiatry. *Convuls. Ther.*, **13**, 83–91.

LaBar, K. S., Gatenby, C., Gore, J. C., LeDoux, J. E. and Phelps, E. (1998). Human amygdala activation during conditioned fear acquisition and extinction: a mixed-trial fMRI study. *Neuron*, **20**, 937–45.

Levy, F. (1991). The dopamine theory of attention deficit hyperactivity disorder (ADHD). *Aust. N. Z. J. Psychiatry*, **25**, 277–83.

Luna, B., Merriam, E. P., Minshew, N. J. et al. (1999). Response inhibition improves from late childhood to adulthood: eye movement and fMRI studies. (Cognitive Neuroscience Society Annual Meeting Program 1999.) *J. Cogn. Neurosci. Suppl.*, p. 57.

Malonek, D. and Grinvald, A. (1997). Vascular regulation at sub millimeter range. Sources of intrinsic signals for high resolution optical imaging. *Adv. Exp. Med. Biol.*, **413**, 215–20.

Mazziotta, J. C., Toga, A. W., Evans, A., Fox, P. and Lancaster, J. (1995). A probabilistic atlas of the human brain: theory and rationale for its development. *Neuroimage*, **2**, 89–101.

McIntosh, A. R., Grady, C. L., Ungerleider, L. G., Haxby, J. V., Rapoport, S. I. and Horwitz, B. (1994). Network analysis of cortical visual pathways mapped with PET. *J. Neurosci.*, **14**, 655–66.

Muzik, O., Ager, J., Janisse, J., Shen, C., Chugani, D. C. and Chugani, H. T. (1999). A mathematical model for the analysis of cross-sectional brain glucose metabolism data in children. *Prog. Neuropsychopharmacol. Biol. Psychiatry*, **23**, 589–600.

Pascual-Leone, A., Tarazona, F., Kennan, J., Tormos, J. M., Hamilton, R. and Catala, M. D. (1999). Transcranial magnetic stimulation and neuroplasticity. *Neuropsychologia*, **37**, 207–17.

Paus, T., Jech, R., Thompson, C. J., Comeau, R., Peters, T. and Evans, A. C. (1997). Transcranial magnetic stimulation during positron emission tomography: a new method for studying connectivity of the human cerebral cortex. *J. Neurosci.*, **17**, 3178–84.

Pennington, B. F. and Ozonoff, S. (1996). Executive functions and developmental psychopathology. *J. Child Psychol. Psychiatry*, **37**, 51–87.

Rauch, S. L., Shin, L. M., Whalen, P. J. and Pitman, R. K. (1998). Neuroimaging and the neuroanatomy of PTSD. *CNS Spectrums* **3** (Suppl. 2), 30–41.

Rosen, B. R., Buckner, R. L. and Dale (1998). Event-related functional MRI: past, present, and future. *Proc. Natl. Acad. Sci. USA*, **95**, 773–80.

Sergent, J., Zuck, E., Levesque, M. and MacDonald, B. (1992). Positron emission tomography study of letter and object processing: empirical findings and methodological considerations. *Cereb. Cortex*, **2**, 68–80.

Solanto, M. V. (1984). Neuropharmacological basis of stimulant drug action in attention deficit disorder with hyperactivity: a review and synthesis. *Psychol. Bull.*, **95**, 387–409.

Teicher, M. H., Polcari, A., English, C. D. et al. (1996). Dose dependent effects of methylphenidate on activity attention, and magnetic resonance measures in children with ADHD. *Soc. Neurosci. Abst.*, **22**, 1191.

Thatcher, R. W. (1996). Multimodal assessments of developing neural networks: integrating fMRI, PET, MRI, and EEG/MEG. In *Developmental Neuroimaging: Mapping the Development of Brain and Behavior*, eds. R. W. Thatcher, G. R. Lyon, J. Rumsey and N. Krasnegor,. San Diego, CA: Academic Press.

Thompson, P. M., Schwartz, C. and Toga, A. W. (1996). High-resolution random mesh algorithms for creating a probabilistic 3D surface atlas of the human brain. *Neuroimage*, **3**, 19–34.

Thompson, P. M., MacDonald, D., Mega, M. S., Holmes, C. J., Evans, A. C. and Toga, A. W. (1997). Detection and mapping of abnormal brain structure with a probabilistic atlas of cortical surfaces. *J. Comput. Assist. Tomogr.*, **21**, 567–81.

Turjanski, N., Sawle, G. V., Playford, E. D. et al. (1994). PET studies of the presynaptic and postsynaptic dopaminergic system in Tourette's syndrome. *J. Neurol. Neurosurg. Psychiatry*, **57**, 688–92.

Vaidya, C. J., Austin, G., Kirkorian, G. et al. (1998). Selective effects of methylphenidate in attention deficit hyperactivity disorder: a functional magnetic resonance study. *Proc. Natl. Acad. Sci. USA*, **95**, 14494–9.

Vitiello, B. and Jensen, P. S. (1997). Medication development and testing in children and adolescents. Current problems, future directions. *Arch. Gen. Psychiatry*, **54**, 871–6.

Zametkin, A. J., Liebenauer, L. L., Fitzgerald, G. A. et al. (1993). Brain metabolism in teenagers with attention deficit hyperactivity disorder. *Arch. Gen. Psychiatry*, **50**, 333–40.

Zametkin, A. J., Nordahl, T. E., Gross, M. et al. (1990). Cerebral glucose metabolism in adults with hyperactivity of childhood onset. *N. Engl. J. Med.*, **323**, 1361–6.

Glossary

This glossary comprises a partial list of technical terms used in nuclear medicine (i.e., PET and SPECT) and nuclear magnetic resonance (i.e., fMRI and MRS). The term 'nuclear' in nuclear medicine and NMR refers to two different aspects of the technique. Nuclear medicine measures events occurring at the level of electron or proton of the nucleus, and NMR exploits the electromagnetic characteristics of the nucleus as a charged spinning object.

Table G.1 contrasts the characteristics of the functional neuroimaging techniques described in this book.

The glossary was developed based on the *Dictionary and Handbook of Nuclear Medicine and Clinical Imaging* (Iturralde, 1990) and a glossary for fMRI developed by Robert L. Savoy and provided by the Massachusetts General Hospital's Department of Radiology as part of their 1998 visiting fellowship program in fMRI, headed by Bruce R. Rosen and Robert L. Savoy.

Table G.1. Characteristics of functional neuroimaging techniques

	Spatial resolution	Temporal resolution	Specifics
Positron emission tomography (PET)	4–5 mm	Variable (1 to 90 min)	Integrated brain activity. Cerebral blood flow and metabolism. Neurotransmitter and enzymatic systems
Single photon emission computed tomography (SPECT)	6–9 mm	Variable (like PET)	Like PET, but, fewer tracers, and limited absolute quantitation; possibility of scanning hours after injection of the tracer
Functional magnetic resonance imaging (fMRI)	2–5 mm	40–200 ms	Integrated brain activity (related to cerebral blood flow): relative measures
Magnetic resonance spectroscopy (MRS)	^{1}H-MRS 3–12 ml ^{1}H-MRSI (imaging) < 1 ml	Variable: minutes (depending on magnetic field strength and other technical parameters)	Brain chemistry (neuronal markers: gamma-aminobutyric acid and glutamate signal)
Magnetoencephalography (MEG)	8–10 mm	< 1 ms	Average neuronal activity at the cortical level mostly

Terms

N-Acetylaspartate A brain chemical identified in imaging and used as a marker of neuronal involvement in a process.

Acquisition delay time The time elapsed between the end of the radiofrequency pulse and the beginning of data acquisition in an NMR experiment.

Acquisition rate Sampling rate or digitizing rate: number of data points acquired per second.

Acquisition time The time during an NMR or PET/SPECT experiment in which data are acquired and digitized. Its length can be a limiting factor, particularly in NMR studies.

Annihilation (PET) The event that occurs when a positive electron (positron) interacts with a negative electron. Both particles disappear and their energy is transferred into electromagnetic radiation (usually as two photons, each of 511 KeV energy emitted in opposite directions).

Antiparticle That particle (known or hypothetical) for which interaction with a given particle results in their mutual annihilation (e.g., electron–positron, proton–antiproton).

Attenuation The process (absorption and scatter) by which a beam of radiation is reduced in intensity when passing through matter.

Attenuation correction Attenuation correction compensates for photons that have been absorbed in the patient, never reaching the detector. Because activity located deeper in the body is attenuated more than activity near the surface, an emission tomographic transaxial slice appears lower in counts in the center and higher near the edges (also called 'hot rim' artifact). A transmission scan (qv) provides the necessary data to correct for attenuation.

Axial resolution The smallest distance that can be resolved along the length of the ultrasound beam (limited by the transmitted pulse length), or along the z axis of the body in PET/SPECT.

B_0 The main static magnetic field.

B_{max} The total number of receptors per unit volume of tissue (i.e., concentration). The term is an adaptation of the classical V_{max} (maximal reaction velocity) used in equilibrium enzyme kinetics. Because a basal level of receptor occupation by endogenous neurotransmitter is believed to be present at all times, an estimate of B_{max} is rarely – if ever – the end result in a PET study analysis.

B'_{max} The total number of available receptor sites per unit volume (as if counted at steady state). Because of the omnipresence of endogenous neurotransmitter, this term is usually the receptor density parameter that is estimated in PET.

Binding potential (BP) Index of receptor binding activity. Because of limitations in parameter identification, BP is often the only parameter that can be reliably estimated from dynamic PET data. $BP = B_{max}/K_d$ (or B'_{max}/K_d) where B_{max} is a measure of the total number of receptors (B'_{max} is a measure of the number of receptors available to be bound, i.e., not occupied by endogenous ligands) and K_d is the equilibrium constant of dissociation. Note, a change in BP cannot be assigned to a change in either B'_{max} or K_d without additional a priori knowledge.

BOLD effect (blood oxygen level-dependent effect) The change in T_2^* that is induced by changes in the amount of oxygenated hemoglobin (Hg) in the venous circulation of the brain. Because oxygenated Hg has a much smaller magnetic susceptibility (qv) than deoxygenated Hg, and because neural activity alters the amount of oxygenated Hg in the venous blood, the susceptibility of the blood decreases, T_2^* increases, and, therefore, the intensity in T_2^*-weighted images increases.

Cerebral blood flow (CBF) Strictly, blood flow is in milliliters per minute. By convention, however, CBF refers to blood flow per mass of tissue (i.e., ml/min per g tissue).

Cerebral metabolic rate of glucose (CMRGlu) Rate of glucose utilization in the brain per unit mass of tissue (μmol/min per g tissue). Rates in varying areas of the brain (regional CMRGlu; rCMRGlu) can be normalized to rates in a particular area used as a reference value.

Chemical shift (δ) The changes in Larmor frequency (qv) caused by the contiguous environment. Nuclei experience slightly different local magnetic fields because of their immediate chemical environments. The protons are influenced not only by nuclei to which they are directly attached but also by nuclei that are one or two bond lengths away. For example, hydrogen nuclei in water and hydrogen nuclei in fat experience different magnetic fields and, therefore, have different Larmor frequencies. These frequencies are used to encode position in MRI and make possible the differentiation of different molecular compounds and different sites within the molecules in high-resolution NMR spectra. The amount of the shift is proportional to magnetic field strength and is usually specified in parts per million (ppm) of the resonance frequency relative to a standard.

Coil Single or multiple loops of wire (or other electrical conductors) designed either to produce a magnetic field from current flowing through the wire (e.g., radiofrequency gradient coil) or to detect a changing magnetic field by voltage induced in the wire (receiver coil).

Coincidence (PET) The occurrence of counts in two or more detectors simultaneously or within an assignable time interval.

Coincidence loss (PET) The loss of events caused by their occurring within a span of time too short to be resolved by the electronic circuit. Also referred to as dead time loss, counting loss, or resolving time loss.

Computed tomography (CT) Use of a computer and data processing from X-rays, radionuclides, or NMR to produce body section images of (i) tissue densities from absorption coefficients when X-rays are transmitted (X-ray CT); (ii) origin of emitted photons when radionuclides are administered and photons emitted (radionuclide emission CT); (iii) tissue T_1 and T_2 values, as well as quantities of magnetically polar nuclei such as hydrogen (NMR).

Convolution A mathematical operation used in image processing that describes a filtering process in real space.

Coronal (frontal) plane Passes longitudinally through the body from side to side at right angles to the sagittal median plane and divides the body into front and back parts.

Counting loss *See* coincidence loss.

Count rate The rate at which decay events are recorded by a detector. Also, the absolute rate (counts per second) of decay events for a standard source.

Dead time Time during which the receiver is unable to register the signal in a pulsed NMR spectrometer. The time interval following a radioactive event in which the detecting apparatus remains unresponsive to further events. Same as pulse resolving time.

Decay Disintegration of radioactive atoms. What remains are different elements. For instance, an atom of polonium decays to form lead, ejecting an alpha particle in the process. In a mass of a particular radioisotope a number of atoms will disintegrate or decay every second, and this number is characteristic of the isotope concerned. Exponential decay, as that of radioactive substances, decreases exponentially with time in accordance with the equation $A = A_0 e^{-\lambda t}$ where A and A_0 are the activities present at times t and zero, respectively, and λ is the characteristic decay constant.

Dephasing In the context of MRI, dephasing refers to the loss of net magnetization in the transverse plane because the individual nuclei are precessing (or wobbling) at different rates. Whereas the rate at which magnetic orientation of the individual nuclei returns to the longitudinal direction is relatively slow (T_1) the rate at which the transverse magnetization disappears is relatively rapid (T_2^*) because the individual nuclei get out-of-phase with each other, and their magnetization vectors cancel.

Disintegration A spontaneous process in which the nucleus of an atom changes its form or its energy state by emitting either a particle or electromagnetic radiation, or by electron capture.

Distribution volume (DV) The volume of tissue into which a mass, x, of ligand will distribute if x distributes into a unit volume of blood plasma. A commonly estimated measure of receptor binding activity, it is the natural outcome of a Logan-plot analysis of dynamic PET data and is equal to binding potential (BP) + 1.

Dosimetry The measurement of the quantity of radiation absorbed by a substance or a living organism.

Echo In MRI, this refers to the regrowth of the transverse component of magnetization after it has disappeared through dephasing. The echo is, in fact, the NMR signal that is normally recorded and analyzed in MRI.

Echo planar imaging (EPI) (NMR) A technique of planar imaging in which a complete planar image is obtained from one selective excitation pulse (single saturation pulse). The free induction decay is observed while rapidly switching the y gradient field in the presence of a static x gradient field. The Fourier transform of the resulting spin echo train can be used to produce an image of the excited plane. It requires gradient power supplies of greater strength than are needed for more conventional imaging strategies. Its advantage is speed.

Emission computed tomography (ECT) Tomographic projections are a series of planar images taken at different angles around the patient. These images are then back-projected into transaxial images. The transaxial images can then be reoriented to produce sagittal, coronal, or oblique angle images.

Epoch In fMRI, this term is often used to refer to a portion of a single fMRI run during which the stimulus presentation and/or response task is unchanged. ("Unchanged" does not mean that the stimulation is necessarily static, but that it is treated as a single type of stimulus.)

Ernst angle The flip angle that yields the most signal for a given time to repetition (TR) and time to inversion (TI).

Field of view (FOV) The area that can be "seen" by an optical system. In PET/SPECT, it defines the volume from which emitted activity may be detected. In MRI, its dimensions are independently controlled by the frequency-encode and phase-encode gradients.

Filtering A process used extensively on nuclear medicine images to reduce statistical noise and to enhance edges for edge detection. It is also used in the reconstruction of tomographic images. Filtering can be performed in either the spatial domain or frequency space.

Flip angle Amount of rotation of the macroscopic magnetization vector produced by a radiofrequency pulse, with respect to the direction of the static magnetic field.

Fluorodeoxyglucose (FDG) Used to examine transport

across the blood–brain barrier and phosphorylation rates with glucose.

Fourier transform analysis Mathematical procedure to separate out the frequency components of a signal from its amplitudes as a function of time. Used in tomographic image reconstruction. In MRI, it permits the analysis of a mixture of NMR signals at slightly different frequencies into their component frequencies (specified by the frequency-encode gradient).

Free induction decay (FID) Transient nuclear signal induced in the NMR coil after a radiofrequency (rf) pulse has excited the nuclear spin system in pulsed NMR techniques. This is referred to as a FID signal because the signal is induced by the free precession of the nuclear spins around the static field after the rf pulse has been turned off. A plot of this signal as a function of time looks like an exponentially damped sinusoid at the Larmor frequency. The FID can be converted to a series of peaks (spectrum) by a mathematical process (Fourier transformation).

Frequency encoding Refers to the use of a magnetic field gradient to cause different rates of precession (different Larmor frequencies) along the direction of the gradient during the time that data are acquired. The frequency composition of the collected data (as determined by Fourier analysis) will correspond to different spatial locations.

Functional magnetic resonance imaging (fMRI) Procedures in which a subject undergoes sensory stimulation while brain imaging is used to detect responses.

Gradient Change of the individual components of a vector quantity along a given spatial coordinate. The amount and direction of rate of change in space of some quantity such as magnetic field strength.

Gradient coils (Gx, Gy, Gz) Current-carrying coils designed to generate a desired gradient magnetic field. The coils, themselves, are normally labeled x, y, and z to indicate the orientation of the magnetic fields that they generate. In the most common case of an axially oriented image, the z gradient coil is used for slice selection, the x gradient coil is used for frequency encoding of the image, and the y gradient coil is used to generate the magnetic fields that permit phase encoding. In general, however, combinations of these coils are used to generate the slice-select, frequency-encode, and phase-encode directions in order to permit imaging in planes other than the axial plane (such as coronal, sagittal, and arbitrary oblique planes). The gradients are responsible for the acoustic noise when current runs through the wires.

Gyromagnetic ratio (magnetogyric ratio, γ) Constant of proportionality relating the angular frequency of precession of a nucleus to the magnetic field strength. It has a value that is both constant and specific to a particular isotope. It is defined by the Larmor equation.

Hann filter A common low-pass filter, also called a Hanning filter, used in nuclear medicine image processing.

Hexamethyl-propyleneamine oxime (HMPAO) Labeled with ^{99m}Tc, this is a probe used to assess perfusion and regional blood volumes with SPECT and other techniques.

Homogeneity In NMR, the homogeneity of the static magnetic field is an important criterion of the quality of the magnet. It can be improved by the use of shim coils. Homogeneity requirements for NMR imaging are generally lower than the homogeneity requirements for NMR spectroscopy.

Interpulse time Time between successive radiofrequency pulses used in pulse sequences. Particularly important are the inversion time (T_1) in inversion recovery, and the time between a 90° pulse and the subsequent 180° pulse to produce a spin echo, which will be approximately one half the spin echo time (TE). The time between repetitions of pulse sequences is the repetition time (TR).

Inversion An excited state in which the net magnetization vector is in a direction opposite to that of the main field (NMR).

Inversion recovery Rate of recovery as the nuclei return to equilibrium magnetization (after their magnetization was inverted by radiofrequency pulse). The rate of recovery depends upon T_1 (NMR).

Inversion recovery sequence Pulse sequence in which the magnetization is inverted by means of a 180° radiofrequency (rf) pulse, and the recovery from this inversion is monitored by means of a 90° rf pulse applied after a delay time τ. This sequence is commonly used for measurement of T_1 (NMR).

Inversion time (TI) *See* time to inversion.

Isotropic voxel A volume element with equal dimensions in x, y, and z.

Larmor equation The equation defining the resonance condition in magnetic resonance phenomena (rotational frequency). The Larmor equation is $\omega_0 = \gamma B_0$, where ω_0 is the Larmor frequency in radians per second, γ is the gyromagnetic ratio, and B_0 is the magnetic field (induction) strength.

Larmor frequency (ω_0) Resonant frequency defined by the Larmor equation. Expressed in hertz (f_0) or radians per second (ω_0); $\omega_0 = 2\pi f_0$. It is the rate at which a given nucleus precesses in a magnetic field of a given strength (frequency at which magnetic resonance can be excited). This rate is proportional to the field strength. By varying the magnetic field across the body with a gradient magnetic field, the corresponding variation of the Larmor frequency can be used to encode position. For protons (hydrogen nuclei), the Larmor frequency is 42.58 MHz/T.

Longitudinal relaxation (spin-lattice relaxation) Gradual recovery of the net magnetization (M_0) owing to the main magnetic field (B_0) after a radiofrequency excitation pulse has flipped the longitudinal magnetization by some angle. For example, after a saturation pulse has flipped the longitudinal magnetization by 90° (thus transforming the longitudinal magnetization to transverse magnetization), the gradual recovery of longitudinal magnetization by virtue of the individual nuclei realigning themselves with B_0 is called longitudinal relaxation.

Longitudinal relaxation time (T_1, spin-lattice relaxation time) The exponential time constant that characterizes the growth or decay of the component of magnetization parallel to the external field; this process occurs by interaction of the nucleus with its entire surroundings (hence spin-lattice relaxation). It provides a measure of the time for spinning nuclei to realign with the external magnetic field. The magnetization in the z direction will grow after excitation from 0 to about 63% of its final thermal equilibrium value in a time of T_1. Therefore, as a convention, T_1 refers to the relaxation time along the longitudinal z axis (T_1 is time of recovery of 63% of the initial magnetization along the z axis).

Lumped constant (PET and FDG) Constant that corrects for the differences between glucose and fluorodeoxyglucose (FDG) in transport across the blood–brain barrier and in phosphorylation. A standard value, measured once in separate groups of normal subjects, is used.

Magnetic gradient Amount and direction of the rate of change of field strength in space; employed to select the imaging region and to encode the NMR response signal spatially.

Magnetic resonance Absorption or emission of electromagnetic energy by nuclei in a (static) magnetic field after excitation by suitable radiofrequency radiation: the frequency of resonance is given by the Larmor equation.

Magnetic susceptibility Denotes the intensity of the magnetization produced in a substance by an applied magnetic field. Paramagnetic substances have positive susceptibility, and diamagnetic substances have negative susceptibilities.

Nuclear magnetic resonance (NMR) The absorption and emission of electromagnetic energy tuned to the Larmor frequency of a nucleus precessing in a magnetic field (H_0). The frequency ω_0 of the magnetic resonance is the same as the frequency of the Larmor precession of the nuclei in the magnetic field and is proportional to the strength of the field. Thus, $\omega_0 = \gamma H_0$, where γ is a characteristic constant, called the gyromagnetic ratio, for a given nucleus. Mobile protons in molecules can be aligned by a magnetic field. If an additional high-frequency magnetic field is applied to disturb this condition and is then removed, the protons return to their original state and emit signals while doing this. The strength of the signal is proportional to the local concentration of the mobile protons. These signals are then used, usually with some type of computer processing, to produce an image (MRI) or to identify the spectrum of chemical substances.

Nuclear magnetic resonance imaging (NMRI or MRI) Creation of tomographic images based on the differences in NMR signal from different places in a body. The immediate practical application involves imaging the distribution of hydrogen nuclei (protons) in the body. The image brightness in a given region usually depends on both the spin density and the relaxation times, with their relative importance determined by the particular imaging technique employed. Motion, such as blood flow, also affects image brightness.

Nuclear magnetic resonance spectroscopy (NMRS or MRS) Technique to detect species of atomic nuclei in a sample (e.g., brain) and to identify the compounds in which they are bound. The technique is based on the stimulation and detection of resonance electromagnetic radiation in the radiofrequency range emitted characteristically by certain magnetically susceptible atomic nuclei. This occurs when a sample is placed in a strong magnetic field B_0 and excited by a pulse of electromagnetic energy B_1 of appropriate frequency. The resonance frequency of the emitted radiation is characteristic of the atomic nucleus and the nature of its immediate chemical environment; its exact value is proportional to the magnetic field B_0. NMRS, in contrast to nuclear magnetic resonance imaging, depends upon the creation of a homogeneous magnetic field (B_0) throughout the entire volume of the sample. In NMRS, small shifts in resonance frequency are observed. The chemical shifts are characteristic of molecular bonding patterns adjacent to the susceptible nucleus. They also yield other information; for example, they can indicate the presence of ion complexes. Not all atoms give rise to NMR signals. Those which do and are of biological importance include ^{1}H, ^{19}F, ^{31}P, and ^{13}C, listed in order of decreasing NMR sensitivity.

Nuclear spin Intrinsic property of certain nuclei that produces an associated characteristic angular momentum and magnetic moment.

Nuclide Atom having specified numbers of protons and

neutrons in its nucleus. Isotopes are the various forms of a single element and, therefore, are a family of nuclides with the same number of protons. Nuclides are distinguished by their atomic mass and number as well as by their energy state. Approximately 1250 different nuclides are recognized at present, each being a distinct species of nucleus with its own characteristic nuclear properties. Of these, 280 are naturally occurring stable nuclides, while the remainder (radionuclides) undergo spontaneous radioactive decay.

Paramagnetic substances These have a small but positive magnetic susceptibility (magnetizability). The addition of a small amount of paramagnetic substance may greatly reduce the relaxation time of water.

Partial voluming (partial volume effect) The alteration in pixel values that occurs when the structure being imaged has a spatial extent that is similar to or smaller than the resolving capabilities of the imaging device. The result is that the value in a particular pixel reflects a mixture of tissues.

Phantom A container of radioactivity, often made of perspex, in the shape of an organ of flat drums used in positron emission tomography. Phantoms are used to calibrate the scanner (measure absolute activity).

Phase encoding Use of a magnetic field gradient to cause different rates of precession for a brief period of time, resulting in phase differences across space in the direction of the gradient.

Pixel (picture element) A single number in a two-dimensional array of numbers that is used to create an image. In MRI, a pixel in the image of a single slice through the body corresponds to a voxel in that body.

Planes of the body The median sagittal plane passes longitudinally through the body from front to back and divides it into right and left halves; the transverse or transaxial plane passes horizontally through the body at right angles to the median plane and divides the body into upper and lower portions; the coronal or frontal plane passes longitudinally through the body from side to side, at right angles to the median plane, and divides the body into front and back parts.

Poisson distribution If random discrete events occur over a period of time, then the relative frequency or probability of a particular number of events N happening in a given short interval is given by the Poisson distribution.

Poisson noise High-frequency random noise associated with Poisson noise (statistical count fluctuations). Reduction of this noise is performed by applying low-pass (smoothing) filters.

Positron A transitory nuclear particle similar to the electron but positively charged.

Positron emission tomography (PET) A procedure used for the study of regional tissue physiology and biochemistry. It is based on the in vivo detection and imaging of positron-emitting radioisotopes that are introduced as tracer elements into the physiological systems of interest. The tracer tag should not perturb the behavior of the molecule.

Precession Slow gyration (wobbling) of the axis of a spinning body (e.g., nuclei) so as to trace a cone; it is caused by the application of a circulatory force (torque) that tends to change the direction of the rotation axis. Similar to the effect of gravity on the motion of a spinning top or gyroscope.

Profile slice A slice through an image by one or two lines, generating a histogram curve that shows count values along the line or between the two lines.

Proton density (ρ) In the context of NMR, the number of hydrogen atoms per unit volume. Images based on proton density are generated using a long time to repetition (TR) and a short time to echo (TE) (e.g., spin-echo, TR = 1800 ms, TE = 20–40 ms). A spin density-weighted image has a low contrast, since hydrogen content differences between tissues are small.

Pulse sequence programming Specification of the signals being sent to the radiofrequency (rf) transmit coil, slice-selection coil, frequency-encoding coil, and phase-encoding coil. This programming is complex. For example, the rf excitation pulse cannot be at a single frequency if it is to work in conjunction with the slice-selection gradient to define a slice of tissue that will be excited. In particular, the Fourier spectrum of the excitation pulse should be tuned to the range of frequencies that correspond to the different Larmor frequencies created by the slice-select gradient, over the spatial extent desired for imaging.

Pulse 180° (π pulse; inversion pulse) Radiofrequency pulse designed to rotate the macroscopic magnetization vector 180° in space as referred to the rotating frame of reference. If the spins are initially aligned with the magnetic field, this pulse will produce inversion (NMR).

Pulse 90° ($\pi/2$ pulse; saturation pulse) Radiofrequency pulse designed to rotate the macroscopic magnetization vector 90° in space as referred to the rotating frame of reference, usually about an axis at right angles to the main magnetic field. If the spins are initially aligned with the magnetic field, this pulse will produce transverse magnetization and a free induction decay (NMR).

Quantum number Refers to the number of values of the angular momentum or spin of nuclei that have a magnetic moment. For example, the quantum number of the

^{1}H nucleus is 1/2, and when placed in a magnetic field, it can exist in only two energy states.

Readout gradient Refers to the "G-frequency-encode" because the actual NMR data collection takes place when this gradient is in use.

Radiofrequency (rf) Wave frequency group intermediate between auditor and infrared range. The rf used in NMR studies is commonly in the megahertz (MHz) range. The principal effect of rf magnetic fields on the body is power deposition in the form of heating, mainly at the surface; this is the main area of concern for safety limits.

Radiofrequency pulse A short burst of radiofrequency (rf) electromagnetic radiation. Rotation of the magnetization vector can be caused by controlling the duration and amplitude of the rf pulse.

Radionuclide A nuclide of artificial or natural origin that exhibits radioactivity. For example, ^{131}I is a radionuclide, whereas ^{127}I is a stable nuclide. Radionuclides are radioactive nuclides.

Receiver coil Coil, or antenna, positioned within the magnet bore to detect the NMR signal: sometimes also used for excitation.

Reconstruction image An image representing a two-dimensional slice of a structure; reconstructed from data obtained by means of any of the tomographic techniques.

Recovery time The time, following detection of a pulse, that must elapse before a second pulse can be detected. Also called resolving time or coincidence time.

Reference region A region of the brain that is assumed to be devoid – or nearly devoid – of receptors. Taken together with receptor-rich regions, the reference region data can often be used to analyze dynamic receptor–ligand data without the need for an arterial input function.

Region of interest (ROI) Outlined area on a computer-processed image defined automatically or manually to obtain the accepted events (e.g., radioactive counts in PET) in that area. Time activity curves result when the ROI is sequentially measured in multiple images of a study. Sometimes ROI is used informally to indicate a subset of voxels in a three-dimensional data set. In NMRS, a volume of interest in single voxel acquisition is usually 1 to 12 ml, and a single spectrum from that region takes 2–10 min to be obtained (in contrast to spectroscopic imaging).

Relaxation rates These are inversions of relaxation times (NMR): spin-lattice relaxation rate $R_1 = 1/T_1$. Spin-spin relaxation rate $R_2 = 1/T_2$.

Relaxation times After excitation, nuclei tend to return to their equilibrium distribution in which the longitudinal magnetization is at its maximum value and oriented in the direction of the static magnetic field, the value of the transverse magnetization being zero. On cessation of the radiofrequency (rf) excitation pulse, the longitudinal magnetization M_z returns toward the equilibrium value M_0 at a rate characterized by the time constant T_1; any transverse magnetization decays towards zero with a time constant T_2 (or T_2^* in the real situation) (NMR).

Repeated free induction decay Another term for saturation recovery (qv). A sequence in which 90° pulses are repeated for excitation and measurement. It results in partial saturation if the period between the 90° pulses is of the order of T_1 or less and gives a T_1-weighted signal. Generally the term is only applied where the signal is detected as a free induction decay (and not as an echo) (NMR).

Repetition time (TR) See time to repetition.

Rephasing gradient Gradient magnetic field applied for a brief period after a selective excitation pulse, in the opposite direction to the gradient used for the selective excitation. The result of the gradient reversal is a rephasing of the spins (which will have become out of phase with each other along the direction of the selection gradient), forming an echo by "time reversal", and improving the sensitivity of imaging after the selective excitation process (NMR).

rf coils Coils that transmit the radiofrequency (rf) electromagnetic energy used to flip $M_{longitudinal}$ into $M_{transverse}$ and to receive the NMR signal generated by the rf pulse. Transmission and reception can be obtained by either a single coil or two separate coils. The reason to use separate coils is that the requirements are different. A transmitter coil needs to be able to send its rf energy uniformly anywhere in the body. The receiver coil may only need to pick up signal from a small portion of the body in some cases. For example, a "surface coil" is sometimes used to receive the signal. It has better signal-to-noise near its center than a receiver coil designed to detect signals uniformly throughout a larger portion of the body.

Run In the context of functional MRI, a run refers to a single, continuous collection of images.

Sagittal plane Passes longitudinally through the body from front to back, dividing it into right and left halves.

Saturation After exposure to a single radiofrequency pulse, if T_2 is much shorter than T_1, then the net transverse magnetization will disappear before significant repolarization of the spins occurs. During this time the sample is said to be saturated (NMR).

Saturation recovery The repeated free induction decay in

NMR sequence using images for which the pixel values are proportional to nuclear density and have a T_1 dependence that varies with the repetition time of the sequence.

Sequence delay time The time between the last pulse of a pulse sequence and the beginning of the next identical pulse sequence. It is the time allowed for the nuclear spin system to recover its magnetization and is equal to the sum of the acquisition delay time, data acquisition time, and the waiting time (NMR).

Sequence repetition time This is the time between the beginning of a pulse sequence and the beginning of the succeeding identical pulse sequence.

Shim coils Coils carrying a relatively small current that are used to provide auxiliary magnetic fields to compensate for inhomogeneities in the main magnetic field of an NMR system.

Shimming Correction of inhomogeneity of the magnetic field over a volume of interest. Inhomogeneity is produced by imperfections in the NMR magnet or the presence of external ferromagnetic objects. Shimming may involve changing the configuration of the magnet, adding shim coils, or adding small pieces of steel.

Signal averaging Technique to improve signal-to-noise ratio (SNR) (sensitivity of the NMR experiment) by averaging repeated scans over a few minutes through the same region of interest. The noise tends to decrease because of its random nature, whereas the signal reinforces itself.

Slice selection The region whose electromagnetic vector will be flipped can be limited to a slice by applying a gradient in the longitudinal direction while the initial saturation radiofrequency pulse is presented.

Smoothing The purpose of smoothing is to enhance an image by reducing high-frequency phenomena, such as statistical noise, while preserving the overall form of the data. However, since edges within an image or large gradients in a curve are dominated by high-frequency components, the effect of smoothing is to reduce or "average out" such features. Smoothing can be applied successfully to both images (spatial representation) and curves (temporal representation) from radionuclide images. For example, in many "dynamic" studies, temporal (i.e., between corresponding pixels in several frames) or spatial (i.e., between adjacent pixels within a frame) smoothing is usually implemented prior to viewing the data in cine mode. It is important to understand that if the image data have been smoothed, then subsequent data extraction or display may be modified by the smoothing algorithm.

Spatial frequency filtering Technique for eliminating in an image the higher spatial frequencies, assumed to be noise; employs Fourier transform analysis (qv).

Spatial resolution The ability of an instrument to image two separate line or point sources of radioactivity as separate entities. The smaller the distance between the two sources, the better the spatial resolution. A measure of spatial resolution is the point spread function (PSF) or the line spread function (LSF) and the derived system transfer function (STF).

SPECT Single photon emission computed tomography.

Spectroscopic imaging Acquisition of NMR spectra from multiple volumes simultaneously (each contiguous volume of 1–2 ml each); takes typically about 20 to 40 min to complete.

Spin coupling The diffusion of magnetic moments owing to actual movement of the associated molecule and/or chemical exchange.

Spin density The density of resonating spins in a given region in SI units of molecules per cubic meter. For water, there are about 1.1×10^5 mol/m^3 hydrogen, or 0.11 mol/cm^3. True spin density is not imaged directly but is calculated from signals received with different interpulse times.

Spin echo The reappearance of an NMR signal arising from refocusing or rephasing the various components of magnetization in the x, y plane. This usually results from the application of the 180° pulse after decay of the initial free induction decay. It can be used to determine T_2 without contamination from inhomogenous effects of the magnetic field (e.g., time to repetition (TR) spin-echo sequence 1800 to 2500 ms; time to echo (TE) 80 to 120 ms). Most ^{1}H MRS uses a spin echo with a long TE (>100 ms), which permits the measurement of three to four compounds present in the brain at relatively high concentrations (e.g., N-acetylaspartate (NAA), creatine (Cr) and phosphocreatine (PCr)). Short TE (<20 ms) permits the observation and quantification of other metabolies (e.g., glucose, *myo*-inositol, glutamate, glutamine, gamma-aminobutyric acid (GABA)).

Spin-lattice relaxation time *See* longitudinal relaxation time.

Spin-spin broadening Increased line width of the NMR spectra caused by interactions between neighboring dipoles. The line width of a peak from its intrinsic T_2 time is typically <1 Hz, whereas the line width from field inhomogeneity may be from 5 to 10 Hz. The term T_2^* refers to the combined effect of the intrinsic T_2 of the peak and the magnetic field inhomogeneity that affects the field width (NMR).

Spin-spin relaxation time *See* transverse relaxation time.

Spin-spin splitting Splitting in the lines of an NMR spectrum arises from the interaction of the nuclear magnetic moment with those of neighboring nuclei.

Surface coil NMR A simple, flat, radiofrequency receiver coil placed over a region of interest will have an effective selectivity for a volume approximately subtended by the coil circumference and one radius deep from the coil center. Such a coil can be used for simple localization of sites for measurement of chemical shift spectra, especially of phosphorus, and blood flow studies. Some additional spatial selectivity can be achieved with gradient magnetic fields.

T_1 *See* longitudinal relaxation time.

T_2 *See* transverse relaxation time.

T_2^* ("T.two-star") The characteristic time constant for loss of phase coherence among spins oriented at an angle to the static magnetic field inhomogeneities, ΔB, and spin-spin transverse relaxation with a resultant more rapid loss in transverse magnetization and NMR signal. NMR signal can still be recovered as a spin echo in times less than or of the order of T_2 ($1/T_2^* = 1/T_2 + \Delta\omega/2$; $\Delta\omega = \gamma\Delta B$).

T_1-**weighted MRI** An MR image generated using imaging parameters that cause contrast to be primarily based on differences in T_1 times for different tissues. (Short time to repetition (TR) and time to echo (TE) are used for T_1 weighting, e.g., TR 400–600 ms, TE 10–30 ms.) Tissues with short T_1 times are bright in T_1 weighted images. The T_1 contrast is best to delineate anatomic structures, differentiate white and gray matter, and detect subacute hemorrhage.

T_2-**weighted MRI** An MR image generated using imaging parameters that cause contrast to be primarily based on differences in T_2 times for different tissues. (Long time to repetition (TR) and time to echo (TE) are used for T_2 weighting, e.g., TR 1800–2500 ms, TE 80–120 ms.) Tissues with long T_2 times are bright in T_2-weighted images. These images have strong contrast between normal brain tissue and areas with high water content, for example cerebrospinal fluid and pathologic tissue (i.e., tumors, inflammation, cysts, demyelinating processes). High iron content decreases MR signal, especially on T_2-weighted images. Gradient-echo sequences do not allow true T_2 weighting to be obtained (because of the absence of a refocusing radiofrequency pulse); rather a T_2^* contrast is obtained that corresponds to spontaneous signal decay along the xy plane and depends on magnetic field inhomogeneities. The T_2^* contrast is widely used in functional MRI.

Talairach coordinates A system for specifying locations in individual brains. It yields three coordinates (x, y, z) based on a rigid rotation of the brain to an orientation specified by anatomic landmarks and followed by a piecewise linear transformation of the brain in six sections that preserve continuity. It is the most widely used system for comparing brains between individuals. (It was first developed and presented by J. Talairach in 1967.)

Time to echo (TE) The time (milliseconds) between presentation of the saturating radiofrequency pulse that flips $M_{\text{longitudinal}}$ by 90° and the time that an echo is detected (because of a refocusing pulse.) The total echo time (TE) affects the peak's intensity as a function of T_2.

Time to inversion (inversion time, TI) The time (milliseconds) between the center of the first inversion pulse and the middle of the saturating (90°) pulse in an inversion recovery pulse sequence.

Time to repetition (TR) The time (milliseconds) between presentation of the radiofrequency pulse that flips $M_{\text{longitudinal}}$ and the start of the succeeding sequence (NMR signal). It affects a peak's intensity as a function of T_1.

Tesla The preferred (SI) unit of magnetic flux density or field strength. One tesla (1 T) is equal to 10 000 Gauss.

Time-activity curve A histogram of the change in the count rate as a function of time.

Transmission scan Detection of radiation transmitted through the body from a source on one side of the body to the detector on the opposite side; it provides an image of body absorption densities much like a radiograph but generally lacking the detailed resolution and produces data to be used in the calculation of attenuation correction (PET).

Transverse magnetization ($M_{\text{transverse}}$) Component (M_{xy}) of the net magnetization vector orthogonal to the direction of the main field (longitudinal, B_0), whose precession, at the Larmor frequency, generates the NMR response signal. In the absence of externally applied radiofrequency energy, M_{xy} decays to zero with a characteristic time constant T_2, or more strictly T_2^*.

Transverse relaxation time T_2 (spin-spin relaxation time) The exponential time constant that characterizes the decay of confinement of magnetization to perpendicular to the external field. It is the rate at which nuclei reach equilibrium (go out of phase, lose phase coherence, with each other) and measures the gradual loss of magnetization in the plane perpendicular to the external magnetic field (B_0). Starting from a nonzero value of the magnetization in the xy plane, the xy magnetization will decay so that it loses 63% of its initial value in a time T_2. Protons attached to large macromolecules have short T_2 values and are observed as broad, short peaks, whereas protons attached to small metabolites have longer T_2 values and are observed as narrow, tall peaks in the proton spectrum. See also T_2^*.

Transverse (transaxial) plane Passes horizontally through the body at right angles to the median sagittal plane and divides the body into upper and lower portions.

References

Iturralde, M. P. (1990). *Dictionary and Handbook of Nuclear Medicine and Clinical Imaging.* Boca Raton, FL: CRC Press.

Index